PRINCIPLES OF
SURGERY

Fifth Edition

Companion Handbook

NOTICE

Medicine is an ever-changing science. As new research and clinical experience broaden our knowledge, changes in treatment and drug therapy are required. The editors and the publisher of this work have checked with sources believed to be reliable in their efforts to provide information that is complete and generally in accord with the standards accepted at the time of publication. However, in view of the possibility of human error or changes in medical sciences, neither the editors nor the publisher nor any other party who has been involved in the preparation or publication of this work warrants that the information contained herein is in every respect accurate or complete. Readers are encouraged to confirm the information contained herein with other sources. For example and in particular, readers are advised to check the product information sheet included in the package of each drug they plan to administer to be certain that the information contained in this book is accurate and that changes have not been made in the recommended dose or in the contraindications for administration. This recommendation is of particular importance in connection with new or infrequently used drugs.

PRINCIPLES OF
SURGERY
Fifth Edition

Companion Handbook

Editor-in-Chief

SEYMOUR I. SCHWARTZ, M.D.
Professor and Chair
Department of Surgery
University of Rochester
School of Medicine and Dentistry

Associate Editors

G. Tom Shires, M.D.
Professor and Chair
Department of Surgery
Cornell University Medical College

Frank C. Spencer, M.D.
Professor and Director
Department of Surgery
New York University School of Medicine

WITH

Wendy Cowles Husser, M.A.
University of Rochester
School of Medicine and Dentistry

McGRAW-HILL, INC.
Health Professions Division

New York   St. Louis   San Francisco   Colorado Springs
Auckland   Bogotá   Caracas   Hamburg   Lisbon
London   Madrid   Mexico   Milan   Montreal   New Delhi
Paris   San Juan   São Paulo   Singapore   Sydney
Tokyo   Toronto

PRINCIPLES OF SURGERY, FIFTH EDITION
COMPANION HANDBOOK

234567890   DOCDOC   987654321

ISBN 0-07-055839-6

This book was set in Sabon by Monotype Composition Company, Inc. The editors were J. Dereck Jeffers and Mariapaz Ramos-Englis; the production supervisor was Annette Mayeski. The cover was designed by N.S.G. Design. R.R. Donnelly & Sons was printer and binder.

Front cover art courtesy of Yale Historical Library.

Library of Congress Cataloging-in-Publication Data

Principles of surgery handbook / [edited by] Seymour I. Schwartz.
      p. cm.
   To be used in conjunction with: Principles of surgery / editor-in
-chief, Seymour I. Schwartz. 5th ed. c1989
   ISBN 0-07-055839-6
   1. Surgery—Handbooks, manuals, etc.   I. Schwartz, Seymour I.,
date   . II. Principles of surgery.
   [DNLM: 1. Surgery—handbooks.   WO 39 P957]
RD37.P75   1991
617—dc20
DNLM/DLC
for Library of Congress   90-5824
                                                              CIP

CONTENTS

CONTRIBUTORS

James T. Adams, M.D., Professor of Surgery, Department of Surgery, University of Rochester School of Medicine and Dentistry, Rochester, New York

Carl H. Andrus, M.D., Clinical Associate Professor, Department of Surgery, University of Rochester School of Medicine and Dentistry, Rochester, New York

James Cerilli, M.D., Professor of Surgery and Director of Transplantation, Department of Surgery, University of Rochester School of Medicine and Dentistry, Rochester, New York

Mark S. Davenport, M.D., Resident in Plastic Surgery, University of Rochester Medical Center, Rochester, New York

Brent Dubeshter, M.D., Assistant Professor, Department of Oncology in Obstetrics and Gynecology, University of Rochester School of Medicine and Dentistry, Rochester, New York

Erdal Erturk, M.D., Assistant Professor, Department of Urology, University of Rochester School of Medicine and Dentistry, Rochester, New York

David V. Feliciano, M.D., Professor of Surgery and SICU Director, Strong Memorial Hospital, Department of Surgery, University of Rochester School of Medicine and Dentistry, Rochester, New York

Walter H. Halloran, M.D., Cardiothoracic Fellow, University of Rochester Medical Center, Rochester, New York

Valluvan Jeevanandam, M.D., Instructor and Fellow, Department of Surgery, Columbia University, New York, New York

Ronald Kirshner, M.D., Clinical Associate Professor, Department of Surgery, University of Rochester School of Medicine and Dentistry, Rochester, New York

Barbara Klatchko, M.D., Attending Surgeon, Bryn Mawr Hospital, Bryn Mawr, Pennsylvania

David A. Krusch, M.D., Assistant Professor of Surgery, Department of Surgery, University of Rochester School of Medicine and Dentistry, Rochester, New York

John R. Morton, M.D., Professor of Surgery, Department of Surgery, University of Rochester School of Medicine and Dentistry, Rochester, New York

Kenneth Ouriel, M.D., Assistant Professor of Surgery, Department of Surgery, University of Rochester School of Medicine and Dentistry, Rochester, New York

Peter J. Papadakos, M.D., Senior Instructor, Anesthesiology, University of Rochester Medical Center, Rochester, New York

James L. Peacock, M.D., Assistant Professor of Surgery and Oncology, Department of Surgery, University of Rochester School of Medicine and Dentistry, Rochester, New York

Webster H. Pilcher, M.D., Adjunct Instructor, Departments of Surgery and Neuroendocrinology, University of Rochester School of Medicine and Dentistry, Rochester, New York

Thomas C. Putnam, M.D., Clinical Associate Professor of Pediatrics and Surgery, Department of Surgery, University of Rochester School of Medicine and Dentistry, Rochester, New York

Randy N. Rosier, M.D., Associate Professor of Orthopaedics, Oncology, and Biophysics, Department of Orthopaedics, University of Rochester School of Medicine and Dentistry, Rochester, New York

Harry C. Sax, M.D., Assistant Professor of Surgery and Co-Director Nutritional Support Service, Deparment of Surgery, University of Rochester School of Medicine and Dentistry, Rochester, New York

David B. Schwartz, M.D., Ph.D., Cardiology Fellow, Peter Bent Brigham Hospital, Boston, Massachusetts

Seymour I. Schwartz, M.D., Professor and Chair, Department of Surgery, University of Rochester School of Medicine and Dentistry, Rochester, New York

PREFACE

This handbook has resulted from the need of students and houseofficers to be able to carry a book with them for easy reference when there is limited access to the companion large textbook. This portable handbook is not meant to supersede the textbook and should be used in conjunction with the 5th edition of *Principles of Surgery*, published in 1989. The preparations of the contributors to the handbook were based solely on the chapters from the 5th edition and are meant to be concise synopses of the work of those original authors.

1 ENDOCRINE AND METABOLIC RESPONSES TO INJURY

The response to injury is quite variable, with multiple factors involved in determining the specific response and its intensity. Three things must occur for the response to be elicited: The stimulus must be perceived at the central nervous system; the information is then integrated and an appropriate output determined; the output at the end organ ensues based on signals leaving the central nervous system. Each of these points will be examined in more depth.

INPUT

For the stimulus to be received, *neurologic* routes must be intact. For example, paraplegics do not have the expected elevated cortisol response to an injury as do normally innervated patients. In an experimental model of cord section, burn below the level of the cord lesion does not cause the same changes in cortisol and vasopressin levels as does a similar burn applied above the lesion. The types of anesthetics used in a patient may have similar results. A general anesthetic does not block the stimulus from reaching the central nervous system, and vasopressin release is stimulated. The use of local anesthetics or a spinal anesthetic blocks this response.

Because injury often is associated with loss of effective circulating volume, there are direct effects from volume receptors. Afferent signals from high-pressure baroreceptors as well as stretch receptors at the heart exert a tonic down-regulation over the release of many hormones. When effective circulating volume decreases, this inhibition is released. Cortisol secretion in response to ACTH is elevated, and increased conversion of angiotensinogen to angiotensin occurs. Glucagon is stimulated to be released by the pancreas with inhibition of insulin. All these changes lead to retention of fluid in an attempt to restore blood volume.

The body also has specific chemoreceptors that react to decreases in oxygen delivery. Hypovolemia as associated with shock will result in lower blood flow through the chemoreceptors. This will increase the extraction of oxygen by the chemoreceptor tissue, thus activating the chemoreceptor and inducing hyperventilation. This hyperventilation may marginally increase oxygenation, improving oxygen delivery.

As with any injury, pain and emotional arousal lead to increases in the secretion of various hormones including vasopressin, ACTH, the endogenous opiates, catecholamines, cortisol, and aldosterone. Many of these are mediated by the catecholamine release, leading to the "fight or flight response." This further causes alterations in levels of glucose and amino acids. These individual substrates then have direct effects. Leucine, a branched chain amino acid, stimulates secretion of insulin and also increases hepatic protein synthesis. Because many amino acids such as phenylalanine and tyrosine are precursors for neurotransmitters such as epinephrine, alterations in their levels can cause changes in the overall neurotransmitter milieu at the central nervous system.

The hypothalamus has a specific set point to temperature. Significant injury results in decreases in core temperature. Hormonal output in response causes shivering and vasoconstriction.

INTEGRATION

Once the signals have reached the brain, it is incumbent on the central nervous system to integrate and determine an appropriate output. This is a very complex concept which involves interaction of many different areas and parameters. This proposal for ACTH secretion is outlined in Fig. 1-1. Multiple stimuli from baroreceptors, from stretch receptors in the heart, and from painful stimuli that are received through the spinal cord are integrated in the pons. Output then ensues from the hypothalamus and the periventricular nuclei. This delineation for other hormones is not as well determined. Integration in and of itself is determined not only by the type of input but also by the rate in which the input reaches the brain. For example, a patient who loses 30 percent of blood volume over 1 h will elicit different and more acute changes than a patient who has lost a similar volume of blood over 1 day (see Fig. 1-2). The timing of the arrival of stimuli may also affect output. Broken ribs cause acute pain and shock of initial injury, followed a short time thereafter by increasing hypovolemia from ongoing blood loss and eventual hypoxemia due to splinting. These stimuli are reaching the integration centers over a different time course and with different intensities. Thus the output would be graded. Concomitant intoxication with ethanol appears to further modify these outputs, not only by directly affecting

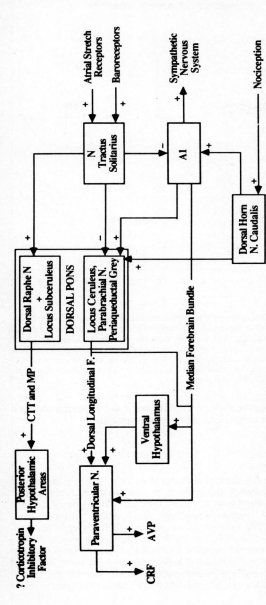

Fig. 1-1. The proposed neural organization for the control of ACTH and vasopressin in response to hemodynamic change and nociception. Three principal areas of the hypothalamus receive signals from the principal pontine areas, projecting through the areas defined in the midbrain to inhibit or facilitate release of vasopressin and of corticotropin releasing factor (CRF) by the median eminence and thus of ACTH. Thus, the principal pathways from atrial and carotid receptors to the median eminence for control of release of CRF and vasopressin are multiple. Symbols: N, nucleus; F, fasiculus; +, stimulates; −, inhibits.

3

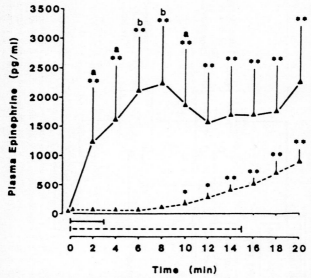

Fig. 1-2. Plasma epinephrine concentrations in response to graded blood loss in the cat at rapid and slow rates of hemorrhage: 30% hemorrhage, rapid rate = Δ——Δ ($n = 8$), slow rate = Δ - - - Δ ($n = 8$). The horizontal bars under each figure represent the period of blood removal for each hemorrhage magnitude, $*p < 0.05$, $**p < 0.01$ vs. control group. a. $p < 0.05$; b. $p < 0.01$ vs. slow rate of hemorrhage. (From: *Bereiter DA et al: Am J Physiol 1986, with permission.*)

metabolic parameters at the liver but also by altering changes in catecholamines and other neurotransmitters.

OUTPUT

Assuming that the signals have been appropriately generated and have reached the brain to be integrated, efferent output and organ response is then expected. Three forms of this output take place: autonomic, local tissue response, and hormone. The autonomic response is generated in an area of the brain separate from the hormonal or hypothalamic response. Output from the autonomic system changes levels of sympathetic and parasympathetic nervous tone, not hormones. Changes of inflammation at the site of the injury including factors generated from the white cells and macrophages can cause a local response. The hypothalamic-pituitary axis secretes multiple hormones which fall into four different classes: the derivatives of cholesterol (such as cortisol and aldosterone); the arachidonic acid pathways (including the prostaglandins and leukotrienes); proteins (including glycoproteins, like thyroid-stimulating hormone and follicle-stimulating hormone); and the small polypeptides (vasopressin).

Outputs work at the cellular surface level. If it is advantageous for the cell to produce a specific protein, the message to do so is first reached at the cellular membrane level. A hormone messenger is bound by a receptor and transported to the nucleus, turning on the appropriate segment of DNA to cause RNA transcription and eventually protein synthesis. Cyclic AMP (cAMP) is the central messenger in these pathways (see Fig. 1-3).

HORMONAL RESPONSES

Cortisol shifts amino acids out of the muscles and into the liver where they are used for gluconeogenesis and protein synthesis. It increases lipolysis and potentiates epinephrine, one of the counterregulatory hormones seen in stress and sepsis. In certain states of severe stress and in those patients whose adrenals have been previously suppressed from exogenous steroid administration, a syndrome of acute adrenal insufficiency can develop. These patients will present with hypoglycemia, hyponatremia, hyperkalemia, and shock. Fevers are often common. Untreated, acute adrenal insufficiency often leads to death.

Because the postinjury state is associated with hypermetabolism, it would seem logical that *thyroid hormone* would be elevated. In fact, this is not the case. In many situations thyroid hormone levels are decreased. Specifically the conversion from T_4 to T_3 is impaired, in part due to cortisol. Excessive amounts of T_4 are converted to the biologically inactive compound reverse T_3, this being characteristic of injury. *TSH* secretion does not appear to be elevated.

Growth hormone is under the same control mechanisms as other pituitary hormones. Growth hormone secretion is stimulated by decreased circulating volume, hypoglycemia, and decreased concentrations of fatty acids. There are a few things that down-regulate growth hormone secretion other than its own level. Growth hormone increases plasma glucose along with fatty acids and ketone bodies. Of great interest are the anabolic activities of growth hormone. Recent studies have shown that even with the provision of hypocaloric

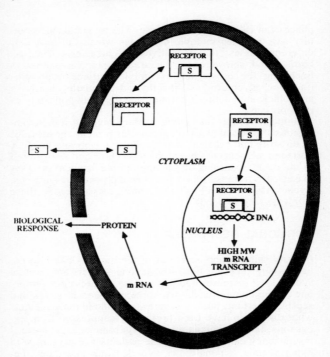

Fig. 1-3. The mechanism of action of steroid hormones. Steroids, which permeate the cell membrane freely, bind to cytosolic receptors and are then translocated to the nucleus, where the receptor hormone complex interacts with DNA to modulate transcription.

nutritional support, supplemental growth hormone can ensure positive nitrogen balance.

The *gonadotrophins,* sex hormones, and prolactin are increased after trauma, although the significance of these physiologic changes is uncertain.

The last 20 years have brought an increased understanding of the body's own pain control mechanisms. The *enkephalins* (endorphins) are polypeptides which are found to bind the same receptors as morphine and other opiates. These endogenous opiates have cardiovascular side effects similar to those of morphine and can be blocked by naloxone.

One of the most potent stimuli to fluid retention is *vasopressin* (ADH), a polypeptide synthesized in the hypothalamus. It is transported to the neurohypophysis, where it is

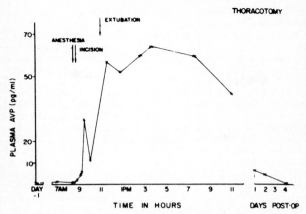

Vasopressin levels before, during, and after surgery.

Fig. 1-4. Plasma vasopressin concentrations during thoracotomy. (From: *Haas M, Glick SM: Arch Surg 113:597, 1978, with permission.*)

then released. Changes in effective circulating volume are the most potent stimuli for vasopressin release. As little as a 10 percent decrease in effective circulating volume causes a 300% increase in vasopressin concentration. Vasopressin is also stimulated by operative trauma and has been found to have four phases (see Fig. 1-4). In phase one, vasopressin has the normal preoperative levels. During the period of overnight fasting prior to surgery vasopressin begins to rise. The incision itself causes a dramatic increase, with elevations of ADH that remain up for several days. As the operative trauma fades and operative fluids are mobilized, vasopressin returns to normal by the fifth day.

A syndrome of inappropriate secretion of vasopressin (SIADH), is associated with head injury. It manifests as low urinary output with a high osmolality and dilutional hyponatremia. More commonly, a syndrome of diabetes insipidus develops, in which the absence of vasopressin allows large amounts of dilute urine. Plasma osmolality is high.

Another hormone intimately involved in fluid and electrolyte regulation is *aldosterone*. Cells in the adrenal gland synthesize and secrete aldosterone in response to several different stimuli, including angiotensin II, ACTH, and an elevation in serum potassium concentrations. Aldosterone acts at the kidney with resorption of sodium and chloride at the expense of potassium.

The *catecholamines* are released in response to injury, fear, and hypoglycemia. Heart rate, glycogenolysis, and glyconeogensis, are stimulated. There are responses at both the alpha and beta receptors, mediated by the amount and type of catecholamines secreted.

The *kidney* is the central organ in fluid and blood pressure control. Within the juxtaglomerular apparatus lies the *renin-angiotensin* system. These receptors not only sense concentrations of tubular fluid but also respond to beta-adrenergic stimulation by the catecholamines. Renin is secreted, which converts a renin substrate produced in the liver to angiotensin I. Angiotensin I is then changed to angiotensin II by a pulmonary-converting enzyme. This active form is a vasoconstrictor and also increases heart rate and contractility. Because angiotensin II is also a stimulator of aldosterone, fluid and sodium is retained. Not surprisingly, plasma concentrations of angiotensin II are elevated immediately after injury.

Glucose control is complex, mediated by insulin and glucagon. The release of insulin after injury is biphasic. Early on, the high levels of catecholamine suppress insulin, leading to an increase in plasma glucose. Later, insulin resistance develops; although more insulin is being secreted, its effect at the end-organ is not as efficient. This explains why patients who have had trauma or stress or are septic have hyperglycemia, which is difficult to control. Once the organism has survived the initial phase of trauma and is now becoming anabolic, insulin resistance lessens and storage of carbohydrate, protein, and lipids is promoted. Glucagon response is different from insulin response. Initially down regulation after trauma occurs, followed over the ensuing 10 h by a gradual rise. The synthesis and secretion of glucagon by the pancreatic alpha cells has multiple controls including concentrations of glucose, amino acids, and fatty acids, and the autonomic nervous system activity. Insulin and glucagon, in general, coexist in a ratio appropriate to maintain euglycemia. In various disease states this ratio is altered. Insulin is anabolic overall, whereas glucagon tends to be catabolic because of its ability to mobilize fatty acids, increasing ketogenesis and glucose production.

The *eicosanoids* are derived from arachidonic acid, a fatty acid which exists in the cellular membrane layer. By reaction with oxygenases they traverse one of several pathways to form either prostaglandins or leukotrienes. There are several families of prostaglandins and they tend to have opposing roles. For example, prostaglandin E produces bronchodilation, whereas prostaglandin F causes bronchoconstriction. By the same token, the balance between prostaglandins and thromboxane balances platelet aggregation and vasoconstriction. The prostaglandins are major components in the inflammatory response, and this explains why the cyclooxygenase inhibitors such as aspirin have an effect on bursitis, arthritis, and tenosynovitis. Leukotrienes are produced by a variety of cells, predominantly white cells, producing postcapillary leakage with broncho- and vasoconstriction. It is felt that they may serve an important role in the pathophysiology of shock.

Other mediators and effectors after injury include the *kallikrenes,* which are local vasodilators and produce pain; *serotonin,* a neurotransmitter formed from tryptophan; *histamine,* which has long been implicated in the pathophysiology of tissue injury; and the somatomedins, which are a family of polypeptides that stimulate proteoglycan synthesis. *Interleukin-1* has been under intense investigation recently as a mediator produced by macrophages. This has been shown to produce a cascade effect in response to trauma and sepsis. Interleukin-1 appears to stimulate protein synthesis and increased production of acute phase proteins. It is likely that interleukin-1 is the trigger for many of the other cascades resulting in the organism's response to sepsis. This is a similar situation for *tumor necrosis factor* (cachectin), which can cause hemorrhagic necrosis of tumors and may be responsible for the wasting associated with chronic illness.

METABOLIC CHANGES INDUCED BY INJURY

Although the area of nutrition will be further explored in later chapters, a basic discussion is in order here. The average individual utilizes 1800 calories a day. The nervous tissue and blood cells require 180 g/d glucose. There is also obligate need for amino acids for protein synthesis and fatty acids for lipid synthesis. During fasting, the body's preexisting supplies are utilized. During the first 24 h of fasting, glycogen is available in the liver and can be broken down to form free glucose. However, after this period of time, glyconeogenesis must take place, with amino acid skeletons being the primary fuel. As fasting is adapted over an extended period of time the organism begins to burn more ketone bodies, with an increasing lipolysis. Thus the initial response to fasting is one of relative hypoglycemia with a falling insulin level, and a gradual increase in glucagon levels (see Fig. 1-5). The amino acids that are utilized enter the Krebs cycle as gluconeogeneic, ketogenic, or mixed amino acids. During

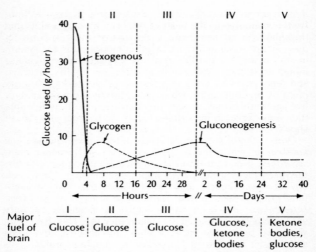

Fig. 1-5. The five phases of glucose homeostasis. This represents the origin of blood glucose in a 70-kg man who ingests 100 g of glucose and then fasts for 40 days. Phase I is the absorptive phase in which the 100 g of glucose enters the circulation by absorption from the gut. Phase II is the postabsorptive phase in which glucose is stored as glycogen in response to increased secretion of insulin and decreased secretion of glucagon. Phase III represents early starvation in which the fall in blood sugar leads to a decrease in insulin secretion and an increase in glucagon and catecholamine secretion. The latter results in an increase in gluconeogenesis and glycogenolysis. Phase IV is intermediary starvation in which hepatic glycogen stores have been depleted and the sole source of glucose is gluconeogenesis. Phase V represents prolonged starvation in which ketone bodies become the primary fuel, thereby resulting in a decrease in gluconeogenesis. (From: *Ruderman NB: Annu Rev Med 248, 1975, with permission.*)

starvation the protein supplied predominantly comes from the muscle as the largest source of amino acid skeletons. On a per organ basis, however, the liver loses a larger proportion of its protein pool than does the skeletal muscle. Over a 5- to 6-week period of starvation the body becomes primarily a ketone utilizer. There remains, however, an obligate protein loss from amino acids for glucose production for the brain and for essential protein synthesis.

Water and electrolytes are similarly affected by starvation. Sodium losses of 300 meq/day ensue initially, gradually adapting to retention. Total body water also decreases.

The injured organism acts differently from the starved

organism. In both cases, a generalized catabolism is seen. Energy expenditure is elevated in injury from 10 to 30% after fracture and up to 100% with large third degree burns. In contradistinction, patients who have been starved for a long period of time have a decrease in base-line energy expenditure.

Glucose metabolism is also different in injury as opposed to starvation. Long starvation leads to a generalized hypoglycemia with increased lipolysis and decreased insulin levels. In severe injury, glucose concentrations are elevated markedly. It is suggested that this high level of glucose is a source of energy for the brain and may offer some survival advantage. This elevated glucose concentration is due to both end-organ insulin resistance and to glucose release due to catecholamines. As the acute trauma has passed an anabolism ensues, insulin resistance lessens, and repair takes place. Protein metabolism during injury manifests as initial loss of skeletal muscle mass. Amino acid skeletons are shunted to the liver for glucose formation and acute phase protein synthesis. When the amino acid skeleton is broken down for use other than for protein, nitrogen is released as a waste product. Therefore, an increase in nitrogen excretion in the urine is consistent with catabolism of skeletal muscle. Urinary nitrogen loss after injury is correlated with extent. Normally, about 13 g nitrogen is excreted daily in the urine; however, after injury, this can rise to as high as 50 g/day. Realizing that every gram of nitrogen is equivalent to 6.25 g protein, skeletal muscle losses of approximately 300 g/day can be found. The balance between nitrogen intake and nitrogen loss normally is slightly positive in the nonstressed organism. Exogenous provision of calories and protein is supportive in the resolving phase of injury. Wound healing additionally requires vitamins A and C, along with zinc, thiamine, and riboflavin. Supplementation may be advantageous in this situation.

Fluid and electrolytes are eventually replenished by renal mechanisms. The initial decrease in renal blood flow leads to resorption of salt and water. Changes in aldosterone and renin secretion cause water and salt to be resorbed in an isotonic fashion. The development of hyponatremia postoperatively is due, therefore, to the provision of hypotonic fluids.

Blood volume is restored by both exogenous isotonic fluids and endogenous movement of interstitial fluids into the effective circulating volume. A fall in capillary pressure first allows protein-free fluid to move into the vascular space. Protein redistribution occurs thereafter. Cellular size then decreases as fluid moves out along the osmotic gradient.

SUMMARY

The endocrine and metabolic responses to injury are many and varied. For a response to ensue, three things must happen: sensation, integration, and output. The output may take the form of hormonal changes or neurologic impulses. Injury initially causes a down regulation (ebb), followed by a hyperdynamic phase (flow), then settles into long-term anabolism and repair. Support of the surgical patient in the perioperative period involves replacement of fluid and electrolyte losses and the provision of adequate exogenous protein and nutrients to aid tissue repair.

2 FLUID, ELECTROLYTES, AND NUTRITIONAL SUPPORT

ANATOMY OF BODY FLUIDS

Total body water comprises 50% to 70% of body weight. It is divided into an intracellular component approximating 40% of body weight and an extracellular component that is 5% of body weight as intravascular fluid volume and 15% as interstitial fluid. There is a water exchange of 2000 ml/day, which is a balance of an intake of 1500 ml orally and 500 ml from food, with an output of 250 ml in stool, 600 ml insensible losses, and 800–1500 ml urine.

Total body stores of salt are primarily in the extracellular volume. The normal salt intake is 50–90 meq/day. Output is highly variable, with excretion in the urine from 10–80 meq/day, intestinal excretion 0–20 meq/day, and sweat as high as 300 meq/h in very hot environments. Increased sodium losses are also seen in patients with fistulas, diarrhea, and protracted vomiting.

CHANGES IN BODY FLUIDS

The changes in body fluids may be divided into three categories: changes in volume, changes in concentration, and changes in composition.

Volume

Volume deficit is the most common problem in surgical patients. Causes include loss of gastrointestinal fluids from vomiting or fistulas, hemorrhage, and the third spacing of fluids into the interstitium from injury and infection. Clinically, the patients will manifest signs of orthostatic hypotension, decreasing urine output, and a mild temperature decrease. Treatment is centered on replacement of intravascular volume in the form of isotonic electrolyte fluids.

The other end of the spectrum is that of fluid overload which can be iatrogenic from excessive administration or secondary to underlining medical diseases, such as renal failure, cirrhosis, and heart failure. The physical signs include a generalized edema with weight gain, and pulmonary basilar rales from left-sided heart failure. Distended neck veins are due to elevated right-sided pressures. Patients in fluid overload are treated based on their underlying physical state. In a healthy patient, merely reducing the infusion rate will allow the body to correct itself. Patients with underlying medical conditions, such as heart failure or kidney disease may require diuresis, salt restriction, and, in extreme cases, dialysis.

Concentration

It is important to note that abnormal concentrations may occur in the presence of normal, excess, or deficient total body amounts of solute. Thus, in each state one must determine whether solute replacement will be required. Hyponatremia is due to either excessive free water or salt losses greater than water losses. Clinically, lethargy may ensue due to cerebral edema, as well as hypertension from increased intracranial pressure in extreme cases. Acute and precipitous drops in serum sodium concentrations will elicit seizures. In symptomatic patients, small volumes of hypertonic (3%) NaCl are administered. In less severe situations, free water restriction and normal saline infusions are adequate to restore serum sodium concentrations toward normal.

Hypernatremia is caused by excessive free water loss or salt replacement. These patients are thirsty, tachycardic, and febrile. Therapy is centered on replacement of free water and, if excessive salt losses are documented, sodium supplementation.

Potassium is a central ion in nervous system conduction and muscular contractility. Hypokalemia is due to multiple causes. These include losses from vomiting and diarrhea. Additionally, iatrogenic hypokalemia from diuretic use is quite common, especially when inadequate potassium replacements are given. During acute metabolic alkalosis, potassium is driven into the cell in exchange for hydrogen ions to buffer the alkalosis. This can cause symptomatic hypokalemia. The initial clinical signs can be of a nonspecific weakness which progresses in severe cases to flaccid paralysis. The major concern is cardiac arrhythmia, especially when patients are on digitalis, which heightens myocardial sensitivity to hypokalemia. EKG changes begin with flattened T waves, which may then progress to ventricular arrhythmias. Potassium can be replaced at a rate not to exceed 40 meq/h; however, in severe cases where arrhythmias are present, replacement rates of up to 2 meq/min can be achieved with careful EKG monitoring. Hypokalemia is a very common problem, and it is often very difficult to handle cardiac patients because they are on both potassium-losing diuretics and digitalis preparations.

Hyperkalemia is another life-threatening imbalance of potassium, which can be induced by renal failure, tissue necrosis, or metabolic acidosis as potassium moves out of the cells. Iatrogenic causes include excessive administration of potassium in the face of renal insufficiency, often in patients who are inadequately resuscitated from hypovolemia. The patients will present with nausea and vomiting. EKG changes progress to peaked T waves, with cardiac arrest always a possibility. Immediate therapy of the acutely hyperkalemic patient involves the intravenous administration of 1 amp sodium bicarbonate, 10 units regular insulin, and 1 amp $D_{50}W$, which will temporarily drive potassium into the cells. Intravenous calcium gluconate (1 g) does not lower potassium levels per se, but reduces its affect on the heart, and may prevent arrhythmia. In less acute situations, Kayexalate, a binding resin, is given orally or as an enema. If other measures fail, dialysis is a final mode of therapy.

Calcium's primary role is in muscle contraction and neurologic transmission through the sarcoplasmic reticulum. Causes of hypocalcemia include hypoparathyroidism, usually the sequela of neck and thyroid surgery; acute alkalosis, which lowers the ionized or active portion of calcium; pancreatitis, due to sequestration of calcium with fat necrosis; and high gastrointestinal losses, especially in patients with short gut syndromes and diarrhea. In the case of acute hypovolemic shock, blood transfusions can bind calcium in the EDTA used as a preservative, but the blood must be given very rapidly, greater than 500 ml in 10 min, for this to become clinically evident.

In general, the signs of hypocalcemia are neurologic with circumoral numbness, carpopedal spasm (Trousseau's sign), and irritability of the masseter muscle when tapping on the facial nerve (Chvostek's sign). An EKG in the hypocalcemic patient will show prolongation of the QT interval. In extreme states of calcium deprivation, seizures may occur. Symptomatic patients are supplemented with 1 g calcium gluconate slowly.

Depending on etiology, long-term therapy includes vitamin D and oral calcium supplements. It is not uncommon to have a coexisting magnesium deficiency in patients who are hypocalcemic; this should be investigated. Due to the widespread availability of screening tests, more and more cases of hypercalcemia are being detected in asymptomatic patients.

The primary causes of hypercalcemia are hyperparathyroidism and bony metastasis, especially from breast, lung, and prostate cancer. An iatrogenic cause is that of the milk-alkali syndrome. Many patients who are hypercalcemic from hyperparathyroidism are asymptomatic or have very mild mental status changes that are nonspecific, such as fatigue and headache. Gastrointestinal complaints will include nausea, vomiting, weight loss, and thirst. Patients with metastases often have bone pain. Renal calculi are common in patients with primary hyperparathyroidism.

The phrase "Stones, bones, abdominal groans, mental moans" is a mnemonic device used to accurately recall the symptoms of patients with hypercalcemia due to hyperparathyroidism. When the acutely hypercalcemic patient presents, immediate therapy to lower calcium is achieved by hydration with calcium-wasting diuretics such as lasix. Over the long term, mithramycin and steroids have been useful, although their effects are not notable for several days. In patients with documented hyperparathyroidism, either primary or secondary from renal failure, parathyroidectomy should be considered.

The changes in concentration of magnesium often parallel those of calcium. Hypomagnesemia is often seen in patients who are malnourished, and especially in those whose malnutrition stems from prolonged starvation and alcoholism. Pancreatitis and diarrhea with fistula losses are additional gastrointestinal causes. Because a coexistent calcium deficiency is common, the signs are very similar, with hyperactive tendon reflexes, delirium, and seizures. Therapy is aimed at a reduction of losses with supplementation by magnesium sulfate in symptomatic patients. It may take several weeks for total body stores to be repleted, even in the face of normal serum magnesium levels.

Hypermagnesemia is most commonly seen in renal failure and may be exacerbated by the provision of magnesium-containing antacids. These patients will show lethargy and weakness and on EKG widening of the QRS complex with an increased PR interval. If possible, hydration is indicated along with withholding of exogenous magnesium. Dialysis can be used in anuric or symptomatic patients.

Composition

The composition of extracellular fluids affects acid base status. When examining the acid base equilibrium, three key measurements are that of pH, P_{CO_2}, and serum bicarbonate.

In each case a primary defect is noted with the body's subsequent attempt at compensation.

Hypoventilation leading to increases in the plasma tension of CO_2 in turn leads to *respiratory acidosis*. This is primarily due to respiratory depression from either narcotics or CNS injury. Patients with primary pulmonary disease such as COPD will also retain CO_2, although they may not become acutely acidotic because of the slow onset of this retention. The body will attempt to compensate for this by renal retention of bicarbonate with a mild metabolic alkalosis. In acute cases of respiratory acidosis, mechanical ventilation will correct the elevated P_{CO_2}.

Patients who are hyperventilated with reduction of the plasma levels of carbon dioxide develop a *respiratory alkalosis*. In general, this is a ventilatory support rate that is too high. Anxiety or pain may cause a central alkalosis due to increased respiratory rate. The kidneys will attempt to compensate with bicarbonate excretion or retention of organic acids. Because alkalosis is so acute, in general, the secondary compensations do not come into effect. Therapy includes adjustment of the ventilator or treatment of the primary CNS etiology.

The development of a *metabolic acidosis* can be due to two primary defects, either an excessive loss of bicarbonate or accumulation of fixed acids leading to *widened anion gap*. Patients with diarrhea or pancreatic fistula who are losing excessive amounts of bicarbonate will develop a metabolic acidosis with a *normal gap*. Shock causing an anaerobic metabolism with increases in lactate in turn causes widened anion gap acidosis, as does ingestion of aspirin. The body will compensate initially by hyperventilating, in an attempt to reduce the P_{CO_2}. The kidneys, where possible, will retain bicarbonate. Therapy such as resuscitation from shock or dialysis of exogenous ingestion is aimed at treating underlying defects. Exogenous bicarbonate supplementation is appropriate only in a normal anion gap acidosis where bicarbonate losses are increased.

Metabolic alkalosis can have two primary defects, either an excessive loss of acids or gain in bicarbonate. Causes of the former include vomiting of gastric contents, especially when associated with gastric outlet obstruction due to peptic ulcer disease ("GOO-PUD"). Similarly, diuretics such as lasix and thiazides cause excessive excretion of chloride leading to alkalosis. Excessive administration of antacids can cause a gain in bicarbonate. The body will make initial attempts to decrease ventilation, but this is limited by the development of hypoxemia. The renal excretion of bicarbonate is a minor compensatory mechanism. In severe alkalosis

TABLE 2-1. Respiratory and Metabolic Components of Acid-Base Disorders

Type of acid-base disorder	Acute (uncompensated)			Chronic (partially compensated)		
	pH	P_{CO_2}*	Plasma $HCO_3^{-\dagger,\ddagger}$	pH	P_{CO_2}*	Plasma $HCO_3^{-\dagger,\ddagger}$
Respiratory acidosis	⇊	⇈	N	↓	⇈	↑
Respiratory alkalosis	⇈	⇊	N	↑	⇊	↓
Metabolic acidosis	⇊	N	⇊	↓	↓	↓
Metabolic alkalosis	⇈	N	⇈	↑	↑ ?	↑

* Respiratory component.
† Metabolic component.
‡ Measured as standard bicarbonate, whole blood buffer base, CO_2 content, or CO_2 combining power. The *base excess value* is positive when the standard bicarbonate is above normal and negative when the standard bicarbonate is below normal.

correction of the underlining defect is vital. In cases of GOO-PUD, the concomitant potassium loss may obligate urinary hydrogen losses in the face of alkalosis, the so-called paradoxical aciduria. This should indicate that replacement of not only volume but also potassium is required (see Table 2-1).

FLUID AND ELECTROLYTE THERAPY

Fluid deficits may be classified as mild to severe; mild deficits are associated with the 4% loss of body weight, and severe deficits greater than 10%. The initial replacement of fluid deficits should be with the balanced, isotonic electrolyte solution until urine output increases to the rate of ½ to 1 ml/kg of ideal body weight per hour. A decrease in a resting tachycardia indicates adequate replenishment.

Base-line needs of fluid are approximately 1000 ml/day as an obligate urinary excretion of catabolic end products and 600 ml/day of insensible losses. As previously noted, sodium and potassium are utilized in varying amounts and their additional losses need to be considered. A solution of 5% dextrose with 70 meq sodium chloride and 20 meq potassium chloride per liter (D_5W ½NS plus 20 meq KCl) running at a rate of 75 ml/h is a reasonable base-line fluid for maintenance in the average adult.

TABLE 2-2. Composition of Gastrointestinal Secretions

Type of secretion	Volume (mL/24h)	Na (meq/L)	K (meq/L)	Cl (meq/L)	HCO$_3$ (meq/L)
Salivary	1500	10	26	10	30
	(500–2000)	(2–10)	(20–30)	(8–18)	
Stomach	1500	60	10	130	
	(100–4000)	(9–116)	(0–32)	(8–154)	
Duodenum		140	5	80	
	(100–2000)				
Ileum	3000	140	5	104	30
	(100–9000)	(80–150)	(2–8)	(43–137)	
Colon		60	30	40	
Pancreas		140	5	75	115
	(100–800)	(113–185)	(3–7)	(54–95)	
Bile		145	5	100	35
	(50–800)	(131–164)	(3–12)	(89–180)	

Additional losses are factored in and can take the form of intraoperative deficits from evaporation and third-space losses. These may run as high as 1000 ml/h during the time that the abdomen is open. Postoperative fistulas and ongoing nasogastric drainage should be replaced on a milliliter for milliliter basis with the appropriate electrolyte solution. One way to determine what fluids should be given is to directly measure the sodium, potassium, and chloride in the various fistula or nasogastric drainages. Additionally, fevers, delirium tremens, or peritonitis increase fluid needs (see Tables 2-2 and 2-3.)

NUTRITIONAL SUPPORT

All patients who will not be able to eat within 7 days should be considered for supplemental nutrition. Patients with preexisting malnutrition must be evaluated and intervention started earlier.

The question of enteral versus parenteral nutrition can be summed up by the quotation, ''If the gut works, use it.'' In fact, the majority of patients can be supported enterally, especially with the advent of small bore nasoenteric tubes. By introducing these tubes through the pylorus into the duodenum, the problem of gastric atony can be overcome. The use of enteral support preserves the gut mucosa, and its integrity is increasingly important. Enteral support is especially appropriate in burns where early utilization of the gut may decrease metabolic rate, head trauma or major neurologic catastrophes, pulmonary disease, and multiple long bone fractures. The major risk of enteral feedings is the risk

**TABLE 2-3. Composition of Parenteral Fluids
(Electroylte Content, meq/L)**

Solutions	Cations				Anions		Osmolality, mO
	Na	K	Ca	Mg	Cl	HCO₃	
Extracellular fluid	142	4	5	3	103	27	280–310
Lactated Ringer's	130	4	3	—	109	28*	273
0.9% sodium chloride	154	—	—	—	154	—	308
D₅ 45% sodium chloride	77	—	—	—	77	—	407
D₅W	—	—	—	—	—	—	253
M/6 sodium lactate	167	—	—	—	—	167*	334
3% sodium chloride	513	—	—	—	513	—	1026

* Present in solution as lactate that is converted to bicarbonate.

of aspiration. *Patients whose airway cannot be protected must be fed distal to the pylorus or via a formal gastrostomy or jejunostomy.*

One of the major advances in the care of surgical patients over the last 20 years has been the advent of total parenteral nutrition (TPN). This modality is lifesaving in many previously fatal conditions. Efficacy of TPN has been specifically demonstrated in the short-gut syndrome, due to vascular accident or congenital defect; intrinsic small bowel disease; systemic sclerosis (scleroderma) with gastrointestinal tract involvement; and prolonged ileus secondary to trauma where enteral feedings are unsuccessful. The use of TPN in patients with cancer cachexia is controversial. In the absence of other therapy in the form of radiation, chemotherapy, or surgery, TPN serves to feed only the tumor and not the host. Specialized forms of utilizing different amino acid formulations have been shown to be efficacious in acute renal failure and hepatic encephalopathy, although the expense associated with these specialized formulas limits their use. TPN must not be initiated in patients who have major fluid and electrolyte abnormalities until these are corrected by conventional means.

Complications associated with TPN are technical, metabolic, and infectious. Placement of central lines is preferably via the subclavian route, in the well-hydrated, sedated patient. A roll along the spine and steep Trendelenberg positioning further opens the route to the subclavian vein. Technical complications such as pneumothorax, hemothorax, or injury to the thoracic duct occur during 4% of insertions. Air embolism is a potentially fatal complication.

Metabolic complications can be protean, including hyperglycemia that can lead to hyperosmolar nonketotic coma. In patients on long-term TPN, serious deficiency states of trace

TABLE 2-4.   **Correlation of Increased Energy Expenditure and Urinary Nitrogen Excretion After Injury and Illness**

	% Increase above basal energy expenditure	Daily urinary N excretion per kg
Normal	—	0.09
Elective, major surgery	24	0.21
Skeletal trauma	32	0.32
Blunt trauma	37	0.32
Head trauma/steroids	61	0.34
Sepsis	79	0.37
40% thermal injury	132	0.37

SOURCE: Adapted from Long CL et al: *J Parenter Enteral Nutr* 3:452, 1979.

metals and vitamins also develop as well as fatty acid deficiencies.

Up to 20% of patients suffer serious infectious complications related to central venous cannulation. The primary pathogens include the gram-positive cocci and yeast and can lead to endocarditis.

Determination of the appropriate amounts to be fed can be via direct or indirect means. A metabolic chart directly determines oxygen consumption and carbon dioxide production in a specific patient. From these can be extrapolated a basal energy expenditure. A metabolic chart is not available in all centers, and the use of the Harris-Benedict equation with Long's stress factors is appropriate in estimating basal energy expenditure (BEE).

$$BEE \text{ (men)} = 66.47 + 13.75(W) + 5.0(H) - 6.76(A) \text{ kcal/day}$$
$$BEE \text{ (women)} = 65.51 + 9.56(W) + 1.85(H) - 4.68(A) \text{ kcal/day}$$

where W = weight in kg; H = height in cm; and A = age in years. Stress of trauma and sepsis will increase these numbers (see Table 2-4).

In parenteral nutrition calories are given primarily as glucose, although intravenous fat solutions may provide up to 40% of daily calories. Protein is given as crystalline amino acids and in the absence of increased losses can be provided at a rate of 1.5 g/kg/day. In some situations, protein is expressed as grams of nitrogen. The conversion is that 1 g nitrogen is equivalent to 6.25 g protein. Standard amino acid mixtures provide a balance of essential and nonessential amino acids in a final concentration of 4–5%. Disease-specific solutions for renal or hepatic failure vary these ratios to meet special needs of the patient. Glucose control is maintained with supplemental insulin added to the total parenteral nutrition. In average patients supplemental insulin is not needed; however, in septic, diabetic, or highly stressed patients, supplemental insulin is often required because of end-organ resistance. The development of glucose intolerance in a previously euglycemic patient who has been on TPN for a long period signals the advent of sepsis.

Vitamins and trace elements are added daily to prevent deficiency states. Electrolytes in the form of sodium, potassium, magnesium, calcium, and phosphorous are added and adjusted based on serum levels and anticipated losses.

Some patients do not have the absorptive surface area to support themselves enterally. In this instance the use of TPN infused at night in the home environment has been lifesaving and has allowed many of these patients to carry on a normal lifestyle. Surgically implanted catheters that are tunneled and exited a distance away from the subclavian vein have allowed long-term central venous access with low infectious complications.

3 HEMOSTASIS

BIOLOGY OF HEMOSTASIS

Hemostasis is a complex process that prevents or terminates blood loss from the intravascular space, provides a fibrin network for tissue repair, and, ultimately, removes the fibrin when it is no longer needed. Four major physiologic events participate in this process.

Vascular Constriction   This is the initial response to injury, even at the capillary level. Vasoconstriction begins prior to platelet adherence, as a reflex response to various stimuli. It is subsequently linked to platelet plug and fibrin formation. The vasoconstrictors thromboxane A_2 (TxA_2) and serotonin are released during platelet aggregation. Local physical factors (e.g., surrounding muscle tissue) may also contribute to the control of bleeding from vascular injury.

Platelet Function   Platelets normally number 150,000–400,000/mm³, with an average life span of 10 days. They contribute to hemostasis by two processes. *Primary hemostasis* is a reversible process that is not affected by heparin administration. Platelets adhere to the subendothelial collagen of disrupted vascular tissue. This process requires von Willebrand factor (vWF), a protein congenitally absent in von Willebrand disease. The platelets expand and initiate a release reaction, recruiting additional platelets. The resulting aggregate forms a plug sealing the disrupted vessel. Adenosine diphosphate, TxA_2, and serotonin are the prominent mediators in this process. Opposing these mediators are prostacyclin and PGE_2, which are vasodilators and inhibit aggregation. The second process by which platelets act, which is irreversible, involves fibrinogen-dependent degranulation. Platelet factor 3 is released, acting at several points in the coagulation cascade.

Coagulation   Coagulation refers to a cascade of zymogen activation that ultimately results in the cleavage of fibrinogen to insoluble fibrin that stabilizes the platelet plug. The *intrinsic* pathway involves components normally present in the blood, while the *extrinsic* pathway is activated by tissue lipoprotein. The two pathways converge at activated factor X (Xa) which, in turn, cleaves prothrombin to thrombin. All the coagulation factors except thromboplastin, factor VIII, and Ca^{2+} are synthesized in the liver. Factors II, VII, IX, and X are vitamin K dependent.

Fibrinolysis The patency of blood vessels is maintained by lysis of fibrin deposits and by antithrombin III (which neutralizes several of the proteases in the complement cascade). Fibrinolysis is dependent on plasmin, which is derived from the precursor plasma protein plasminogen. Plasmin lyses fibrin, the fragments of which interfere with platelet aggregation.

TESTS OF HEMOSTASIS AND BLOOD COAGULATION

The most valuable part of this assessment is a careful history and physical examination. Specific questions should be asked to determine if there was

- untoward bleeding during a major surgical procedure,
- any bleeding after a minor operation,
- any spontaneous bleeding,
- any family history of bleeding difficulties.

The history should include a list of medications and underlying medical disorders (malignancy, liver or kidney disease) that may affect normal hemostasis. Laboratory studies also provide important clues of hemostatic ability.

Platelet Count Spontaneous bleeding rarely occurs with a platelet count of less than $40,000/mm^3$. Platelet counts in this range are usually adequate to provide hemostasis following trauma or surgical procedures if other hemostatic factors are normal.

Bleeding Time This assesses the interaction between platelets and a damaged blood vessel and the formation of a platelet plug. Deficiencies in platelet number, platelet function, and some coagulation factors will yield a prolonged bleeding time.

Prothrombin Time (PT) This test measures the extrinsic pathway of blood coagulation. Thromboplastin, a procoagulant, is added with calcium to an aliquot of citrated plasma and the clotting time determined. The test will detect deficiencies in factors II, V, VII, X, or fibrinogen.

Partial Thromboplastin Time (PTT) A screen of the intrinsic clotting pathway, the PPT will determine abnormalities in factors VIII, IX, XI, or XII. This test has a high sensitivity; only extremely mild deficiencies in factor VIII or IX will be missed. The PTT, used in conjunction with the PT, can help place a clotting defect in the first or second stage of the clotting process.

Thrombin Time (TT) This screen detects abnormalities in fibrinogen and will detect circulating anticoagulants and inhibitors of anticoagulation.

Tests of Fibrinolysis Fibrin degradation products (FDP) can be measured immunologically. Falsely positive results may be seen in liver disease, kidney disease, thromboembolic disorders, and pregnancy.

EVALUATION OF THE SURGICAL PATIENT AS A HEMOSTATIC RISK

Preoperative Evaluation of Hemostasis Rapaport has suggested four levels of concern (given the patient's history and the proposed operation) that should dictate the extent of preoperative testing.

- Level I: The history is negative and the procedure is relatively minor, e.g., breast biopsy or hernia repair. No screening tests are recommended.

- Level II: The history is negative and a major operation is planned, but significant bleeding is not expected. A platelet count, blood smear, and PTT are recommended to detect thrombocytopenia, circulating anticoagulant, or intravascular coagulation.

- Level III: The history is suggestive of defective hemostasis and the patient is to undergo a procedure in which hemostasis may be impaired, such as operations using pump oxygenation or cell savers. This level also applies to situations where minimal postoperative bleeding could be detrimental, such as intracranial operations. A platelet count and bleeding time should be done to assess platelet function. A PT and PTT should be used to evaluate coagulation, and the fibrin clot should be checked to screen for abnormal fibrinolysis.

- Level IV: These patients have a history highly suggestive of a hemostatic defect. The same tests suggested for level III should be checked and a hematologist should be consulted. In case of an emergency, assessment of platelet aggregation and a thrombin time are indicated to detect dysfibrinogenemia or a circulating anticoagulant.

Patients with liver disease, obstructive jaundice, kidney failure, or malignancy should have a platelet count, PT, and PTT checked preoperatively.

CONGENITAL DEFECTS IN HEMOSTASIS

Classical Hemophilia (Factor VIII Deficiency)

Classical hemophilia (hemophilia A) is a sex-linked recessive disorder in which there is a failure to synthesize normal factor VIII. The incidence is approximately 1:10,000 to 1:15,000. Spontaneous mutations account for almost 20% of the cases. Clinical expression of the disease is highly variable.

The severity of the clinical manifestations is related to the degree of factor deficiency. Spontaneous bleeding and severe complications are the rule when virtually no factor VIII activity can be detected. Concentrations in the range of 5% of normal may produce no spontaneous bleeding, yet there may be severe bleeding with trauma or surgical therapy.

Significant bleeding is usually first noted when the child is a toddler. At that time the child may be subject to bleeding into joints, epistaxis, and hematuria. Intracranial bleeding, associated with trauma in half the cases, accounts for 25% of deaths. Hemarthrosis is the most characteristic orthopedic problem. Retroperitoneal bleeding or intramural intestinal hematoma may also occur, causing nausea, vomiting, or crampy abdominal pain. Upper gastrointestinal examination may demonstrate uniform thickening of mucosal folds ("picket fence" or "stack of coins" appearance).

Treatment   Plasma concentration of factor VIII necessary to provide hemostatic integrity is normally quite small (as little as 2–3%). Once serious bleeding begins, however, much higher levels (30%) of activity are required to achieve hemostasis. The half-life of factor VIII is 8–12 h; after an initial posttransfusion its half-life is approximately 4 h. One unit of factor VIII is considered to be the amount present in 1 mL normal plasma. Cryoprecipitate concentrates of factor VIII contain 9.6 units/mL. The amount of activity suggested to be repleted varies according to the severity of the lesion. The amount of material can be calculated from the formula:

$$\frac{\text{Patient's weight (kg)} \times \text{desired rise of factor VIII}}{\text{Total units of factor VIII in dose}} \begin{array}{c} \text{(\% average normal)} \end{array} = R$$

where R represents the rise of factor VIII observed in the patient's plasma for every unit of transfused factor VIII per kilogram of body weight. Half that amount is subsequently administered every 4–6 h to maintain a safe level.

Wet-frozen cryoprecipitate is preferred for replacement in patients with mild hemophilia, since it provides the lowest risk of viral hepatitis. Factor VIII concentrates are preferred in severe disease. In mild hemophilia A and mild von Willebrand disease, dDAVP, a synthetic derivative of vasopressin, has been used to produce a dose-dependent increase in all factor VIII activities and release plasminogen activator. Following major surgical treatment of a hemophiliac, transfusion replacement of factor VIII should be continued for at least 10 days. Even relatively minor procedures should be supplemented with factor VIII to achieve levels above 25–30%.

Christmas Disease (Factor IX Deficiency)

Factor IX deficiency is clinically indistinguishable from factor VIII deficiency. It is also inherited as an X-linked recessive disease with variable expression. The severe form of the disease has a level of less than 1% of normal activity. Half the patients belong to this group.

Treatment   All patients require substitution therapy when major or minor surgery is performed. Current therapy involves the administration of factor IX concentrate. The initial half-life is shorter than that of factor VIII; its subsequent half-life is much longer (18–40 h). A variety of factor IX concentrates are available. Konyne contains 10–60 units/mL of factor IX, but has been associated with thromboembolic complications. Newer preparations have had additional clotting factors removed, and the incidence of thromboembolic events is lower. During severe hemorrhage, treatment should be directed to achieving levels of 20–50% of normal for the first 3–5 days and then maintaining a plasma level of 20% for approximately 10 days. Plasma activity should be monitored during the course of therapy. The development of antibodies occurs in about 10% of patients.

von Willebrand Disease

von Willebrand disease occurs with the same frequency as true hemophilia. This disorder is usually transmitted as an autosomally dominant trait, but recessive inheritance may occur. The disease is characterized by a decrease in the level of factor VIII:C (procoagulant) activity that corrects the clotting abnormality in hemophilia A. Characteristically, patients with this disease have a prolonged bleeding time, but this is less consistent than the factor VIII:C reduction. A given patient may have an abnormal bleeding time on one occasion and a normal bleeding time on another. Ristocetin fails to cause platelet aggregation in about 70% of patients with this disease.

Clinical Manifestations Clinical manifestations are usually minimal until trauma or surgery makes them apparent. Spontaneous bleeding is often limited to the skin or mucous membranes. Epistaxis and menorrhagia are relatively common. Serious bleeding following minor surgery is not uncommon.

Treatment Treatment is directed at correcting the bleeding time and factor VIII R:WF (the von Willebrand factor). Only cryoprecipitate is effective (10–40 units/kg every 12 h). Replacement therapy should start 1 day prior to surgery, and the duration of therapy should be the same as that described for classical hemophilia.

ACQUIRED HEMOSTATIC DEFECTS

Platelet Abnormalities

Thrombocytopenia, the most common abnormality of hemostasis in the surgical patient, may be due to a variety of disease processes or massive blood loss. Thrombocytopenia may also result from the administration of heparin. This complication has been reported in 0.6% of patients receiving heparin and is thought to be immune mediated. The lowest platelet counts occur after 4–15 days of initial therapy and after 2–9 days in patients receiving subsequent courses.

Abnormalities in platelet number may also be accompanied by abnormalities in function. Uremia affects bleeding time and platelet aggregation. Defects in platelet aggregation and secretion occur in patients with thrombocytopenia, polycythemia, or myelofibrosis.

Treatment A count greater than 50,000/mm^3 requires no specific therapy. Thrombocytopenia due to acute alcoholism, drug effect, or viral infection will generally correct within 1–3 weeks. Severe thrombocytopenia may be due to vitamin B$_{12}$ or folate deficiency. This condition is usually responsive to the appropriate nutrient therapy. In patients with idiopathic thrombocytopenia or lupus erythematosus, a platelet count of less than 50,000/mm³ may respond to steroid therapy or plasmapheresis. Splenectomy alone should not be performed to correct thrombocytopenia associated with splenomegaly due to portal hypertension.

Prophylactic platelet administration is not routinely required following massive blood transfusions. One unit of platelets contains approximately 5.5×10^5 platelets and would be expected to increase the circulating platelet count by 10×10^9/L in a 70-kg man. In patients refractory to standard platelet transfusion, the use of HLA-compatible platelets has proved effective.

Acquired Hypofibrinogenemia-Defibrination Syndrome (Fibrinogen Deficiency)

This is rarely an isolated defect, because deficiencies in factors II, VI, VIII, and platelets will usually accompany this state. The majority of patients with acquired hypofibrinogenemia suffer from intravascular coagulation (disseminated intravascular coagulation, DIC). DIC is caused by the introduction of thromboplastic material into the circulation. This syndrome has been seen with retained dead fetus, separation of the placenta, and amniotic fluid embolism. Defibrination has been observed in association with extracorporeal circulation, disseminated carcinoma, lymphoma, and a variety of infections (including both gram-negative and gram-positive sepsis).

It is difficult to distinguish DIC from secondary fibrinolysis because both show prolongation in the thrombin time, PTT, and PT. The combination of a low platelet count, a positive plasma protamine test, reduced fibrinogen, and increased fibrinogen degradation products (taken in the context of the patient's underlying disease) is highly suggestive of the syndrome.

The prime consideration in treatment is relieving the underlying medical problem. The use of intravenous fluids is indicated to maintain volume. If there is active bleeding, hemostatic factors should be replaced with fresh frozen plasma, cryoprecipitate, and platelet concentrates as needed. Most studies show that heparin is not indicated in acute forms of DIC but is indicated for purpura fulminans or venous thromboembolism. Fibrinolytic inhibitors may be used to block the accumulation of degradation products. They should not be used without prior effective antithrombotic treatment with heparin.

Fibrinolysis

The acquired hypofibrinogenemic state in the surgical patient may also be due to pathologic fibrinolysis. This can be seen in patients with metastatic prostatic carcinoma, shock, sepsis, hypoxia, neoplasia, cirrhosis, and portal hypertension. A reduction in fibrinogen and factors V and VIII is seen, since they all are substrates for the enzyme plasmin. Thrombocytopenia is not an accompaniment of the purely fibrinolytic state. Treatment of the underlying disorder (if identified) is warranted. ϵ-Aminocaproic acid (EACA), an inhibitor of fibrinolysis, may also be useful.

Myeloproliferative Diseases

Thrombocytopenia can be treated by standard therapy for the underlying disease. Ideally, the hematocrit should be kept below 48% and the platelet count less than 400,000/mm³. In a study with polycythemic patients undergoing major surgical procedures, 46% had complications perioperatively, including a 16% mortality (80% in whom the disease was not under control). Hemorrhage is the most common complication in this group, followed by thrombosis and infection. Preoperative use of antiplatelet agents (aspirin, dipyridamole) and anticoagulants has been suggested in these patients.

Liver Disease

Advanced liver disease may result in decreased synthesis in the coagulation factors II, V, VII, X, and XIII. Also, there may be increased fibrinolysis due to the failure of the liver to clear plasminogen activators.

Anticoagulation and Bleeding

Spontaneous bleeding may be a complication of anticoagulant therapy, with an incidence proportional to the degree of anticoagulation. Surgical therapy may be necessary in patients receiving anticoagulant therapy. The risk of thrombotic complications is increased when anticoagulant therapy is suddenly discontinued, and may be due to a "rebound phenomenon." When the clotting time is less than 25 min in the heparinized patient or when the PT is less than 1.5 times control, reversal of anticoagulant therapy may not be necessary. If an emergent surgical procedure is necessary, anticoagulation can be reversed. Heparin can be reversed with protamine sulfate (1 : 1.28 mg). Bleeding is infrequently related to hypoprothrombinemia if the prothrombin concentration is greater than 15%. Coumadin can be discontinued several days prior to surgery. If emergency surgery is required, parenteral vitamin K_1 can be used. Reversal may take up to 6 h, so fresh frozen plasma may be needed.

LOCAL HEMOSTASIS

The goal of local hemostasis is to prevent the flow of blood from incised or transected blood vessels. The techniques may be classified as mechanical, thermal, or chemical.

MECHANICAL The oldest mechanical device to effect closure of the bleeding point or to prevent blood from entering the area of disruption is digital pressure. The finger has the advantage of being the least traumatic means of hemostasis. Diffuse bleeding from multiple transected vessels may be controlled by mechanical techniques, including direct pressure over the bleeding area, pressure at a distance, or generalized pressure. Direct pressure is preferable and is not attended by the danger of tissue necrosis associated with a tourniquet. Gravitational suites have been used to create generalized pressure.

The hemostat represents a temporary mechanical device to stem bleeding. Ligature replaces a hemostat as a permanent method of hemostasis of a single vessel.

THERMAL Cautery effects hemostasis by denaturation of proteins, which results in coagulation of large areas of tissue. Cooling has also been applied to control bleeding, and acts by increasing the local intravascular hematocrit and decreasing the blood flow by vasoconstriction. Cryogenic surgery uses temperatures between -20 and $-180°C$.

CHEMICAL Some act as vasoconstrictors, others are procoagulant, and others have hygroscopic properties that aid in plugging disrupted blood vessels. Epinephrine is a vasoconstrictor, but because of its considerable absorption and systemic effects, it is generally used only on areas of mucosal oozing. Local hemostatic materials include gelatin foam, cellulose, and micronized collagen.

TRANSFUSION

Approximately 14% of all inpatient operations include blood transfusions. Blood provides transportation of oxygen to meet the body's metabolic demands and removes carbon dioxide.

Replacement Therapy Banked whole blood is stored at 4°C and has a storage life of up to 35 days. Up to 70% of transfused erythrocytes remain in the circulation 24 h posttransfusion; 60 days posttransfusion, approximately 50% of the cells will survive.

Banked blood is a poor source of platelets. Factors II, VII, IX, and XI are stable in banked blood. Factor VIII rapidly deteriorates during storage. During the storage of whole blood, red cell metabolism and plasma protein degradation result in chemical changes in the plasma including increases in lactate, potassium, and ammonia, and a decrease in pH.

Typing and Cross Matching Serologic compatibility is routinely established for donor and recipient A, B, O, and Rh groups. As a rule, Rh-negative recipients should be transfused only with Rh-negative blood. In the patient receiving repeated transfusions, serum drawn less than 48 h before cross matching should be used. Emergency transfusion can be performed with group O blood. If it is known that the prospective recipient is group AB, group A blood is preferable.

Fresh Whole Blood This term refers to blood given within 24 h of its collection.

Packed Red Cells and Frozen Red Cells Packed cells have approximately 70% of the volume of whole blood. Use of frozen cells markedly reduces the risk of infusing antigens to which the patients have previously been sensitized. The red cell viability is improved and the ATP and 2,3-DPG concentrations are maintained.

Platelet Concentrates Platelet transfusions should be used for

• thrombocytopenia due to massive blood loss replaced with stored blood.

• thrombocytopenia due to inadequate production.

• qualitative platelet disorders.

Isoantibodies are demonstrated in about 5% of patients after 1–10 transfusions, 20% after 10–20 transfusions, and 80% after more than 100 transfusions. HLA-compatible platelets minimize this problem.

Fresh Frozen Plasma and Volume Expanders Factors V and VIII require plasma to be fresh or freshly frozen to maintain activity. This risk of hepatitis is the same as that of whole blood or packed red cells. In emergency situations, Ringer's lactate can be administered in amounts 2–3 times the estimated blood loss. Dextran or Ringer's lactate with albumin can be used for rapid plasma expansion.

Concentrates Antihemophilic concentrates are prepared from plasma with a potency of 20–30 times that of fresh frozen plasma. The simplest factor VIII concentrate is plasma cryoprecipitate. Albumin may also be used as a concentrate (25 g has the osmotic equivalent of 500 mL), with the advantage of being hepatitis-free.

INDICATIONS FOR REPLACEMENTS OF BLOOD OR ITS ELEMENTS

Volume Replacement The most common indication for blood transfusion in the surgical patient is the restoration of circulating blood volume. The hematocrit can be used to estimate blood loss, but up to 72 h is required to establish a new equilibrium after a significant blood loss.

In the normal person, reflex mechanisms allow the body to accommodate up to moderate-size blood losses. Significant hypotension develops only after about a 40% loss of blood volume.

Loss of blood during operation may be estimated by weighing the sponges (representing about 70% of the true loss). In patients who have normal preoperative blood values, replacement recommendations are shown in Table 3-1.

Improvement in Oxygen-Carrying Capacity Transfusion should be performed only if treatment of the underlying anemia does not provide adequate blood counts for the patient's clinical condition. In general, raising hemoglobins above 10 g

TABLE 3-1

Percent of total blood volume loss	Replace
20%	Crystalloid solutions
20–50%	Crystalloids and red cell concentrates (RBCs)
Above 50%	Crystalloids, RBCs, and albumin or plasma
Continued bleeding above 50%	Crystalloids, RBCs, FFP, and albumin or plasma

provides little additional benefit. A whole blood substitute, Fluosol-DA, provides oxygen-carrying capacity in the absence of blood products.

Replacement of Clotting Factors   Supplemental platelets or clotting factors may be required in treatment of certain hemorrhagic conditions. Fresh frozen plasma is used in the treatment of a coagulopathy in patients with liver disease, but its efficacy is very low. The rigid use of PT and PTT to anticipate the effect of FFP is not justified. If fibrinogen is required, a plasma level greater than 100 mg/dL should be maintained.

Massive Transfusion   This term refers to a single transfusion of greater than 2500 mL or 5000 mL over a 24-h period. A variety of problems may accompany the use of massive transfusion, including thrombocytopenia, impaired platelet function, deficiency in factors V, VIII, and XI, and the acid load of stored blood products.

With large transfusions, a heater may be used to warm the blood, since hypothermia may result in decreased cardiac output and an acidosis.

COMPLICATIONS

Hemolytic reactions from blood group incompatibilities are usually manifest by a sensation of warmth and pain along the site of transfusion, flushing in the face, pain in the lumbar region, and constricting pain in the chest. The patient may additionally experience chills, fever, and respiratory distress. In anesthetized patients, two signs of reaction include abnormal bleeding and continued hypotension in the face of adequate replacement. The morbidity and mortality of hemolytic reactions is high, and includes oliguria, hemoglobinuria, hypotension, jaundice, nausea, and vomiting. The transfusion should be stopped immediately if a transfusion reaction is suspected. Samples of the recipient and donor blood should be sent for comparison with pretransfusion samples. Renal function should be monitored following a suspected transfusion reaction. Renal toxicity is affected by the rate of urinary excretion and the pH. Alkalinization of the urine prevents precipitation of hemoglobin.

Febrile and Allergic Reactions   These occur in approximately 1% of transfusions. They appear as urticaria and fever occurring within 60–90 min of the start of the transfusion. Occasionally the reaction is severe enough to cause anaphylactic shock. Treatment consists of antihistamines, epinephrine, and steroids, depending on the severity of the reaction.

Transmission of Disease   Posttransfusion viral hepatitis is the most common fatal complication of blood transfusion. Other viral illnesses may be transmitted (CMV, HIV, etc.) as well as several bacterial species.

Additional, less-frequent, complications include:

- Embolism: Volumes of less than 200 mL are generally well tolerated by normal adults.
- Volume overload: The patient's risk is related to underlying cardiac reserve.
- Bacterial sepsis: Gram-negative organisms and *Pseudomonas* predominate.
- Thrombophlebitis: More commonly seen with prolonged infusions.

4 SHOCK

Shock implies inadequate tissue perfusion. The low-flow state is the final common denominator, although there are multiple etiologies. It results from dysfunction of four separate but interrelated systems: the heart, blood volume, arteriolar resistance (afterload), and venous capacitance (preload).

The clinical signs and symptoms of shock that are associated with surgical patients are those of hypovolemia. In most young, healthy patients, an initial restlessness and anxiety from catecholamine releases is seen. The classic signs of hypovolemic shock are not seen until 30% of blood volume has been lost. In this situation, the patient is hypotensive, tachycardic, and diaphoretic.

In lesser forms of shock, arterial blood pressure is maintained by increased peripheral vascular resistance and mild tachycardia in an attempt to increase cardiac output. Because the heart is working harder, it also consumes more oxygen, and blood is shunted away from the periphery to the heart and brain. Mild forms of hypovolemia are well tolerated by the body as extracellular fluid moves into the intravascular space causing hemodilution. This is a fairly slow process. During rapid hemorrhagic shock the hematocrit will not change, because whole blood has been lost and the body has not yet had time to move fluid down the osmotic gradient yielding to hemodilution.

Clear biochemical changes evolve during shock: the pituitary-adrenal response to stress; the responses of end-organs to reduction in their perfusion; and the failing function specifically within the organ.

The immediate effect along the pituitary axis is that of increased sympathetic and hormonal tone from catecholamine and cortisol release. This causes the well-known stress responses including negative nitrogen balance and retention of sodium and water. Over the longer term, the low-flow state delivers inadequate volumes of oxygen and blood to the peripheral tissues. With this is an obligate anaerobic metabolism with the production of lactic acid, and a shift of intracellular pH. In fact, peripheral pH, as monitored by blood gases, may not reflect the degree of cellular acidosis in the initially shocked animal.

Extent of organ failure is dependent on the duration and severity of shock. It may be as simple as mild renal failure from transient hypovolemia or as severe as multisystem organ failure with progression to death. The overall causes of this are unclear, although they appear to be related to exaggeration and eventually loss of the normal homeostatic mechanisms as the body attempts to compensate for decreased circulating volume.

PATHOPHYSIOLOGY

Studies of body fluid compartments after hemorrhagic shock revealed that in addition to the volume of blood lost, a deficit in extracellular fluid was seen equal to that of plasma. Restoration of the shed blood alone was inadequate for resuscitation. When an adequate volume of isotonic solution was infused along with shed blood, mortality was dramatically reduced. Thus, the body's compensatory response of shifting extracellular fluid to the intravascular space may be detrimental in the long term if adequate resuscitation is not carried out. Cellular swelling with fluid replacement leads to changes in membrane potential, as cells gain sodium water and chloride while losing potassium. With these alterations in electron potential cell failure eventually ensues as the formation and utilization of high-energy ATP is interrupted.

During severe shock, kidney function essentially stops. The kidneys are able to tolerate the diversion of blood to essential organs such as heart and brain for a period of approximately $1\frac{1}{2}$ h. Thereafter acute damage occurs, with the development of tubular necrosis. This is the most common form of renal insufficiency seen in patients who have been resuscitated from hypovolemic shock. Acute tubular necrosis is characterized by azotemia with a rise in blood urea nitrogen. This may or may not be associated with decrease in urine output once resuscitation has been completed. Glomerular filtration rate, even in the face of adequate urine output, is low. The acute tubular necrosis seen after hemorrhagic shock is associated with inappropriately high urinary excretions of sodium with a fractional excretion of sodium $[(U_{Na}/P_{Na})(P_{cr}/U_{cr}) \times 100]$ being greater than 1. In the oliguric surgical patient, this is an excellent marker to differentiate from patients who may be inadequately resuscitated or have postobstructive azotemia where the fractional excretion of sodium will be less than 1.

As patients are being more successfully resuscitated from severe hypovolemic shock, secondary organ failures are becoming more apparent. Adult respiratory distress syndrome (ARDS) is a common sequela of patients who have undergone severe trauma. It is also known as "shock lung,"

"Da Nang lung," or traumatic wet lung. On x-ray, the appearance is that of pulmonary edema; however, with interventional cardiac monitoring it has been seen that cardiac filling pressures are normal. Thus, an inappropriate capillary leak has developed. These patients are hypoxemic even in response to elevation of inspired oxygen concentration. This suggests a further ventilation perfusion imbalance with shunting of deoxygenated blood away from ventilated areas. The lungs become increasingly stiff. Pulmonary capillary wedge pressures and other evidence of left-sided cardiac failure are absent. Many of these patients will present initially with a decreased P_{CO_2} as they hyperventilate in an attempt to improve their oxygenation.

The pathophysiology of ARDS involves a fall in effective resting lung volume. There is less air remaining in the lungs after normal expiration due to replacement by fluid. The lack of an increase in peripheral oxygenation with the provision of 100% inspired oxygen not only suggests that this is a diffusion problem, but also confirms shunting. This appears due to a breakdown in the normal response mechanisms. In the normal lung, when an alveolus becomes plugged by mucus, the decrease in resting oxygen tension causes a vasoconstriction of the capillary serving that alveolus, thereby avoiding perfusion of unventilated alveoli. In ARDS significant shunt develops nonetheless. (See Figs. 4-1 and 4-2.)

The etiology of ARDS remains an area of intense research. There are multiple causes (see Table 4-1); however, overall end point is the same: leaky capillary syndrome in the face of normal filling pressures with ventilation perfusion mismatch.

Management of this syndrome is aimed at supporting the patient. Intubation and mechanical ventilation should be considered early especially if Pa_{O_2} has dropped to less than 65 torr. The effect of mechanical ventilation is to increase the functional residual capacity through increases in tidal volume and the institution of positive end expiratory pressure (PEEP). This will recruit collapsed or partially collapsed alveoli and may improve ventilation perfusion mismatch. PEEP is not entirely benign. Levels above 20 cmH_2O are associated with tension pneumothorax. Patients should also have their oxygen-carrying capacity maximized by keeping their hemoglobin near 10 gm%. There is no evidence that diuretics will help improve oxygenation unless patients are concomitantly fluid-overloaded. Antibiotics are not necessary unless an organism has been cultured and patients show other signs of pneumonic sepsis. Finally, the underlying cause of ARDS, be it hypovolemic shock or untreated sepsis, must be treated.

PULMONARY GAS EXCHANGE
CONTRIBUTING FACTORS

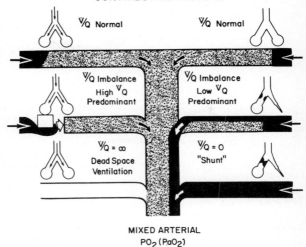

MIXED ARTERIAL
PO_2 (PaO_2)

Fig. 4-1. Diagrammatic representation of ventilation/perfusion ratio ($\dot{V}/Q$) abnormalities.

OXYGEN TRANSPORT

No discussion of shock is complete without a brief examination of oxygen transport. The hemoglobin molecule picks up oxygen in a sigmoid configuration along the oxygen-hemoglobin dissociation curve. In the normal patient this curve is 50% saturated (P_{50}) at an oxygen pressure of 27 mmHg. It rapidly increases beyond that and moves toward full saturation in the range of 70–80 mmHg. This curve can be shifted to the right, in which case oxygen is more easily unloaded from the blood. A leftward shift at the curve causes oxygen to bind more tightly. (See Fig. 4-3.) A shift to the left is associated with a decrease in the P_{50}. An increased P_{50} or rightward shift is advantageous.

Various factors alter hemoglobin oxygen affinity. (These are shown in Table 4-2). The compound 2,3-DPG is present in the red cells. Old banked blood as given in transfusions often is very low in 2,3-DPG, with a decrease in P_{50}.

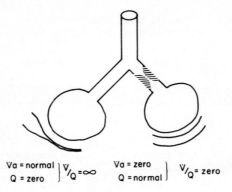

$$V_a = \text{normal} \atop Q = \text{zero} \Big\} \, V/_Q = \infty \qquad V_a = \text{zero} \atop Q = \text{normal} \Big\} \, V/_Q = \text{zero}$$

Fig. 4-2. Diagrammatic representation of mismatched ventilation and perfusion.

THERAPY

Therapy for shock is aimed at replacement of preexisting deficits through the rapid infusion of isotonic fluid solutions and blood. The development of acidosis during resuscitation from shock merely indicates inadequate resuscitation and should be treated with additional fluids, not bicarbonate. There appears to be no advantage to the use of "colloid" solutions such as albumin over that of crystalloid. Hypotension is treated through continued fluid replacement. Vasopressors do not have a role in the therapy of hypovolemic shock, as they serve only to further constrict an already highly vasoconstricted state and further worsen peripheral perfusion. There appeared to be early support for the use of vasodilators to improve peripheral perfusion during shock. However, their clinical usefulness in patients has not been proved. Although early studies suggested that there is adrenocorticoid depletion in hemorrhagic shock, in the normal patient steroids have no place during resuscitation.

OTHER FORMS OF SHOCK

It is important to differentiate hemorrhagic shock from other forms of shock such as cardiogenic, neurogenic, or septic. With the availability of direct measurements of cardiac output and filling pressures, this differentiation is more straightforward.

TABLE 4-1. Disorders Associated with (Causing) Adult Respiratory Distress Syndrome

Blood-borne or vascular source of injury	
Trauma (soft tissue or skeletal)*	Drug overdoses:
Sepsis*	Heroin, methadone,
Fat embolism	ethchlorvynol, acetylsalicylic
Pancreatitis	acid, propoxyphene
Shock	Drug idiosyncratic reaction
Multiple transfusions:	Thrombotic thrombocytopenic
Microemboli	purpura
Leukoagglutinin reaction	Leukemia
Disseminated intravascular	Venous air embolism
coagulation	Head injury
Surface burns	Paraquat
Miliary tuberculosis	Cardiopulmonary bypass/
	hemodialysis
Inhalation or airway source	*Direct or physical source*
Aspiration of gastric contents*	Lung contusion
Diffuse infectious pneumonia:*	Radiation
viral, mycoplasma,	High altitude
Legionnaires', pneumocystis	Hanging
Near-drowning*	Reexpansion
Irritant gas inhalation: NO_2, Cl_2,	
SO_2, NH_3	
Smoke inhalation	
O_2 toxicity	

* Common cause of ARDS.

Cardiogenic Shock

In contrast to hypovolemic shock, cardiogenic shock is due to fluid levels exceeding that which the heart can handle. This is usually because of primary pump failure from loss of muscle wall contractility due to ischemic cardiomyopathy. The filling pressures in this patient, in contrast to those of the patient in hemorrhagic shock, are high; cardiac output, however, continues to be low. The body will try to compensate as it would in hemorrhagic shock. Peripheral vascular resistance is elevated. This may, in fact, compound the problem by making it harder for the heart to eject its volume. Tachycardia can ensue, but the already diseased heart cannot always respond. Oxygen delivery to the tissues is decreased and extraction increased. These patients respond to diuretics and inotropic agents that increase contractility and decrease afterload (systemic vascular resistance), such as dobutamine. Digitalis will improve contractility and can slow rapid ventricular rates due to atrial fibrillation.

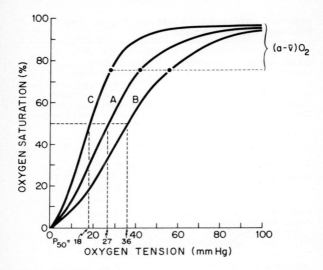

Fig. 4-3. Oxygen-hemoglobin dissociation curves in *(A)* normal, *(B)* rightward-shifted, and *(C)* leftward-shifted positions. The P_{50} value denotes the position of the curve along the horizontal axis and represents the oxygen tension (in mmHg) necessary to saturate 50 percent of available hemoglobin with oxygen. Note that as the curve moves toward the left, the arteriovenous oxygen difference, $(a-\bar{v})$ O_2, can be maintained only by decreasing venous oxygen tension. (Adapted from: *Shappell SD, Lenfant CJM: Anesthesiology 37:127, 1972, with permission.*)

Septic Shock

So-called warm shock is the response to toxins released from pathologic organisms. In contrast to hemorrhagic and cardiogenic shock, cardiac output is elevated, often to hyperdynamic levels. Systemic vascular resistance is down, leading to a low blood pressure. The patient's extremities appear warm and well perfused. Because of dysfunction at a cellular level, however, oxygen extraction is impaired, leading to a narrowing of the arteriovenous oxygen difference. Other signs of infection, including hyperpyrexia and leukocytosis, aid in the diagnosis. Therapy involves finding and correcting the underlying infection. Volume expansion and inotropic agents that raise systemic vascular resistance are adjunctive to treating the primary cause.

TABLE 4-2. Factors that Alter Hemoglobin/Oxygen Affinity

Increase P_{50}	Decrease P_{50}
By direct effect:	By direct effect:
Increases [H^+]	Decreased [H^+]
temperature	temperature
P_{CO_2}	P_{CO_2}
DPG, ATP	DPG, ATP
Hb conc	Hb conc
Ionic strength	Ionic strength
Abnormal hemoglobin	Abnormal hemoglobin
Aldosterone	Carboxyhemoglobin
	Methemoglobin
By increasing DPG:	By decreasing DPG:
Decreased [H^+]	Increased [H^+]
Thyroid hormone	Decreased thyroid hormone
Pyruvate kinase deficiency	Hexokinase deficiency
Increased inorganic phosphate	Decreased inorganic phosphate
Cortisol	Cell age (old)
Cell age (young)	

SOURCE: Adapted from Shappell SD, Lenfant CJM: Adaptive, genetic and iatrogenic alterations of the oxyhemoglobin dissociation curve. *Anesthesiology* 37:127, 1971.

Neurogenic (Spinal) Shock

The sudden loss of vascular tone, as seen after a spinal cord injury, leads to venous pooling with decreased return to the right heart as well as vasodilation of the arterial tree. Blood pressure is decreased, but these patients do not manifest reflex tachycardia. Extremities are warm. Treatment is moderate volume expansion to fill the increased venous pool, and vasopressors such as neosynephrine to increase arterial tone. Isolated head injuries do *not* cause neurogenic shock.

Tension Pneumothorax, Pulmonary Embolism, and Cardiac Tamponade

All three are associated with decreased output due to impaired filling of the heart. Although they present a picture similar to that of cardiogenic shock, they must be promptly recognized and treated specifically.

In tension pneumothorax, the mediastinal shift causes kinking of the vena cava at the level of the right atrium. Venous return is cut off, with a resultant hypotension. Pneumothorax can be clinically recognized by tracheal deviation, elevated neck veins, and hyperresonance of the

TABLE 4-3.   Characteristics of the Different Forms of Shock*†

	CO	SVR	CVP	PCWP	A-VDO$_2$
Hemorrhagic	↓	↑	↓	↓	↑
Cardiogenic	↓	↑	↑	↑	↑
Septic	↑ ↑	↓	NL *or* ↓	NL *or* ↓	↓
Spinal	NL *or* ↓	↓ ↓	↓	NL *or* ↓	↑ *or* NL
Tension Pneumothorax	↓	↑	↓	↓	↑
Pulmonary Embolism	↓	↑	↑	↓	↑
Tamponade	↓	↑	Equalized pressures		↑

* CO, Cardiac output; SVR, systemic vascular resistance; CVP; central venous pressure; PCWP, pulmonary capillary wedge pressure; A-VDO$_2$, arteriorvenous O$_2$ difference (extraction).

† ↓, Decreased; ↑, increased; NL, normal.

involved chest cavity. The pneumothorax must be relieved by insertion of a 14-gauge needle in the second interspace anteriorly, followed by tube thoracostomy. *Tension pneumothorax is a clinical diagnosis; if one waits for radiographic confirmation prior to therapy, it is often too late.*

Pulmonary embolism causes hypotension by decreasing blood flow to the left side of the heart. This is a combination of mechanical factors in large emboli and a compensatory vasoconstriction of the pulmonary bed in smaller multiple emboli. In the patient with a Swan-Ganz catheter, there is dramatically elevated central venous pressure with a low or normal pulmonary capillary wedge pressure. Sudden onset of hypoxemia aids in diagnosis.

In cardiac tamponade, mechanical inhibition of cardiac expansion during diastole prevents adequate filling. It is characterized by equalization of cardiac chamber pressures. Clinically, Beck's triad of muffled heart tones, hypotension, and elevated CVP should raise suspicion of the diagnosis. Therapy is aimed at relieving tamponade through pericardiocentesis or by operative intervention.

SUMMARY

The characteristics in various forms of shock are outlined in Table 4-3. Prompt recognition and institution of corrective therapy is vital to overall survival.

5 INFECTIONS

BACKGROUND

Infection is the result of invasion of the body by pathogenic microorganisms and reaction of the host tissues to organisms and their toxins. The external and internal surfaces of the body are colonized with a variety of microorganisms that do not cause harm until a break in the normal barriers of host resistance occurs. Only a few of the many thousands of microorganisms known in nature are actually pathogenic to human beings. The other organisms constitute the normal flora and themselves provide natural resistance against invasion by pathogenic species.

Over 80 years have passed since the theories of aseptic technique in surgery have been applied. Nonetheless, infections continue to be a great problem in the practice of surgery as much now as in the past. As newer and more powerful antibiotics evolve, different organisms and modes of resistance arise.

Nosocomial infections are those which result from transmission of pathogens to a previously uninfected patient from a source in the hospital environment. These are hospital-acquired infections which may represent especially resistant organisms due to their residence in an environment containing broad-spectrum antibiotics. Staphylococci continue to be the most prevalent organisms that cause nosocomial infections.

An *autoinfection* occurs when an infection arises from pathogens that reside within patients themselves. Alternatively, an *iatrogenic* infection occurs when the infection is secondary to treatment by a physician or nurse, such as insertion of urinary or venous catheters.

Virulence of a particular pathogen refers to its power to invade tissue and cause illness. This term is quantitated by the smallest dose of bacterial strain that will produce disease in a specified host. Usually this kind of assessment is done in experimental animals and does not necessarily reflect human disease.

Carriers are healthy people who may harbor pathogenic bacteria but are not clinically affected. A common example is the presence of resistant staphylococci in the nasopharynx of hospital workers, which can be transmitted and cause infection through contact with patients but cause no illness in the carriers themselves.

Opportunistic bacteria are nonpathogenic under ordinary circumstances but may become pathogenic when host-parasite equilibrium is upset. Disturbances in this equilibrium are usually secondary to deficiencies of host resistance. *Host resistance* is the ability of the body to keep bacteria outside of the skin and mucosal surfaces, and, failing this, to localize and destroy invading microorganisms. The critical components of host-resistance are: (1) intact skin and mucous membranes, (2) a system of circulating phagocytic cells, (3) antibodies, and (4) the ability to form a local tissue reaction (hyperemia and leukocytosis).

The virulence and pathogenicity of bacteria are related to their ability to produce toxins. *Exotoxins* are specific, soluble proteins produced by certain bacteria that cause cytotoxic effects remote from the actual area of the infection. Examples of exotoxin-producing organisms are *Clostridium tetani* and *Streptococcus pyogenes*. *Endotoxins* are complex lipopolysaccharides that are a part of the bacterial cell wall in gram-negative organisms. These lipopolysaccharides are released from the cell and incite dramatic systemic response in the hosts, including fever, tachycardia, and hypotension.

Diagnosis

The clinical signs of infection are redness, swelling, heat, and pain. Loss of function is another clinical parameter that is often seen with infection. Other nonspecific signs include fever, tachycardia, and chills. Leukocytosis provides general laboratory evidence of infection. Differentiation of the white blood cell count will commonly demonstrate a "left shift" when greater than 85% of the white blood cells seen on peripheral smear are immature granulocytes.

Exudate is the extracellular fluid that commonly accumulates and signifies the presence of an infection. This fluid should be examined by the physician for color, odor, and consistency, all characteristics which can help categorize the causative organism. In addition, a Gram stain of the exudate is an essential procedure for adequate treatment. In some cases of infection a biopsy of involved tissue will be necessary for diagnosis. This is especially true for granulomatous infections such as tuberculosis or blastomycosis.

Culture of exudative fluid is the next step toward diagnosis and treatment of infection. Cultures for aerobic and anaerobic organisms must be obtained and handled properly to ensure reliable results. Good cultures of exudative fluid are the most important diagnostic maneuver in treatment of surgical infections.

Blood cultures are used as a diagnostic step for infection of unknown source. In order to increase the yield of information from blood cultures they should be done frequently in patients with clinical sepsis. Commonly, however, blood cultures fail to capture causative organisms in a transient bacteremia. Chills and fever, the usual signs provoking blood cultures, frequently lag 30–90 min behind the actual bacteremia. For this reason frequent, random blood cultures are often necessary to diagnose septicemia of an unknown source.

Surgical Treatment

The principles of surgical treatment for established infection begin with debridement of necrotic and injured tissue. These tissues harbor foreign objects and multiple microorganisms, and they have poor blood supply and therefore decreased host resistance. Second, drainage of abscesses to remove infected fluid is essential. Removal of foreign bodies that are a nidus for infection is a third important principle of surgical treatment. Other supportive measures in the treatment of surgical infections include immobilization of the infected region, elevation to promote venous and lymphatic drainage, and relief of swelling and pain. Moist heat is applied to increase local blood supply and facilitate exudation.

Antibiotic Therapy

Judicious and precise utilization of antibiotics is essential in treatment of surgical infections. Success of antibiotic therapy depends on adequate blood supply to the infected region. For this reason, abscesses are usually less responsive to systemic antibiotic treatment. Alternatively, cellulitis and systemic infection can be treated effectively with antibiotics.

An important principle of antibiotic utilization is to acquire all blood, body fluid, and tissue cultures prior to initiating antibiotics. The presence of antibiotics in these specimens will hinder growth in culture.

Hyperbaric oxygen therapy has emerged as a new treatment for selected infections. This modality increases oxygen tension in plasma, lymph, and tissue fluids as much as 15–20-fold. Infections by obligate anaerobic organisms such as clostridia are the principal target for hyperbaric oxygen therapy.

Common Surgical Infections

Cellulitis is inflammation of the skin and subcutaneous tissue that is usually caused by hemolytic streptococci. This type of infection is generally nonsuppurative. The skin appears red, hot, and indurated.

Lymphangitis is a variant of cellulitis that refers to inflammation of lymphatic pathways and appears clinically as streaking redness usually along the extremities. Hemolytic streptococci are the causative organisms. Lymphangitis is treated with rest, immobilization, and elevation of the extremity, and antibiotics.

Erysipelas denotes a spreading cellulitis and lymphangitis with unusually distinct lines of demarcation between infected and normal tissue. This type of infection is treated in a manner similar to lymphangitis.

An *abscess* is a localized collection of pus. Treatment generally requires incision and drainage of purulent fluid. Antibiotics are adjunctive but not primarily therapeutic.

Impetigo refers to multiple small intraepithelial abscesses. Streptococci and staphylococci are the most common bacteria.

Another type of abscess is a *furuncle*. This abscess occurs in sweat glands or along hair follicles and is generally larger than the abscess of impetigo.

Carbuncles are larger extensions of a furuncle into underlying subcutaneous tissue. These are generally caused by *Staphylococcus aureus*. However, gram-negative bacilli and streptococci can be found coincidently.

Bacteremia is defined as bacteria in the circulating blood with no indication of toxemia or clinical manifestations. Bacteremia is usually transient and may last only a few moments, and the reticuloendothelial system localizes and destroys these organisms under favorable conditions.

Septicemia is a diffuse infection in which bacteria and their toxins are present in the bloodstream. Septicemia may arise directly from invasion of organisms into the circulation but, as a rule, is secondary to a focus of infection within the body. The mechanisms of entrance of bacteria into the bloodstream are: (1) direct extension into an open vessel, (2) release of infected emboli, and (3) discharge of infected lymph into the bloodstream.

Toxemia is defined as the presence of toxins circulating in the blood, though the microorganism producing the toxin may not be present. Toxemia is usually associated with infection by toxin-producing bacteria such as clostridia. Ingestion of botulinum toxin or staphylococcal enterotoxin may cause profound toxemia without any infection at all.

TABLE 5-1

Cellular site of inhibition	Bacteriocidal	Bacteriostatic
Cell wall synthesis	Penicillins Cephalosorins Vancomycin	
Barrier function of cell membrane	Amphotericin B Polymyxin	Nystatin
Protein synthesis in ribosome	Aminoglycosides	Tetracycline Chloramphenicol Erythromycin Clindamycin
DNA replication	Griseofulvin	

ANTIBIOTIC THERAPY

Antibiotics are chemotherapeutic agents which act primarily upon parasitic organisms and not upon the host. These agents can be broadly classified as bacteriostatic or bacteriocidal. *Bacteriostatic* agents prevent growth of bacteria but do not actually destroy them; *bacteriocidal* agents actively kill bacteria. The biologic mode of action varies among groups of antibiotics. Many antibiotics inhibit synthesis of bacterial cell wall, while others interrupt protein synthesis by the bacterial ribosomes. Other types of antibiotics interfere with DNA replication within the bacteria, and some impair barrier functions of cell membranes. Table 5-1 is a list of various antibiotics and their classification according to cellular function.

The fundamental principles that govern utilization of antibiotics are: (1) use of an agent which is effective against the infecting organism, (2) adequate contact between the drug and the organism, (3) absence of toxic side effects of the drug, and (4) augmentation of host defenses to maximize antibacterial effects. Cultures should always be taken before initiation of antibiotic therapy if possible. Subsequent changes in antibiotic therapy can be made when culture and sensitivity reports become available. Clinical judgment is called upon to administer antibiotics on an empiric basis prior to these laboratory reports. Many infections may be polymicrobic and therefore will require a combination of antibiotics to cover the probable pathogens.

Antibiotic therapy unavoidably causes changes in the resident microflora of the host. *Colonization* is defined as the quantitative appearance of changes in the microflora which are induced by antibiotic therapy. *Superinfection* is a new microbial disease introduced or potentiated by antibiotic therapy. Superinfection is frequently the result of colonization.

Antibiotic Prophylaxis

Chemoprophylaxis is the treatment of potentially contaminated wounds. The use of prophylactic antibiotics, however, is only an adjunct and not a substitute to good surgical technique, the ultimate prophylaxis against surgical infection. The need for prophylactic antibiotic therapy in addition to good surgical technique is based on the risk of contamination. Clean operations have minimal risk and no antibiotics are necessary. Clean contaminated operations designate operations that allow exposure or contact of the interior of the respiratory, urinary, or gastrointestinal tracts. Contaminated procedures are those complicated by gross spillage of intestinal contents, or wounds secondary to trauma. Dirty wounds are those that are in contact with an established prior infection such as an intraabdominal abscess or perirectal abscess.

Aside from the degree of contamination in a particular operation, host-risk factors can increase the possibility of postoperative infection. Special risk groups include those patients who are malnourished, obese, elderly, and have immunodeficiency. The presence of shock and/or poor blood supply to the operative region also increases the risk for infection. Prophylactic antibiotics should be considered in these cases.

In general, prophylactic antibiotics should be started early enough to allow adequate tissue and body fluid levels during the procedure. Frequently, intraoperative administration of an antibiotic is necessary to maintain adequate tissue levels. The length of the operative procedure and the serum half-life of the chosen antibiotic are critical factors for obtaining successful chemoprophylaxis.

Table 5-2 is an abbreviated list of procedures which usually benefit from antibiotic prophylaxis.

Intestinal Antisepsis

Prophylaxis against intraabdominal wound infection in intestinal surgery requires reduction of the normal intestinal flora. One standard method is that devised by Nichols and Condon. This regimen includes a liquid diet for 2 days followed by a vigorous mechanical bowel preparation the day before surgery. Neomycin and erythromycin base, which are unabsorbed through the gastrointestinal tract, are given 1 g each

TABLE 5-2

Cardiovascular	Coronary artery bypass, bowel replacement
Orthopaedic	Hip prosthetic
OB/GYN	C-Section, hysterectomy
Biliary tract	Age greater than 70, common bile duct stones, obstructive jaundice, acute cholecystitis
Gastrointestinal tract	Colonic procedures, gastric resection, oropharyngeal procedures
Urologic	Any patient with prior bacteriuria

at 1, 2, and 11 o'clock on the evening before surgery. This method of intestinal antisepsis has been shown to reduce the incidence of postoperative complications related to bacteria but does not protect against errors of surgical skill or judgment.

Antimicrobial Agents

It is important to use an antibiotic agent for a sensitive microorganism not simply to treat a particular disease. Accurate laboratory culture and sensitivity reports are critical for good antimicrobial therapy. The white blood cell count is important in evaluating the response to antibiotic treatment. Various antibiotic agents that are useful in surgical practice are described below.

Penicillins Penicillins are antimicrobial agents that block synthesis of the bacterial cell wall peptides. The beta-lactam ring is essential for this antibacterial material activity. Bacteria which produce beta-lactamase are resistant to penicillin. There are several groups of penicillins: (1) Penicillin G offers good gram-positive coverage but is susceptible to beta-lactamase. (2) Methicillin and nafcillin are uniquely resistant to beta-lactamase but have much less gram-positive coverage. (3) Ampicillin, carbenicillin, and ticarcillin have a broader spectrum than most penicillin agents with both gram-positive and gram-negative coverage. They are, however, susceptible to beta-lactamase. (4) Penicillin-V and cloxacillin are forms of penicillin that are suitable for oral intake. (5) Mezlocillin and piperacillin are new extended-spectrum penicillins that have greater activity against gram-negative organisms. These agents are particularly effective against *Pseudomonas, Serratia,* and *Klebsiella.*

Cephalosporins These agents are related to penicillins and are also bacteriocidal. Instead of a 6-aminopenicillanic acid nucleus they have a nucleus of 7-aminocephalosporanic acid. They are arranged in generations based on expanding activity against gram-negative bacteria.

First-generation cephalosporins have good gram-positive coverage but are poor against anaerobes and only moderately effective against gram-negative organisms. These agents, however, are much cheaper than higher generations of cephalosporin and remain common in clinical practice.

Second-generation cephalosporins have higher gram-negative coverage and anaerobic coverage. They are especially effective against *Bacteroides fragilis*. This spectrum makes second-generation cephalosporin especially useful for treatment of intraabdominal sepsis, particularly when combined with aminoglycosides.

The third-generation of cephalosporins have an even broader spectrum of coverage against gram-negative bacteria. They are especially useful against nosocomial pathogens. These agents have a better stability against beta-lactamase. The disadvantages of third-generation cephalosporins are their lesser coverages against anaerobes and staphylococci. Also, these agents are comparatively expensive.

Erythromycin Erythromycin is a macrocyclic lactone. It is active against gram-positive bacteria. The mechanism of action is bacteriostatic rather than bacteriocidal. The drug functions by inhibiting bacterial protein synthesis. Erythromycin in base form is generally well tolerated but can cause some gastrointestinal disturbance. This form of the drug is useful for intestinal antisepsis. Erythromycin is the agent of choice for treatment of mycoplasma infections and Legionnaire's disease.

Tetracyclines These agents are also bacteriostatic. They are broad-spectrum oral antibiotics with activity against *Treponema, Myobacterium, Chlamydia,* and *Rickettsia.* Tetracyclines should be avoided in children and patients with renal failure.

Chloramphenicol This broad-spectrum agent is bacteriostatic in nature. It has been used for treatment of typhoid fever, *Salmonella,* and meningitis resistant to penicillin. Side effects include aplastic anemia, which is rare but can occur. Also, circulatory collapse can occur in premature infants given this drug, a phenomenon called "Gray syndrome."

Aminoglycosides These agents are bacteriocidal and have activity against both gram-negative and gram-positive organisms. They inhibit protein synthesis by attaching to messenger RNA. The toxicity of aminoglycosides includes both renal and ototoxicity. Serum creatinine levels and creatinine clearance should be carefully monitored during administration of these agents.

Aminoglycosides have been shown to have synergism with beta-lactam antibiotics, such as cephalosporin or carbenicillin against *Klebsiella* and *Pseudomonas,* respectively. Aminoglycosides are categorically among the most valuable agents available for treatment of life-threatening infections by enteric gram-negative bacteria. Resistant strains of various gram-negative bacteria have evolved. Generally, amikacin or netilmicin is reserved for treatment of severe nosocomial infections by gram-negative pathogens.

Polymyxins These agents are basically polypeptides that are effective against *Pseudomonas aeruginosa.* They must be given parenterally. Because of their toxicity, which includes paresthesias, dizziness, nephrotoxicity, and respiratory arrest, these agents are used much less commonly today.

Lincosamides Clindamycin is the primary member of this group. They function primarily against anaerobic infections. Also, gram-positive pulmonary infections are adequately treated with clindamycin. The major side effect is pseudomembranous colitis, which is manifested by bloody diarrhea secondary to a necrotizing toxin produced by *Clostridium difficile. C. difficile* is resistant to clindamycin and becomes the predominant clostridial flora of the intestine during either oral or parenteral administration of this agent.

Vancomycin This antibiotic is bacteriocidal for gram-positive microorganisms, including staphylococci, streptococci, and clostridia. It is especially useful for multiresistant gram-positive organisms. In oral form vancomycin is good for treatment of clostridial difficile overgrowth. The principal side effect is ototoxicity. In addition, serum half-life is prolonged in renal failure.

Metronidazole This is an antibiotic effective against ameba, trichomonades, and giardiasis. Coverage is also excellent against anaerobic organisms. This drug readily crosses the blood-brain barrier and has been effective in treating some brain abscesses. Metronidazole is also an alternative to vancomycin for treatment of *C. difficile.*

Imipenem This drug is carbapenem, which has the broadest antibacterial spectrum of any beta-lactam antibiotic available. The drug is given in combination with cilastatin, which inhibits renal tubular metabolism of imipenem, and prevents formation of nephrotoxic compounds. Imipenem can be used alone for treating mixed bacterial infections which otherwise would require a combination of multiple antibiotics.

Antifungal Agents

Amphotericin B is the only antifungal antibiotic which is effective in treatment of systemic mycotic infections. Amphotericin B alters the permeability of the fungal cell wall, which causes cytolysis. The drug can be administered intravenously or topically. It is absorbed poorly from the gastrointestinal tract. The toxic side effects include fever, chills, nausea, vomiting, and headache. Renal dysfunction and permanent damage to the kidney are toxic effects brought on by long-term continued use.

Griseofulvin is a topical and oral form of antifungal therapy. It is useful for treating superficial fungal infections of skin and hair or nails. Long-term treatments with this agent are well tolerated.

Nystatin also damages the fungal cell membrane and is fungistatic. This agent is not absorbed by the GI tract. Nystatin is generally used as a prophylactic and therapeutic agent for gastrointestinal candidiasis secondary to broad-spectrum antibacterial therapy.

Flucytosine inhibits nucleic synthesis in fungi. It is absorbed well and has low toxicity. Flucytosine is useful for treatment of cryptococcus and candidiasis but generally is used in combination with amphotericin B.

Sulfonamides

These agents represent the first antibacterial agents discovered. They are bacteriostatic and are especially useful for treatment of urinary tract infections due to *Escherichia coli*. Also, sulfonamide derivatives have been important in the topical treatments of severe burn wounds. The activity of these compounds is inhibited by pus, which is rich in amino acids and purine made available by the breakdown of protein and nucleic acids. These breakdown products inactivate sulfonamides.

Sulfisoxazole and sulfamethoxazole are used for treating urinary tract infections. Mafenide is a topical creme for treatment of burn wound infections. Pain from tissue necrosis is a significant side effect of this topical treatment.

Sulfamethoxazole combined with trimethoprim is useful for the treatment of severe urinary tract infections, bronchitis, and pneumonia caused by *Pneumocystis carinii*. This drug is also primary treatment for resistant strain of *Salmonella*.

STREPTOCOCCAL INFECTIONS

Streptococci are the dominant aerobic flora of the mouth and pharynx. They are gram-positive organisms that are organized in short chains. Some streptococci are anaerobic. Streptococci can be divided into those that produce a soluble hemolysin and those that do not when cultured on blood agar. A clear zone of hemolysis on blood agar is beta hemolysis. Most human infections with streptococci are beta-hemolytic. There are numerous groups of beta-hemolytic streptococci. These groups are identified by antisera to a carbohydrate antigen on the cell wall. Ninety percent of human infections are group A (*Streptococcus pyogenes*). These organisms produce streptokinase and hyaluronidase, enzymes that enhance their virulence. Streptococcal pharyngitis, scarlet fever, and rheumatic fever are the principal illnesses that result from group A beta-hemolytic streptococci.

Other groups of streptococci are much less virulent. One exception, however, is group D streptococci, also known as *S. faecalis*. These bacteria are members of the category of organisms called enterococci. They are virtually always present in the colon, terminal ileum, and upper jejunum.

Alpha hemolysis on blood agar is caused by streptococci that create a greenish-brown color on the culture plate. Most of these organisms are *S. viridans*. They are usually associated with chronic diseases or are nonpathogenic. However, they are the commonest cause of subacute bacterial endocarditis in patients who have congenitally deformed or rheumatically damaged heart valves.

Erysipelas

Erysipelas is a superficial spreading cellulitis caused by streptococci. The cellulitis and associated lymphangitis have sharply defined and irregular red borders. The toxins induced by hemolytic streptococci cause the cellulitic reaction. Generally this reaction follows minor skin injuries that allow invasion by streptococci on the surface. The classic lesion of erysipelas is a butterfly erythema centered around the nose and extending to both cheeks. Penicillin is usually effective; however, the erythema disappears slowly despite eradication of the offending organism.

Necrotizing Fasciitis

Necrotizing fasciitis is a life-threatening infection that is relatively rare. This type of infection causes necrosis of the superficial fascia of the abdominal wall or perineum. There is generally a severe associated systemic toxicity. Although 90% of these infections have beta-hemolytic streptococci, this disease is more of a clinical entity than a specific bacterial infection. Multiple organisms are usually cultured. Rarely will gram-negative enteric pathogens be cultured alone.

Necrotizing fasciitis may follow minor abdominal trauma or operations such as appendectomy or colon resection. Diabetics are distinctly susceptible to this syndrome.

Clinical manifestations of necrotizing fasciitis include superficial and widespread fascial necrosis. This is usually heralded as cellulitis and edema of the abdominal wall. The wound exudate is usually serosanguineous in nature. Upon exploration the fascia is necrotic, dull gray in color, and stringy in character. Gram stain of this material is important for appropriate antibacterial therapy. Other principles of therapy include debridement through multiple linear incisions. First-line antibiotic treatment generally includes ampicillin, aminoglycosides, and clindamycin. Repeated debridements are often necessary.

Streptococcal Myonecrosis

Streptococcal myonecrosis resembles clostridial gas gangrene. Usually there is an incubation period of 3–4 days followed by swelling, edema, and purulent wound exudate. Pain in the involved region becomes severe. The infected muscle appears soft, purplish, and gangrenous. There is a sour odor to the seropurulent discharge. The muscle becomes gangrenous as opposed to necrotizing fasciitis, in which the fascia is affected. Treatment involves incision and drainage, antibiotic therapy, and supportive measures.

Meleney's Ulcer

Anaerobic or microaerophilic streptococci can cause a chronic burrowing skin ulcer which is called *Meleney's ulcer*. These ulcers usually begin as a superficial lesion following minor trauma. Commonly they occur after excision of a lymph node in the neck, axilla, or groin. Slow, progressive enlargement of the lesion occurs over months or years. Treatment consists of debridement, drainage of sinuses, and penicillin therapy. Skin grafting is often necessary.

STAPHYLOCOCCAL INFECTIONS

Staphylococci are normal inhabitants of the skin. Infection by staphylococci is characterized by suppuration (formation of pus). Gram stain of these organisms reveals gram-positive cocci in clusters. Usually these bacteria produce beta hemolysis on blood agar culture plates. Only two staphylococci species are important clinically. *Staph. aureus* is the most pathogenic species. These organisms are distinguished by their production of coagulase and fermentation of mannitol. In addition, their virulence is characterized by the ability to produce hemolysins and enzymes.

Staph. epidermidis is becoming recognized as an important cause of opportunistic infection following surgical procedures, especially those in which foreign materials and prostheses are used. Endocarditis can occur from staph epidermidis infection following open heart surgery. This organism is coagulase-negative.

Skin is the most common site of staphylococcal infections. They usually begin in hair follicles or sebaceous glands. The resultant infections are generally small abscesses commonly called furuncles or carbuncles. These infections are manifested by pain, swelling, and induration of the surrounding skin. The abscess contains a characteristic thick, yellow pus that is not foul smelling.

Staphylococci are the primary cause of wound sepsis in otherwise "clean" surgical incisions. Virulent and resistant strains of staphylococci may be carried by hospital personnel. The consequent nosocomial infections can be difficult to treat with standard antibiotics.

Treatment of staphylococcal skin infections, whether they are primary or secondary to surgical incision, is wide drainage. Fulminating septicemia can arise from severe wound infections. This syndrome is manifested by high fever, leukocytosis, toxemia, and evidence of irritation of the central nervous system. The mortality rate is high if these infections are untreated.

Staphylococcal Enteritis

The utilization of oral broad-spectrum antibiotics can lead toward overgrowth of staphylococcal organisms, particularly *Staph. aureus*. This produces a clinical syndrome of nausea, vomiting, diarrhea, abdominal distention, and fever. The diarrhea can be perfuse, watery, and usually nonbloody. This disease is also called pseudomembranous enterocolitis. Stool cultures may reveal a pure culture of *Staph. aureus*. Treatment consists of discontinuation of oral antibiotics, institution of oral vancomycin, and supportive measures. Intramuscular administration of cortical steroids has also been advised. Resolution of the illness depends on reestablishment of normal bacterial flora.

Peptococci

Peptococci are anaerobic staphylococci that are found in similar sites with bacteroides, clostridia, and aerobic gram-negative bacilli. They are generally part of the normal flora but are relatively nonpathogenic. They can be found in wound infections, abscesses, and septicemias of other causes.

CLOSTRIDIAL INFECTIONS

Clostridia are large, gram-positive, rod-shaped microorganisms. They are obligate anaerobes and generally live in soil or the intestinal tracts of humans and animals. These organisms produce an exotoxin that causes putrefaction and tissue necrosis, the classic characteristics of gas gangrene. *Clostridium perfringens* is the most important pathogen of this group. Various toxins are produced by *C. perfringens*. The most important of these is lecithinase, which causes necrosis and hemolysis. Other toxins which contribute to the pathogenicity of *C. perfringens* include collagenase, hyaluronidase, and deoxyribonuclease.

Clostridial cellulitis   This is manifest by infections that cause crepitus and gas in the skin and subcutaneous tissues. The cellulitis is foul smelling with a seropurulent discharge from the depths and crevices of the wound. Usually, the infection extends along the fascial planes but does not involve intact, healthy muscle.

Clostridial myonecrosis   This is a rapidly progressive infection that is generally called *gas gangrene*. Crepitance and edema of the soft tissues are noted. These infections occur with large wounds of muscle that are contaminated with *C. perfringens*. High-velocity missile wounds are characteristic of this type of injury. Contamination by soil, clothing, or foreign bodies predisposes to clostridial myonecrosis. Progression of infection into uninjured tissue is promoted by the products of bacterial metabolism. The true finding of clostridial gas gangrene occurs with an overall incidence of less than 2%, although 4–40% of wounds may be contaminated with clostridia.

C. septicum is another organism which causes myonecrosis, but is particularly related to malignancy and immunosuppression. In a patient with evidence of clostridia myonecrosis or sepsis and no external source, the cecum or distal ileum should be considered a likely site of a malignancy.

Treatment of clostridial infections includes early surgical debridement and drainage. As little as a 24-h delay can be fatal. Multiple longitudinal incisions should be made for adequate drainage and debridement. Antibiotics including penicillin G and tetracycline are the most effective adjuncts to operative treatment. Antitoxin has no benefit and should not be used. Hyperbaric oxygen may be helpful as an adjunctive therapy.

Gastrointestinal enteritis Clostridia, coliforms, bacteroides, and enterococci are the most abundant flora in strangulated or obstructed bowel loops. Biliary tract infections with clostridia are probably secondary to transportation of organisms through portal circulation and excretion into bile. Abdominal wall gangrene occurs from clostridial contamination of the wound during operations on the lower intestinal tract. Systemic infections occur with rapid onset and require early operative drainage and antibiotic therapy.

Pseudomembranous colitis This gastrointestinal infection occurs during antibiotic therapy, particularly regimens which utilize clindamycin, although other agents have been implicated as well. The colitis is caused by *C. difficile,* which overtakes normal flora. The toxin produced by *C. difficile* causes watery diarrhea, fever, leukocytosis, and abdominal pain. Sigmoidoscopy will reveal yellowish, white, exudative plaques which are called pseudomembranes. Stool cultures often demonstrate *C. difficile*. Ampicillin, clindamycin, and cephalosporins are the most common causes of this syndrome. Any antibiotic, however, can be the cause.

To treat pseudomenbranous colitis, stop the offending antibiotic and begin oral vancomycin. Oral metronidazole can be an alternative to vancomycin. Cholestyramine has been shown to help bind the toxin. Isolate the patients to prevent nosocomial cross-contamination.

Urogenital Infections These can result after nephrectomy, prostatectomy, or other procedures which instrument the urogenital system. Contamination of the postabortal uterus is promoted by residual necrotic tissue. This setting favors multiplication of clostridia and can be diagnosed by the finding of gram-positive rods on Gram stain.

Tetanus   This is a disease which results from toxin produced by *C. tetani* at a traumatized site. The syndrome of tetanus is usually not associated with gas gangrene. The organisms producing tetanus exotoxin need favorable anaerobic conditions. *C. tetani* is found in soil and intestinal tracts of humans and animals. Penetrating wounds from rusty nails or thorns commonly predispose this infection. In most cases the injury is mild, and even healed, before toxemia develops.

The average incubation period for tetanus is 7–10 days after injury. In unusual cases reflex spasms may begin as early as 24 h after the onset of symptoms. Trismus is generally the first symptom. Pain and stiffness in the neck, back, and abdomen follow. Occasionally dysphagia appears early. The characteristic anxious expression in which the eyebrows and the corners of the mouth are drawn up is called *risus sardonicus*. Severe spasms may begin with a sudden jerk. Every muscle in the body is thrown into intense, tonic contraction. Flexion of the chest and abdomen occurs. These spasms could last several seconds or several minutes. Frequent spasms lead to rapid exhaustion and death from asphyxiation. Aspiration pneumonia is a common contributory cause of death. Exposure and subsequent survival of this illness does not confer immunity on the host.

Immunizations.   Prophylaxis with tetanus toxoid is the best means of preventing tetanus. Standard immunization begins at age 7 with 0.5 mL tetanus toxoid given intramuscularly. This is repeated after 4–6 weeks, and repeated a third time after 6–12 months. All three of these injections are required for completion of immunity. Antibody levels are usually safe at approximately 30 days after the initial dose.

Treatment.   Treatment of tetanus begins with thorough cleansing and debridement of the wound in order to remove necrotic tissue and foreign bodies. Penicillin is the antibiotic of choice. Tetracycline can be used for those who are allergic to penicillin. Systemic administration of muscle relaxants and pentothal are used in severe spasms. Respiratory control and pulmonary toilet are important in severe cases.

Prophylaxis.   The American College of Surgeons Committee on Trauma recommends the following general guidelines for management of wounds with reference to tetanus prophylaxis.

1. Adequate prophylaxis will be determined by the attending physician.

2. Meticulous surgical care must be provided immediately.
3. Human tetanus immune globulin must be considered individually for each patient. Passive immunization with human tetanus immune globulin (TIG) is not indicated if the patient has had two or more injections of toxoid in the past.
4. Routine booster injections every 10 years. Specific guidelines include:
   a. Fully immunized patients who have had a booster within 10 years require no additional treatment for nontetanus-prone wounds. If the wound is tetanus-prone a booster injection of 0.5 mL adsorbed toxoid should be given if more than 5 years have elapsed since the last dose.
   b. Patients with a history of full immunization but whose previous booster was greater than 10 years prior should receive 0.5 mL tetanus toxoid for all penetrating wounds.
   c. Patients with immunization histories of one injection or less or an unknown history should receive 0.5 mL tetanus toxoid for nontetanus-prone wounds. For tetanus-prone wounds in this setting injection of 250 units of human TIG in a different site should be added to the injection of 0.5 mL tetanus toxoid.

Botulism   *Botulism* results from ingestion of the exotoxin formed by *Clostridium botulinum*. This organism grows in improperly sterilized or inadequately preserved foods. The illness is manifested by gastrointestinal symptoms, diploplia, blurred vision, dysphagia, and motor paralysis. Wound botulism is suspected in patients who have no specific food history and develop signs of descending paralysis. Treatment of the wound is routine as described above. Respiratory care and assisted ventilation may be required. Equine trivalent antitoxin should be given after testing for sensitivity to equine serum.

GRAM-NEGATIVE INFECTIONS

Gram-negative organisms are usually found in the gastrointestinal tract. Prior to World War II these organisms were only rarely pathogenic in humans. Improved efficacy of treating gram-positive organisms has potentiated more infections with gram-negative bacteria. In addition, impaired host defenses and surgical procedures which introduce foreign objects have allowed these lesser virulent species to establish infections.

There are three families of gram-negative bacilli: *Pseudomonas, Enterobacteriaciae, and Bacteroides.*

Pseudomonas

These gram-negative organisms are strict aerobes and occur on skin surfaces. They are opportunistic pathogens which can cause serious and lethal infections. Frequently they occur along ventilator equipment, indwelling intravenous and urinary catheters, and other invasive foreign objects. Intravenous drug abusers are prone to pseudomonal osteomyelitis.

These bacteria produce an endotoxin which is not as toxic as enteric gram-negative organisms. Pseudomonas also produces an exotoxin similar to hemolysin and protease.

Treatment of pseudomonal infections is primarily with tobramycin or gentamicin, usually in combination with carbinocillin or ticarcillin. Resistant strains of *Pseudomonas* are becoming more common.

Enterobacteriaciae

Escherichia coli   These bacteria are facultative anaerobes. They are the most common organisms of intestinal flora. Their pathogenic characteristics include the ability to produce toxins, both endotoxin and exotoxin. The endotoxin associated with *E. coli* infection is very potent and can produce profound circulatory shock. *E. coli* can cause a variety of infections including wounds, intraabdominal abscess, urinary tract infection, meningitis, peritonitis, or endocarditis. Treatment generally includes an amino glycoside plus ampicillin.

Salmonella   These bacteria are enteric pathogens that are transmitted by food and water. They typically cause gastroenteritis or typhoid fever. Multiplication within the lymphoid tissue of the intestine causes ulceration, hemorrhage, and perforation. Treatment includes ampicillin or chloramphenicol.

Klebsiella   These are opportunistic pathogens in the *Escherichia* family. These organisms are usually hospital-acquired infections. They can cause severe pneumonia, endocarditis, urinary tract infections, or wound infection. *Enterobacter* and *Serratia* are gram-negative organisms that are similar to *Klebsiella.* They are usually nonpathogenic but can cause hospital-acquired infections. *Serratia marcescens* produces a characteristic red pigment. Treatment of these gram-negative organisms principally includes amino glycosides.

Proteus This is another member of the *Enterobacteriaciae* family, distinguished by its ability to produce the enzyme urease. These organisms all occur in abscesses and also in burns. Indole-negative proteus is usually treated with ampicillin; indole-positive species require aminoglycosides.

Acinetobacter These are gram-negative aerobes that are opportunistic organisms capable of causing infections in compromised patients. Again, aminoglycosides are the appropriate therapy.

Anaerobic Bacteria

Obligate anaerobes occur on skin and all mucous membrane surfaces. They predominate as normal flora within the oral cavity. Also, anaerobic bacteria are predominant in the large intestine, where they outnumber aerobic organisms 1000:1. Anaerobic bacteria that can invade the trachea and lungs include peptostreptococci, peptococci, *Bacteroides melaninogenicus,* and fusobacteria. Anaerobic intraabdominal infections are generally caused by *B. fragilis*. This organism can also cause gynecologic infections involving the vagina, uterus, and contiguous structures.

The clinical signs of an anaerobic infection are foul-smelling discharge, the presence of gas in surrounding tissues, and evidence of necrosis of the involved tissues. The failure to grow bacteria on aerobic cultures of the infected fluid is good empiric evidence of an anaerobic infection. More than 90% of intraabdominal abscesses or female pelvic infections will have some associated anaerobic organism.

Bacteroides This organism is gram-negative and behaves as an obligate anaerobe. *Bacteroides* can penetrate tissue and the bloodstream. This kind of invasion occurs in patients with chronic illnesses or malignant disease, or in conjunction with cystoscopy and surgical treatments. *Bacteroides* infections are characterized by spiking fevers, jaundice, and leukocytosis. Elderly and immunocompromised patients have a high mortality with bacteroides infections. Typically, there is a foul-smelling, purulent exudate which is an indication of anaerobic sepsis. Gram stain will reveal gram-negative organisms and frequently there will be no growth on standard cultures.

Treatment of *Bacteroides* infections utilizes the same principles of other surgical infections. Surgical drainage and excision of necrotic tissue is key. Appropriate antibiotics include penicillin G if the primary source is thought to be oropharyngeal. Clindamycin or metronidazole are the drugs of choice if a gastrointestinal origin is speculated.

PSEUDOMYCOTIC INFECTIONS

Actinomycosis

This disease is caused by anaerobic organisms that are true bacteria and resemble fungi. For this reason they are called pseudomycoses. Actinomyces are residents of oral flora and when involved with infection cause a dense fibroblastic reaction. Hyphae that resemble sulphur granules are often seen in microscopic examination of the pus from these infections. Treatment consists of penicillin G or tetracycline in addition to surgical drainage.

Nocardiosis

These are aerobic inhabitants of the soil which cause a rare but progressive disease manifest by pulmonary infection. Treatment consists of sulfadiazene for 4–6 months or alternatively ampicillin.

FUNGAL INFECTIONS

Mycoses

Mycoses are fungal infections that are generally the result of opportunistic pathogens. However, some mycotic infections are secondary to true pathogens. These include *Blastomyces, Paracoccidioides, Histoplasma,* and *Cryptococcus.* The opportunistic fungal pathogens are *Mucor, Rhizopus, Aspergillus,* and *Candida.*

In general, fungal diseases are suspected in chronic illnesses where no other cause can be established. Symptoms of fungal infection may include skin lesions, low-grade fever, weight loss, or chronic pulmonary infection. Often, serologic tests can help confirm the suspicion of fungal infection.

A tender, swollen joint, draining subcutaneous abscess, or ulcerative oropharyngeal lesion are all clinical examples of fungal infection.

Blastomycosis   *Blastomyces dermatitidis* is a fungus that grows as a single budding yeast or as a mold. These organisms are nonencapsulated and multinucleated yeast cells. Usually they begin as pathogens in the lungs and clinically resemble tuberculosis or possibly carcinoma. Skin lesions may appear later and are characterized as ulcerated and crusting. Treatment for blastomycosis is uniformly amphotericin B.

Histoplasmosis *Histoplasma* are dimorphic fungi that are present in soil containing feces from birds and bats. They are endemic along the Mississippi and Ohio valleys. Pulmonary infection is the first clinical sign of invasion by histoplasmosis. The symptoms typically are fever, cough, chest pain, and pleurisy. Dissemination throughout the body can involve the reticuloendothelial system, frequently the spleen. Histoplasma infections often coexist in patients with tuberculosis, leukemia, or Hodgkin's disease. The primary treatment is systemic administration of amphotericin B.

Coccidioidomycosis *Coccidioides* are dimorphic fungal organisms that are found in soil and are endemic to the southwest United States. They spread through airborne release of spores and eventually are inhaled by human beings. Pulmonary infection is established with clinical symptoms that resemble influenza. Disseminated disease may appear years later. The treatment for active infection includes amphotericin B, although therapy is usually reserved for disseminated infections involving bone, skin, or subcutaneous tissues.

Cryptococcosis Cryptococci are encapsulated yeast cells with a distinctive polysaccharide capsule. They reside in dust and bird feces. Transmission to human beings is usually by inhalation. Disease from *Cryptococcus* is usually manifested by CNS infection, commonly cryptococcal meningitis. Treatment utilizes flucytosine and amphotericin B. These infections almost always occur as opportunistic infections in immunocompromised patients.

Sporotrichosis *Sporothrix* are dimorphic fungi that are generally transmitted to human beings by inoculation from thorns or splinters. They cause skin and subcutaneous infections that spread into lymph channels and nodes. Treatment incorporates oral potassium iodide and intravenous amphotericin B.

Mucormycosis *Mucor* and *Rhizopus* are opportunistic saprophytic fungi that invade the compromised host. They cause brain and lung abscesses. Uncontrolled diabetes is a potentiator of the life-threatening infection caused by these fungi. Also, steroids, broad-spectrum antibiotics, and malnutrition are predisposing factors. Treatment includes systemic administration of amphotericin B. Commonly, surgical debridement of rapidly progressive infections is necessary.

Aspergillosis *Aspergillus* are opportunistic, saprophytic fungi that generally cause pulmonary infections. Bronchial aspergillomas are also known as "fungus balls." Systemic aspergillosis can occur and has a very poor prognosis. Treatment is systemic amphotericin B.

Candidosis *Candida albicans* is a dimorphic fungus that affects mucous membranes. The clinical sequelae are thrush in the oropharyngeal cavity, vulvovaginal candidosis, and systemic candidemia. Immunosuppressed patients are prone to systemic *Candida*. Also, patients receiving steroids, broad-spectrum antibiotics, and hyperalimentation, and patients with burns are equally susceptible to *Candida*. Topical nystatin for oral, skin, or vaginal surfaces is appropriate prophylaxis. Amphotericin B is used for systemic treatment.

PRINCIPLES OF ASEPSIS

The purpose of asepsis in surgery is to prevent access of bacteria to surgical wounds. The accomplishment of asepsis begins with sterilization of instruments, gowns, gloves, sutures, and dressings that come in contact with the surgical wound. Second, disinfection of the skin at the surgical site is accomplished by application of antiseptic agents. These principles are considered in more detail below.

Sterilization "Sterilization" means the destruction or elimination of all microorganisms. This can be done with physical or chemical agents.

Steam is the most reliable modality for sterilization. Steam under pressure will destroy all forms of life. Generally, 15 pounds of steam per square inch for 15–45 min is adequate. Autoclaves that have the capability for vacuum pumping can sterilize instruments in a shorter time, as little as 3 min.

Dry heat can be used for sterilization of glassware. Approximately 6 h in a hot-air oven at 120°C is necessary.

Gas sterilization with ethylene oxide is used for delicate instruments. Exposure to gas for as long as 3–6 h is necessary for adequate sterilization.

Radiation sterilization using electron accelerators can be used for special circumstances.

Chemical sterilization is generally used for anesthetic and dental equipment. These instruments are submerged in 2% aqueous glutaraldehyde or isopropyl alcohol.

Degerming of skin This applies to both the surgical site and the surgeon's hands. Scrubbing with antiseptic soap temporarily diminishes bacteria but can not eradicate all bacteria.

Hexachloraphene disinfects skin slowly and decreases the number of bacteria over a process of days. The soap leaves an antibacterial film that is easily removed by other soaps. This is not very effective against gram-negative organisms. Hexachloraphene can be absorbed and cause encephalopathy in infants.

Iodophors are agents that contain iodine and detergent. Approximately 1% of the soap is iodine. Free iodine is bacteriocidal and acts more rapidly than hexachloraphene.

Cholohexidine kills gram-positive, gram-negative, and fungal organisms. The onset of action is rapid. Toxicity is minimal.

Alcohol combined with iodine kills gram-positive and gram-negative organisms. The action of alcohol is very rapid, and brief contact with the skin is adequate.

6 TRAUMA

GENERAL CONSIDERATIONS

Trauma ranks overall as the fourth leading cause of death in the United States today. Over 140,000 deaths occur each year from accidents, and there are an estimated 140 million bed days of annual disability. The Centers for Disease Control found that over 4 million years of future work life are lost each year to injury, vs. 2.1 million to heart disease and 1.7 million to cancer.

Categories of Patients

There are three categories of patients, according to immediacy of injury. Patients in the first category are those whose injuries interfere with vital physiologic functions. Examples would be patients who have obstruction of an airway, those whose respiration is compromised due to a hemothorax or pneumothorax, or those with internal bleeding. Patients in the first two groups require urgent intervention in the emergency room, while patients in the latter group will require urgent thoracotomy or laparotomy in the operating room to control hemorrhage.

A second category of trauma patients includes those who will require surgical procedures within 1–2 h after admission to the hospital. These patients have frequently suffered truncal trauma from either blunt or penetrating injuries, but their vital signs are stable on first presentation. Preparation for surgery includes type and cross match of blood, appropriate x-rays, and continual observation by a physician until the patient is transferred to the operating room.

The third group of patients includes those who have occult injuries that are missed on first examination in the emergency room. Examples would be patients with small pneumothoraces, small bleeding lacerations of the spleen or liver, blunt rupture of the small intestine, etc. Even with appropriate x-rays and continued clinical evaluation, some of these injuries may be missed for hours or days.

Initial Resuscitation of the Severely Injured Patient

The trauma resuscitation room in the emergency center should contain standard equipment such as an overhead operating room light, oxygen lines, cardiac monitor and defibrillator, and a portable carriage that is suitable for an operating room table in an emergency situation. Bags of intravenous fluid should be hanging and ready to be immediately infused into the injured patient. Cabinets in the room should include equipment for endotracheal intubation, tracheostomy, thoracocentesis, tube thoracostomy, venous cutdown, central line insertion, pericardiocentesis, and diagnostic peritoneal lavage.

AIRWAY A variety of airway maneuvers are necessary in managing patients with major trauma. It is often useful to have a pegboard near the head of the emergency room table that allows for rapid retrieval of a laryngoscope, cuffed endotracheal tubes of various sizes, tracheostomy tube, cricothyrotomy tube, and an Ambu bag. It is also necessary to have some type of suction available in the resuscitation room to remove pulmonary secretions, foreign bodies, and blood from the upper respiratory tract.

Breathing Once a patient has an adequate airway in place, failure of one or both sides of the chest to show signs of ventilation should make the examiner suspicious that a major thoracic injury is present. If a pneumothorax is questionable, an 18-gauge needle may be inserted into the chest in the second or third intercostal space in the anterior axillary line and aspiration done to reveal the presence of air. This would be necessary only in a patient with a life-threatening tension pneumothorax in whom time is not available for a chest x-ray. The presence of any type of pneumothorax is treated with the insertion of a chest tube and underwater seal and drainage.

The presence of a hemothorax may significantly impair ventilation also. For this reason, tube thoracostomy is once again performed, frequently with an anterior chest tube placed in the second interspace in the midclavicular and a posterior chest tube placed in the eighth interspace in the posterior axillary line. The chest tubes inserted should be #36 French so that adequate drainage is maintained. Thoracotomy is rarely indicated in patients with hemothoraces unless greater than 1000 mL is removed through the tubes within the first 30–60 min or if there is continued bleeding of 100–200 mL/h for several hours.

A patient with an open chest injury or so-called sucking chest wound is best managed by immediately covering the open wound with whatever material is available, such as a large Vaseline gauze bandage. A chest tube is then inserted at a separate site to help relieve the pneumothorax. Operative intervention is usually necessary to reconstruct the defect in the chest wall.

Paradoxical motion of the chest wall is indicative of a flail chest caused by segmental fractures of several ribs in sequence. Currently approximately two-thirds of patients, even those with underlying pulmonary contusions, can avoid intubation or tracheostomy if their pain is controlled and if they are given adequate pulmonary toilet.

Ruptured Bronchus   This relatively rare injury presents with respiratory distress, hemoptysis, cyanosis, and a massive air leak. Immediate tube thoracostomy is necessary to relieve the associated pneumothorax; bronchoscopy and open thoracotomy in the operating room are necessary to localize and repair the bronchial defect.

SHOCK AND HEMORRHAGE   Hypovolemic shock is treated once the patient's airway and breathing problems are controlled. Two 18-gauge or larger intravenous catheters are started in peripheral veins and a balanced salt solution such as Ringer's lactate is given until partial typing and cross matching of blood is completed. Shock resulting from a blood loss of 750 mL can usually be corrected by rapid administration of 2 L Ringer's lactate solution over 15–20 min. Blood loss in excess of 750 mL usually requires the administration of whole blood in addition to a balanced salt solution. If the patient initially responds to 1–2 L balanced salt solution as evidenced by improving blood pressure and decreasing pulse rate, but then subsequently becomes hypotensive, blood administration is usually necessary. In a patient with exsanguination, un-cross-matched type O, Rh-negative blood is administered without hesitation.

External bleeding from an extremity is best controlled by direct finger pressure or the application of a pressure dressing to the bleeding wound or vessel. Tourniquets are not routinely used outside the operating room. Even with temporary control of hemorrhage from finger pressure or the application of a pressure dressing, the patient should be taken to the operating room expeditiously to attain hemostasis.

OTHER LIFE-THREATENING INJURIES   Patients with a small atrial perforation from a penetrating wound or blunt atrial rupture may slowly develop a cardiac tamponade while being observed in the emergency room. In a patient with either mechanism of injury to the chest, clinical signs pathognomonic for a cardiac tamponade are: progressive rise in venous pressure, decreased pulse pressure, paradoxical pulse, occasional cyanosis, and decreased heart sounds. When the diagnosis is suspected and the patient is rapidly deteriorating, a pericardiocentesis performed with an 18-gauge needle inserted at the xiphocostal angle is indicated. Because of the large number of false-positive and false-negative examinations with pericardiocentesis, many trauma centers have chosen to use the technique of subxiphoid pericardial window under local anesthesia in the operating room to confirm the diagnosis of a cardiac rupture. If the diagnosis is confirmed, immediate thoracotomy is indicated to repair the cardiac wound.

A contained rupture of the descending thoracic aorta just beyond the left subclavian artery is usually suspected from widening of the superior mediastinum on an upright chest x-ray in the emergency room. If the patient has this finding or the history of the injury is strongly suggestive of deceleration from a high rate of speed, immediate aortography is necessary to rule out this highly lethal injury.

OTHER MANEUVERS   As part of the early resuscitation and evaluation of the multiply injured patient, nasogastric intubation is usually indicated. Exceptions would include those patients with penetrating wounds of the face and head, complex facial injuries, or suspected cervical spine fractures. An esophageal or gastric injury from penetrating or blunt trauma is suggested by finding bright red blood in the nasogastric tube drainage. Gastric intubation prevents gastric dilatation during tracheal intubation and aids in the prevention of postoperative distention of the small bowel.

A bladder catheter is also usually inserted in multiply injured patients to monitor for the presence of hematuria as well as to follow the urinary output during and immediately after resuscitation. Gross hematuria is evidence of urinary tract injury and is usually evaluated by performing both a retrograde cystogram and an intravenous pyelogram. In patients with a penetrating wound but no hematuria, an intravenous pyelogram is frequently performed in case an urgent nephrectomy is required during the subsequent emergency operation. The purpose of the preoperative intravenous pyelogram is to document the presence of both kidneys.

Primary Survey of the Injured Patient

Once the patient's ABCs are stabilized, the patient is rapidly examined to diagnosis any other injuries. Unconscious patients should have an airway established at this point if it has not been done previously. The frequent association of cervical spine injuries and cranial injuries mandates that a lateral x-ray of the cervical spine be performed early in such patients, as well. As hypotension rarely results from a closed head injury, the patient with hypotension and a head injury should always be quickly evaluated for intrathoracic or intraabdominal bleeding.

Penetrating wounds of the abdominal wall are explored to determine if they have truly penetrated the peritoneal cavity. This is usually done with stab wounds because the tract of a gunshot wound is frequently easier to assess. When local wound exploration reveals penetration of the anterior or flank peritoneum by a stab wound but the patient has no hypotension or peritonitis, diagnostic peritoneal lavage is used to assess the presence of intraperitoneal injuries. In contrast, for gunshot wounds in which physical examination or x-ray strongly suggests a peritoneal traverse of a missile, laparotomy is always mandated because most gunshot wounds that enter the peritoneal cavity cause major visceral or vascular injuries.

If fractures of the extremities are present, early immobilization may prevent additional nerve and blood vessel injury and conversion of a closed fracture to an open one. If no major intracranial or thoracoabdominal injuries are present, the fracture can then be managed as a priority. If there is absence of distal arterial pulses in the fractured extremity after reduction, an immediate arteriogram is necessary. Fractures in the pelvis at two separate sites are best treated with external pelvic fixation. This allows for early mobilization and pain relief and may be a factor in controlling bleeding.

Any penetrating injury in an extremity in the proximity of a major artery should be evaluated for possible arterial injury. The yield of arteriography with such proximity of injury to an artery is approximately 3–15 %, and the decision to perform arteriography is best made by an experienced trauma surgeon.

Secondary Survey

Once the patient is stabilized, a more comprehensive, head-to-toe examination should be performed. When there is still suspicion of occult blood loss, a diagnostic peritoneal lavage in the abdomen coupled with further x-rays of the chest may reveal the site. In patients with penetrating wounds, further x-rays may also be indicated to help predict the course of the missile.

Prophylactic Antibiotics and Tetanus Prophylaxis

Prophylactic antibiotics are given preoperatively to all patients sustaining penetrating wounds to the abdomen. These may be discontinued if exploratory celiotomy is negative for injury to the gastrointestinal tract. Coverage should be against both aerobes and anaerobes and should always be given preoperatively or intraoperatively.

Any patient with a penetrating wound should be reimmunized against tetanus with an injection of tetanus toxoid booster. In unimmunized patients the wound is debrided, and 250 units of tetanus immune globulin is administered. Previously immunized patients who are taking steroids or are undergoing immunosuppressive therapy such as chemotherapy should also receive human immune globulin. Severely contaminated wounds should be left open or converted to open wounds when feasible.

PRINCIPLES IN THE MANAGEMENT OF WOUNDS

Local Care of Wounds

On the trunk, stab wounds of soft tissues are explored in the emergency room with a gloved finger or under local anesthesia by extending the length of the laceration to determine the direction and extent of the wound. The wound is then irrigated with copious amounts of saline solution. If the wound does not penetrate the peritoneal cavity, a small soft-rubber Penrose drain is inserted and the wound is left open for drainage. Gunshot wounds are debrided externally and left open for drainage, also. In the extremities, major vessel bleeding should be controlled by application of a dry sterile pressure dressing. An x-ray may be indicated to rule out the presence of a foreign body, but immediate surgery is necessary to control the hemorrhage in the operating room. When major hemorrhage is not occurring, vigorous irrigation of the wound, finger exploration, and closure is indicated in the emergency room. Antibacterial soaps or detergent materials are not used to irrigate the wounds of the extremity when muscle, tendon, or blood vessels are visible because severe chemical irritation of these structures may occur.

With all soft tissue wounds, tissue that is dead or has a poor blood supply, or is heavily contaminated should be removed if at all possible. This is particularly true of subcutaneous fat and muscle. The wound is then irrigated with copious quantities of saline solution. Many factors su contamination, blood supply of the remaining tissue, host resistance, presence of shock, tissue tension, and dead space will have to be considered before such a large open wound is closed in the emergency room.

One troublesome wound is the puncture injury caused by a rusty nail in the foot. The patient should be administered antibiotics to prevent secondary infection and to aid in the prevention of tetanus. Conservative debridement is performed if only the skin and subcutaneous tissue are involved. Human tetanus immune globulin in a dose of 250 mL is given to the unimmunized patient. The wound is left open whether the patient has been previously immunized or not.

Power mower injuries may result from flying objects as well as directly from the mower blade itself. Most of these wounds in the hands or fingers are best left open at the first operation because of the high incidence of secondary infection. Systemic antibiotics and tetanus prophylaxis are given, and skin grafting and reconstruction should be delayed.

Emergency Celiotomy

A midline incision is used for exploratory celiotomy in patients with abdominal trauma. Tissue should be kept moist and gently handled during the operative procedure. Before closure, any intraabdominal drains, such as those placed for hepatic or pancreatic injuries, are brought out through a separate stab wound in a direct route. Drainage of the free peritoneal cavity is not attempted.

In a patient without major colonic or purulent contamination, a midline incision is usually closed with number 0-Prolene. Sutures should be staggered at varying intervals from the edge of the midline fascia, and the strongest repair is felt to be simple, interrupted sutures. Regardless of the type of suture or method of placement, the fascia should be loosely approximated and not strangulated. When extensive contamination of the peritoneal cavity is present such as from a shotgun wound or massive injury to the colon, or when the patient has been on steroids or has associated intraabdominal infection, the best closure for the abdominal wound is a through-and-through closure. Other indications for this type of closure include chronic pulmonary disease, obesity, and/or chronic debilitating disease. Closure of this type is usually performed using large nonabsorbable or absorbable sutures and adjustable bridges or German silver wires swaged on a large cutting needle. This rapid closure may also be indicated in patients at the end of a lengthy operation or when reoperation for problems such as gastrointestinal bleeding or intestinal obstruction is necessary in the first few weeks after the original operation. The large full-thickness sutures are left in place for 3 weeks.

Antibiotics

Sepsis is the second most common cause of death in patients sustaining penetrating abdominal trauma. Burke has clearly demonstrated that the administration of antibiotics in the preoperative period is necessary to lower the postoperative incidence of infection.

A variety of antibiotic regimens have been used in patients with penetrating abdominal trauma involving the gastrointestinal tract. With closure of all gastrointestinal injuries, irrigation of the enteric and fecal debris out of the peritoneal cavity, and debridement of nonviable tissue, the use of either a single cephalosporin antibiotic or combinations of antibiotics with both aerobic and anaerobic coverage will keep the rate of formation of postoperative intraabdominal abscesses to a minimum.

Even with appropriate surgical technique and antibiotics, intraabdominal abscesses occur, especially when the patient has received a gunshot wound to the colon. An early diagnosis of an intraabdominal abscess is usually made by a CT scan. When the abscess is in the periphery of the abdomen, percutaneous drainage has a 75 to 80% chance of success.

Intraperitoneal irrigation with antibiotic solutions after removal of particulate debris is usually not necessary if appropriate blood levels are obtained by the administration of intravenous antibiotics. As previously noted, the skin and subcutaneous tissue of the midline incision should be left open for delayed primary closure when extensive enteric or fecal contamination has been present during a trauma laparotomy.

BITES AND STINGS OF ANIMALS AND INSECTS

Rabies

In the U.S. an estimated 2 million human beings are bitten by animals yearly, and half a million are bitten by dogs. Any mammalian animal may carry rabies; however, the animals most frequently reported infected are skunks (45%), raccoons (26%), and bats (15%). It is also accepted that wildlife species account for 91% of the rabies in this country. Only two human cases of rabies occur each year in the United States.

Rabies Control   Wild and exotic animals who are to be kept as household pets must first be quarantined for a minimum of 90 days after capture and vaccinated at least 30 days prior to being released to an owner. Annual vaccination is also recommended.

Dogs and cats bitten by a known rabid animal should be destroyed immediately. If the owner refuses to have this done, the unvaccinated animal should be placed in strict isolation for 6 months and vaccinated 1 month before being released. If the animal has been vaccinated within the previous 3 years it should be revaccinated immediately and confined for 90 days.

Diagnosis   Most bites from domestic animals are provoked attacks. Previous vaccination of a domestic animal is over 90% effective in preventing transmission of the disease. Also, bites from rodents seldom require specific rabies prophylaxis.

The likelihood that rabies will result from a bite varies with its extent and location. Severe or high-exposure bites are considered to be those that include multiple or deep puncture wounds or any bites of the head, face, neck, hands, or fingers. Mild bites are considered to be scratches, lacerations, or single bites on areas of the body other than the head, face, neck, hands, or fingers. Open wounds, such as abrasions, suspected of being contaminated with saliva also belong to this category.

The direct focus inhibition test of brain material is the recommended technique to diagnose rabies. If a human being has been bitten by a suspect animal, but the direct focus inhibition test is negative, the microscopic examination of mice brain tissue for Negri bodies after intracerebral inoculation is still one of the most useful tests.

Management of Biting Animal   Domestic animals that bite a person should be captured and observed for symptoms of rabies for 10 days. If none develops, the animal may be assumed to be nonrabid. If the animal dies or is killed, the head (keep refrigerated) should not be damaged but should be sent promptly to a public health laboratory for examination.

Patient Management   For mild exposure of a person who has demonstrated an antibody response to antirabies vaccination received in the past, two IM doses (1.0 mL each) of human diploid cell vaccine (HDCV), one immediately and one 3 days later, are recommended. If it is not known whether an exposed person has had antibody previously demonstrated, the complete postexposure antirabies treatment with human rabies immune globulin for five doses may be necessary. If antibody can be demonstrated in a serum sample collected before vaccine is given, treatment can be discontinued after at least two doses of HDCV.

Individuals in avocations or vocations with frequent contact with dogs, cats, or any of the high-risk animals should be considered for preexposure prophylaxis. Three 1-mL injections of HDCV are given intradermally in the deltoid area on days 0, 7, and 21 or 28. Serologic testing is not necessary after preexposure prophylaxis. Patients given this dosage do not begin to respond for 7 days and do not obtain significant titers for 10–14 days.

Postexposure Prophylaxis It is generally accepted that the postincubation period for rabies in human beings ranges from 10 days to 1 year; however, most cases occur within 20–90 days from exposure. When an individual is bitten, local care of the animal bite should consist of thorough irrigation with copious amounts of saline, cleansing with a soap solution, debridement, leaving the wound open, and administration of the appropriate antibiotic and tetanus toxoid.

For passive immunization after a bite, human rabies immune globulin (HRIG) in combination with HDCV is considered the best exposure prophylaxis. HRIG is given in a dose of 20 units per kilogram of body weight and is recommended for most exposures classified as severe, for all bites by rabid animals or those expected of having rabies, for unprovoked bites by wild carnivores and bats, and for nonbite exposure by animals suspected of being rabid. The HRIG is given only once as early as possible following exposure and is accompanied by five intramuscular 1.0-mL doses of HDCV.

When the HDCV is given in the five injections mentioned above, actual primary immunization can be completed by giving a sixth dose 90 days after the first dose.

In patients continuously exposed to the risk of rabies, booster doses of HDCV should be given at 2-year intervals. A previously immunized person who is exposed to rabies should receive two doses IM of 1 mL HDCV, one immediately and one 3 days later.

Side effects to the HDCV vaccine have included warmth, redness, pain, swelling, and itching at the injection site in approximately 15–25% of patients. Rarely have systemic reactions including hives and anaphylaxis occurred.

When patients who are receiving immunosuppressive agents such as corticosteroids must undergo postexposure prophylaxis, it is especially important that the serum be tested for antibody to ensure that an adequate response has developed. Also, it should be remembered that pregnancy is not considered a contraindication to postexposure prophylaxis. In patients with a history suggesting hypersensitivity to HDCV, antihistamines and epinephrine should be available should an anaphylactic reaction occur.

If a patient develops rabies, the first manifestation is 2–4 days of prodromal symptoms before the patient reaches the so-called excited stage. Paresthesias in the region of the bite is an important early symptom. Other symptoms noted with the onset of clinical rabies include headaches, vertigo, stiff neck, malaise, and severe pulmonary symptoms. The patient may also have spasms of the throat muscles with dysphagia, drooling, maniacal behavior, and convulsions followed by coma, paralysis, and death. The primary treatment is intensive respiratory support, including the insertion of an airway, pulmonary care, and treatment of cardiac arrhythmias and seizures. Intensive nursing care as well as treatment of cardiopulmonary and neurologic complications has resulted in several survivors in the U.S.

Snakebites

Incidence   Approximately 8000 persons are bitten each year by poisonous snakes in the U.S., with over 98% of bites occurring on the extremities. Children less than 10 years of age account for 35% of snakebites. Since 1960, an average of 14 victims per year have died in the U.S. as a result of snakebites, with five states accounting for 70% of these deaths—Texas, Georgia, Florida, Alabama, and Southern California.

In North America poisonous snakes are members of the family *Crotalidae,* or pit vipers, or of the family *Elapidae,* or coral snakes. Rattlesnakes are responsible for approximately 70% of all deaths due to snakebites, while death from the bite of a copperhead is extremely rare.

Poisonous vs. Nonpoisonous Snakes   The pit vipers are named for the characteristic heat-sensitive pit that is located between the eye and the nostril on each side of the head. Also, pit vipers have elliptical pupils rather than the round pupils of harmless snakes. In contrast, the coral snake does have a round pupil and lacks the facial pit. Pit vipers have well-developed fangs and a single row of subcaudal plates. Nonpoisonous snakes have teeth rather than fangs and have a double row of subcaudal plates. To distinguish the poisonous coral snake from related snakes of the same color, it should be remembered that the nose of the coral snake is black and that coral snakes have red rings next to yellow rings.

The venom of poisonous snakes contains hyaluronidase, which enhances the rapid spread of venom by way of the superficial lymphatics. Other toxic products in venom include neurotoxins, hemorrhagic and thrombogenic toxins, hemolytic toxins, cytotoxins, and anticoagulants.

Clinical Manifestations   Pain from the bite of a poisonous snake is excruciating and probably the symptom that most easily differentiates poisonous from nonpoisonous snakebites. Poisonous snakebites usually inflict one or two fang marks which are rapidly surrounded by swelling, tenderness, pain, and ecchymoses. If no edema or pain is present within 30 min of injury, the pit viper probably did not inject any venom. If venom has been injected, hemorrhagic vesiculations, bullae, and petechiae may appear after 8 h, with swelling progressing for a full 24 h. Systemic symptoms include muscle fasciculations that are especially noticeable in the perioral region after a rattlesnake bite. Other systemic symptoms include hypotension, weakness, sweating and chills, dizziness, and nausea and vomiting.

Rattlesnake bites are characterized by an injection of venom less than 50% of the time. Systemic symptoms frequently occur early and are associated with defects in blood coagulation, injuries to the intimal lining of vessels, damage to the heart muscle, and alterations in respiration. Pulmonary edema and hemorrhagic complications frequently occur with major envenomation, and both bleeding and clotting times are usually prolonged.

The coral snake contributes to only 3% of all bites and 1.5% of all deaths from poisonous snakes. After envenomation the patient may notice blurred vision, drowsiness, sweating, paresthesias around the mouth, and nausea and vomiting.

Laboratory Evaluations   Blood should be immediately drawn for typing and cross matching and sent for tests such as a complete blood count, platelet count, prothrombin time, partial thromboplastin time, urinalysis, blood sugar, BUN, and electrolytes. Additional tests include a fibrinogen level, red cell fragility, clotting time, and clot retraction time.

Local Treatment   The involved extremity should be immobilized, and a venous-lymphatic obstruction tourniquet should be applied proximal to the bite. If the bite has occurred within the last hour, incision and suction of the bite may be of benefit. Approximately 50% of subcutaneously injected venom can be removed when the suction is started within 3 min. Also, a 30-min period of suction extracts about 90% of the venom. The incision over the fang marks should be

¼-in. long and ⅛–¼-in. deep, longitudinal, and not cruciate. The suction is applied with a suction cup; however, if this is not available, mouth suction can be used as long as the individual performing the maneuver does not have any mucosal defects in his or her mouth.

Another option is to perform excision of the entire area of the bite including the skin and subcutaneous tissue if the bite has occurred within 1 h. This is rarely indicated, as medical therapy is effective in most patients if given soon after the bite.

The tourniquet may be removed as soon as an intravenous infusion is started, when antivenin is ready for administration, and if the patient is not in shock. Cryotherapy, a popular form of treatment in the past, is mentioned only to be condemned because it clearly increased the rate of amputation.

Systemic Treatment In 1954, a polyvalent Crotalidae antivenin became commercially available. It covers all the pit viper bites in North America and is rarely indicated for copperhead bites. Because antivenin contains horse serum, its administration require prior skin testing.

The antivenin for coral snakebites is different. A North American coral snake (*Micrurus fulvius*) antivenin has been developed. It effectively treats *Micrurus* coral snakebites but is not effective in treating bites of *Micruroides,* the genus native to Arizona and New Mexico. Coral snake antivenin can be obtained from either state health departments or the U.S. Public Health Service National Communicable Disease Center in Atlanta, Georgia. When individuals such as reptile handlers in the zoo are bitten by exotic snakes, the zoo usually carries the appropriate antivenin. Otherwise, information can be obtained from the Antivenin Index Center of the Oklahoma Poison Information Center, Oklahoma City, Oklahoma, (405) 271-5454.

The timing of antivenin administration depends upon the snake involved. With bites by the pit vipers in the United States, 30% of which result in no envenomation, the antivenin should be withheld until a physician can determine if it is indicated.

There is a grading system for severity of envenomation, which is described as follows: Grade 0—one or more fang marks, minimal pain, less than 1 in. surrounding edema, and no envenomation. Grade I—minimal envenomation. There is moderate to severe pain around the fang marks and 1–5 in. surrounding edema and erythema in the first 12 h after the bite. Grade II—moderate envenomation. There is severe pain in the area of the fang marks with 6–12 in. edema and erythema in the first 12 h after the bite. Possible systemic symptoms. Grade III—severe envenomation. Severe pain in the areas of the fang marks, with more than 12 in. surrounding edema and erythema in the first 12 h after the bite. Systemic involvement usually includes generalized petechiae and ecchymoses. Grade IV—very severe envenomation. Systemic involvement is always present, and symptoms may include renal failure, blood-tinged secretions, coma, and death. Local edema may extend beyond the involved extremity to the ipsilateral trunk.

Antivenin is usually not required for grades 0–I envenomation. Grade II may require 3 or 4 ampules, and grade III usually requires 5–15 ampules. If symptoms increase, several ampules may be required during the first 2 h. Because children are smaller, they receive relatively larger doses of venom, which places them in a higher risk group. Thus, the smaller the patient, the greater the required dose of antivenin. Antivenin is usually given in a dosage of 3–5 vials in an intravenous drip of 500 mL normal saline solution or 5% glucose solution. If severe systemic symptoms are already present, 6–8 vials are added. The dose of intravenously administered antivenin can be more easily titrated with response to treatment, and the amount administered is based on improvement in signs and symptoms, not on weight of the patient. Antivenin is administered until severe local or systemic symptoms improve.

If too much time has elapsed for excision to be effective and the patient is allergic to horse serum, a slow infusion of 1 ampule of antivenin and 250 mL 5% glucose solution may be given in a 90-min period with constant monitoring of the blood pressure and electrocardiogram. If an immediate reaction occurs, the antivenin is stopped, and a vasopressor such as epinephrine and perhaps an antihistamine may be required.

The incidence of serum sickness is related to the volume of horse serum injected. Of patients receiving 100–200 mL horse serum, 85% will have some degree of sensitivity in 8–12 days following injection.

Other systemic therapy such as steroids remains controversial, as the major effect appears to be a decreased incidence of serum sickness. Respiratory problems are treated with endotracheal intubation, while acute renal failure may require renal dialysis. On occasion, fascial planes in the extremity may become very tense and require fasciotomy. Numerous coagulopathies have been reported, and the administration of blood, fibrinogen, and vitamin K may be required. Antibiotics are also started immediately to prevent secondary infection, and tetanus toxoid is administered.

Stinging Insects and Animals

HYMENOPTERA The arthropods of the order Hymenoptera include the honey bee, bumblebee, wasps, yellow and black hornet, and the fire ant. The venom of these stinging insects is just as potent as that of snakes and causes more deaths in the U.S. yearly than are caused by snakebites.

Other than the bee, insects in this group retain their stinger and are in a position to sting repeatedly, each time injecting some portion of the venom sac contents. In contrast, the bee has a barbed stinger that cannot be withdrawn. As the bee attempts to escape, it is disemboweled; the stinger with the bowel, muscles, and venom sac is left behind and rhythmically contracts for as long as 20 min.

Symptoms of a bite from one of these insects consist of localized pain, swelling, generalized erythema, headache, blurred vision, apprehension, petechial hemorrhages of skin and mucous membranes, sweating, severe nausea, asthma, angioneurotic edema, vascular collapse, and possibly death from anaphylaxis. Fatal cases may manifest glottal and laryngeal edema, pulmonary and cerebral edema, and intraventricular hemorrhage. Death apparently results from a combination of shock, respiratory failure, and CNS changes and usually occurs 15–30 min after the bite.

Affected persons should be taught to remove the venom sac if a bee has been the causative agent. Highly sensitive individuals may find it necessary to carry an emergency kit which contains a tourniquet, sublingual isoproterenol, epinephrine hydrochloride aerosol for inhalation, and tweezers to remove the stinger and venom sac. Patients such as this should be taught to give themselves an epinephrine injection of 0.3–0.5 mL 1:1000 solution intravenously. Antihistamines may also be intravenously administered.

It has been noted that 50% of patients who have a severe generalized reaction to stings had no previous history of a severe reaction. Patients with a history of severe local or systemic involvement following insects stings should be desensitized. Venom immunotherapy is safe and is highly effective within a few weeks.

STINGRAY Approximately 750 persons each year are stung by stingrays; however, during the past 60 years, only two deaths in this country have been attributed to the venom of the stingray.

As the spine enters the flesh of the victim, the sheath surrounding the spine ruptures and venom is released. As the spine is withdrawn, fragments of the sheath may remain in the wound. Pain is usually immediate and severe and increases to a maximum in 1–2 h.

Copious irrigation with water to wash out any toxin and fragments of the spines and sheath should first be performed. Because the venom is inactivated when exposed to heat, the area of the bite should be placed in water as hot as the patient can stand without injury for 30–60 min. After soaking, the wound may be further debrided and treated appropriately.

PORTUGUESE MAN-OF-WAR   The tentacles of this coelenterate are covered with thousands of stinging cells known as nematocytes. Each nematocyte consists of a small sphere containing a coiled, hollowed thread that is activated by touch. This thread is uncoiled with such force that it can penetrate skin and even rubber gloves. The sting produces extreme pain and often signs of clinical shock; however, no deaths have been reported.

Symptoms include severe nausea, gastric cramping, constriction and tightness of the throat and chest, and intense burning pain.

Immediate treatment is to apply a substance of high alcohol content such as rubbing alcohol to the involved area. This is followed by the application of a drying agent, such as flour, baking soda, talc, or shaving cream. The tentacles may then be removed by shaving. Alkaline agents such as baking soda are then applied to the involved area in order to neutralize the toxins, which are acidic.

BLACK WIDOW SPIDER   The most common biting spider in the U.S. is the black widow spider (*Latrodectus mactans*). The spider is black and globular with a red hourglass mark on the abdomen. The venom is primarily neurotoxic, and its action appears to center around the spinal cord. The bite causes severe muscular pain and stiffness, nausea, vomiting, and headache. The most severe symptoms last 24–48 h and are characterized by generalized muscle spasms in the trunk and thighs. Less commonly, the patient may have hypertension, hyperreflexia, and urinary retention. Treatment has consisted of narcotics for the relief of pain and a muscle relaxant such as methocarbamol or intravenous calcium gluconate. Although an antivenin is available, it is rarely required.

NORTH AMERICAN LOXOSCELISM   The brown recluse spider (*Loxosceles reclusa*) has a darker violin-shaped band over the dorsal cephalothorax. This spider is native to the south central U.S. and is found both indoors and outdoors.

The initial bite may go unnoticed or be associated with a mild stinging sensation with pain not occurring for 6–8 h. Typically, there is a zone of hemorrhage and induration and a surrounding halo of erythema. As the central ischemia turns dark, eschar forms by the 7th day and the area sloughs by the 14th day. Approximately 3 weeks is required for the lesion to heal. Patients may have systemic symptoms such as fever, nausea, vomiting, and arthralgias, and these are particularly severe in children. The two principal systemic effects, hemolysis and thrombocytopenia, have been responsible for deaths.

Immediate excision with primary closure has been advocated as the treatment of choice. This is usually not possible, since patients can rarely be certain that they have been bitten by a brown recluse spider. In recent years the drug dapsone in a dose of 100 mg daily has been given for 14 days followed by surgical excision, if needed. There are numerous significant side effects including hemolytic anemia, methemoglobinemia, and rashes. It has also been suggested that one should obtain blood for G6PD levels and hematocrit before dapsone therapy.

PENETRATING WOUNDS OF THE NECK AND THORACIC INLET

In patients with penetrating wounds between the clavicles and angle of the mandible, exploration is warranted for those with obvious signs of vascular or visceral injuries such as a pulsatile hematoma, external bleeding, subcutaneous air, hemoptysis, or difficulty swallowing. Many other patients will be asymptomatic after sustaining a wound penetrating the platysma muscle. In order to describe the management of these patients, it is helpful to use Monson's division of the neck into three zones: zone I—below a horizontal line 1 cm above the claviculomanubrial junction; zone II—between zone I and the angle of the mandible; zone III—between the angle of the mandible and the base of the skull. There are two schools of thought on the management of patients with penetrating wounds in zone II. In many centers mandatory exploration is performed for platysma penetration in zone II, and 50% of the explorations are negative. Other centers have recently pursued vigorous workups to rule out carotid and vertebral arterial injuries using arch aortography and to rule out esophageal injuries using barium esophagograms and flexible and rigid endoscopy. The accuracy of arteriography is extraordinarily high, while the sensitivity for barium swallow and rigid esophagoscopy to rule out injury to the esophagus is less so. For surgeons working in hospitals caring for a limited number of traumatized patients, routine exploration probably remains the safest approach to the management of penetrating neck injuries.

Treatment in the Emergency Room

The ABCs are taken care of in the usual fashion, recognizing that an emergent cricothyroidotomy or tracheostomy may be necessary if a laryngotracheal injury or a large cervical hematoma is present. Large bore intravenous lines are started in the extremities, with crystalloid solutions given originally followed by type-specific blood. In the most severe instances of shock, type O, Rh-negative low-titer unmatched blood is infused rapidly. X-rays of the neck and chest are important to track the course of the missile and rule out an associated thoracic problem such as a pneumothorax. On rare occasions, penetrating wounds involving the upper chest and zone I may require an emergent left or right anterolateral thoracotomy in the emergency room to gain proximal control of hemorrhage from laceration or penetration of either subclavian artery.

In more stable patients, penetrating injuries in zone I and zone III are usually studied with arteriography in order to determine if a major arterial injury is present in either of these difficult-to-expose anatomical areas. In contrast, symptomatic patients with injuries in zone II usually undergo early exploration.

Anesthetic Management

Awake intubation is preferred in patients with wounds to the neck proper because difficulties imposed by cervical hematomas or upper-airway edema may delay adequate oxygenization in paralyzed patients. Disruption of existing hemostasis by retching or struggling with intubation can be controlled by external pressure.

Technique of Operation

The anterior neck, anterior chest and shoulders, and one lower extremity (to allow for harvesting of a saphenous vein if necessary) are prepared and draped. The most commonly utilized incision is an oblique one along the anterior border of the sternocleidomastoid muscle. This incision can be extended down into a median sternotomy. With wounds in the supraclavicular area of zone I, a supraclavicular incision may be more appropriate. With bilateral injuries a collar incision may be useful.

The tract of the missile is carefully followed and injuries to major structures are repaired.

Vascular Injuries

The primary controversy in treating vascular injuries in any of the zones of the neck is what to do with patients with carotid artery injuries and severe preoperative neurologic deficits. It is concluded from available data that vascular reconstruction is advisable in patients with mild deficits and in those with recent severe deficits in which prograde flow is present preoperatively. In patients with hemiplegia or coma and no prograde flow, either ligation or reconstruction can be performed, with a dismal prognosis in either group.

The operative technique is to obtain proximal and distal control of the vessel before entering the hematoma, if this is possible. Shunts are rarely needed for repairs of the carotid arteries in the neck as long as the patient's blood pressure is maintained and operation is performed expeditiously.

Injuries of the internal jugular vein are repaired by lateral venorrhaphy, if possible; however, unilateral ligation is well tolerated.

The other major vascular injury to the neck from penetrating wounds is that to the vertebral arteries. One study has shown that three quarters of these patients have no clinical findings or arterial injury other than a penetrating wound or a stable hematoma. Because the frequency of untoward sequelae of vertebral injuries is unknown, the indications for operations in asymptomatic patients are not clear. Late complications of vertebral artery injuries such as pseudoaneurysms or vertebral-jugular fistulas can generally be treated by an interventional radiologist.

Other vascular injuries that are technically difficult to expose include those in the thoracic inlet. Specific vessels here include the innominate artery, the subclavian arteries, the proximal common carotid arteries, and adjacent veins. These patients will generally present with exsanguinating hemorrhage externally or into the pleura cavity, with a contained hematoma in the thoracic inlet that may be visible on a chest x-ray, or with a penetrating wound alone. Wounds of the common carotid artery can generally be exposed through the previously described oblique cervical incision on the appropriate side. With suspected or confirmed injury to the proximal subclavian arteries, a horizontal supraclavicular incision with subperiosteal resection of the median half of the clavicle adequately exposes the area. Extension to a median sternotomy is necessary to expose the innominate artery. Exposure of the proximal left common carotid artery also usually requires an extension to a median sternotomy. On occasion, the combination of a high anterolateral thoracotomy, upper median sternotomy, and supraclavicular incision on the same side may be necessary to expose injuries to the proximal left carotid artery, left subclavian artery, or left innominate vein. This so-called trapdoor incision actually does not fold back unless all the ribs involved in the flap are broken; however, it does open farther than the routine thoracotomy or supraclavicular incision and allows for better exposure of the named vessels. Vascular injuries in all these areas are preferably repaired by lateral arteriorrhaphy or resection with end-to-end anastomosis. When graft interposition is required, autogenous material is preferred.

Larynx and Trachea

Patients with injuries to these structures present with respiratory distress, hoarseness, hemoptysis, and subcutaneous emphysema. Whenever a patient presents with a laryngeal or tracheal injury, a tracheostomy may be necessary before transfer of the patient to the operating room. In more stable patients, laryngoscopy is preformed preoperatively if the patient is hoarse or if the wound is near the thyroid gland or larynx.

Tracheal wounds are usually obvious during operative exploration; but, if the injury cannot be identified, the endotracheal tube cuff should be deflated to increase intratracheal pressure and enhance the air leak. Clean lacerations of the trachea or larynx are generally closed using synthetic absorbable sutures. Tracheostomy is not often indicated when a moderate lateral repair is performed, but may be necessary when a large defect is present or when an end-to-end anastomosis has been required.

Pharynx and Esophagus

The clinical findings suggesting pharyngeal or esophageal injury are hematemesis, dysphagia, and subcutaneous emphysema. Confirmation of an esophageal perforation is usually made with routine x-rays, a barium swallow, or endoscopy.

Repair is usually accomplished with a two-layer closure. Drainage is generally performed in case a small leak occurs. When there is massive loss of esophageal tissue, it may be necessary to perform a cutaneous esophagostomy for feeding purposes and a cutaneous pharyngotomy for salivary drainage.

Nerve Injuries

Injuries to the brachial plexus, phrenic nerves, and the cranial nerves can occur with penetrating wounds to the neck. Whenever possible, severed or lacerated nerves are debrided and repaired primarily using interrupted fine silk sutures on the perineurium.

Salivary Glands

Debridement, hemostasis, and simple drainage provide effective treatment for most penetrating wounds of these structures. When the major duct of the parotid gland is injured, it may be repaired with fine silk over a ureteral catheter stent. Persistent salivary fistulas can occur postoperatively and may respond to irradiation in adults.

Miscellaneous Injuries

Injuries to the thyroid gland require only debridement of devitalized tissue, hemostasis, and adequate drainage. The thoracic duct is generally ligated if it is perforated. If leakage from this structure does occur postoperatively, incision and drainage with the application of a bulky pressure dressing for a few days will usually effect closure of the lymphatic fistulae.

ABDOMINAL TRAUMA

Blunt Trauma

Evaluation Patients with blunt abdominal trauma most commonly have injuries to the spleen, liver, kidneys, and bowel. As many of these patients have multiple injuries to the head and chest or are unconscious because of alcoholism, drug abuse, and shock, difficulties in diagnosis arise.

Clinical Manifestations Information about the patient and the accident scene can be obtained from the paramedics, witnesses, family, police, and patient. Factors such as rapid deceleration, impact forces, and seatbelt restraints make abdominal viscera prone to injury. Physical examination is misleading in approximately 30–40% of patients, and it should be remembered that extraabdominal injuries are present in

70% of those patients with abdominal trauma who were admitted alive.

Abdominal pain and tenderness, when present, are very reliable findings. Abdominal rigidity, involuntary guarding, and rebound tenderness are all very suggestive of intraperitoneal injury.

If the patient presents with signs of intraabdominal hemorrhage, resuscitation is performed as previously noted, starting with a crystalloid solution such as Ringer's lactate while blood typing and cross matching is being performed. Blood loss in the range of 30–40% of the blood volume must be present in order to produce sustained marked hypotension with a systolic blood pressure consistently below 60–70 mmHg.

Diagnostic Procedures Sudden acute blood loss may not be adequately reflected by early hemograms. Serum electrolytes are rarely abnormal after trauma, but the serum potassium level is extremely important to know if operation is contemplated. Abnormal amylase levels may be seen in patients with injuries to the duodenum, upper small bowel, and pancreas.

Routine x-rays such as an abdominal flat plate are usually not too helpful in patients with blunt abdominal trauma. An intravenous pyelogram is useful, however, in evaluation of the genitourinary system when hematuria suggests an injury.

Diagnostic peritoneal lavage, first described by H. D. Root et al. in 1965, has a 96–98% accuracy in evaluating patients with possible intraperitoneal injuries after blunt abdominal trauma. The technique is performed in patients with closed-head injuries, altered consciousness, spinal cord injuries, or equivocal abdominal findings. It is not recommended for patients with gunshot wounds to the lower chest or abdomen, stab wounds to the back, previous abdominal procedures, presence of dilated bowel, or late pregnancy. The open technique is the safest, but newer approaches such as use of the percutaneous Lazarus-Nelson catheter have been successful. A peritoneal tap that detects >10–20 mL blood is considered to be positive, and no peritoneal lavage is indicated. If no blood is aspirated, 1 L of either Ringer's lactate or normal saline is rapidly infused into the peritoneal cavity of adults. The patient is turned from side to side in order to further mix the blood and fluid; however, this step is not performed when pelvic or spinal fractures are present. The empty intravenous fluid bottle is then lowered and the fluid siphoned out of the peritoneal cavity. Quantitative analysis of the fluid with results >100,000 RBC/mm^3 or 500 WBC/

mm^3, or the detection of bile, bacteria, food fibers, or amylase is considered to be a positive study. It should be remembered that diaphragmatic injuries as well as those involving the duodenum, kidney, or major vessels in the retroperitoneum are frequently not detectable by diagnostic peritoneal lavage.

The other most helpful study in evaluating patients with blunt abdominal trauma is abdominal CT scanning. This technique is used only in stable patients and is most accurate when enhanced CT or CT performed after the ingestion of gastrointestinal dye and the injection of intravenous dye is performed. Numerous studies attest to the increasing accuracy of this technique in evaluating patients with injuries to solid organs after blunt abdominal trauma. Injuries to the retroperitoneal duodenum have also been diagnosed with reasonable accuracy. Injuries to the small bowel have been missed in many centers, and this is an area of continuing concern.

Arteriography is occasionally indicated after blunt abdominal trauma to assess potential injury to the renal artery or to diagnose localized arterial bleeding in a small subset of patients with severe pelvic fractures. If a specific bleeding point can be identified on a pelvic arteriogram, therapeutic embolization is indicated.

Penetrating Trauma

Stab Wounds Three methods of evaluation for patients with stab wounds of the abdomen have evolved in recent years. These include routine exploration of all patients, selective management based on evolving signs on a physical examination, or exploration following demonstration of probable injury to intraabdominal viscera or vascular structures on diagnostic peritoneal lavage.

Mandatory operation is recommended for patients with abdominal stab wounds and signs of peritonitis, unexplained shock, loss of bowel sounds, evisceration of omentum or a viscus, evidence of blood in the stomach, bladder, or rectum, or evidence of visceral injury such as a pneumoperitoneum or visceral displacement on an x-ray film. In the absence of any of these findings, some centers have chosen to use selective management in which a patient without obvious indication for surgery is observed for 24–48 h and reevaluated repeatedly. In Nance and Cohn's study, 4.8% of 210 patients initially observed subsequently required an operation when manifestations of visceral injury developed.

Another option is to first perform local wound exploration

in the emergency room to verify that the peritoneum has been penetrated in the asymptomatic patient. If the peritoneum has not been penetrated then the wound can be irrigated and either packed open or closed and the patient discharged immediately. In the patient with documented penetration of the peritoneum from an abdominal stab wound, diagnostic peritoneal lavage can be performed with an accuracy of approximately 94–95% in ruling out intraperitoneal injury.

In stab wounds below the nipples, the diaphragm and intraperitoneal structures are injured in approximately 15% of patients. It is also true that stab wounds of the flanks and back may involve intraperitoneal structures; however, many of these patients are asymptomatic, and repeated physical examinations coupled with blood counts have decreased the incidence of negative laparotomies from wounds in these locations.

Gunshot Wounds The incidence of visceral injury in patients with abdominal gunshot wounds is 95–98% as compared to 30–40% patients with abdominal stab wounds. Therefore, a missile wound with probable peritoneal traverse on physical examination or x-rays is treated with early operation. Many authors feel that any bullet passing in proximity to the peritoneal cavity also requires exploratory celiotomy, as the blast effect may injure intraabdominal organs. It should also be noted that gunshot wounds below the nipples and above the costal margins may involve the peritoneal cavity in approximately 45% of patients and, therefore, laparotomy is mandatory for wounds in such a location in many centers at the present time.

OPERATIVE APPROACH Patients with exsanguinating abdominal hemorrhage from either blunt or penetrating trauma are occasionally resuscitated with left anterolateral thoracotomy and clamping of the descending thoracic aorta in the emergency room. This maneuver may be lifesaving in less than 5% of patients with abdominal trauma, but should be used judiciously because it requires opening another major body cavity, increases afterload on the heart, may affect spinal cord blood flow, and is certainly ineffective in controlling major venous bleeding. Immediate transfer to the operating room is indicated in all these patients. A midline abdominal incision is used in all patients who undergo celiotomy after abdominal trauma. It gives access to all parts of the abdomen and may be readily extended into either side of the thorax or continued superiorly as a median sternotomy. It also may be rapidly closed, which is of great importance in decreasing the anesthesia and operative time in severely injured patients.

Stomach

Penetrating injuries to the stomach occur frequently, while blunt rupture is rare except immediately after the patient has finished a meal.

Diagnosis   The diagnosis of gastric injury is generally made by observing the course of a penetrating wound or by seeing bloody returns in the nasogastric tube. In the operating room most gastric perforations from blunt trauma are large and associated with excessive contamination of the upper abdomen. Hematomas along the greater or lesser curvature of the stomach should be opened in any patient with a penetrating wound because they may cover an occult perforation.

Treatment   Gastric wounds are repaired by placing a continuous locked absorbable suture through all layers of the gastric wall because of the extensive blood supply. An outer inverting row of interrupted nonabsorbable mattress sutures is then placed. Copious irrigation of food particles out of the peritoneal cavity is mandatory to decrease the incidence of postoperative intraabdominal abscesses.

After operation, nasogastric tube suction should be maintained for several days until the danger of postoperative gastric dilatation decreases.

Major complications after repair of gastric injuries include hemorrhage, leakage, or the development of intraabdominal abscesses.

Duodenum

Blunt rupture has been missed on many occasions in the past and will lead to a mortality rate of 40% in patients who are not operated on within the first 24 h of injury. It is difficult to diagnose because the injury is frequently retroperitoneal, and duodenal fluid may cause minimal irritation. Such an injury should be suspected in any patient who receives a direct blow such as from a steering wheel to the upper abdomen or lower chest.

Diagnosis   Plain x-rays of the abdomen may show air along the right kidney or along the right psoas muscle margin. If air is not present in the retroperitoneum but there is still suspicion that a rupture exists, it may be helpful to inject air into the nasogastric tube to produce or enlarge an air collection to make it more detectable. The next step would be to give the patient a water-soluble radiopaque contrast medium to see if extravasation can be demonstrated. In recent years enhanced CT has been useful in making a diagnosis of a ruptured retroperitoneal duodenum.

In patients with either blunt or penetrating trauma, perforations or rupture of the duodenum have been missed because of inadequate exposure or lack of persistence on the part of the surgeon. In any patient with a retroperitoneal hematoma near the duodenum or one in whom there is crepitation or bile-stained fluid along the lateral margins of the duodenum, the entire retroperitoneal duodenum should be exposed by performing a Kocher maneuver. The third and fourth portions of the duodenum are visualized by mobilizing the cecum, right colon, hepatic flexure of the colon, and the mesenteries of these organs up to and including the ligament of Treitz. When a patient is suspected of having a missed injury of the duodenum, reexploration will usually reveal elevation of the posterior peritoneum with glassy-appearing edema, fat necrosis over the ascending and transverse colon, and a retroperitoneal phlegmon.

Treatment   A simple perforation of the duodenum is closed with a continuous locking 3-0 absorbable suture through all layers of the wall, followed by an outer layer of nonabsorbable interrupted mattress sutures in the seromuscular layer. When more extensive duodenal perforations or ruptures are present, options for management include an anastomosis of the open end or side of a defunctionalized Roux en Y jejunal loop over the duodenal defect, complete division of the duodenum and an end-to-end anastomosis, or division of the duodenum, closure of both ends, and a gastroenterostomy. On rare occasions even a pancreaticoduodenectomy may be necessary to manage extensive devitalizing trauma to the duodenum and periampullary regions.

Tenuous closures of the duodenum, very severe injuries of the duodenum, or combined pancreaticoduodenal injuries may be repaired with adjuncts such as the Berne duodenal "diverticulization" procedure. In this operation, the gastric antrum is removed, the duodenal stump is closed, and a vagotomy and a gastrojejunostomy are performed. A tube duodenostomy is added to reduce the possibility of disruption of the duodenal suture line. Extensive drainage of the pancreatic duodenal injury is performed as well. The biliary tract is drained by inserting a T tube into the common duct or by performing a tube cholecystostomy. Alternative methods for diversion of gastric contents away from the severely injured duodenum include pyloric exclusion with gastrojejunostomy and triple-tube decompression as described by Stone and Fabian. In the former procedure, a distal gastrotomy is made on the greater curvature of the antrum. The pylorus is then closed with a polypropylene suture, and an antecolic gastrojejunostomy is performed. The pyloric exclusion will usually stay closed for approximately 3 weeks and should lower the fistula rate when severe duodenal or combined pancreaticoduodenal injuries are present. Stone's approach includes the insertion of a gastrostomy tube and twin jejunostomy tubes, one passing retrograde into the duodenum, and one passing antegrade into the jejunum for feeding. Stone and Fabian report a series of 321 patients with duodenal wounds and the most recent 237 were all managed with the triple-tube approach. Only one duodenal fistula (0.5%) occurred in 210 surviving patients.

In the opinion of most surgeons, drainage of some type is usually used near a closure of a large duodenal defect.

Postoperative Care   Nasogastric tube decompression is routinely used after the repair of duodenal injuries. If a fistula forms, a sump drain should be inserted into the drain tract for continuous active suction of the fistulous tract. Also, central intravenous hyperalimentation should be added. A reasonable trial of conservative treatment should last several weeks before operative closure of the fistula is considered. If this is necessary, the fistula is exposed at its origin from the duodenum and a Roux en Y defunctionalized limb of proximal jejunum is brought up to the fistula and anastomosed to it.

INTRAMURAL HEMATOMA OF THE DUODENUM   Blunt upper abdominal trauma may rupture blood vessels in the submucosal layer of the duodenal wall, leading to a sausage-shaped mass and either partial or complete duodenal obstruction. Plain films of the abdomen may show an ill-defined right upper quadrant mass and obliteration of the right psoas shadow. Felson and Levin have shown that an upper gastrointestinal tract series is generally diagnostic, showing dilation of the duodenal lumen with the appearance of a "coiled spring" in the second and third portions of the duodenum due to the crowding of the valvulae conniventes by the hematoma.

It has become increasingly evident that when there is no indication of perforation of the duodenum, most patients with an intramural hematoma can be treated conservatively with nasogastric suction and intravenous hyperalimentation for a period of several weeks, after which the duodenal hematoma usually resolves.

Small Bowel

Eighty percent of bowel injuries occur between the duodenojejunal junction and the terminal ileum, with approximately

10% each in the duodenum and the large intestine. With blunt trauma, the small bowel can be crushed between the veterbral column and steering wheel or ruptured by shearing and tearing forces applied to the abdomen. Penetrating injuries, particularly from knives and low-velocity missiles, will usually cause perforations in adjacent segments.

Treatment Single small perforations of the small bowel may be closed safely with a single layer of interrupted nonabsorbable mattress sutures that include and invert the seromuscular and submucosal coats of the bowel. Two small perforations that are very close together may often be repaired by converting the wounds into one and closing the resulting defect as a single linear wound. Long linear lacerations of the small bowel lumen also should be closed with a single row of nonabsorbable sutures after ligating any persistent bleeders with nonabsorbable sutures. Such longitudinal lacerations should preferably be closed in a transverse direction. When extensive blast injuries or contusions are present, the damaged segment of the small bowel should be resected. This is also true if there are multiple wounds in a short segment of bowel.

Colon

The mortality rate for wounds of the colon was 37% in World War II, but decreased to approximately 15% during the Korean war. The majority of military injuries of the colon have been exteriorized as colostomies; however, recent experience in civilian life with perforating wounds from knives and low-velocity missiles has challenged this traditional approach.

Etiology Blunt injuries of the colon are rare and many will be the result of instrumentation during the process of sigmoidoscopy, the administration of enemas, or sexual behavior. Inadvertent penetration of the colon or rectum may occur during difficult operations in the pelvis, as well as from external forms of violence such as guns and knives.

Diagnosis Rectal examination and sigmoidoscopy should occupy a prominent place in the examination of patients suspected of having a colorectal injury. Abdominal x-rays are taken to determine if there is a perforation with leakage of air into the free peritoneal cavity. Contrast studies of the colon should be employed rarely and cautiously in view of the high morbidity and mortality associated with leakage of barium and feces into the free peritoneal cavity.

Treatment Small wounds located on the antimesenteric border with minimal tissue destruction and minimal or no peritoneal soiling (including those of the left colon), and without associated injuries in other abdominal viscera, may often be adequately managed by primary two-layer closure. High-velocity missile wounds associated with shock, extensive fecal contamination, and significant associated injuries should rarely if ever be closed primarily. An alternative form of therapy when primary closure is desired, but the patient's condition makes observation of the repair mandatory, is exteriorization of the repair. This technique is useful primarily in wounds of the descending colon and sigmoid and has been used with much less frequency than in former years. In recent years, 75–90% of colon injuries have been repaired primarily. Only the most destructive wounds that are large and ragged in nature should be exteriorized as a colostomy. Whenever there is some question about the safety of primary closure of a colon repair, a proximal diverting loop colostomy can be performed.

Localized wounds of the right colon in which there is some concern about primary repair may often be managed by primary closure with the adjunct of appendicostomy. In this technique primary repair of the cecum and an appendectomy is followed by the insertion of a decompression tube through the stump site of the appendix.

Extraperitoneal perforations of the rectum are best treated by the creation of a double-barrel proximal colostomy and presacral drainage posterior to the rectum. Even in those instances where the rectal wound has been closed and diverting colostomy has been performed, presacral drainage is necessary. Serious perineal injuries are treated in a similar manner, as sepsis can be avoided by early fecal diversion. Early closure of the colostomy is indicated in patients who have completely recovered and have no distal colon injury.

Liver

About 80% of liver injuries occur as a result of penetrating trauma, while only 15–20% occur from blunt trauma. In recent years the overall mortality rate of patients with hepatic trauma has been about 10–15%. Much of this depends on the etiology of the hepatic wound, as stab wounds have mortality of only 1% while major hepatic injuries requiring resection may have a mortality of 45–50%.

Treatment The Pringle maneuver and compression is applied in patients with major hepatic injuries. There is general agreement that in the normothermic liver, blood flow to the liver can be completely occluded with safety for periods in excess of 15 min and probably longer without causing any hepatocellular damage.

Drainage Alone Drainage with a closed suction drain is employed in patients in whom hepatic hemorrhage has spontaneously ceased by the time the abdomen is opened. With more extensive hepatic wounds, several Penrose drains in addition to closed suction drains are used. The Penrose drains may be inserted after the lateral ½ or ⅔ of the right 12th rib is removed to allow for dependent drainage. The Penrose drains are left in place for 5–10 days, thereafter being slowly removed over a 3-day period.

Suture, Hemostatic Techniques, and Drainage Wounds involving the outer 2–3 cm of the parenchyma may be sutured shut using interrupted sutures of 2-0 or 0 chromic on a blunt 2-in. "liver needle." These sutures are placed 2 cm back from the edges of the wound margin. If the sutures tear through as they are tied, a bolster of vascularized omentum is preferable. With more superficial wounds, microcrystalline collagen powder or Avitene may be used in selected patients.

The use of liver sutures to obtain hemostasis in both the entrance and exit sites of long gunshot tracts in the liver is controversial. Placement of the liver sutures at both ends of the tracts stops bleeding arising from the subcapsular area, which is the usual source. In several studies, this maneuver has been effective in controlling hemorrhage from the tract. If blood continues to ooze between the liver sutures or if there is an increase in the size of the liver within 10 min after placement of the sutures, the tract will have to be directly opened.

Extrahepatic artery ligation is used when a Pringle maneuver controls intrahepatic hemorrhage, but a direct search of a liver laceration discloses no discrete arterial bleeder.

Large lacerations in the liver in which selective ligation has controlled hemorrhage are best filled with a piece of vascularized omentum as an autogenous pack.

Resection Resectional debridement is used for ragged liver injuries caused by shotgun wounds, rifle wounds, or severe blunt trauma. The margins of resectional debridement should be 2–3 cm beyond the point of injury, and bleeding during debridement is controlled by digital parenchymal compression and/or temporary occlusion with a Pringle maneuver. Small oozing at the completion of the resectional debridement can be controlled by the insertion of a viable pack of omentum into the crack of the liver.

Anatomic hepatic lobectomy to control bleeding is reserved for patients in whom hepatic suturing is unsuccessful, resectional debridement or hepatotomy with intraparenchymal hemostasis is precluded by the anatomic location of the injury, or if occlusion of the hepatic artery fails to control hemorrhage. If more extensive exposure is necessary to complete a hepatic resection, a median sternotomy is performed rather than a right thoracoabdominal incision. If compression will control bleeding from the injured parenchyma, then preliminary hilar dissection of the ipsilateral hepatic artery, portal vein, and bile duct is performed. These structures are suture ligated and divided and the resection performed using the finger fracture technique through the liver substance. As the middle hepatic vein demarcates the right from the left lobe of the liver, the line of resection should keep to the right or left of this vein depending upon whether a right or left lobectomy is being performed. The Lin hepatic compression clamp may be useful in performing resections. A T tube is not indicated after injury to the liver.

When a patient has hemorrhage from the retrohepatic vena cava or posterior hepatic veins, one of several vascular isolation techniques should be considered. The first of these employs occlusive vascular clamps across the aorta just below the diaphragm, on the porta hepatis, and across the inferior vena cava above and below the liver. An alternative technique is the insertion of a #9 endotracheal tube or #36 chest tube through the right atrial appendage of the heart down into the infrarenal inferior vena cava in combination with a Pringle maneuver. With inflation of the balloon of the endotracheal tube or the tightening of a Rumel tourniquet around the suprarenal vena cava in the abdomen, as well as tightening of the Rumel tourniquet around the inferior vena cava next to the heart, blood flow from the lower half of the body will be diverted through the shunt rather than through the retrohepatic vena cava. Walt found a survival rate of 20% in reviewing 60 patients from several institutions in whom the shunt was used. It was felt that most of these patients would not have survived without the shunt. Another method of controlling hemorrhage from the retrohepatic vena cava or major hepatic veins has been to insert a Foley catheter into the exposed laceration.

Under rare circumstances it may be worthwhile to compress the injured lobe of the patient who has a coagulopathy. Dry laparotomy pads are generally used and are best placed over a steridrape so as to prevent the packs from adhering to any raw hepatic surface. The packs are generally removed 1–2 days after the original operation when the patient's condition is stable. The "second-look" operation is valuable, since it permits further debridement of nonviable tissue, irrigation of the perihepatic spaces, and insertion of clean perihepatic drains.

SUBCAPSULAR HEMATOMA A subcapsular hematoma may resolve spontaneously, expand and burst with delayed intraperitoneal bleeding, cause a hepatic abscess, or decompress into the biliary tree and cause hematobilia. The present recommendation is to watch these hematomas in stable patients who have a contained hematoma on a CT scan. Very large palpable hematomas generally do poorly, and operation may be preferable in this subgroup of patients. If continued intrahepatic hemorrhage is suspected, hepatic arteriography with selective embolization of a bleeding site in the injured lobe may be worthwhile.

HEMATOBILIA This rare problem is characterized by a triad including upper or lower gastrointestinal hemorrhage, obstructive jaundice, and colicky abdominal pain. While ligation of the extrahepatic arteries was performed in the past to control this postoperative problem, selective embolization of the offending artery is now the preferred technique.

Complications Major nonfatal complications occur in approximately 20% of patients with hepatic injuries. These range from pulmonary problems in the chest to intraabdominal perihepatic abscesses with an incidence of 4.5–20%. Patients with major lobar resections may be expected to have some postoperative bilirubin elevation which should resolve over a 3-week period.

Gallbladder

Penetrating or avulsion injuries of the gallbladder are best managed by cholecystectomy; however, when the patient is unstable a tube cholecystostomy can be performed. In the postoperative period a cholangiogram is performed through the cholecystostomy tube. If this shows that the gallbladder and biliary ducts are normal, the cholecystostomy tube is removed.

Porta Hepatis

When the hepatic artery and portal vein are involved with a penetrating injury to the porta hepatis, the mortality rate is quite high because of massive hemorrhage. If the patient has survived to be surgically explored, no active bleeding from the subhepatic region may be noted initially. With further dissection, clots that may have formed and tamponaded major bleeding sites may be dislodged from the portal vein, hepatic artery, or their branches. At this point a Pringle maneuver should be applied proximally as well as another vascular clamp placed on the hepatoduodenal ligament as near the liver as possible. Vascular structures in the porta hepatis are generally repaired with 5-0 permanent suture after dissection of the area of injury. With injuries to the extrahepatic biliary ducts, incomplete disruptions can be managed with a primary repair with or without T-tube stenting. Complete transections usually lead to devascularization of some tissue, and a primary end-to-end anastomosis can be performed only with excessive tension. Therefore, a Roux en Y choledochojejunostomy or end-to-side choledochoduodenostomy is preferred.

With blunt injuries to the biliary tree, diagnosis may be delayed if biliary leakage is minimal. Eventually, the onset of ascites, jaundice, and inanition will alert the physician to the missed diagnosis. Complete transection of the extrahepatic biliary duct from blunt trauma is preferably treated with a Roux en Y choledochojejunostomy. Choledochoduodenostomy is also an alternative, but leakage from this repair will result in a lateral duodenal fistula.

Portal Vein

Approximately 90% of portal vein injuries occur because of penetrating trauma, and most are associated with other visceral and vascular injuries such as to the inferior vena cava, liver, pancreas, and stomach.

Once proximal and distal vascular control have been obtained, the preferred repair of a penetrating wound to the portal vein is a lateral venorrhaphy with permanent suture. When more extensive injuries are present, the insertion of an autogenous vein graft to bridge the defect in the portal vein has been used with success, on occasion. If necessary, ligation can be performed; however, acute splanchnic hypervolemia will result in peripheral hypovolemia. These patients should receive tremendous amounts of blood and fluid in the postoperative period to maintain circulating volume.

Pancreas

Approximately 70% of pancreatic injuries are caused by penetrating trauma, while 30% result from blunt trauma.

Diagnosis As pancreatic injuries resulting from penetrating trauma are usually part of a multiple-injury complex, the diagnosis is made at surgery in these patients.

In patients with blunt trauma these injuries may be occult because of the lack of abdominal pain and the nonspecific nature of elevation of the serum amylase level. Even with a complete transection of the pancreas, only 65% of patients have elevated serum amylase levels. Routine abdominal x-rays may show obliteration of the psoas muscle margin or displacement of the stomach, but are rarely helpful. CT scanning has become much more helpful in recent years to make the diagnosis of these occult injuries. Another option is to perform an endoscopic retrograde cholangiopancreatogram when the diagnosis is suspected but no other x-ray findings are present.

Surgery Simple pancreatic contusions without capsular or ductal disruption and without persistent hemorrhage require no suturing or debridement. These injuries are drained with the sump drain placed directly at the site of the pancreatic contusion and brought out along a short direct tract at the tip of the 12th rib. As septic complications have occurred around open drain tracts in some patients, closed sump drainage is now preferred in some institutions.

When the pancreas is transected to the left of the mesenteric vessels, distal pancreatectomy with or without splenectomy is the preferred treatment. In resecting the distal pancreas the cut edge is beveled in a fish-mouth fashion. The transected duct of Wirsung in the remaining proximal gland is ligated with a transfixion suture of fine, monofilament nonabsorbable material such as Prolene. An alternative approach is to use the autostapler once the vessels have been ligated proximally. Approximately 25% of patients undergoing a distal pancreatectomy develop an intraabdominal abscess.

Should the transection of the pancreas be to the right of the mesenteric vessels, a Roux en Y anastomosis to the distal pancreas with oversewing of the end of the proximal segment may be used. This anastomosis is accomplished using permanent sutures placed approximately 1 cm apart in a single-layer fashion. The rationale for performing such an operation is that approximately half the patients who require 80% resection of the pancreas after trauma develop hyperglycemia and one half of that group require insulin.

Mild injuries to the pancreas and duodenum are treated in the appropriate fashion for each organ; however, proximal diversion techniques such as the Berne duodenal diverticulization or pyloric exclusion with gastrojejunostomy are frequently added.

Pancreaticoduodenectomy is rarely indicated except when the head of the pancreas is crushed or the entire duodenal segment is devascularized. Mortality is 25–30% in most series and is reserved for those patients with hemodynamic stability at the onset.

Complications   Pancreatic fistulas are the most common complication, and most close within 1 month. Intravenous hyperalimentation may be useful in such patients because it maintains excellent nutrition and nitrogen balance without stimulating the pancreas. A pancreatic pseudocyst is relatively rare if the pancreas has been explored and managed appropriately. Pancreatic fistulas may lead to the presence of abscesses in the lesser sac and subphrenic areas. Most patients who develop these have associated injuries to the gastrointestinal tract and the spleen.

Mortality   The mortality following stab wound to the pancreas is 5%, gunshot wounds 22%, and blunt trauma 19%.

Spleen

Diagnosis   Only about 30–40% of patients with splenic injury present with a systolic blood pressure below 100 mmHg. Physical signs that may be helpful include Kehr's sign, which occurs only when the patient is in a supine or head-down position. Also, many patients with splenic rupture have a leukocytosis of more than 15,000. In recent years computerized tomography has replaced radionuclide scanning in patients with possible occult lacerations of the spleen.

Delayed rupture of the spleen is now considered to be a relatively infrequent phenomenon but probably represents rupture of the splenic capsule from continued intrasplenic hemorrhage.

Management   Because of the significant rate of overwhelming postsplenectomy infections (OPSI) in children and a reasonably well-documented but much lower rate of the same problem in adults after splenectomy, both operative splenic repair and nonoperative therapy have become popular in both pediatric and adult centers in recent years. The major problem with nonoperative management in adults has been the data suggesting that as many as 30% of patients may have an injury in addition to the splenic injury. Another concern is that continued transfusion for the nonoperative patient may increase the risk of non-A, non-B hepatitis, which may be of greater danger to the patient than acquiring the relatively rare entity of OPSI later in life.

Should operative therapy be chosen, splenorrhaphy can be performed by the application of topical hemostatic agents, suture repair, or partial splenectomy for devascularizing injuries. Contraindications to splenic salvage procedures include patient instability, splenic avulsion or extensive fragmentation, extensive hilar vascular injury, or failure to attain splenic hemostasis.

Operative Technique Splenectomy is performed in the usual fashion after mobilization and hilar ligation of the splenic artery and vein. Controversy continues concerning the role of postoperative drainage after splenectomy. If such drains are to be placed, it is best to remove them as early as possible.

After splenectomy in children, most authors advocate prophylactic penicillin therapy until the child is 5 years of age, and some have recommended that protection be extended into the teenage years. Pneumococcal vaccination is recommended following splenectomy, also. This should protect against 80–85% of the pneumococcal strains leading to sepsis. The mortality after splenectomy primarily depends on the presence of associated injuries, mechanism of injury, age of the patient, and presence of shock at admission, and averages approximately 10%.

Retroperitoneal Hematoma

Diagnosis Abdominal pain occurs in approximately 60% of patients and back pain in about 25%. Occasionally a tender mass is palpable, as well as dullness to percussion over the flanks. The Grey-Turner's sign may be noted in the flanks and back after several hours but is not a helpful clue to early diagnosis. The presence of a pelvic fracture on an x-ray is highly suggestive of the presence of a retroperitoneal hematoma. Another helpful x-ray finding is obliteration of the psoas shadow.

Treatment The retroperitoneum has been divided into three areas in an attempt to clarify the various problems encountered. Area I is the upper central area and is best opened in patients with either blunt or penetrating injuries. Area II consists of the right and left flanks. It is opened only in patients with penetrating wounds, but is not opened in patients with blunt trauma when preoperative x-ray evaluation shows no major injury to the kidney. If Gerota's fascia is to be opened, midline control of the renal artery and vein is obtained. Area III consists of the pelvis, and this hematoma is not opened unless there is strong suspicion of injury to a major named vessel that can be reached by the surgeon.

With major pelvic hematomas not amenable to the usual selective surgical techniques, insertion of large pelvic packs or postoperative selective arteriography with embolization may be necessary for vascular control.

Inferior Vena Cava

The infrarenal inferior vena cava is the most susceptible and most often injured portion of the inferior vena cava. Most injuries are secondary to penetrating wounds.

Diagnosis Penetrating wounds involving the inferior vena cava usually involve other retroperitoneal vascular structures or intraabdominal viscera; hence, there is little question that operation is indicated.

Treatment Patients actively bleeding at the time of operation have a mortality of approximately 80%, while those who are tamponaded have a mortality of only 15–20%. Exposure of the inferior vena cava is obtained by reflecting the right colon, duodenum, and head of the pancreas medially. When standard techniques of vascular control do not work, the insertion of a balloon catheter or grabbing the edges of the laceration with Allis clamps may be helpful. When there are multiple caval wounds requiring complicated repairs or if the patient is profoundly hypotensive, infrarenal ligation can be performed. Ligation above the renal veins, however, should not be performed. Wounds to the inferior vena cava behind the liver are best approached using one of the transatrial vascular shunts previously described for hepatic injuries.

Complications and Mortality On occasions, iliofemoral venous thrombosis has occurred after repair. The mortality in patients with isolateral injuries to the inferior vena cava was 11% in one series, but 67% of the patients with more than one major vessel injury died.

Female Reproductive Organs

Most injuries to the uterus result from penetrating wounds, and no cases of blunt rupture of an unenlarged uterus from blunt trauma have ever been recorded. Rupture of the pregnant uterus due to blunt trauma is rare, but has occurred. It should be noted that the most common cause of fetal death in an automobile accident is maternal death. Therefore, early diagnosis and therapy of the uterine rupture in the mother is imperative for fetal survival.

Treatment Most patients present with abrupt massive intraperitoneal hemorrhage, and urgent celiotomy is necessary for control. Wounds of the uterus and adnexa are repaired by figure-of-eight chromic catgut sutures without drainage in most instances. If hysterectomy is necessary, it is best to leave the vaginal cuff partially open because of the likelihood of abscess formation. On rare occasions it may be necessary to perform bilateral-in-continuity ligation of the hypogastric arteries when there is massive, uncontrollable hemorrhage from the female pelvic organs.

It is of interest that approximately 80% of patients with uterine injuries during pregnancy can deliver per vagina subsequently without problem.

Abdominal Wall

A rectus abdominis hematoma is below the umbilicus in over 80% of cases. To distinguish this mass from intraperitoneal masses, patients should be requested to raise their heads against resistance; the mass should disappear if it is intraperitoneal and remain the same if it is in the abdominal wall.

7 BURNS

SCOPE OF THE PROBLEM IN THE U.S.

1. More than 2 million persons burned annually and 100,000 hospitalized
2. Second only to motor vehicle accidents as cause of accidental death, affecting particularly children, young adults
3. Hospital and medical costs now greater than $1,000,000,000/ year.

ETIOLOGY

1. Depth of injury dependent on intensity and duration of heat application, conductivity of tissue
2. Temperature below 45°C rarely produces significant cellular injury; increasingly severe cellular injury occurs between 45°C and 50°C; denaturation of protein and tissue destruction occurs above 50°C
3. Burns in young children common, many secondary to child neglect or child abuse
4. 60,000 injuries and 3000 deaths per year in the U.S. from chemical injury
5. Electrical injuries produce 1500 deaths per year in the U.S.; cutaneous injury usually restricted to entrance-exit sites; nerve, blood, muscle conduct current well, sustain maximum damage; secondary myoglobinuria indicates degree of muscle damage

IMMEDIATE THERAPY

1. *Maintenance of airway and ventilation*
   a. Adequate ventilation the first priority
   b. Thermal injury confined to upper airway with soft tissue edema of pharynx in first 48 h
   c. Smoke inhalation occurs with indoor fire, produces chemical pneumonitis, diminished oxygen exchange, occasionally CO_2 retention
2. *Intravenous fluid resuscitation*
   a. Massive shift of fluid, electrolytes from intravascular and extravascular space into cells during first 24 h

    b. Fluid requirements determined by area, depth of burn

    c. Fluid requirements by Parkland formula:
4 ml/kg body weight/percent burn in first 24 h, given ½ in first 8 h, ½ in second 16 h

    d. Monitor initial fluid replacement by inserting Foley catheter and maintaining urinary output between 30–70 mL/h, increasing or decreasing rate of fluid administration accordingly

    e. When diuresis begins in 24–72 h, switch to glucose in water to maintain serum sodium at 140 meq/L and add a colloid such as albumin

    f. During diuresis maintain urinary output between 30–100 mL/h

    g. Central venous catheter or Swan-Ganz catheter not routine; indicated in occasional patient, especially elderly individual with poor cardiac reserve; if necessary catheter can be inserted through burned tissue

3. *Pain control*

    a. Full-thickness burns destroy nerve endings, are not painful

    b. Partial thickness burns painful, require small doses of a narcotic such as morphine intravenously during initial management

4. *Antibiotics*

    a. Deeper burns relatively avascular, have early growth of gram-positive organisms, later colonization with gram-negative organisms

    b. Prophylactic antibiotic therapy not indicated, will not prevent bacterial growth in wound

    c. Parenteral antibiotics do not penetrate burn eschar well, are used for control of systemic sepsis

    d. Topical antibiotics used to control growth of organisms in burn wound

5. *Tetanus*

    a. Burn wound provides excellent culture medium for anaerobic organisms; appropriate tetanus protection required

6. *Escharotomy*

    a. Deep burn wound denaturizes protein, produces tourniquet effect; recognized by slow capillary refill, neurologic deficits, diminished flow rates by ultrasonic Doppler

    b. Tourniquet effect treated by escharotomy through full length and depth of burn; can be done without anesthesia and with minimal blood loss

    c. Fasciotomy rarely indicated even with severe thermal injury, may be required with electrical injury

7. *Gastric decompression*

a. Large area burn regularly complicated by paralytic ileus
b. Early nasogastric decompression prevents later problems
c. Gastric pH monitored from nasogastric drainage; acidity neutralized with instillation of antacids through nasogastric tube
d. H_2 blockers indicated only if antacid instillation does not prevent gastric erosion and hemorrhage

8. *Appropriate transfer*
   a. Certain patients require transfer to burn treatment facility for optimal care:
      if burn greater than 20% of body surface area
      if full-thickness burn greater than 10% of body surface area
      if age of patient below 5 or greater than 60
      if severe inhalation injury present
      if severe electrical injury present
      if significant preexisting illness present
   b. Transfer in first 48 h after controlling airway, initiating intravenous fluid replacement, inserting Foley catheter and nasogastric tube, performing any necessary escharotomies

THERAPY OF BURN WOUND

1. Remove only loose eschar initially
2. Burns usually covered with sterile dressings, but dressing care not essential; exposure of wounds with patient lying on clean sheet appropriate for any area and preferred treatment for facial and perineal burns
3. If patient is stable, it is appropriate to perform early (within 72 h) tangential excision of full-thickness and deep partial-thickness burns down to viable bleeding tissue with immediate skin grafting
   a. This procedure requires clean wound (less than 10^4 organisms per gram of tissue), major blood replacement, prolonged anesthesia, experienced physician and nursing care; should be done in burn treatment center experienced with technique
4. Topical chemotherapy used to control gram-negative burn wound colonization: mafenide acetate, silver sulfadiazine, povidone-iodine among appropriate agents, but mafenide acetate produces local pain and carbonic anhydrase inhibition, silver sulfadiazine produces skin rash, povidone-iodine produces eschar desiccation

5. Growth of bacteria in wounds best monitored by periodic quantitative burn wound culture
6. Skin grafts should be isografts when unburned skin areas available; cadaver allografts or pigskin xenografts may be used as dressings or as temporary grafts until isograft donor sites available
7. With limited skin areas available for donor sites grafts should be meshed to permit spreading over a wider area, better contouring to grafted area
8. Various synthetic skins being used currently as dressings; a bilayer artificial skin being tested with the deeper layer being incorporated by body into neodermis, which will later accept skin isograft

GENERAL THERAPEUTIC CONSIDERATIONS

1. Major burns characterized by hypermetabolic response with resting metabolic rate approaching twice normal
2. Patient with major burn loses large amounts of water by evaporative loss, but energy requirements not decreased by reducing water loss, changing environmental temperature or humidity
3. Hypermetabolic state associated with increase in body temperature controlled by a change in hypothalamic temperature center
4. Total daily energy requirements in severely burned patient approximate 40 calories per percent burn plus 25 calories per kilogram body weight
5. Posttraumatic catabolism results in weight loss, poor wound healing, negative nitrogen balance
6. During first postburn month nitrogen intake in excess of 20 g/m² of body surface required; replacement of nitrogen and calories must be started early and pursued vigorously
7. In almost all patients calories and nitrogen can and should be supplied by enteral route, usually through enteral feeding tube

REHABILITATION

1. After recovery from major burn, patient frequently troubled by major scarring, especially facial scarring, by limitation of joint motion secondary to severe contractures, by major psychologic problems
2. Scar hypertrophy can be minimized by use of elastic

pressure garments during convalescence because pressure produces better alignment of dermal collagen
3. Contractures with loss of joint function common after severe burn, can be minimized by use of appropriate splints and early vigorous physical therapy
4. Psychologic problems with thermal injury may be prevented or controlled by appropriate psychiatric management

COMPLICATIONS

1. *Smoke inhalation syndrome*
   a. May develop from exposure of lower respiratory tract to chemicals, especially aldehydes, after exposure to fire in closed space
   b. Symptoms frequently delayed 24 h or more
   c. Diagnosed by presence of carbonaceous sputum coughed up by patient or visualized during fiber-optic bronchoscopic examination
   d. Treated by humidified air and oxygen, repeated irrigation of tracheobronchial tree by fiber-optic endoscopy with intubation and mechanical ventilation as required
2. *Burn wound sepsis*
   a. Host resistance to infection markedly diminished; deep burns avascular; systemic antibiotics not effective in controlling bacterial growth in wound
   b. Multiplying bacteria may lead to septicemia, one of principal causes of death after thermal injury
   c. Topical antibiotics have reduced but not eliminated burn wound colonization
   d. Early excision of eschar decreases potential for burn wound sepsis; when this is not feasible, subeschar administration of appropriate antibiotics may be useful
3. *Distant septic complications*
   a. Bronchopneumonia, suppurative thrombophlebitis, suppurative chondritis among major complications
   b. Bronchopneumonia managed by usual respiratory support, systemic antibiotics
   c. Suppurative thrombophlebitis treated by excision of infected vein
   d. Because cartilage has poor blood supply, suppurative chondritis requires surgical excision of infected cartilage

4. *Gastrointestinal complications*
    a. Stress ulcer or hemorrhagic gastritis no longer common lethal complication after burn injury due to maintenance of neutral gastric pH, better nutritional support, control of systemic sepsis
    b. In rare instances with major bleeding important to prevent prolonged shock; early celiotomy with control of hemorrhage, vagotomy, and hemigastrectomy should be done despite high operative mortality

SPECIAL PROBLEMS

1. *Long bone fractures*
    a. In patients with burns and multiple injuries including long bone fractures, treat fractures by skeletal traction rather than casts over burn injuries
2. *Burn injury of joints*
    a. With open joint, necessary to remove cartilage and perform arthrodesis
3. *Facial burns*
    a. No dressings used except for burns of ears
    b. Eyelid burns require use of artificial tears, tarsorrhaphy to protect globe
    c. Facial scars after burns often difficult to improve, should be managed conservatively for a prolonged period; pressure mask may be useful

MORBIDITY AND MORTALITY

1. Improved through the years, but both morbidity and mortality remain significant
2. Infection remains the major problem, with over half of deaths due to septic complications
3. Presence of inhalation injury increases mortality significantly but usually leaves no permanent residual pulmonary problems in survivors
4. National Burn Information Exchange reports that LA_{50}, the area of injury associated with 50% mortality, varies with age:

0–4 years	67% total burn or 51% full-thickness burn
5–34 years	76% total burn or 53% full-thickness burn
35–49 years	67% total burn or 43% full-thickness burn
60–74 years	38% total burn or 25% full-thickness burn
over 74 years	22% total burn or 14% full-thickness burn

5. Multidisciplinary team management allows many patients with major burns to resume full, productive lives

8 WOUND HEALING AND WOUND CARE

Wound healing is the restoration of physical integrity of both external and internal structures by synthesis of scar tissue. The process of fibrous tissue synthesis, however, can be detrimental, even to the extent of destroying the organism that it sought to preserve. Examples of these potentially fatal processes are deformity of valve leaflets during healing of rheumatic fever valvulitis, development of posthepatic cirrhosis, and development of esophageal stenosis after swallowing a corrosive agent. Therefore, the understanding of principles of wound healing is important not only for care of injuries and postsurgical wounds, but also for primary treatment of many disease processes.

With the possible exception of the liver, regeneration in human beings is limited to simple tissues such as epithelial cells. The healing process in all other complex tissues such as skin, deep organs, and nervous system requires epithelialization and fibrous tissue synthesis. Epithelialization is the fundamental process that seals the wound, whereas fibrous tissue synthesis provides structural strength. When tissue is missing, an additional process called wound contraction moves tissue edges into closer approximation so that epithelialization and fibrous protein synthesis can accomplish their objectives. Therefore, the principles of wound management revolve around a detailed understanding of epithelialization, fibrous protein synthesis, and the biology of wound contraction. In addition, some knowledge of the milieu, or so-called ground substance, in which these events occur is important.

WOUND CONTRACTION

Wound contraction is a dynamic term applied to the centripetal movement of skin edges in the process of healing where loss of skin is permanent. This term should be distinguished from *wound contracture,* which is actually the end result of wound contraction.

The end results of wound contraction can be predicted by grasping the edges of an open wound and manually coapting them. If it is not physically possible to coapt edges of a wound by reasonable external force then natural processes also will not be effective. The effectiveness of wound contraction is related to the amount of skin available in a given area of the body for stretch. Wound contraction across margins of a joint will result in movement of the joint to an extreme position causing a "contracture."

A great deal of scientific investigation has gone into understanding wound contraction. The interruption of the integrity of the skin seems to be the initiating stimulus. Approximately 4 days elapse before movement of the wound edges is actually measurable. Although this time period is called the lag phase, a great deal of cellular work is ongoing. Contraction of a wound does not appear to stop immediately with closure. Some wounds that are coapted immediately still have some considerable contraction. Also, closure of wounds with a free skin graft or pedicle flap does not stop the contracting process. The ultimate configuration of the scar produced by a contracting wound is the result of variations in the rate of movement of different segments as well as the firmness of attachment of different areas of skin to moveable and immoveable structures. One practical example is the contraction and stenosis of an ileostomy. If the skin hole for the ileostomy is made as a perfect circle, wound contraction and subsequent stenosis will be minimal.

Wound contraction does not seem to be affected or related to the rate of collagen synthesis. Biochemical manipulation to suppress collagen synthesis or interfere with cross linking does not change the rate of wound contraction in experimental wounds. Contraction is suppressed, however, by poisons such as potassium cyanide that interfere with living cells. The area of living cells most critical to wound contraction forms a picture frame distribution around the margins of the wound. Excision of central tissue in the wound does not affect the rate of contraction.

Within the picture frame area the strategic location of highly specialized cells called myofibroblasts has been discovered. These cells have smooth muscle–like contracting powers that provide a great deal of the machinery for wound contraction. In addition, granulation tissue between two wound edges has been shown to have elastic properties that produce tension between the wound edges and assist in contraction.

The phenomenon of wound contraction is one of the most predictable and powerful of all biologic reactions and must be positively reckoned with in the management of wounds where tissue has been lost. The myofibroblasts involved in this process have been shown to contain contractile proteins such as actin and can be inhibited by colchicine and vinblastine, which interfere with microtubule formation. These agents have been tested clinically for their ability to control wound contraction in human beings.

EPITHELIALIZATION

Epithelialization is the regeneration of epidermis across an area of denuded skin. This is the first sign of wound repair and occurs long before any evidence of fibrous tissue synthesis. The first function of epithelialization is to provide a watertight seal of the wound. The layer of cells in the epidermis is essential for maintaining a watertight seal but provides very little structural strength. The surrounding fibrous protein framework is required to give strength to a scar. A wound that has healed only by epithelialization will stop ''weeping'' and be safe from bacterial invasion as long as the epithelial layer is intact, but the slightest trauma literally will wipe off what is hardly more than a gelatinous film. The second important reason to understand the process of epithelialization is that the potential for development of cancer in certain types of wound scars is related to the variations of cell division and cell movement that occur in this phase of wound healing. A histologic sample taken from a 5-day-old normal healing wound can be interpreted as a fibrosarcoma if none of the historical details is available. Healing is dependent on processes such as mitosis, pleomorphism, disorganization, and loss of polarity, all of which resemble the uncontrolled growth of a malignant neoplasm. The difference is, however, that some controlling influence brings order out of disorder in the healing wound. Neoplasms fail to evolve in order, and factors of control never appear.

Cell division and ameboid movement cease only when cells are surrounded by other cells of their own type. Collisions of dissimilar cells result in repulsion, whereas collisions of similar cells result in two cells sticking together. As increasing portions of the circumference of the cell membrane become satisfied by attaching to cells of similar lineage, the remaining unsatisfied sides become the exploring or searching surfaces. Failure to achieve complete surface contact with other cells results in a continued state of embryonic activity. These mechanisms are thought to be the stimulus for epithelial cells to overcome injury and develop embryonic kinetics following creation of a wound. The recognition of the similarity of these processes to malignant growth insinuates that any wound that is prevented from healing is potentially a malignant neoplasm. Radiation energy or specific chemicals applied to wounds have been associated with occurrence of squamous cell malignancy for these reasons. Also, a postphlebitic leg ulcer may become a chronic nonhealing ulcer that can develop cancer over a long period of time.

Theoretically, it should be possible for a wound of any size to be epithelialized. In clinical practice there is a limit to the size of the area that can become epithelialized naturally.

In incised and sutured wounds, epithelialization produces a watertight seal in 24 h even though there is a dip where the cells have migrated into the crevice. Epithelialization also occurs along the path of a suture to the extent that a completely epithelialized tract may be produced or a small cyst formed after sutures are removed. Epithelialization across the surface of a wound that has not been coapted involves similar movement of epithelial cells but over a much more hazardous terrain. The early escape of blood and serum in open wounds produces a scab. The regenerating epithelium moves beneath the scab, literally detaching it from the underlying surface as it seals the wound. The protective influence of a scab to prevent trauma, drying, or contact with caustic material is important for secondarily healing wounds. Successful epithelialization occurs only if the cumulative effect of physical manipulation, such as drying or bacteriocidal agents, does not exceed the finite capacity of available cells to divide, dedifferentiate, and move across the surface.

Some factors have been found to enhance cellular events that occur during wound healing. Epidermal growth factor is a polypeptide chain that has been extracted from a number of tissues. Local application of epidermal growth factor enhances accumulation of cells in experimental wounds. As yet, epidermal growth factor has not been shown to be of any clinical value in the treatment of wounds in human beings.

GROUND SUBSTANCE

The term ''ground substance'' usually refers to a continuous, nonfibrillar matrix including water and electrolytes through which metabolites diffuse between blood vessels and cells. Ground substance is the milieu in which the processes of wound healing occur. Various histochemical reactions have been identified, many of which include mucopolysaccharide. A great deal of attention has been focused on acid mucopolysaccharides and their function in wound healing. The nonsulfated mucopolysaccharides (hyaluronic acid and chondroitin) are the main component of the structuralist gel fraction of ground substance. The sulfated mucopolysaccharides (chondroitin sulfate, heparitin sulfate) are most closely associated with fibrillar elements of connective tissue. Mucopolysaccharides appear to have a role in polymerizing reactions that are important in organizing collagen fibrils.

Ground substance is most important in the phenomenon of healing because of its relation to collagen synthesis and remodeling. Chemical bonds that are important in the development of strength and orientation of collagen fibers are linked to presence of mucopolysaccharides in ground substance.

COLLAGEN

The essence of healing is fibrous protein synthesis. The principal fibrous protein in healing wounds is collagen. Collagen is an extracellular protein that is synthesized by a specialized fibroblast. Actually, the fibroblasts synthesize tropocollagen, a molecule approximately 15 Å in width and 2800 Å in length. Tropocollagen is soluble in salt solution.

Collagen molecules are expressed as different subtypes. Type I collagen is the most prevalent type in the mature vertebrate organism. Type II collagen is limited to cartilage and is found primarily in human articular and costal cartilages. Type III collagen is found in association with Type I collagen and is most prevalent in tissue undergoing remodeling or fetal organogenesis. Type III collagen also appears to be an important component of tissues with an unusual degree of elasticity such as the aorta, esophagus, and uterus.

The amino acids found only in collagen and used to identify it in analytical procedures are hydroxyproline and hydroxylysine. Multiplication of the amount of hydroxyproline in a tissue specimen by a factor of 7.8 determines the amount of collagen present. Collagen is unique in respect to its content of hydroxyproline. Hydroxylation of proline and lysine is important in transport of collagen molecules across cell membranes. Also, these specialized amino acids are involved in formation of various intra- and intermolecular cross links that give collagen molecules their characteristic rigidity.

A critical stage in construction of collagen is the hydroxylation of proline to produce hydroxyproline. Metabolic defects that hinder this metabolic step have been identified in collagen deficiency diseases such as scurvy. In ascorbic acid deficiency, an accumulation of proline-rich precursors and deficiency of hydroxyproline-containing polypeptides occurs.

Another enzymatic step important in normal assembly of collagen is catalyzed by procollagen peptidase. This enzyme removes the nonhelical terminal extensions from both ends of the collagen molecule. A type of Ehlers-Danlos syndrome has been found to be the result of persistent pro-α chains.

Intracellular cross links of various types are the backbone of strength in the collagen molecule. The most important cross links are covalent ester bonds. One example is oxidative deamination of lysine by lysyl oxidase. Other types of cross links, such as electrostatic interactions and Van der Waals, are also involved.

Collagen molecules lie next to each other in a staggered overlapping formation. This staggered arrangement yields a typical repeating axial of 640 Å. Collagen molecules assembled under normal physiologic conditions will have 640-Å repeating periods. On various laboratory preparations that alter the conditions of a ground substance or electrostatic charges, the characteristic 640-Å density can be changed.

Cross linking, among other factors, is a function of aging; the older a specimen of collagen becomes, the firmer and more numerous the cross links are. Maturation increases the number and strength of cross links. Alternatively, the age of collagen can be estimated by its solubility, a manifestation of cross linking. Variations in cross linking are partially responsible for the final appearance, texture, and elasticity of human scars.

The production of collagen fibers by specialized fibroblasts is just the beginning of strength accrual in the wound. The most important factor in gain of strength is the physical weave of the fibers after they are produced. The old concept of collagen as a static, adynamic substance is erroneous. Actually, collagen in wound scar is a relatively dynamic structure that is undergoing constant remodeling and replacement. After 42 days of wound healing there is no measurable increase in the amount of collagen, yet the scar continues to gain strength for at least 2 years. Turnover of collagen in a healing is extensive. Most newly synthesized collagen is replaced as the scar matures.

Lathyrism is a syndrome of altered collagen metabolism. The term is derived from a disease caused by excessive ingestion of certain peas in the genus *Lathyrus*. The active fraction that produces altered collagen metabolism is beta-aminopropionitrile. The primary effect of beta-aminopropionitrile is to block the formation of inter- and intramolecular cross links during all stages of collagen aggregation. As a result cross linking of collagen fibrils is very unstable and most of the collagen produced is soluble. Mature animals with this disease will develop hernias or die suddenly of dissecting aneurysms. Clinical implications of using this agent are exciting. Because some of the effects of fibrous tissue healing in specialized organs, such as liver or heart, can be more ruinous to health than the disease that preceded healing, the demonstration that some control over deep scar formation is possible is an exciting one. Penicillamine, another lathy-rogenic agent, as well as a copper chelator previously used to treat Wilson's disease, is being used to treat arthritis and undesirable scar tissue in human beings.

Remodeling of scar tissue necessarily requires the presence of an enzyme capable of digesting collagen, so-called colla-genase. Collagenase activity has been discovered in human tissues, particularly in epithelium-containing structures. The most uniformly positive tissue for collagenase activity is cutaneous scar. A high level of activity in scar can be found as long as 30 years after initial wounding. Retarded wound healing may be the result of excessive collagenolysis. Serum, cysteine, and progesterone have been shown to inhibit tissue collagenase acting at neutral pH. Progesterone in ophthalmic concentrations is the agent of choice in treating corneal injury, particularly alkali burns in which delay of tissue collagenase activity is the cause of rupture of the globe.

Scar tissue is a product of opposing forces of collagen synthesis and collagen destruction. The maximum amount of total collagen in a healing wound is found by the 42nd day. Human keloids probably represent an abnormality of the equilibrium between collagen synthesis, deposition, and degradation.

Further examples of collagenase activity are the classic descriptions of scurvy. These wounds did not just fail to heal; they actually disrupted months after they had healed perfectly. Synthesis of new collagen is blocked during as-corbic acid deficiency, while collagenolytic activity probably proceeded normally, a possible explanation for dehiscence of an old scar.

Collagen diseases represent abnormal amounts of collagen in abnormal places, but they are not specific diseases of the collagen molecule or fibril itself. The collagen in such diseases as rheumatic fever, dermatomyositis, and scleroderma is more accurately considered the scar from a primary wound or inflammatory process. On the other hand, destruction of collagen and diseases such as rheumatoid arthritis are par-tially the result of excessive tissue collagenase activity. Therefore, the concept of the collagen system as a dynamic, constantly remodeling one opens the door for investigation of a large number of diseases.

SEQUENCE OF EVENTS: SUMMARY

Sealing the wound, regaining tensile strength, and acquiring a scar that is functionally acceptable are the principal events of wound healing. Long-term processes such as remodeling of collagen are not the most immediate concerns of the physician and his or her patients. The basic process by which an incised and sutured wound properly heals is called "healing by primary intention." A wound in which tissue has been lost so that healing must occur by contraction and epithelialization is called "healing by secondary intention."

The chronologic processes of healing are more conveniently studied during secondary healing. The first event after full-thickness skin loss is that normal elasticity of the skin and external tension produced in some areas by muscle enlarge the defect. The skin defect, therefore, may have little relation to the size or shape of the fragment of tissue that was removed. Second, a clot will form quickly. The clot then contracts and dehydrates to form a scab. A scab serves a useful purpose in providing limited protection from external contamination, satisfactory maintenance of internal hemostasis, and a surface beneath which cell migration and movement of wound edges can occur. The cellular events that occur in this time period leading to cell migration are essentially those of controlled inflammation. This period is often called the "lag" phase, which gives an inaccurate connotation that there is nothing of importance happening.

How well a wound heals is related to the amount of inflammation present. Perfusion of capillaries, release of various amines, changes in capillary wall permeability, and accumulation of white blood cells and connective tissue cells are well-known changes in general inflammation that are also important in providing the best milieu for wound repair.

Approximately 12 h after injury has occurred, epithelial migration, the first clear-cut sign of rebuilding, occurs. Epithelialization is complete in a few hours in a primary wound; in a secondary healing wound migration of cells progresses more slowly, so that days or even weeks elapse before epithelialization is complete. Wound contraction begins 4 or 5 days later and generally assists epithelialization in coverage of the wound.

In the center of the wound after the scab or eschar has been removed and before epithelium has covered the surface a great amount of activity takes place. The surface becomes granular and bright red in color. This process is the formation of *granulation tissue* and is secondary to extravagant proliferation of richly perfused capillary loops. The loops of blood vessels impart a granular appearance to the surface. Granulation tissue is a good defense against invasion by surface contaminants. Surface infection can occur, however, changing the fiery red granular dots to a purple, soggy, gray-black cluster that impedes the possibility of epithelialization.

Collagen synthesis probably begins about the 3rd or 4th day after injury. Visible signs of collagen deposition do not occur until the 7th day. At that time, the young collagen fibrils resemble a gel in a laboratory beaker, with no purposeful orientation or polarity. As fibrogenesis proceeds, purposefully oriented fibers become thicker and a dense, compact scar results.

Contraction of the wound is a major influence; it exerts full potential before scar tissue synthesis is complete. Wounds surrounded by mobile and redundant skin have a very small central scar because of contraction.

Wounds closed primarily are held together by the effects of vascularization and epithelialization up until the 5th day. These effects are adequate to hold wound edges together if not under excessive tension. The wound rapidly increases in strength over the following 12 days secondary to collagen synthesis. Gains in tensile strength are small but detectable thereafter for almost 2 years. The strength of a scar never quite reaches that of unwounded skin despite continual remodeling.

WOUND CARE

The key to deciding when a wound should be closed is an understanding of the difference between contamination and infection. This requires the ability to recognize signs of inflammation. A contaminated wound can be converted to a clean wound with subsequent immediate closure. An infected wound cannot be surgically debrided and closed without high risk of failure.

The strength of the bacterial inoculum and the ability of a substrate to combat invasion are the principles for deciding when to close the wound. Quantitative measures of the number of bacteria in tissue samples have shown that concentrations greater than 10^5 organisms per gram of tissue are likely to cause abscess and wound breakdown following secondary closure.

Once the decision has been made to close a laceration, the surrounding skin should be prepared with a suitable antiseptic and local anesthetic injection. One guiding principle is never to put anything in a wound that could not be tolerated comfortably in the conjunctival sac. Caustic solutions that are capable of sterilizing the skin will also destroy delicate cells on the surface of the wound. Removal of surface contaminants in wounded tissue can be accomplished by a copious stream of saline to flush foreign bodies and undesirable organisms out of the wound cavity. Surgical excision of affected tissues is required when devitalized or contused tissue fragments are still attached to the wound.

Selection of proper suture materials correlates with the biology of the healing process. Absorbable sutures are used when infection is known to be present or when debridement has been difficult. Plain gut sutures are solubilized within 10 days. Gut sutures treated with chromium salts will remain intact for weeks.

Before suture is selected the questions should be asked: What is the suture required to do? How long does it need to work? Sutures in weak tissues such as fat, epithelium, liver, or kidney, are used to obliterate potential cavities and provide hemostasis, or as a fine-adjustment leveling device on delicate repairs of skin. Absorbable sutures are satisfactory for these functions. Conversely, fascial closure should be done with a permanent suture such as silk or some synthetic substance.

The width of a wound following closure of the subcutaneous tissue is a predictor of the width of the final cutaneous scar. One way to reduce widening of a scar after skin sutures are removed is to place permanent sutures in the fibrous protein layers of the skin to bring the edges together. This is accomplished by subcuticular or intradermal suture of silk or synthetic material. Although permanent subcuticular sutures will not completely eliminate secondary widening of a scar, such sutures will reduce the extent of transverse remodeling in many wounds.

Sutures should be removed when adequate tensile strength to hold the wound edges together has developed. The rate of healing is variable in different parts of the body and under different conditions in a single individual. The wound must be examined; sometimes one or two sutures must be removed to see if the skin edges are sufficiently adherent to permit removal of all sutures. Resorption of excess collagen, development of pliability, and the fading of undesirable color are called "maturation" of the scar. This occurs more rapidly in old people than in the young. Because of the continual maturation of scars it is seldom wise to attempt surgical improvement of the scar in less than 6 months; often natural improvement will continue for as long as 12 months. If scar tissue is elevated slightly above the level of surrounding skin, abrasion of that area with sandpaper or rotating brush will produce a smooth, denuded surface over which new epithelium will spread in a more even plane.

Protection of wounds from physical, chemical, or bacteriologic complications is the best aid a physician can get to accelerate normal healing. Topical vitamin A can correct the inhibition of epithelialization caused by steroid therapy. Vitamin A does not accelerate epithelialization, however, over normal expectation.

Choosing the proper dressing material involves a clear understanding of the objectives for dressings on open wounds. The first layer of dressing is usually made of fine-mesh gauze, so that granulation tissue will not penetrate the interstices and cause hemorrhage when the dressing is removed. Dry gauze is a perfectly satisfactory dressing for subsequent layers of most wound surfaces. Sponges and cotton are used to make the dressing conform to a desired shape and immobilize the wound in part.

Infected wounds have considerable drainage and therefore must be dressed often to provide suitable drainage and removal of infected tissue. Although it is common practice to use a wet dressing on infected wounds, there is no inherent advantage to such, and continuous moisture of wounds favors maceration of skin and subsequent growth of bacteria or fungi. The objective of wound dressings is to keep wound secretions from accumulating and retarding repair by enzyme activity. This can be accomplished by dry dressing, which will absorb secretions better.

SKIN GRAFTS

Skin grafts are classified as free grafts or pedicle grafts. Free grafts are completely separated from the donor site in one stage. They may be full thickness, in which the entire epidermis and dermis is transferred, or split thickness, which means that the entire epidermis and only a portion of the dermis are transferred. Successful "take" of a free graft refers to a pink appearance that occurs between the 3rd and 5th day after transfer. This signifies adequate vascular connections that develop between the recipient bed and the transplant.

Diffusion is not as important in the take of a skin graft as the mechanical barriers such as pus, blood, or fat, which prevent vascular connections from developing. Thicker grafts are more likely to fail, especially if mechanical factors interfere with the graft-wound interface. Therefore, thin skin grafts are used for recipient sites that are less than ideally prepared. Thicker grafts are reserved for surgically produced wounds under optimal conditions.

The dermis is the portion of skin that provides the qualities ʹuch as strength, flexibility, and appearance that are desirable. Therefore, the importance of these qualities determines the thickness of the skin graft or the amount of dermis which should be transferred. Following transfer of skin, epithelial cells migrate out of deep glands and hair follicles to reepithelialize the donor site and the recipient site.

Split-thickness skin grafts have a tendency to develop deep pigmentation after transfer. It is important to warn patients who have recently had split-thickness skin grafts placed on exposed areas of the body that protection from solar radiation is advisable for at least 6 months.

Skin grafts can also function as biological dressings. Xenografts of porcine skin, human allografts of split-thickness skin, and human amnion are all examples of biologic dressings that can prevent metabolic and infectious complications of large wounds. Porcine xenografts have the disadvantage of expense and biologic crossing of major histocompatibility loci. Human amnion obtained from the delivery room is a good alternative for biologic dressings.

A pedicle flap is a transfer of skin on a direct vascular connection. This connection may be in situ or supplied by direct vascular anastomosis. Thick pedicle flaps do not actually add more blood supply. The important vessels of a pedicle flap are in the subdermal plexus. Underlying fat does not add any appreciable blood supply.

Following transfer of a flap circulation must be observed carefully for the first 48 h, as signs of impending circulatory embarrassment occur before irreversible thrombosis and cell death. Failure of pedicle flaps is most often related to venous thrombosis rather than arterial insufficiency. Signs of impending venous thrombosis include development of a sharp line of color differentiation. Besides adequate venous drainage other factors that lead to complications are too much tension, poor dressing, hematoma, or infection.

Smoking has been shown to adversely affect circulation in pedicle flaps. Heparin and low-molecular-weight dextran have been beneficial in dangerously compromised circulation.

A myocutaneous pedicle flap involves transfer of intact muscle, subcutaneous tissue, and overlying skin as a single unit rotated on the relatively narrow vascular supply of the muscle. Examples are from the pectoralis major, latissimus dorsi, and gracilis muscles.

A free flap is a transfer of muscle, subcutaneous tissue, and skin to a distant site with microvascular suture of feeding blood vessels. These have been very successful in covering surface defects in the lower leg and foot.

A recent development that has reduced the need for distant pedicle flaps is local tissue expansion with an implanted inflatable device. Gradual stretching of the skin for 4–6 weeks can be accomplished with such a device so that local rotation flaps become possible in the areas where local skin is not sufficient to resurface the defect. The high cost of donor site mutilation, length of time required for transfer, and adynamic features make the pedicle flap second choice to a free graft if a free graft can be used.

9 ONCOLOGY

Oncology is the study of neoplastic diseases. Neoplasms are altered cell populations characterized by excessive proliferation of cells that are unresponsive to normal control mechanisms. Malignant neoplasms exhibit uncontrolled proliferation and impair the function of normal organs by local tissue invasion and are also characterized by metastatic spread to distant anatomic sites. In contrast, benign neoplasms do not invade locally or metastasize to other sites.

Neoplastic disease is the second most frequent cause of death in the United States. Approximately 3 out of every 10 persons living today has or will develop cancer. Forty percent of those who have cancer will survive for at least 5 years with some kind of treatment.

EPIDEMIOLOGY

Although there has been a decrease in mortality from certain neoplasms, the overall cancer death rate is continuing to show a slow, steady increase. Lung cancer represents the leading cause of cancer nationwide. The mortality rate from lung cancer has increased steadily and represents the most dramatic change for any cancer site.

Pancreatic cancer death rates have also steadily increased through the years. Other cancers, such as stomach and uterus, have had a striking reduction in mortality over the past three decades. Earlier detection and improved treatment are part of the explanation for this decline.

The most frequent sites of cancer in men are lung, colon and rectum, and prostate. In women, the most common cancer sites are lung, breast, and colon and rectum.

The incidence of various types of cancer does not necessarily correlate with the death rates of the same neoplasms. Five-year survival rates are best in patients with cancer of the skin, cervix, uterus, and bladder. Conversely, the lowest survival occurs in patients with pancreatic cancer. Overall, the leading cause of cancer death is lung cancer.

Females tend to have a greater number of 5-year survivals with cancer for a given site than males. The reasons for this observation are unknown.

ETIOLOGY

Chemical carcinogens were one of the first mechanisms discovered for the etiology of cancer. In 1775 Percival Pott, an English surgeon, described cancer of the scrotum frequently occurring in chimney sweeps. Subsequent studies through the years have demonstrated that hydrocarbons isolated from coal tar are carcinogenic agents. Now, a variety of chemical agents have been found that are capable of inducing neoplasms in experimental animals and in human beings. These chemicals are called *carcinogens*.

Aromatic amines are known to cause tumors of the urinary tract. Benzene has been associated with acute leukemia. Coal tar, pitch, creosote, and anthracene have been associated with cancer of the skin, larynx, and bronchus. Mesotheliomas occur very frequently in miners and shipworkers exposed to asbestos.

Some carcinogens are physical rather than chemical in nature. The primary physical carcinogen is ionizing radiation. Radium dial painters, who commonly licked brushes containing radioactive material, have developed bone cancers. Cancer of the thyroid is frequently associated with neck irradiation in early childhood. Also, survivors of atomic bomb detonations have shown an increased incidence of leukemia.

Ultraviolet light is another example of a physical carcinogen. Farmers and sailors have an increased incidence of skin cancer from excessive exposure to sunlight, as do fair-skinned people living in tropical regions.

Another example of a physical carcinogen is mechanical irritation. Chronic irritation is associated with the development of cancer as exemplified with malignant degeneration in old burn scars, called a Marjolin's ulcer.

Viruses that have become increasingly implicated as primary etiologic agents of cancer—particularly hepatocellular carcinoma, adult T-cell leukemia, Burkitt's lymphoma, and cervical cancer—have all been linked with a number of viruses occurring in human beings. Investigation of these tumor viruses has led to the discovery of oncogenes that have been found to induce cell transformation.

Hereditary factors are of major importance in the etiology of cancer. The patterns of colon cancer in family members with familial polyposis, as well as familial patterns associated with breast cancer, have contributed evidence to the importance of genetic factors. Certain families seem to have an increased incidence of neoplastic diseases. For example, a dominant inheritance for such diseases as retinoblastoma, lipomatosis, and colonic polyposis has been described.

Geographic factors are also influential in the development of cancer. Striking racial and regional differences in the occurrence of specific types of cancer can be found. Incidence of cancer of the stomach is very high in Scandinavia, Iceland,

and Japan, but quite low in North America. Primary cancer of the liver is predominant in South and West Africa. Cancer of the nasopharynx, which is quite uncommon in North America, is very frequent in China.

Other examples of geographic differences in cancer incidence include a very low rate of colorectal cancer in black Africa, a low incidence of prostate and breast cancer in Japan, and a low incidence of cancer of the uterine cervix in Israel.

Migration of populations will usually cause a shift toward the patterns of cancer incidence of the host country. For example, a Japanese native who migrates to the U.S. will have a low risk of stomach cancer and, if he or she is a smoker, a high risk of lung cancer.

Socioeconomic factors are also attributed to the etiology of cancer. Cancer of the stomach and cervix are three to four times more frequent in lower socioeconomic groups. On the other hand, cancer of the breast, leukemia, and multiple myeloma are more frequent in high socioeconomic groups.

Oncogenes are segments of DNA that can cause the cell to enhance or decrease essential products associated with growth and differentiation, and subsequently cause the cell to exhibit unrestricted growth and dissemination; all characteristics of cancer. These genetic fragments have been discovered as constituents of tumor viruses. Many of these tumor viruses have been classified scientifically in great detail. The oncogenes contained within these viruses are derived from normal cellular genomes found in mammals, fish, birds, or invertebrates. The viral oncogene is not an exact copy of the cellular oncogene. The general theory is that cellular oncogenes are normal genes that regulate growth and differentiation. Alteration of the cellular oncogene itself or of its regulation results in abnormal growth and differentiation of the cell. Perhaps the transforming viruses do not actually contain oncogenes but integrate near the cellular oncogenes and cause molecular alterations that allow abnormal growth.

One example is the *ras* oncogene. This gene codes for a series of proteins called P21 protein. The P21 proteins are thought to be intimately involved with regulation of cell proliferation. A point mutation in the *ras* gene results in a mutant P21 protein, which gives the cell a growth-promoting signal in some way. Experimentally, a variety of carcinogens can cause such a mutation in the *ras* gene. The *ras* cellular oncogene has been associated with human bladder, lung, and kidney cancers. Other examples of oncogenes associated with cancer are the *src* and *myc* oncogenes. These have been associated with Burkitt's lymphoma, neuroblastoma, and retinoblastoma. Laboratory testing for amplification of the *myc* gene has correlated closely with tumor progression and has been used as a determinate of response to tumor therapy. In a similar fashion, amplification of the HER-2/*neu* oncogene has been correlated with prognosis in breast cancer.

It is likely that most cancers are the result of multiple factors. For example, in carcinoma of the lung it may be that in addition to heavy cigarette smoking, a specific genetic background, suitable male hormonal factors, and a virus are required to actually cause a carcinoma. For these reasons efforts to identify all the causative factors of cancer and to educate people about these factors must be continued.

BIOLOGY

A cancer cell is a progeny of a normal cell that has lost its cellular mechanism for controlling proliferation. Almost all malignant neoplasms seem to arise from a single cell that has undergone malignant transformation to form a malignant clone. Cancer cells generally proliferate faster than normal cells except for leukocytes or cells of the intestinal mucosa. As the tumor mass grows, however, the proliferative rate increases. Therefore, the proportion of cells undergoing mitosis is much greater when there are only a few cancer cells present than when there is a large tumor mass. This observation may account for the relative resistance of large tumor masses to therapies directed at mechanisms of proliferation.

Malignant cells tend to revert to more primitive cell types, that is to dedifferentiate. The normal orderly tissue patterns of growth are lost and replaced by random piling up of malignant cells. These morphologic changes are the basis for histopathologic or cytologic diagnosis of cancer.

Changes in the chemical architecture of the cellular membrane of malignant cells are associated with the loss of contact inhibition through proliferation and intracellular adhesiveness. No single biochemical alteration has yet been defined that is absolutely characteristic of malignant transformation.

The reversion of cell function to an embryonal state produces distinctive embryonal substances whose presence in the adult may be used to diagnose cancer. The carcinoembryonic antigen associated with gastrointestinal cancers and α-fetoglobulin associated with hepatoma are thought to be examples of this type. The genes responsible for production of these substances acquire the ability to be expressed when cells undergo dedifferentiation. Another example of variable genetic activity in cancer cells is the production of parathyroid-like hormones in bronchogenic carcinomas.

Growth Rates If one assumes that a cancer begins from a single cell, it takes about 30 exponential divisions to produce a 1-cm nodule. At 45 exponential divisions, the patient is apt to be dead from the shear bulk of the malignant tumor.

The growth rate of tumors can be expressed by tumor doubling time, i.e., the time it takes the tumor to double in volume. Tumor doubling time is an accurate method for comparing biologic aggressiveness of neoplasms.

Semilogarithmic paper is used to plot tumor dimensions against the time in days. The slope of the line along these points represents the rate of tumor growth. This result usually varies between 20 and 100 days. The measurement of tumor doubling time can be helpful in determining prognosis or evaluating response to chemotherapy. In biologic terms, the tumor doubling time represents the balance between intrinsic proliferative rate of the tumor cell and the patient's inhibiting defense mechanism.

Most human tumors have been present in the body for at least 1 year and many as long as 10 years prior to clinical detection. A long period of time occurs between the inception of neoplastic transformation and the development of clinical cancer.

IMMUNOBIOLOGY

Interest in the immunology of neoplastic disease began when tumor-specific antigens were conclusively demonstrated in mouse sarcomas. Mice were presensitized with a transplant of tumor tissue that was allowed to grow for a time and then was excised. These immunized animals were then resistant to challenge with further transplants of the same neoplasm. Challenge with large numbers of tumor cells, however, usually overwhelmed the immunologic defense and progressive tumor growth was observed. Subsequently, tumor-specific antigens have been demonstrated. Fundamental questions persist, however, concerning the expression of tumor-specific antigens by human tumors, the host response to these antigens, and the ability to manipulate the response to achieve regression.

Once a tumor-specific antigen is recognized the important

effectors in the immune mechanism include tumor antigen–specific antibodies, mononuclear phagocytes, natural killer cells, and cytotoxin T lymphocytes. The major antibody classes associated with tumor immunity are IgM and IgG. Binding of antibody to the tumor target cell does not by itself result in gross suppression or destruction. It serves only as a recognition signal for cytolytic effectors.

The classic complement system is composed of a group of serum proteins, most of which are β-globulins. A cascade of component activation results in the release of C3A and C5A. These compounds, called *anaphylatoxins,* cause neutrophil activation, increased vascular permeability, and smooth muscle contraction. Subsequent compounds of the complement system are responsible for attacking the cell membrane target and causing osmolysis of the cell.

Monocytes and macrophages are very efficient cytotoxic effectors in the immune system. The so-called K cell, a poorly defined lymphocyte of uncertain lineage, is quite active. Monocytes and macrophages are found in the spleen, lymph nodes, and alveoli of the lung. Kupffer cells are specialized macrophages that are found in the liver.

Macrophages help initiate the immune response by serving as antigen-presenting cells. They have a wide range of regulatory, tumoricidal, and bacteriocidal properties. Elaboration of lymphokines such as interleukin-1 (IL-1) is important in lymphocyte activation and the generation of fever. Macrophages also produce tumor necrosis factor that has a broad range of cytocidal and regulatory properties. Activation of macrophages themselves occurs secondary to bacterial products such as endotoxin and antibody-coated targets.

Natural killer cells are large granular lymphocytes capable of killing certain tumor target cells without requiring immunologic memory. The mechanism of NK lysis is not fully understood but does require cell contact and is mediated by cytotoxins. NK cells are probably important in immunologic surveillance and eradication of small numbers of tumor cells.

The cytotoxic T lymphocyte is the only effector with intrinsic immunologic specificity by virtue of its antigen-specific receptor. This receptor can protect foreign antigens associated with Class I major histocompatibility complex. These cytolytic cells induce ultrastructural lesions in the membrane lipid bilayer of target cells. They can be clonally expanded in the presence of interleukin-2 (IL-2).

Suppressor T cells can be induced by tumor antigen also. These cells control the activity of immune reactions. They, in turn, are regulated by countersuppressor T cells. Cyclophosphamide, cimetidine, and indomethacin are agents used to inhibit immune suppression and augment tumor immunity.

Biologic Response Modifiers

Genetic engineering technology has allowed investigation of several immune effectors for manipulation of the immune response to tumors.

IL-1 is a lymphokine produced by activated macrophages. IL-1 induces some T cells to produce IL-2 and others to express IL-2 receptors. This activity is important in the clonal expansion of tumor cell subsets. IL-1 may also have a maturation effect on B lymphocytes and participate in proliferation of these lymphocytes by producing interferon β. In addition, IL-1 initiates the febrile response and causes a release of neutrophils into circulation. IL-1 plays a role in induction of hepatic synthesis of acute phase proteins and induction of skeletal muscle metabolism in periods of stress.

IL-2 is a glycoprotein produced by helper T lymphocytes. This compound was originally called "T-cell growth factor" and has been found in tissue culture to support the long-term proliferation of T cells. IL-2 augments the generation of cytolytic T lymphocytes, natural killer cells, and lymphokine-activated killer cells.

Tumor necrosis factor (TNF) is a polypeptide hormone found in the sera of mice sensitized with BCG and subsequently challenged with bacterial endotoxins. This agent was found to cause hemorrhagic necrosis of certain experimental tumors. A broad range of biologic activities have been described further. Properties of TNF include direct cytotoxicity for certain cells, stimulation of procoagulant activity of vascular endothelial cells, activation of neutrophil adherence and phagocytosis, and induction of fever by direct effect on the hypothalamic thermoregulatory center. TNF is one of the major effector molecules of macrophage-mediated cytotoxicity. It plays a central role in pathogenesis of endotoxin-induced shock, and this agent may account for the wasting and catabolic state associated with chronic illness and cancer.

Interferons (IFNs) were discovered as antiviral agents. There are three major classes of IFN: α, β, γ. IFNα is produced by monocytes and called *leukocyte interferon.* IFNβ is termed *fibroblast interferon.* IFNγ is produced by immune T cells and has been called *immune interferon.* The antitumor effects of interferon are related to expression of interferon receptors by tumor cells. IFNα has been used to treat leukemia, Kaposi's sarcoma, lymphomas, and malignant melanoma. IFNβ has demonstrated some activity against multiple myeloma and lymphoma.

Immune Surveillance

The concept of immunologic surveillance is based on the premise that carcinogenesis occurs frequently as a spontaneous mutation. The purpose of the immune system is to recognize the foreignness of tumor-specific antigens and to mount an immune response capable of eliminating them. A variety of possible ways by which cancer cells evade this surveillance system has been described.

Insufficient antigenicity to evoke an immune response may account for growth of some neoplasms. Tumor cells with strong tumor antigens may be recognized and eliminated, whereas those cells with weak antigens escape detection and destruction.

Antigenic modulation can occur on the surface of the tumor cell, which may account for the heterogeneity of certain neoplasms. For example, the lung metastases of a strongly immunogenic tumor may be antigenically different from the primary tumor and resistant to therapy.

Immunosuppression by irradiation, neonatal thymectomy, chemotherapy, or steroid treatments usually increases frequency and growth rate of neoplasms in experimental animals. Likewise, in human beings, the incidence of cancer increases significantly with advancing years as the immune response diminishes. Patients with congenital immunodeficiency diseases have an incidence of spontaneous cancer 10,000 times greater than the age-matched population.

Immunologic tolerance developed during the fetal or neonatal periods owing to exposure to tumor-specific antigens or oncogenic viruses may account for subsequent lack of protection against tumor growth. This mechanism has been demonstrated in mice infected as neonates with mammary tumor virus that became tolerant to the tumor-specific antigen of this virus-induced neoplasm as adults.

There are a number of well-documented clinical observations that suggest immune defense against cancer in human beings. These include the following: (1) Spontaneous regression of established tumors is a rare but well-documented phenomenon. It is most frequently seen in neuroblastomas, malignant melanoma, and adenocarcinoma of the kidney. Likewise, spontaneous regression of small pulmonary metastases following the surgical removal of the primary tumor has been observed. (2) Recurrence of tumor 10 years after successful treatment of the primary is often manifested by rapid tumor growth and death. This course suggests a host defense that inhibits the tumor growth during the disease-free interval. (3) Microscopic evidence of histiocytic, plasmocytic, and lymphocytic infiltration of tumor resembles that seen in organ transplants that are undergoing rejection.

Fetal Antigens Fetal antigens are produced by normal fetal organs during embryonic development. Their production is repressed shortly after birth. Their occurrence in tumors is thought to be secondary to alterations in the pattern of gene regulation as the result of dedifferentiation and reversion of the cell to a primitive embryonic state.

α-Fetoglobulin is one fetal antigen that circulates in approximately 70% of patients with primary hepatomas. This antigen has also been found in patients with gastric cancer, prostatic cancer, and primitive testicular tumors. Testing for α-fetoglobulin has been useful in the diagnosis of hepatomas.

Carcinoembryonic antigen (CEA) is another tumor-associated antigen occurring in fetal gut, liver, and pancreas. This antigen has been found in a variety of adenocarcinomas of the gastrointestinal tract and pancreas, as well as sarcomas and lymphomas of different histologic types. Elevated CEA levels have been found in patients with a variety of nonmalignant conditions including alcoholic cirrhosis, pancreatitis, cholecystitis, diverticulitis, and ulcerative colitis. For these reasons, the test has not been useful as a serologic screening method for the diagnosis of malignant tumor. However, CEA levels may be of some value for following the clinical course of patients with known malignant disease in order to detect evidence of recurrence prior to its becoming clinically detectable.

Immune Competence

A number of studies have tested the immunologic system of cancer patients. These studies are concerned with humoral antibody production as well as cell-mediated immune reactions. There is no evidence to implicate a defect in humoral antibody production in most cancer patients. On the other hand, cell-mediated immune reactions are significantly impaired in patients with some type of neoplasm. Cancers of the lymphoreticular system are known especially for impairment of cell-mediated immune reaction. In patients with solid tumors, the degree of immunologic impairment seems to vary with the extent of the disease. Many patients with advanced disease are often anergic.

Monoclonal Antibodies

Technical methods for producing monoclonal antibodies have improved greatly. The creation of hybridomas that produce antibodies against a single antigen makes the study of tumor immunology and tumor-specific antigens much more precise. Hybridomas have produced a monoclonal antibody that appears to react with tumor-specific antigens of target cells. These antibodies could be used to develop immunodiagnostic techniques as well as therapeutic techniques. Attempts are being made to link specific monoclonal antibody to cytotoxic antigens such as adriamycin or ricins in order to deliver lethal drugs to a tumor without affecting the normal tissues.

Other applications of immunobiology to cancer therapy include immunoprevention via vaccine prepared from common tumor antigens or tumor viral antigens. Also, immunologic monitoring of cancer patients undergoing treatment could be extremely useful in determining choice of therapy. Eventually, it may become possible to carry out immunologic engineering on patients with defective immune responses.

PATHOLOGY

When confronted with a mass, the clinician must perform a biopsy before he or she can make a specific diagnosis. Pathologists use certain features, such as the arrangement of cells, their relation to surrounding tissue, and the appearance of the nucleus and nucleoli, to sort out inflammatory from neoplastic processes. Certain terms used to describe these microscopic findings include: *anaplasia,* meaning lack of differentiation; *polarity,* referring to the normal orderly alignment of epithelial cells; and *nuclear changes,* including enlargement and density of nuclei. Carcinoma in situ defines lesions that demonstrate many of these changes without evidence of invasion of deeper histologic layers.

One of the most characteristic features of malignant disease is the ability to infiltrate adjacent tissues. A benign tumor grows by expansion but does not infiltrate the surrounding tissue.

The electron microscope has been helpful in diagnosing some tumors such as malignant melanoma and soft tissue sarcomas.

Classification   Many different classifications of tumors exist, but the most useful one is based upon the cell type of tissue of origin. Neoplasms arising from epithelial cells are known as carcinomas. Sarcomas arise from connective tissue and cells of mesenchymal origin such as muscle, skeletal, or vascular tissue. Teratoma signifies a neoplasm in which anaplastic, immature somatic cells are dominant. These tumors occur in the testis, ovary, and mediastinum.

Grading Four grades of malignancy are used to define the degree of differentiation of a tumor. The appearance of the cells, their nuclei, and the number of mitotic figures are characteristics that determine the grade of malignancy. The least malignant tumors are classified as grade 1, and the most malignant as grade 4.

Routes of Spread In general, a malignant tumor may spread by four routes: directly by infiltrating surrounding tissues; via lymphatics; by vascular invasion; or by implantation in serous cavities. Many cancers will spread by more than one route, and an orderly course of metastases cannot be relied upon. Knowledge of the patterns of neoplastic spread is important in planning definitive therapy. Lymph node metastases are first confined to the subcapsular space of the node. Gradually, the tumor cells permeate the sinusoids and replace the parenchyma. Initially, the node may not be enlarged and will appear normal to the naked eye despite involvement with tumor cells. Lymphatic involvement is extremely common in epithelial neoplasms of all types, except basal cell carcinoma of the skin. Sarcomas metastasize to lymph nodes less than 10% of the time.

Vascular spread of cancer cells occurs through direct invasion of the capillaries or by progression through the thoracic duct and entry into the bloodstream. Also, invasion or progression of tumor along the veins is not infrequent. Arteries, however, are rarely invaded. When vascular endothelium is destroyed by tumor a thrombus forms that is likewise invaded by the tumor. The combination of thrombus and tumor may detach to form a large tumor embolus. For this reason vascular invasion by carcinomas and sarcomas is associated with a poor prognosis.

Direct growth of tumor through the wall of an organ allows access of tumor cells to serous cavities. Many tumor cells are capable of growing in suspension without a supporting matrix and thereby can spread within the peritoneal cavity or attach to serous surfaces.

CLINICAL MANIFESTATIONS OF CANCER

The clinical abnormalities produced by advancing neoplastic diseases may be grouped into two categories: those abnormalities that stem directly from the presence of a tumor mass, and those physiologic derangements produced indirectly. Warning signs associated by direct effects of tumor include: change in bowel or bladder habits, a sore that does not heal, unusual bleeding or discharge, thickening or lump in the breast or elsewhere, indigestion or difficulty swallowing, obvious change in a wart or mole, and a nagging cough or hoarseness.

Tumors may have a variety of remote and systemic effects that contribute to morbidity. Cancer patients frequently develop unusual symptoms and physiologic derangements that cannot be attributed to the mechanical presence of primary metastatic disease. For example, the cachexia of carcinomatosis may result from competition between the tumor and the host for basic components of the same metabolic pool. Likewise, the ectopic production of hormones or the secretion of unidentified physiologically active substances are some manifestations of malignant tumors. Toxic substances secreted from the tumor are thought to be another pathway of cachexia.

CANCER DIAGNOSIS   Diagnosis of cancer should proceed in an orderly fashion: careful history, thorough physical examination, examination of blood and urine, and appropriate radiologic examinations.

History   Weight loss, loss of appetite, and/or change in bowel habits are subtle symptoms in the history of a patient that may indicate malignancy. Other indicators are more specific for a given malignancy, such as nipple discharge, changing color of a mole, or difficulty swallowing.

Physical Examination   Physical examination includes a search of the entire skin surface for suspicious lesions. Lymph nodes should be palpated for enlargement. Careful breast examination should be performed. A Papanicolaou's smear from the cervix should be obtained. Rectal examination and proctoscopic examination should be included. For patients with hoarseness an indirect laryngoscopy should be performed.

Laboratory Examination   Laboratory examination should include complete blood cell count, urinalysis, examination of stool for occult blood, and chest radiograph.

Diagnosis of solid tumors rests on locating and performing a biopsy of the lesion. Cancers of the internal organs are more difficult to diagnose and biopsy. Information from CT studies has been very useful. Often, exploratory surgery is required to confirm the diagnosis and obtain a biopsy.

Screening Tests   The chances of detecting cancer in a given annual examination are no more than 1 in 100 even under optimal circumstances. For this reason, most cancer detection tests are not economical or efficient. It is difficult to determine whether mass screening will have an impact on the cure rate for cancer. Most likely, the selection of certain high-risk groups for periodic screening will be the solution.

Biopsy It is imperative to obtain microscopic proof of malignant disease before institution of treatment. Biopsy reports and slides of previous biopsies should be obtained and reviewed prior to treatment as well. Definitive therapy cannot be planned rationally without knowing the nature of the neoplastic lesion.

Needle biopsy is the simplest method for obtaining tissue for histologic examination. This method causes minimal disturbance of the surrounding tissue. The danger of implanting tumor cells in a needle tract during aspiration is extremely small. Considerable experience, however, is required to interpret needle biopsy specimens.

Incisional biopsy involves removing only a portion of a tumor mass for pathologic examination. It is best performed in circumstances where the incisional wound can be encompassed and totally excised at the time of the definitive surgical procedure. This technique is used when needle biopsy fails to establish a diagnosis, a situation usually encountered in deeper subcutaneous or muscular tumor masses. The disadvantages of incisional biopsy are that the removed portion may not be representative of all the involved tissue and the surgeon may seed cancer cells into the operative wound.

Excisional biopsy is the total local removal of the tumor mass. This is used for small discrete masses, 2–3 cm in diameter, when local removal will not interfere with the wider excision required for permanent local control. Excisional biopsy is usually contraindicated for skeletal and soft tissue sarcomas. These biopsies require meticulous hemostasis, since a collecting hematoma may extend tumor cell contamination by infiltration through tissue planes.

Occasionally, lymph nodes are the only tumor mass available for biopsy. Cervical lymph nodes should not be biopsied until a careful search for the primary tumor has been made. This includes indirect laryngoscopy, pharyngoscopy, esophagoscopy, bronchoscopy, and thyroid scan. Supraclavicular nodes are more frequently enlarged from metastases originating in the thoracic or abdominal cavity. Upper cervical nodes, however, are usually due to metastases from laryngeal, oropharyngeal, or nasopharyngeal neoplasms.

STAGING OF CANCER The extent of the patient's tumor by clinical evaluation at the time of initial presentation is called the *clinical stage*. Clinical staging is essential prior to making a decision about therapy. Stage I usually indicates a neoplasm confined to its primary site of origin. Stage II indicates metastases to regional lymph nodes, and stages III and IV indicate distant metastatic spread. Standardization of staging around the world has been accomplished by using the TNM system. T classifies the primary tumor, N classifies the presence or absence of lymph node metastases, and M designates the presence or absence of distant metastases. Within each category subscripts 1–4 are used for classifications that correspond with decreasing prognosis.

The importance of accurate staging and designating a therapeutic program for patients with cancer cannot be overemphasized. When comparing the results of therapy in different centers the validity of evaluation depends on careful staging.

THERAPY

The categories of cancer therapy include surgical resection, radiation therapy, and chemotherapy. Most patients with potentially curable solid tumors are treated with surgery. Radiation and chemotherapy have been added in an attempt to improve overall cure rate. Chemotherapy and immunotherapy represent systemic forms of treatment effective against tumor cells already metastatic to distant organ sites. Treatments that combine surgery, radiation therapy, and chemotherapy will significantly improve cure rates above those achieved with any single therapeutic modality in many types of cancers.

PALLIATION Once the diagnosis of malignant disease has been made and the extent of disease determined, a decision must be made as to whether the patient is curable. If the cancer is localized without evidence of spread, the goal of therapy is to eradicate the cancer and cure the patient. When the cancer spreads beyond local cure, the goal is palliation, i.e., to control the patient's symptoms and to maintain maximum activity for the longest possible time. The most important criterion for incurability is distant metastases. Occasionally, an exploratory celiotomy or thoracotomy may be necessary to determine the nature of equivocal lesions that may represent distant metastases. Also, local extension may be a criterion of incurability. In equivocal situations, after extensive studies have failed to demonstrate metastatic or incurable local extension, the patient deserves the benefit of doubt and should be treated for cure.

CHOICE OF THERAPY Surgery, radiation therapy, and chemotherapy are the most common modalities in the fight against cancer. Immunotherapy is a new modality that currently has a limited role in cancer therapy. A variety of factors must be considered in choosing the appropriate modality for treatment. The patient's general condition and the presence of any coexisting disease must be considered. Also, the psychologic makeup of the patient and the patient's life situation must be considered.

ADJUVANT THERAPY As approximately 60% of malignant tumors ultimately recur, the search continues for modalities of cancer therapy that will treat subclinical metastases at the time of diagnosis. This approach is called *adjuvant treatment* and usually involves chemotherapy or immunotherapy. The rationale for adjuvant treatment rests with the opportunity for cure during an early stage of disease or immediately after surgery when tumor burden is minimal. One example is adjuvant chemotherapy for premenopausal patients with Stage II carcinoma of the breast. Other tumors that seem to respond to adjuvant chemotherapy are Wilms' tumor, osteosarcoma, and ovarian carcinoma.

SURGICAL THERAPY Surgical treatment represents the most frequently used and the most successful single method for cancer therapy currently available. More patients are cured of cancer by surgery than by any other therapeutic modality. Advances in surgical techniques, anesthesia, and supportive care have permitted the development of more radical and extensive operative procedures. Unfortunately, these more radical procedures have often failed to increase cure rates significantly. It would appear, then, that any therapeutic advances in cancer treatment must come from the combination of other modalities with cancer surgery.

Preoperative preparation of patients for cancer surgery is essential. Patients may have poor nutritional status, anemia, electrolyte disorders, or defects in coagulation, which contribute to morbidity and mortality. Every effort should be made to correct these deficiencies before extensive surgical procedures.

Once the decision has been made to proceed with surgical therapy, the operative procedure should be planned carefully. The best and often only opportunity for cure is at the time of the first operation. Enucleation or incomplete excision of tumor masses is never indicated as a therapeutic measure.

Local recurrence of cancer following surgery may be due to incomplete removal or spillage of cancer cells into the operative area. When a preliminary biopsy has been done, the entire operative field should be reprepared after the biopsy incision is closed. The instruments and gloves used during the biopsy are not used again. The importance of this is illustrated by a patient with breast cancer who had a skin graft taken from the thigh to close a skin defect after a mastectomy. Later, tumor nodules having the same histologic characteristics as the primary neoplasm developed on the thigh at the skin graft donor site.

The rate of local recurrence in the suture line following resection of carcinoma of the colon is about 10%. Ligation of the bowel with umbilical tape proximal and distal to the tumor, irrigation of the cut ends of the colon with mercury bichloride solution, and excision of the edges of each end of the bowel are methods that have decreased the recurrence rate to less than 2%. Usually, a local recurrence is associated with systemic disease and is an unfavorable prognostic factor.

Blood-borne metastases are a major factor in the death of patients with most tumors. There is a correlation between prognosis and the presence of tumor cells seen in the blood during the operative procedure. Furthermore, manipulation of the tumor at any time in the surgical procedure can greatly increase the number of cancer cells recovered from the blood. Measures taken to prevent dissemination of tumor cells include: avoiding manipulation of the tumor (no-touch technique), early ligation of the vascular pedicle, and the use of tourniquets on all extremity tumors.

TYPES OF CANCER OPERATIONS

Wide local resection is a common surgical treatment of solid tumors in which an adequate margin of normal tissue is removed with the tumor mass. This treatment is appropriate for low-grade neoplasms that do not metastasize to regional nodes or widely infiltrated adjacent tissues. For example, basal cell carcinomas and mixed tumors of the parotid gland would be treated by wide local resection.

Tumors that infiltrate adjacent tissues should be treated by radical local resection. For these tumors it is necessary to remove a wide margin of normal tissue with the neoplasm. Soft tissue sarcomas and esophageal and gastric carcinomas are examples of tumors that should be treated in this fashion. If the tumor was previously explored but not removed, or if an incisional biopsy was performed, it is extremely important that a wide segment of skin and the underlying tissue beyond the limits of the original incision be removed.

It must be constantly emphasized that malignant neoplasms are not well encapsulated. A pseudocapsule composed of a compression zone of neoplastic cells usually covers the tumor. The surgeon must cut through normal tissue at all times and should never encounter neoplasm or the pseudo-capsule during its removal. Radical resection with en bloc excision of lymphatics is an operation designed to remove the primary neoplasm and the regional lymph nodes draining from the area in continuity with all the intervening tissues. It is important to avoid cutting across involved lymphatic channels because such action greatly increases the possibility of local disease recurrence. The principle of en bloc excision of lymphatics was applied to breast cancer by Halsted at the turn of the century.

The high rate of local cancer recurrence following surgical resection when lymph nodes are grossly involved and the high error rate when palpation is used to assess the extent of the involvement have led to routine dissection of regional nodes close to the primary tumor even though they are not clinically involved.

Surgery of Recurrent Cancer

There is a definite role for surgical resection of localized recurrent neoplasms of low-grade malignancy and slow growth where further resection may produce a long period of remission. Various tumor markers, such as CEA, have been extremely useful for selecting patients likely to benefit from reoperation.

RESECTION OF METASTASES Removal of metastatic lesions in the lung, liver, or brain has occasionally produced a clinical cure. This is especially true if the metastasis is solitary. Those patients with solitary metastasis, or metastases located in one lobe of the liver, are often successfully treated with resection. Approximately 25% of these patients will survive for 5 years. Resection of a solitary pulmonary metastasis provides a higher rate of 5-year survival than resection of primary bronchogenic carcinoma of the lung.

Appropriate selection of patients for surgical treatment of metastatic disease depends also on tumor doubling times. In some studies, tumor doubling times greater than 40 days have received significant palliation from pulmonary resection. In contrast, patients with tumor doubling time of less than 20 days did not significantly benefit from resection of their metastatic lesions.

Isolated Perfusion Technique

Continuous infusion of chemotherapeutic drugs can be carried out with portable infusion pumps attached to a catheter placed in an artery that supplies the neoplastic lesion. This method increases the effectiveness of chemotherapy because of greater concentrations obtainable. Patients with hepatoma have responded well to intraarterial infusion of 5-FU.

Hepatic artery ligation itself may be of benefit in the management of hepatic metastases. Metastases derive their blood supply predominantly from the hepatic artery, whereas normal liver tissue receives blood from the arterial and portal systems.

Hyperthermic infusion with chemotherapeutic agents may be worthwhile in treating satellite or in-transit metastasis from malignant melanoma. Heat itself may be an effective agent against some types of tumor, and when combined with chemotherapy may be an important tool in the treatment of metastatic or recurrent cancers.

Palliative Surgery

Surgical procedures are sometimes indicated to relieve symptoms or to prolong a useful, comfortable life. Such operations improve the quality of life even if they do not prolong it. Examples of palliative procedures are gastrojejunostomy; colostomy; chordotomy to control pain; amputation for painful, infected tumors of the extremities; and colon resection despite the presence of hepatic metastases.

Radiation Therapy

Ionizing radiations are effective in controlling a variety of malignant tumors. Radiation therapy is used in the management of 50–60% of all patients with cancer. The advantage of radiation is the ability to destroy tumors with preservation of anatomic structures. The disadvantage of this method includes the increase of some sequelae with time and the long overall treatment.

Doses of radiation are properly quantified in units of grays (Gy), with 1 Gy equal to 1 joule per kilogram (J/kg) of the absorber. Thus, 1 Gy equals 100 rad and 1 cGy equals 1 rad.

Renewed interest has developed in the direct placement of a range of newly developed radioactive isotopes into selected cancers. Consequently, the radiation oncologist has become more involved with the surgical oncologist as methods of intraoperative delivery of radiation continue to evolve.

The basis of radiation-induced damage of mammalian cells and tissues is considered secondary to ionization of water. In addition, ionization and excitation of intracellular targets provide a direct effect of toxicity. The free radicals produced have a short life span. The presence of oxygen and sulfhydryl compounds modifies the recombination of ionization products.

Radiosensitivity is the measure of susceptibility of cells to injury by ionizing radiation. Radiocurability is related primarily to tumor size, site, and type, and less to radiosensitivity.

Tumor cellular hypoxia decreases the effectiveness of radiation because molecular oxygen must be present for maximal cell killing. Hyperthermia is an attractive adjuvant to radiation therapy because it is effective during the S phase of the cell cycle and is not adversely influenced by hypoxia. Also, the radiosensitivity of cells can be increased by altering the target DNA, such as by replacing thymidine with halogenated pyrimidine analogues (BUdR, IUdR) during cell replication.

Radiation therapy has definite indications and contraindications. The potential for tumor control by radiation therapy is more closely related to tumor size and primary site. As tumors increase in size, the likelihood of radiocurability decreases. Even when seemingly indicated, radiation therapy may be inappropriate because of host factors. These may include general debility or local tissue changes that preclude a high-dose treatment.

Early radiation-induced reactions are usually self-limited. These include anorexia, nausea, fatigue, diarrhea, esophagitis, and hematopoietic suppression. The more important severe sequelae of radiation therapy, such as bowel stenosis and wound necrosis, become evident months or years after treatment. Another side effect of radiation therapy is the risk of carcinogenesis. However, ionizing radiations are weak co-carcinogens in laboratory animals. The therapeutic use of ionizing radiation did not cause any detectable increase in second cancers among 2000 patients with breast carcinoma.

Chemotherapy

The majority of antineoplastic drugs appear to affect either enzymes directly, or substrates of enzyme systems. Usually the effects are on enzymes or substrates related to DNA synthesis. Drugs that act by inhibiting enzymes of nucleic acid synthesis are called *antimetabolites*. Methotrexate is an irreversible inhibitor of the active site of the enzyme dihydrofolate reductase. Another common antimetabolite is 5-FU, which acts as a reversible inhibitor of the enzyme thymidylate synthetase.

Alkylating agents are reactive compounds that substitute

an alkyl group for the hydrogen atom of organic compounds. They primarily affect nucleic acid, especially DNA. Alkylation of DNA molecules interferes with replication in transcription. Examples of alkylating agents are cyclophosphamide and chlorambucil.

A third group of compounds that works primarily on enzyme substrates is the antibiotics. These products are derived from soil fungi. They form relatively stable complexes with DNA and subsequently inhibit synthesis of DNA and RNA. Examples of these drugs are actinomycin D, doxorubicin, and bleomycin.

The fourth class of antineoplastic agents is called the *vinca alkaloids*. They bind to microtubular proteins necessary for cell division and cause death of the cell during mitosis. These agents include vincristine and vinblastine.

There appears to be quantitative differences in the duration of the cell cycle and the sensitivity of cells to drugs during various phases of the cell cycle. Antineoplastic drugs can be divided into those that are phase-specific and phase-nonspecific. Those drugs that can affect multiple phases of the cell cycle are termed *phase-nonspecific*.

Tumor cells appear to be intrinsically unstable and highly susceptible to mutation. This leads to a heterogeneous population of cells within a single tumor. Tumor cell heterogeneity has important implications for cancer treatment. It implies that the larger the size of the tumor, the more likely is the resistance to multiple chemotherapeutic agents. Chemotherapy should be used as early as possible in the natural history of cancer in order to assure the highest probability that the tumor will be homogeneous and sensitive to treatment.

Antineoplastic drugs are incapable of killing all cancer cells at any given exposure. They will kill a variable fraction of cells from a very few up to a maximum of 99%. Since the body burden of tumor cells in a human being with advanced disease may be greater than 10^{12} cells, and since the best one can hope for with a single maximal exposure of tumor cells to a drug is 2 log–cell kill, it is apparent that treatment must be repeated many times in order to achieve even partial control. Studies with experimental animal tumors have conclusively demonstrated the critical importance of drug scheduling in therapy. This is especially true for phase-specific agents.

It is clear that the optimal way to use chemotherapy against most forms of human cancer is to administer combinations of drugs. The successful programs of combination chemotherapy have been designed with the following criteria in mind: (1) only drugs active against the tumor in question are included; (2) drugs included have different mechanisms of action in order to minimize the possibility of drug resistance; and (3) drugs chosen generally have different spectra of clinical toxicity.

A variety of routes can be chosen for administration of antineoplastic agents. Consideration of pharmacologic principles is important in cancer chemotherapy. Besides routes of absorption, transport mechanisms are also important. Interference with binding to serum protein by other drugs significantly alters the efficacy of the antineoplastic agent.

The route of excretion of a drug may be critical. For example, treatment with methotrexate requires careful observation of kidney function.

The most common cause of treatment failure is the development of drug resistance by the tumor cells. Some investigators have successfully used clonogenic assays to predict drug resistance. In these studies human tumors are grown in short-term tissue culture to test for drug resistance.

Adjuvant Chemotherapy

The ineffectiveness of surgical resection alone for many types of cancer has led investigators to the use of chemotherapeutic agents as adjuvant treatment. The theory is that these agents might control microscopic foci of cancer already disseminated in the body. Thus far very few significant benefits have been demonstrated using single agents. Future applications of this strategy using newer agents in combination for prolonged periods of time may result in improved survival.

GUIDELINES FOR CHEMOTHERAPY   The following principles should be guidelines for administering chemotherapy to patients with nonhematologic malignant tumors.

1. The patient should have a histologic diagnosis of a malignant disease that is known to respond in a reasonable percentage of cases in a manner beneficial to the patient.
2. It is absolutely essential that there be adequate facilities to monitor the potential toxicity of the drugs being administered.
3. In order to minimize unwarranted toxicity the physician should diligently search for disease markers to assist in monitoring treatment. Parameters of tumor response should be followed in order to objectively assess the therapy. As a general rule a 50% reduction in the product of the greater and lesser diameters of a given tumor constitutes a partial response.

Some tumors have a remarkably high response rate to chemotherapy and are worthy of special mention. Metastatic choriocarcinoma is curable in 80–90% of women using chemotherapeutic drugs alone. Nearly all forms of testicular cancer are now considered to be highly responsive to chemotherapy using combinations of cisplatin, bleomycin, and vinblastine. The mainstays of therapy for disseminated cancer of the prostate are orchiectomy and estrogen therapy. Estrogen therapy is of major palliative value in controlling pain. The sequential use of optimal surgery, radiation therapy, and chemotherapy has improved the ability to control Wilms' tumor in 80% of children. 5-FU, cyclophosphamide, and methotrexate have greatly improved the response rates for Stage II carcinoma of the breast.

Immunotherapy

Immunotherapy depends on basic antigenic differences between neoplastic and normal cells for its therapeutic effect. The advantage of immunotherapy is the ability to inhibit the proliferation rate of cancer cells without affecting function of normal cells. Immunotherapy is a logical adjunct to the treatment of subclinical microscopic disease following definitive cancer surgery. General immune competence of the host is greatest when the disease is localized and becomes impaired after metastasis. Immunotherapy should complement rather than interfere with currently available methods of cancer therapy. Recombinant DNA technology has increased the availability of purified biologic response modifiers and potentiated the use of these factors, such as interleukin-2 and tumor necrosis factor, as antineoplastic agents.

Active specific immunotherapy is an effort to stimulate the host to generate a specific immune response to its tumor. This method uses vaccines made from tumor cells or tumor antigens. Prior to vaccination the tumor cells must be rendered incapable of proliferation. This can be done by radiation, freezing, or heat treatment. The greater the antigenicity of the vaccine the greater the chance of immunologic reaction and tumor progression. For this reason immunologic adjuvants, such as BCG vaccine, *Corynebacterium parvum,* and Freund's adjuvant, have been used with tumor vaccines to enhance the host immune response. Results of this strategy to date, however, have not been impressive. As knowledge about lymphokines that modulate immune response improves, active immunotherapy may become more effective.

PASSIVE IMMUNOTHERAPY In passive immunotherapy, tumor-specific antiserum is used systemically in an effort to suppress tumor. Only antibodies of certain classes and subclasses can interact effectively with cellular effectors. An example of passive immunotherapy is the use of murine monoclonal antibodies. However, the antigenicity of these antibodies to human hosts has limited their application.

Immunotoxins Immunotoxins are tumor-specific antibodies attached to toxic molecules. Monoclonal antibodies are preferred as the immunologic carrier. A wide range of toxic molecules have been tested and include radioactive isotopes, traditional cancer drugs, and plant and bacterial toxins. So far, the overall therapeutic efficacy of immunotoxins has been unproved.

Adoptive Immunotherapy In adoptive immunotherapy, immune lymphoid cells are transferred to a recipient to mediate tumor destruction. These immune lymphoid cells recognize tumor antigens and are actually classical cytolytic T lymphocytes. The utilization of lymphokine-activated killer cells has been pioneered by Rosenberg and colleagues. LAK cells are cytolytic lymphocytes generated in the presence of interleukin-2 (IL-2). The biochemical nature of tumor-specific recognition by LAK cells is not fully defined. Clinical trials using autologous LAK cells and systemic readministered IL-2 have resulted in clear, objective responses in some patients with bulky metastatic cancer. Great toxicity is seen, however, with combined administration of LAK cells and IL-2.

Nonspecific immunotherapy utilizes certain substances that have the ability to nonspecifically enhance host resistance to viral, fungal, and bacterial agents. These agents stimulate immune response to a wide variety of antigens including tumor antigens. The use of attenuated bovine tuberculous bacillus (BCG) is a recent example of nonspecific immunotherapy. Morton and colleagues have observed that intratumor injection of BCG caused 90% of intradermal metastases from malignant melanoma to regress in patients who were immunologically competent. Uninjected nodules also were observed to regress in approximately 20% of patients.

Other agents that nonspecifically stimulate the immune system are *C. parvum,* bacterial antitoxins, and polynucleotides. Another form of nonspecific immunotherapy involves the use of agents capable of restoring depressed immune responses. These agents include thymic hormones such as thymosin and the antihelminthic drug levamisole. Adjunctive use of levamisole and 5-FU has been shown recently to improve survival following surgery for Duke C adenocarcinoma of the colon.

Hyperthermia

Hyperthermia may have a substantive role in future cancer treatment. Tumor cells are selectively thermosensitive compared with normal cells at temperatures from 42–45°C. Investigators have found that a major factor in cell killing at 45°C is the irreversible damage to cancer cell respiration. This mechanism, combined with an increase in cell wall membrane permeability and the liberation of lysoenzymes, probably accounts for the autolytic cell destruction after hyperthermia. Extensive temperature measurements during hyperthermia in animal and human tumors demonstrate that many tumors selectively retain more heat than normal tissue because their neovascularity is physiologically unresponsive to thermal stress and is incapable of regulating and augmenting blood flow. Extensive vascular thrombosis occurs in tumors at temperatures greater than 45°C. Subsequent resection of tumors has been facilitated in some cases by the avascular nature of the tumor following hyperthermia. Hyperthermia has been combined with radiation therapy to produce a synergistic response.

PROGNOSIS

A number of known factors are important in determining prognosis of cancer. The site of origin of the primary tumors is one of the most important factors. While skin, breast, and thyroid carcinomas are frequently localized and curable, neoplasms of the lung, pancreas, and esophagus spread beyond their primary site and cause death in over 90% of patients.

The stage of disease at the time of initial treatment is of considerable importance in determining survival. Blood-borne metastases to distant sites portends grave prognosis, and few patients are curable at this stage. As a general rule, lymph node involvement sharply reduces survival probability by about one half.

The histologic features of the neoplasm correlate in a general way to prognosis. More undifferentiated neoplasms have frequent mitosis and early spread.

Host immune factors may be an important aspect of prognosis. Patients who have spontaneous depletion of their immune responses have a uniformly poor prognosis.

Finally, the age of the patient may be an important factor affecting prognosis; younger patients tend to carry a poorer prognosis than the same tumors in middle-aged or elderly patients.

10 TRANSPLANTATION

IMMUNOBIOLOGY OF THE ALLOGRAFT

Grafts between individuals of different species (xenografts) are rejected rapidly. Grafts between identical twins (isografts, isogeneic grafts, or syngeneic grafts) or from individuals to themselves (autografts) survive indefinitely.

The rejection of an allograft is elicited by foreign histocompatibility antigens. The ABO blood group antigens will elicit rapid graft rejections in hosts with natural isoantibody. Xenografts are rejected rapidly because tissue incompatibilities are so profound that preformed antibodies may exist in the recipient. Alloantigeneic incompatibilities between members of a species vary, however, and strong antigens can lead to graft rejection within 8 days, while weaker differences will permit graft survival of well over 100 days.

The strongest of the transplantation antigens is the expression of a single chromosomal region called the *major histocompatibility complex* (*MHC*) located on chromosome 6. The presence of HLA antigens on a cell surface can be detected by using antigen-specific antisera, or by measuring the reactivity of host lymphocytes to cellular transplantation antigens from potential graft donors. The antigens that can best trigger the proliferation of allogeneic lymphocytes were designated Class II antigens. The antigens that trigger allogeneic lymphocyte proliferation poorly were designated Class I antigens. Both Class I and Class II antigens can now be detected by specific antisera. The Class I antigens are expressions of those portions of the MHC supergene called HLA-A, HLA-B, and HLA-C. The Class II antigens are expressions of HLA-D, DQ, and DW/DR subloci.

HLA Class I molecules can be detected on the cell surfaces of almost all nucleated cells. In contrast, HLA Class II molecules are found only on cells of the immune system—macrophages, dendritic cells, B cells, and activated T cells. Because of extreme polymorphism, only rarely do two unrelated individuals share all the antigens expressed. Relatives, on the other hand, often share some antigens because each person inherits one chromosome and, hence, one set of HLA antigens from each parent. Typing was thought to be clinically useful because it seemed clear that survival of transplanted organs between family members correlated with the closeness of the HLA antigen match. The clinical results of organ transplantation have not, however, clearly demonstrated the importance of HLA-A and HLA-B identity in organ transplantation between unrelated (cadaver) donor-recipient pairs. This apparent paradox seems caused by the fact that inheritance of the MHC in its entirety is important for graft survival rather than simple sharing of several HLA antigens.

Using the patient's leukocytes and a group of standard antisera, it is possible to characterize most of the strong HLA antigens in both donor and host. Several points about histocompatibility matching deserve emphasis:

1. Recipients receiving grafts, even from donors who are HLA-identical matches with them, will still reject the graft (although more slowly) unless immunosuppressive drugs are utilized. Only an identical twin is truly a perfect match.
2. Even with poor histocompatibility matches between relatives, the results are frequently good, which indicates it is sometimes possible to suppress even great degrees of antigenic incompatibility.
3. Even with a good histocompatibility match, the graft may fail if the host happens to have preformed antibodies against a donor's tissue. These antibodies can be recognized if recipient serum is allowed to react with donor lymphocytes in a cytotoxicity test. This test, called *cross matching,* should be performed with fresh serum as a final test of compatibility prior to transplant. Preformed cytotoxic antibodies to donor tissue cannot be detected by the usual typing procedure itself.
4. The presence of ABH isohemagglutinins will most often lead to the prompt rejection of tissue bearing incompatible blood group substances.
5. Despite the results of tissue typing, a related donor has generally produced better transplant results than an unrelated (cadaver) donor.
6. Tissue typing for unrelated cadaver donors has not been successful, with one exception: HLA identity of all detectable antigens may correlate with a higher incidence of graft success. But such identity is rare.

IMMUNOLOGIC EVENTS IN ALLOGRAFT REJECTION

The immunogens of a grafted organ, being surface components of the cell membrane, are readily available to the recipient's T lymphocytes. For the lymphocyte to become sensitized, however, an accessory cell of the monocyte-macrophage lineage is necessary. In the case of protein antigens, the macrophage efficiently traps an antigen, processes it, and presents it in a form more easily recognized by the T-cell receptor. For this to occur, the responding lymphocyte and the macrophage must share identical Class II antigens on their cell surfaces. This is strong evidence for the importance of self-recognition of cooperating cells in the immune response. The accessory cell also provides a second signal by means of a secreted (monokine) molecule that enhances T-cell responses in its immediate vicinity; the most important monokine is called *interleukin-1 (IL-1)*. In cooperation with antigen binding by the T cell, IL-1 fosters the appearance of receptors for a second lymphokine on the cell surface of the antigen-reactive cell, namely, IL-2 receptors. IL-2 is simultaneously secreted by antigen-responsive helper cells. Interaction of IL-2 with its receptor allows the cell to proliferate and mature.

Cell-Cell Interactions During graft rejection antigen-responsive clones require accessory cells plus interleukin. Also, extensive lymphocyte-lymphocyte interaction is needed for the development of maximum lymphocyte proliferative and cytotoxic activity. The requirement for cooperation between T and B cells was established by showing that neither cell population alone could mount an immune response to certain antigens, whereas mixtures of the two cell types resulted in the production of high levels of antibody. Because B cells are the precursors of antibody-forming cells and T cells do not synthesize readily detectable amounts of immunoglobulin, certain T cells must serve as "helper cells" that assist B cells to differentiate into producers of antibody. An antibody response to the major histocompatibility antigens requires this cooperation, and suspensions of B cells alone in tissue culture will not effectively produce antibodies to these antigens unless T cells are added. Therefore, T-cell recognition of the antigen is necessary for the production of specific antibody by the B cell. Not all T cells can function in this role, only the subgroup of helper T cells (T_H). Also T_H cells are needed for the development of lymphocyte-mediated cytotoxicity. The lymphocytes that produce direct cytotoxicity are also T cells; effector (T_E) or killer cells. The T_H cell is required for the T_E cell to develop fully the capacity to inflict cell damage. Cell-associated histocompatibility antigens are prominent among the antigens that require T_H-T_E cell cooperation for induction of maximum cytotoxicity. There is evidence that yet another T-cell subgroup can inhibit either the development of antibody-producing B cells or the generation of T_E cells, i.e., suppressor T (T_S) cells.

Specifically sensitized T_E cells are present within most rejecting allografts and are capable of inflicting damage. Alloantigenically stimulated T_H cells are there as well and can secrete lymphokines capable of mediating delayed hypersensitivity reactions. But specifically sensitized cells are in the minority and it is likely that a small number of specifically sensitized lymphoid cells initiate a rejection reaction but that the completion of reaction requires many nonsensitized cells as well. Polymorphonuclear eosinophils, leukocytes (PMNs), plasma cells, and unsensitized mononuclear cells are all part of the rejection process; furthermore, there is convincing evidence that antibody can initiate graft destruction in the relative absence of a cellular reaction under appropriate circumstances.

Role of Antibody in Allograft Rejection

There is no doubt that rejection can be mediated by alloantibodies—especially the rejection of vascularized organ allografts. Unlike cell-mediated immunity, where the recognition system is intimately associated with the destruction of the target, humoral antibody must activate other systems in order to effect cell death. Although antibodies bind to allografts, such binding is of no consequence by itself. The combination of antibody with the antigen produces an active complex, which triggers a number of nonspecific effector pathways. The immunologic response, therefore, can be both efficient and discriminatory. Relatively few specifically differentiated cells can produce molecules that will perform the recognition function. Since few cells are committed to each antigen, many more antigens can be discriminated. The antibodies in turn initiate a relatively general effector mechanism that can destroy the graft.

Antigen-antibody complexes activate complement and Hageman factor. Hageman factor in turn produces clotting, activates plasmin, and perhaps directly activates complement. Plasmin in turn can activate C3 to produce, among other effects, chemotactic factors, immune adherence, and opsonization. Activation of Hageman factor also leads to kinin production. Activation of the complement system produces aggregation of platelets and, consequently, initiation of the clotting mechanism. Thrombin formation, in turn, stimulates the production of plasmin from plasminogen. Prostaglandin activity is released following complement activation, and may contribute to vascular permeability, although the significance of this in allograft rejection remains unclear.

An Integrated View of the Rejection of Organ Allografts

A predictable series of events ensues when an unsensitized patient is allografted. The first visible change is a perivascular infiltration of round cells. The original enclaves around small vessels spread, and the interstitial space is further infiltrated. A potpourri of cells accumulates: Cells resembling small lymphocytes are seen, as well as large transformed lymphocytes with basophilic cytoplasm. Large histiocytes or macrophages are just beginning to arrive in numbers. Plasma cells are still relatively scarce: As a terminal product of cellular differentiation, they may require several cell divisions before they appear in the organ.

Antibody and complement are deposited in the area of the capillaries, and some of the infiltrating lymphoid cells are producing immunoglobulins by the third day. Recognition molecules (antibody) as well as sensitized cells are therefore present early in the allograft reaction.

Sensitized lymphoid cells, upon recognizing the foreign tissue, release several mediators of inflammation and cell damage. The release of cytotoxic factors directly injures membranes of adjacent cells. Mitogenic products stimulate division of lymphoid cells, perhaps expanding the immunocompetent population. Activated, phagocytic macrophages are effectively concentrated in the area by migration inhibitory factor and other chemotactic factors. In addition, vascular permeability agents are released. Meanwhile, complement is fixed, thereby producing chemotactic factors, anaphylatoxins, and finally cellular damage when the terminal components are activated. Capillary permeability is increased by anaphylatoxins from the complement chain and probably by kinins. Interstitial edema becomes prominent. At the same time there are several additional inducements to cellular infiltration. The complement cascade generates molecules that produce immune adherence and others that have chemotactic activity. Damaged cells release additional compounds that contribute infiltration by PMNs, as well as other cells. PMNs in turn release vasoactive amines (including histamine or serotonin) and additional vascular permeability-promoting factors. The PMNs squeeze through the enlarged endothelial cell junctions and release proteolytic cathepsins D and E, causing basement membrane damage.

Fibrin and α-macroglobulins are deposited by 7 days.

During this time, lymphoid cells have continued to accumulate and, joined by significant numbers of plasma cells and PMNs, obscure the normal architecture. The round cell population presumably contains many macrophages and other immunologic nonspecific cells at this point. Increasingly frequent mitoses may indicate the production of immunocompetent cells within the graft.

The small vessels become plugged with fibrin and platelets, diminishing the perfusion and preventing function. In this relatively rapid sequence of events the organ has little chance to respond, and the pathologic process is dominated by the host effector pathways.

The morphologic features associated with more chronic rejection become dominated by the response of tissue to injury. A good deal of endothelial cell damage occurs in the allograft and the responses of cellular repair, hypertrophy, and hyperplasia, follow. Endothelial cell damage also elicits repair processes. Aggregations of platelets within the intimal layer are resolved, and the dissolution of the thrombi is accompanied by the infiltration of macrophages and foam cells. The result is a thickened intimal layer with the loss of smooth endothelial lining and the presence of vacuolated cells. The lumen narrows as a result.

Platelets may be of greater significance than PMNs in mediating damage. Immune complexes (which activate complement) will result in platelet adherence and the release of vasoactive substances. Platelet aggregation leads to the release of histamine, serotonin, and other capillary permeability factors that expose more basement membrane; the exposed collagen fibers of the basement membrane further enhance platelet aggregation.

Compromise of the respiration of the cells of vascular organs by vascular endothelial and medial hypertrophy, intravascular aggregations of platelets, and interstitial accumulations of edema and mononuclear cells will have predictable consequences for these cells. They will atrophy, and death may be followed by replacement fibrosis.

Circumventing Rejection

Theoretically, there are a number of methods by which the allograft rejection response can be suppressed, including: (1) destroying the immunocompetent cells prior to transplantation, (2) making the antigen unrecognizable or even toxic to the reactive lymphocyte clones, (3) interfering with antigen processing by the recipient cells, (4) inhibiting lymphocyte transformation and proliferation, (5) limiting lymphocyte differentiation into killer or antibody-synthesizing cells, (6) activating sufficient numbers of suppressor lymphocytes, (7) inhibiting destruction of graft cells by killer lymphocytes, (8) interfering with the combination of immunoglobulins with target antigens, or (9) preventing tissue damage by the nonspecific cells or antigen-antibody complexes.

Antiproliferative Agents

Most traditional immunosuppressive agents act to impair the proliferation of lymphocytes. Such agents include the anti-metabolites, alkylating agents, toxic antibiotics, and x-ray. They inhibit the full expression of the immune response by preventing the differentiation and division of the immuno-competent lymphocyte after it encounters the antigen. All of them, however, fall into one of two broad mechanistic categories. Either they structurally resemble needed metab-olites or they combine with certain cellular components, such as DNA, and thereby interfere with cell function.

Purine Analogs The purine analog azathioprine (AZ) (Imu-ran) has been the most widely used immunosuppressive drug in clinical organ transplantation. Azathioprine is 6-mercap-topurine (6-MP) plus a side chain to protect the labile sulfhydryl group. In the liver, the side chain is split off to form the active compound, 6-MP. The mechanism of action would seem to be similar for these two compounds; however, azathioprine seems to enjoy the advantage of slightly lower toxicity.

The toxicity of azathioprine results from the same mech-anisms. Its primary toxic effect is bone marrow suppression, leading to leukopenia. Although pyrimidine analogs have been studied extensively as immunosuppressants in the laboratory, they have only limited clinical use.

Folic Acid Antagonists The folic acid antagonists, aminop-terin and methotrexate, inhibit the enzyme dihydrofolate reductase, and prevent the conversion of folic acid to tetra-hydrofolic acid. This step is necessary for the synthesis of DNA, RNA, and certain coenzymes; again, proliferating cell systems are most affected.

The usefulness of alkylating agents, which include nitrogen mustard, phenylalamine mustard, busulfan, and cyclophos-phamide, is limited by their toxicity. Even so, cyclophos-phamide has been used with good results in renal transplan-tation. Cyclophosphamide is frequently used in clinical bone marrow transplantation, where it potentiates the effects of radiation and enhances the disruption of DNA. When cyclophosphamide is used, lower doses of radiation are required to deplete the recipient bone marrow population and provide space for donor cells. When leukemia is the indication for bone marrow transplantation, cyclophosphamide will aid in the destruction of these cells. Toxicity is high, however, and predictable reactions occur, principally to rapidly replicating cell populations. Stomatitis, nausea, vomiting, diarrhea, skin rash, anemia, and alopecia are all common reactions.

Antibiotics   The immunosuppressive antibiotics include the inhibitors of nucleic acid synthesis, and chloramphenicol and puromycin, which interfere with cellular protein synthesis. Mitomycin C combines with cellular DNA and hinders replication. None of these agents is clinically useful as an immunosuppressive agent for transplantation.

Cyclosporine   Cyclosporine is a fungal cyclic peptide that represents an entire new class of clinically important immunosuppressive agents. It is not an alkylating, antimitotic, or lympholytic agent. Its action at the molecular level seems highly specific, not just for lymphoid cells, but rather for certain subpopulations of T cells.

Cyclosporine strongly inhibits the formation of cytotoxic T cells in mixed lymphocyte culture, and prophylactic administration is strongly suppressive of allograft rejection. Indeed, rejection or graft-vs.-host disease can sometimes be overcome or reversed. Stopping the drug permits rejection to resume so that cyclosporine plus antigen does not lead to permanent tolerance. Cyclosporine does not appear to affect precursor hematopoietic cells, resting or dividing lymphocytes, or macrophage functions. It acts by interfering with the production of the lymphokine IL-2, which is normally essential for lymphocyte proliferation. Thus the expansion of antigen-responsive clones of T lymphocytes is suppressed. T suppressor cells, however, are not inhibited. Additive immunosuppressive effects can be achieved in combination with ALG, azathioprine, prednisone, irradiation, and other anti-inflammatory drugs.

Cyclosporine has virtually revolutionized clinical transplantation. In combination with modest doses of prednisone, it appears to be of equal clinical utility, or superior, to ALG-azathioprine and prednisone. Its renal toxicity is a serious disadvantage but can usually be controlled by reducing the dose or combining it with conventional immunosuppressive drugs.

Adrenal Corticosteroids   Steroids cross the cell membrane and bind to specific receptors in the cytoplasm of most cells, lymphocytes included. The steroid-receptor complex then enters the nucleus and interacts with DNA in an unknown way. In lymphocytes, DNA, RNA, and protein synthesis are inhibited, as is glucose and amino acid transport. At a sufficient dosage, lymphocyte degeneration and lysis occur. The primary antilymphocyte action of steroids may be to deplete small lymphocytes before they are activated by antigen. Steroids also suppress most of the accessory functions of macrophages including the ability to secrete IL-1. Although B-cell activity and antibody production are relatively unaffected by steroids, many other cell types that participate in graft rejection are damaged. Both macrophage and neutrophil chemotaxis and phagocytosis are inhibited. The accumulation of neutrophils, macrophages, and monocytes at sites of immune and inflammatory activity is reduced. Steroids alone cannot prevent clinical allograft rejection, but, together with other compounds, they are potent in both preventing and reversing rejection reactions.

Steroid toxicity of some degree is frequent and commonly includes a cushingoid appearance. Other characteristic problems are hypertension; weight gain, peptic ulcers, and gastrointestinal bleeding; euphoric personality changes; cataract formation; hyperglycemia; and osteoporosis with avascular necrosis of bone. The appearance and severity of these complications vary considerably. Clinical transplantation will be improved tremendously when present steroid dosages can be reduced.

Antilymphocyte Globulin   A variety of antibody preparations designed to react with immunoresponsive lymphocytes are available, and they are designed to prevent and to treat graft rejection. Heterologous polyclonal antilymphocyte globulins (ALG) are produced when thoracic duct, peripheral blood, lymph nodes, thymus, or spleen lymphocytes are injected into animals of a different species.

The action of heterologous polyclonal ALG seems to be directed mainly against the T cell. ALG therefore interferes most with the cell-mediated reactions–allograft rejection and the graft-vs.-host reaction. ALG can abolish preexisting delayed hypersensitivity reactions and it has a definite, but lesser, effect on antibody production to T-cell-dependent antigens.

Although these preparations have been widely used in clinical transplantation with beneficial results in both the prevention and treatment of organ allograft rejection, monoclonal reagents with more predictable reactivity are becoming available. Such antibodies are the products of cell fusions between antilymphocyte antibody–producing clones of mouse B cells and laboratory myeloma cells. The resulting hybridomas have become rendered immortal, and each cell line produces a single antibody directed to a single antigen on a human lymphocyte. If the target cell is a cell type essential for the immune response, such as a T cell, severe degrees of immunosuppression can be induced in the recipient of the monoclonal antibody. Mouse monoclonal antibody directed against T cells is now available for clinical use in the treatment of rejection.

The toxicity of any heterologous antibody prepared against human tissue depends in part on its cross reactivity with other tissue antigens, and the ability of the patient to make antibodies against the protein itself. Polyclonal ALG can produce anemia and thrombocytopenia despite prior absorption with human platelets and red cell stroma. Monoclonal antibodies have few cross reactions, but fever, chills, nausea, diarrhea, and aseptic meningitis are frequently seen during the intravenous administration of the first few doses. All heterologous globulins can elicit allergic reactions against themselves. These are generally mild and infrequent, but monoclonal antibodies are strongly antigenic so that they are less effective after 1 or 2 weeks of use. Polyclonal antibody preparations seem to be repeatedly effective.

Irradiation

Total body irradiation has limited use in clinical transplantation because the toxicity is too great. Fractionated doses of radiation to the lymphoid tissues (total lymphoid irradiation), similar to those used in the treatment of Hodgkin's disease, can cause profound immunosuppression, and low dosages of azathioprine and prednisone can maintain the effect.

Lymphoid Depletion Unfortunately, thymectomy has not been useful in clinical transplantation. Splenectomy appears to be slightly beneficial in combination with ALG, azathioprine, and prednisone in prolonging human organ allograft survival. Its effect may simply be to reduce the toxicity of the myelosuppressive drugs so that greater doses of azathioprine can be tolerated in splenectomized transplant recipients. Because splenectomy also increases the risk of subsequent infection, it is rarely used in organ transplantation.

Cannulation and drainage of the thoracic duct will deplete the body of a large proportion of its circulating T lymphocytes, and such depletion will lead to prolongation of allograft survival and to lesser decreases in the capacity for antibody synthesis. Thoracic duct cannulation and drainage have been used for clinical immunosuppression with great success, but the procedure is cumbersome.

Adverse Consequences of Immunosuppressive Therapy

Patients who do not have rejection episodes generally do not suffer major complications of immunosuppressive therapy. An immunosuppressive effect can be detected during the first 2 weeks after kidney transplantation. The response of the patient's circulating lymphocyte to either the mitogen phytohemagglutinin (PHA) or to foreign leukocytes is depressed. The T-cell number in cyclosporine recipients is not diminished, but there may be some alteration in the relative proportions of helper and suppressor T cells.

Bacterial and Fungal Infection Most common bacterial infections are now caused by organisms that are normally weakly pathogenic. Antibiotics will eradicate the more aggressive bacteria, but they leave opportunistic organisms free to colonize the susceptible transplant patient. The opportunistic organisms, which are normally eliminated by cellular mechanisms, can now blossom in the face of the relative T-cell depression. Fungi are prominent opportunists, and they can cause cutaneous, mucosal, pulmonary, and central nervous system infections, as well as generalized sepsis. *Candida* infections are probably the most common. The inevitable mucosal candidiasis can be satisfactorily prevented by oral mycostatin.

Aspergillus species are probably the second most common cause of fungal infection and typically produce upper lobe pulmonary cavities and brain abscesses. There have been many reports of hospital epidemics traceable to construction or ventilation problems. *Rhizopus oryzae, Histoplasma capsulatum,* and *Cryptococcus neoformans* also invade the lung; the latter is the most common cause of meningitis. The indolent bacterium *Nocardia asteroides* occasionally infects, producing nodular pulmonary lesions. The protosoan *Pneumocystis carinii,* more commonly seen in patients undergoing cancer chemotherapy, usually causes a diffuse alveolar infiltrate.

Viral Infections Viral infections seem almost ubiquitous among kidney transplant recipients. Infection or antibody response to cytomegalovirus (CMV) is found in 50–90% of patients after renal transplantation. Herpes simplex infection occurs in about 25% and zoster in 10% of graft recipients. Epstein-Barr virus (EBV) commonly infects transplant patients, but most infections are mild. EBV is associated with posttransplant malignancy in rare patients, however.

Antigenic evidence for hepatitis B virus infection can be detected in many transplant patients, and non-A, non-B hepatitis is probably a cause of liver failure in some long-term survivors. Cytomegalovirus (CMV) is the most important infectious illness that afflicts immunosuppressed transplant patients. CMV infection can produce a spectrum of illness typically characterized by fever, neutropenia, arthralgias, malaise, myocarditis, pancreatitis, or gastrointestinal ulceration. The most severe illnesses are acquired as primary infections from latent virus residing in the grafted tissue. Less often, blood transfusions are the vector. Some cases of apparently new infection represent reactivation of latent intracellular viruses. Transplant recipients who do not have antibodies to CMV and who receive grafts from donors who do are at higher risk. The use of antilymphocyte antibody preparations for immunosuppression increases the risk. Recipients of cyclosporine appear to be at lower risk.

Malignancy   Cancer has been an unexpectedly frequent companion of clinical transplantation. The incidence of cancer is not high enough, however, to contraindicate the transplant procedure. A rare cause is the inadvertent transplantation of a cancer from a cadaver donor in whom the cancer was unsuspected. These tumors can sometimes be treated simply by halting immunosuppression therapy and allowing rejection of the tumor tissue, as well as the transplant, to occur.

The more common cancers are primary tumors that appear in the immunosuppressed recipient. Seventy-five percent of the spontaneous cancers are either epithelial or lymphoid in origin. Carcinoma in situ of the cervix, carcinoma of the lip, and squamous or basal cell carcinomas of the skin account for about half of this group, while B-cell lymphomas make up the remainder. It has been estimated that the risks to the transplant recipient of developing cervical cancer, skin cancer, or lymphoma are increased by 4, 40, and 350 times, respectively. The lymphomas are unusual both in their frequency and in their behavior. Almost 50% of the immunosuppressed patients with lymphomas have brain involvement, which occurs in only 1% of nontransplanted related cases of lymphoma. These lymphomas, although initially responsive to radiation therapy, are usually fatal.

Recent evidence suggests that all lymphomas are not true neoplasms. Immunologic analysis has indicated that these tumors secrete several different types of immunoglobulins, i.e., they do not have the monoclonal characteristics of cancer. Most evidence suggests that some may represent uncontrolled B-cell proliferative responses to EBV.

Miscellaneous Complications Gastrointestinal bleeding due to reactivation of a preexisting ulcer or diffuse ulceration of the gastrointestinal tract can be a fatal complication. The relative pathogenetic contribution of progressive uremia and steroid administration is unknown, but when bleeding appears, it can be difficult to control by nonoperative means. Diverticulitis, bleeding, and ulceration are associated with immunosuppressive treatment. A syndrome of acute cecal ulceration with gastrointestinal bleeding is due to cytomegalovirus. Cytomegalovirus underlies sporadic ulcer disease in other enteric locations as well. Cataracts are common, develop slowly, and appear to be independent of the absolute prednisone dosage. Thrombophlebitis may occur in the renal transplant recipient, particularly on the side of the graft where the venous anastomosis may become partially or completely thrombosed. The diagnosis is difficult because swelling of the leg on the side of the transplant site is an occasional sign of rejection. Hypertension can usually be controlled with dialysis or, in rare refractory cases, with nephrectomy.

Hemodialysis can correct the uremic state, but bone disease may actually progress if the stimulus to parathyroid hormone secretion is not effectively eliminated. Parathyroidectomy is sometimes required to help arrest progressive bone disease but is not indicated for hypercalcemia alone after transplant. Parathyroidectomy seems primarily indicated for patients on chronic hemodialysis in whom transplantation is not planned. A disturbing complication of successful renal transplantation is avascular necrosis of the femoral heads and other bones. Its occurrence is most closely correlated with dosage of steroid use. Migratory arthralgia, myalgia, and tendonitis are common, but persistent joint pain and swelling are most often signs of intraarticular infection. Pancreatitis may appear suddenly and unexpectedly in renal allograft recipients, and recurrent bouts may prove to be fatal. It has been attributed variously to corticosteroid therapy, azathioprine, cytomegalovirus, or hepatitis virus. The transplanted kidney is apparently fully capable of manufacturing erythropoietin. Erythremia also may appear, but apparently it is not related to elevated erythropoietin levels. Phlebotomy has been advised for hemoglobin levels greater than 16 g/dL. Since chronic renal failure itself is inhibitory to development, uremic children are usually far behind their peers in size. After successful transplantation their growth response is highly variable and may depend on age, previous growth rate, renal function, and immunosuppressive drug regimen. Many normal children have been born to renal transplanted women despite their use of mutagenic immunosuppressive drugs. The pregnancies of renal transplanted recipients are frequently complicated, however, by toxemia and bacterial and viral infections, particularly of the urinary tract. Another important problem that must be faced is the decreased life expectancy of the transplant recipient. Parenthood is a long-term obligation, and counseling of these patients should include a discussion of these considerations.

HEMOPOIETIC AND LYMPHOID TISSUES

Bone Marrow

Injury to bone marrow by drugs, chemicals, and diseases poses several clinical problems. Bone marrow transplants between identical twins have been successfully carried out in many cases of irradiation exposure, aplastic anemia, and leukemia. Autologous marrow transplantation has also been found useful after planned treatment with toxic levels of alkylating agents.

Marrow allotransplants are far less successful. Marrow is highly immunogenic and will be readily rejected by the immunologically normal host. If, however, the marrow is allotransplanted into an immunologically crippled (irradiated, immunosuppressed) host, a chimera is produced. The problem then becomes not destruction of the marrow by the host, but the maturation of donor marrow stem cells that results in total immunologic competence and rejection of the host by the graft. This graft-vs.-host (GVH) phenomenon is not seen with skin, kidney, heart, and liver grafts, but it is a major unsolved problem in the transplantation of foreign bone marrow, white blood cells, and lymphoid tissues. GVH disease does not occur in bone marrow transplant between identical human twins, and the GVH reaction is less severe if the donor and recipient are identical at the entire HLA locus. A long-range goal in marrow transplantation is the use of these grafts as a means of promoting acceptance of other organs, such as liver, heart, and kidney. Once the foreign marrow is established, a state of relative or complete specific nonreactivity against donor antigens is conferred.

Human bone marrow allotransplantation has enjoyed increasing success. HLA-identical marrow transplants (from matched siblings) are commonly used to treat aplastic anemias, combined immunodeficiency disease, and thalassemia major. The majority of patients enjoy long-term disease-free survival. Marrow transplantation is now used to treat other acquired and congenital disorders of hemopoietic stem cells and congenital enzymatic defects. Transplantation for leukemia is less successful. The best results are achieved in the treatment of chronic myelogenous leukemia in the chronic phase, and for acute nonlymphoblastic leukemia in first remission.

Aside from transplants between identical twins, transplantation with HLA-matched but nonidentical twin marrow is very successful, with the best record of successful engraftment and the least severe GVH disease. The use of non-HLA-matched donors is far less successful. In these patients, marrow allotransplantation requires much larger doses of immunosuppressive cytotoxic drugs. Furthermore, GVH disease in these HLA-mismatched recipients has been difficult to control.

ORGAN TRANSPLANTATION

Pancreas

The discovery of insulin in 1921 was hailed as the cure for diabetes; it controlled the overt symptoms of diabetes and provided an increased life expectancy. As diabetic patients lived longer, however, previously unseen complications developed. Diabetes is responsible for at least 30,000 deaths per year.

Whole Organ

Either whole organ or distal segmental pancreatic transplants will ameliorate experimental diabetes. In addition to the expected problems associated with the control of immunologic rejection and the need for immunosuppressive drugs, there are special technical concerns. The major problem is difficulty in establishing drainage of the pancreatic duct. Theoretically, ligation of the pancreatic duct should result in atrophy of exocrine tissue without affecting endocrine tissue. But in practice a severe inflammatory reaction occurs and leads to a constricting fibrosis that damages even the islets. Filling the ductal system with plastic is an alternative approach to the prevention of exocrine secretion. Unfortunately pancreatic fibrosis remains a problem with this technique as well. Initial attempts used a combined pancreaticoduodenal approach, with the duodenum serving as a conduit for drainage of exocrine enzymes. The use of a short segment of duodenum anastomosed to the bladder seems to be the most successful solution. Graft thrombosis and other complications associated with graft pancreatitis are decreasing in frequency. Despite these problems, more than 1000 clinical transplants have been performed. Usually cadaver organs are used, and most recipients already have diabetic end-stage renal disease; both kidney and pancreas are transplanted at a single operation. Increasingly, however, as success grows pancreas transplantation will be carried out in patients before advanced renal disease occurs. Experience in human beings has shown that functioning vascularized pancreatic allograft will correct the metabolic deficiency in diabetes. The techniques are now safer and more successful, with the best centers reporting 70–80% of the patients off insulin at 6 months posttransplant.

Islet Tissue

It is not necessary to transplant the pancreas in order to cure diabetes; transplantation of the pancreatic islets will suffice. The current technique for isolation of islets from the pancreas involves mechanical disruption, enzymatic digestion, and density-gradient separation. Isolated adult islets infused into the portal vein will produce long-lasting control of diabetes in rats. This technique has also been successfully applied to the autotransplantation of islets in people who require total pancreatectomy for chronic pancreatitis. Clinical islet allotransplantation has been frustrated by the apparent increased susceptibility of islets to allograft rejection. Survival is very difficult to achieve even when immunosuppression that will prolong skin, kidney, or heart allografts is used.

Gastrointestinal Tract

Allotransplantation of the small bowel and stomach has been carried out experimentally. These grafts are rejected in the usual fashion, and within the same general period as kidneys and other organs. Lymphoid tissues within the intestinal wall can initiate a GVH reaction.

Although there is little apparent clinical use for a gastric transplant, there is definite need for transplantation of the small bowel. Infarction of the bowel sometimes requires excision of the entire small bowel, and this leads to nutritional deficiency that requires expensive and cumbersome parenteral alimentation. Patients with various nutritional and mo-

TABLE 10-1. Common Indications for Hepatic Transplantation

Adult	Children
Chronic active hepatitis	Biliary atresia
Alcoholic cirrhosis	Chronic active hepatitis
Primary biliary cirrhosis	Hepatoma
Secondary biliary cirrhosis	Neonatal hepatitis
α-1-Anti-trypsin deficiency	Secondary biliary cirrhosis
Budd-Chiari syndrome	Inborn errors of metabolism
Acute hepatitis B	

tility problems, as well as certain patients with Crohn's disease, might benefit from safe and successful bowel transplantation. A few attempts in human beings have been successful for several months, but no long-term survival has been achieved.

Liver

Liver transplantation has become a highly successful solution to a variety of congenital and acquired hepatic disorders in thousands of patients. A liver transplant may be positioned in the normal anatomic location (orthotopic transplantation) following a total hepatectomy of the recipient. Alternatively, the donor organ can be placed in an ectopic site (heterotopic transplantation) generally with retention of the host's liver (auxillary transplantation). Orthotopic grafts are universally preferred by clinicians because experimental heterotopic grafts have been so unsuccessful.

INDICATIONS FOR LIVER TRANSPLANTATION In theory, liver transplantation is appropriate for any disease that will cause total liver failure (see Table 10-1).

In children the most common indication for transplantation is extrahepatic biliary atresia. Transplantation is technically feasible in infants weighing as little as 5 kg; in patients smaller than this, the portal vein is usually too small to remain patent. Naturally transplantation is contraindicated in any patient with (1) irreversible infection, (2) widespread malignancy, (3) concurrent disease (e.g., myocardial failure, old age) that would seriously impair survival, or (4) a high risk for recurrent disease in the transplant organ. Because active hepatitis also usually recurs, the presence of HBsAg or HBeAg antigenemia is a relative contraindication. The risk of recurrent alcoholism also makes alcoholic cirrhosis a relative contraindication unless the patient has abstained from alcohol for at least 2 years. In patients with sclerosing cholangitis, active ulcerative colitis also rules out liver transplantation.

Preoperative Evaluation of the Recipient Intensive preoperative evaluation is designed to (1) characterize those physiologic defects in hepatic, pulmonary, renal, or cardiac function that will influence the patient's chance of survival; (2) determine whether the transplant is technically feasible for that particular patient; and (3) search out sites of occult infection and malignancy. Attention to respiratory reserve is important, because all patients are respirator-dependent in the early posttransplant period. Hepatitis screening results will determine the need for hyperimmunce globulin to prevent recurrent hepatitis, and unsuspected tumors are sought using α-fetoprotein, hepatic ultrasound, and computed tomography (CT). A coagulation profile is obtained to document functional capacity of the liver and predict the need for correction. An uncorrectible prothrombin time abnormality is a poor prognostic sign. A radionuclide hepatic excretion scan will reveal unsuspected biliary calculi that must be removed from the common bile duct at the time of recipient hepatectomy. An upper gastrointestinal series and upper gastrointestinal endoscopy will reveal the presence of gastric or esophageal varices. Patency of the portal vein system must be determined before transplantation because occlusion of the portal vein contraindicates liver transplant. Most centers prefer that liver donors and recipients are ABO compatible.

Postoperative Management If renal function is satisfactory, cyclosporine and prednisone are preferred for immunosuppression. If renal function is poor, cyclosporine is temporarily omitted and antilymphoblast serum and azathioprine are used.

Monitoring liver transplant function with frequent chemical determination of coagulation parameters is mandatory. Changes in these levels can signal rejection, ischemia, viral infection, cholangitis, or mechanical obstruction. A radionuclide excretory cholangiogram is performed on postoperative day 3 and at weekly intervals. Delayed excretion into the biliary tree can reflect hepatocellular damage during death of the donor, complications of the donor operation, prolonged cold storage, vascular compromise, or rejection. Also, delayed excretion into the biliary tree can reflect rejection, hepatocellular damage from ischemia, or viral infection. Delayed passage into the small bowel can indicate mechanical obstruction or breakdown. A T-tube cholangiogram (performed with gravity) will diagnose breakdown at the site of biliary drainage. During rejection lymphocytes infiltrate portal tracts and central veins, with varying degrees of bile duct epithelial damage; therefore, a percutaneous liver transplant biopsy and culture is the only way to differentiate among rejection, ischemia, viral infection, and cholangitis. Primary nonfunction is first suspected when factor V levels in the plasma fail to return to normal. Intraoperative bleeding results from many causes: Extensive portasystemic shunts are almost always present, and global coagulation defects always exist. Even when hemostasis appears adequate during operation, bleeding is a special hazard in the immediate postoperative period. Thrombotic occlusion of either the hepatic artery or portal vein will cause sudden deterioration of hepatic function. Vena caval stenosis (most often the suprahepatic anastomosis) leads to edema in the lower trunk and renal insufficiency.

Cholangitis of the transplant can be diagnosed only by biopsy. Subclinical and reversible rejection episodes are commonly detected if liver biopsies are carried out at weekly intervals. Rejection may occur at any time in the postoperative period including the first 24 h, but most cases occur at least several weeks after transplantation.

Results The longest-living survivor is well 12 years after transplantation. Currently, a combination of steroids, azathioprine, and cyclosporine are used for the prophylaxis of rejection following liver transplantation with a $> 80\%$ 1-year survival.

Heart

Heterotopic transplants, in which the heart is placed in parallel in the circulation, were done as early as 1905 by Carrel and Guthrie. Orthotopic transplants, in which the donor heart replaces the recipient heart, were first done successfully in dogs by Lower and Shumway in 1959. By 1982 the series at Stanford enjoyed 50% survival at 5 years.

Spectrum of Disease Patients requiring cardiac transplantation can be combined under a diagnosis of congestive cardiomyopathy, a broad category of diverse pathogenesis, defined by histopathology and functional characteristics. The "idiopathic" cardiomyopathies share common end-stage pathology characterized by dilated cardiac chambers, myocardial degeneration, and fibrosis. Ischemic cardiomyopathy is an end-stage manifestation of coronary atherosclerosis. Patients with ischemic cardiomyopathy are generally older and have a higher frequency of associated problems such as diabetes and peripheral vascular disease. Transplantation in childhood is elected for a combination of idiopathic cardiomyopathies and primary congenital lesions, such as hypoplastic left heart syndrome. The age range for all patients transplanted from 1967 through early 1986 is 4 days to 66 years, with a mean age of 40. Fifty-seven percent of all patients transplanted have had idiopathic cardiomyopathy, 40% have had ischemic cardiomyopathy, and 3% have had congenital heart disease or other diagnoses.

Recipient Selection Recipients are selected from among patients with end-stage ventricular failure, clinically NYHA Class III–IV, who are unlikely to survive more than 1 year, and for whom there is no alternative therapy. In all patients with left ventricular failure, regardless of etiology, pulmonary artery pressure (PAP) increases as left atrial pressure rises. A normal donor heart, accustomed to low pulmonary artery pressure and resistance, will fail immediately if placed in a recipient with sufficiently elevated PVR. If the PVR can be reduced to less than 5 WU, the patient is considered an acceptable risk. Pulmonary artery systolic pressure greater than 50 mmHg is reason for concern.

Donor Evaluation About 14,000 people per year in the U.S. could benefit from cardiac transplant. A maximum of 2000 potential heart donors are available each year. Many donor exclusions made are not meant to imply that the heart is not functioning well in the donor but are based on concern about the ability of the donor heart to tolerate ischemia during the cold preservation period; ideally this ischemic period is kept under 6 h. A common scenario is a patient on high-dose dopamine with diabetes insipidus and a low CVP, who can be taken off dopamine after volume replacement. The ECG should be normal, but striking ST-T changes can be associated with cerebrovascular accidents, hypothermia, and electrolyte abnormalities. Echocardiography is extremely helpful under such circumstances, as it is in the evaluation of blunt trauma, to assess contractability and search for focal wall motion abnormalities. Positive serology for HTLV-III or hepatitis B excludes a potential donor.

Recipient Operation To minimize ischemic time, close communication is maintained with the donor team so that implantation can proceed as soon as the donor heart arrives. The patient is placed on total cardiopulmonary bypass. The recipient aorta is cross-clamped just proximal to the innominate artery and the heart is removed by dividing the great vessels at their commissures and separating the atria from the ventricles at the atrioventricular groove. Both atrial appendages are excised. The posterior aspects of both atria are left intact and connected by the interatrial septum. The donor heart is brought onto the field, trimmed appropriately. Size discrepancies are easily accommodated in the atrial suture lines. Significant aortic size discrepancy is quite common, especially when there is a large age difference. The cross clamp is removed, and a spontaneous rhythm is restored. The sinus node of the donor heart becomes the dominant pacemaker. The recipient's intrinsic rhythm frequently persists, producing regular nonconducted contractions of the native atrial tissue. The denervated heart often requires a period of chronotropic support, which is usually provided by isoproterenol infusion or epicardial pacing to maintain a heart rate of 90–110.

Immunosuppression Maintenance immunosuppression consists primarily of oral cyclosporine and prednisone. Complex interactions with other medications are frequently seen, especially with drugs metabolized in the liver. Chronic low-grade rejection not controlled by cyclosporine and not easily detected by routine endomyocardial biopsy might be responsible for the gradual development of myocardial fibrosis in many patients, and for the appearance of severe diffuse coronary artery disease in about 10% of patients after 1 year.

Rejection Rejection is monitored by right ventricular endomyocardial biopsy, done at least weekly in the first month, then less frequently. At the time of each biopsy a right heart catheterization is performed. Most rejection episodes have normal hemodynamics, but a low cardiac output, low mixed venous oxygen saturation, and elevated right atrial or wedge pressures raise suspicion of rejection. The biopsy is performed through the same venipuncture with a flexible biopsy forceps passed into the right ventricle. Myocyte necrosis is considered diagnostic of significant rejection. Inflammatory cell infiltrates are considered abnormal but are usually not treated as rejection in the absence of myocyte necrosis. Subjective signs may include malaise, fatigue, and frank dyspnea or orthopnea. Physical findings are usually absent but can include tachycardia, a ventricular gallop, rales, and edema. Diminution in ECG voltage is correlated with rejection in patients maintained on azathioprine and steroids but is without value in patients on cyclosporine. Echocardiography can add suggestive findings but is not independently diagnostic. Occasionally all the evidence will suggest rejection in the presence of a repeatedly negative biopsy. In such cases, once bacterial sepsis, viral infection, constrictive pericarditis, and tamponade are excluded, a left heart catheterization is likely to show diffuse coronary disease. Rejection episodes unresponsive to the oral pulse are treated with intravenous methylprednisolone, unless they are associated with hemodynamic instability or a low serum cyclosporine level, in which case intramuscular rabbit antithymocyte globulin (R-ATG) is added simultaneously. Uncomplicated rejection associated with an adequate cyclosporine level but failing to respond to intravenous methylprednisolone is treated with R-ATG or OKT-3 as a third stage.

Results   One-year survival with cyclosporine is 79% vs. 66% without cyclosporine and at 5 years the difference is 77% vs. 55%. Although long-term survival appears to be excellent, perioperative mortality remains high. During 1985 there was 12% mortality during the first 30 days. In cyclosporine-treated patients, 30-day mortality was attributed to rejection in 22%, infection in 20%, and "cardiac" and other causes in the majority (58%). In patients treated with cyclosporine, the percentage of mortality due to infection eventually accounts for about 40% of the mortality. Death due to rejection remains relatively stable throughout, at 20–25%. Infectious complications in cardiac transplant recipients are most often pulmonary.

One unfortunate consequence of denervation is that angina cannot occur as a premonitory symptom in patients developing graft atherosclerosis, so that these patients tend to present with sudden death or congestive heart failure. The coronary atherosclerosis seen in cardiac transplants is characteristically diffuse and progressive, frequently occurring in the first 1–2 years, with an incidence of about 10%. The leading suspicion regarding etiology is that the phenomenon reflects chronic low-grade rejection that is poorly detected by conventional means, and raises concern that the incidence may continue to increase. In Stanford's first 106 patients, 97% were restored to NYHA Class I existence. At Columbia Presbyterian, 62% of patients have returned to their previous lifestyle after 6 months, a figure that rises to 100% after 2 years. At the other end of the spectrum, results in infants and children have been disappointing, with 1-year survival of only 49% in the 0–10 age group recorded in the registry.

Heart-Lung

Patients who might benefit from heart-lung transplant have suffered irreversible damage to both the heart and lungs. In pulmonary vascular disease the high-resistance circulatory disorder is primary, while in respiratory diseases chronic disturbance in gas exchange and alveolar mechanics leads to a secondary increase in pulmonary vascular resistance.

Recipient Selection   The rarity of suitable donors makes it mandatory to select only patients with the greatest probability of a good outcome. Results have been best in young patients with end-stage primary pulmonary hypertension (PPH) or Eisenmenger's syndrome. In patients thought to have PPH it is important to exclude chronic pulmonary thromboembolism.

Postoperative Care During the first 2 weeks, before lymphatic drainage is reestablished and ischemic injury has healed, the lungs are kept as dry as possible with vigorous diuresis. Tracheal healing is carefully protected by withholding maintenance steroids for 2–3 weeks. Maintenance cyclosporine treatment is augmented during that period with azathioprine, and frequently with antithymocyte globulin as well. Surveillance for cardiac rejection with endomyocardial biopsies cannot be relied upon to faithfully mirror activity in the lungs. Diagnosis of lung rejection is based on arterial blood gases, chest x-rays, bronchoscopy, and airway cultures. Cardiac rejection in heart-lung transplantation is seen with much lower frequency than in cardiac transplantation ($p < 0.01$).

Results In early 1986, with just 91 cases recorded, 1-year survival was a rather disappointing 54%. The 3-year actuarial survival of 51% provides some reason for optimism. Heart-lung transplant offers an excellent therapeutic alternative in certain diseases for which no other treatment exists, but long-term durability remains uncertain, and the procedure is likely to remain a therapeutic frontier for the rest of the decade.

Single Lung

The first human lung transplant was performed in 1963, and was followed by more than 45 attempts around the world during the next 20 years, without a single long-term success. Bronchial healing seemed to pose an insolvable problem. Single lung transplantation in patients with emphysema set the stage for major ventilation/perfusion mismatch, because of preferential ventilation and air trapping in the highly compliant native lung at the same time that perfusion was directed almost exclusively to the low compliance vascular bed of the transplanted lung. By the end of 1986 seven single transplants had been performed with five long-term survivors. Initial experience focused entirely on patients with pulmonary fibrosis, avoiding patients with emphysema and cystic fibrosis.

It still appears that patients with end-stage pulmonary

disease who have significant right ventricular failure will be operable only with combined heart-lung transplant. Patients with preserved right ventricular function should receive a single lung transplant for pulmonary fibrosis, and double lung transplant for obstructive and septic diseases. Heart-lung transplant should be reserved for patients with pulmonary vascular disease, and possibly for selected patients with nonvascular pulmonary disease and significant right ventricular failure.

Kidney

Transplantation, when successful, offers a greater degree of rehabilitation to the uremic patient than does either hemodialysis or peritoneal dialysis. Children should be transplanted because growth is better after transplantation. Diabetics seem to have fewer problems after transplantation than during dialysis. Older patients without related donors, however, may survive longer on hemodialysis. All patients with HLA-identical sibling donors should certainly be transplanted. In other groups of patients, the indications are less clear and the preference of the individual is the dominant factor. Most patients who have had a transplant—even one that has failed—prefer life with a kidney transplantation to life on dialysis.

A few renal diseases will recur in transplants, but such diseases are only relative contraindications; focal glomerulosclerosis, hemolytic uremia syndrome, membranoproliferative glomerulonephritis of the dense-deposit type, and diabetes are among them.

A number of metabolic diseases (gout, oxalosis, cystinosis, hyperoxaluria, nephrocalcinosis and amyloidosis) have very little in common except for the accumulation within the kidney of abnormal deposits associated with renal failure. Transplants in most of these diseases can be successful, although recurrence after oxalosis is common.

Peripheral neuropathy, uncontrollable hypertension, severe anemia, severe bone disease (especially in children), all should lead to early dialysis and transplantation. Most patients with end-stage renal disease will undergo a period of dialysis prior to transplant. The urinary tract should be evaluated for patency of its outflow and absence of ureterovesical reflux. Tissue typing to match donor and recipient is extremely valuable in family donor selection because HLA identity between siblings occurs 25% of the time and has long-term success rates of 95%. There is controversy whether matching unrelated cadaver donors with recipients will have beneficial consequences for the outcome of renal transplantation. It is important to determine whether a recipient has antibodies against antigens on donor tissue. Patients who have been presensitized by blood transfusion, pregnancy, or previous transplantation can then be identified by serum reactivity against a panel of normal leukocytes bearing known HLA specificities.

Because many patients have preformed antibodies against a potential renal allograft donor, cross matching of the patient's serum to detect antibodies against donor leukocytes must be carried out immediately prior to the transplant. If these preformed antibody barriers are crossed, immediate (hyperacute) or accelerated rejection frequently ensues.

Selection and Evaluation of Living Donors Even mismatched sibling and parent kidneys may survive with better function than do closely matched cadaver kidneys. HLA-identical sibling grafts have better than 95% chance for long-term success.

A living related donor offers other advantages to the recipient; the delay between renal failure and rehabilitation is shorter, posttransplant renal function is usually immediate, and there are fewer rejection episodes, so that smaller doses of immunosuppressive drugs are required. Although a number of successful allotransplants have been carried out across AB isoantibody barriers, it is generally unwise to perform transplants into patients with known preformed isohemagglutinins against the donor blood type. The risk of life to a perfectly healthy donor has been estimated to be 0.05%. Much evidence suggests that no long-term harm results from life with a single kidney. No pressure is exerted to persuade or dissuade potential donors. Donors under the age of 18 should not be used except for identical-twin transplants.

Selection of Cadaver Donor The ideal cadaver kidney donor (1) is young, (2) has remained normotensive until a short time before death, (3) is free of transmissible infection and malignant disease, and (4) has died in the hospital after observation for a number of hours. Under these ideal conditions the donor kidneys can be removed within minutes to minimize the warm ischemia time. Not more than 1 h of warm ischemia time should elapse during donation.

Criteria of Brain Death The exact criteria of brain death vary among institutions; Table 10-2 lists the guidelines for the determination of death reported to the President's Commission for the Study of Ethical Problems in Medicine and Biomedical and Behavioral Research by a panel of medical consultants. It is possible to harvest kidneys at the moment

TABLE 10-2.   Criteria for Determination of Death

An individual with the findings in either section A (cardiopulmonary) or B (neurologic) is dead.

A. Cardiopulmonary
　Irreversible cessation of circulatory and respiratory functions
　1. Absence of responsiveness, heartbeat, respiratory effort.
　2. Irreversibility is recognized by persistent cessation of functions during an appropriate period of observation and/or trial of therapy.
B. Neurologic
　Irreversible cessation of all functions of the entire brain, including the brain stem.
　1. Cessation is recognized when evaluation discloses findings of *a* and *b.*
　　a. Cerebral functions are absent.
　　b. Brain stem functions are absent.
　2. Irreversibility is recognized when evaluation discloses findings of *a* and *b* and *c.*
　　a. The cause of coma is established and is sufficient to account for the loss of brain functions.
　　b. The possibility of recovery of any brain functions is excluded.
　　c. The cessation of all brain function persists for an appropriate period of observation and/or trial of therapy.

of death and preserve them in iced solutions or by perfusion for more than 24 h until the transplant recipients are ready. Kidneys can now be preserved by hypothermic perfusion for more than 48 h. The development of preservation also allows for more careful typing, matching, shipping, and sharing of organs between various centers.

Recipient Technique   It is rarely necessary to remove the kidneys from most patients. Removal of the patient's diseased kidneys may be considered to control hypertension, to eliminate a source of infection, or eliminate the nephrotic syndrome. The renal artery and vein are anastomosed to the iliac vessels. Urine usually appears within a few minutes of completion of the vascular anastomoses in related living donor kidneys. Ureteroneocystostomy is usually used for establishing urinary tract continuity.

Prophylactic Immunosuppression   Immunosuppressive management centers now consist of cyclosporine and prednisone. Because of cyclosporine's nephrotoxic properties, ALG or azathioprine or both are sometimes employed until renal function approaches more normal levels. Then ALG is stopped and cyclosporine started. Most centers are currently individualizing the concurrent use of all four of these drugs, but cyclosporine has replaced azathioprine as the backbone of the regimen. A higher dose of prednisone is used for rejection episodes. Some centers reserve the use of ALG or monoclonal antilymphocyte antibodies to treat steroid-resistant rejection episodes.

COMPLICATIONS   Renal Failure   The most serious complication of renal transplantation is the failure of the graft to initiate or maintain function. The functional failure of the kidney is best examined in relation to the time after transplantation. The kidney may (1) never function, (2) have delayed onset of functions, (3) fail to function after a brief or prolonged time, or (4) gradually lose its function over a period of months or years. In each phase, four general diagnoses should be considered: (1) ischemic damage to the kidney; (2) rejection of the kidney by reactions directed against histocompatibility antigens on the kidney; (3) technical complications; and (4) the development of renal disease, either a new disease or recurrence of the original.

Early Anuria and Oliguria   Early anuria or oliguria is a major diagnostic problem. The possibilties include (1) hypovolemia, (2) thrombosis of the renal artery or renal vein, (3) hyperacute rejection of the kidney, (4) ischemic renal damage (ATN), (5) compression of the kidney (by hematoma, seroma, or lymph), and (6) obstruction of the urinary flow.

If an obstructed catheter has not caused the oliguria, one must rule out hemorrhage and hypovolemia combined with compression or displacement of the kidney. Restoration of the blood volume will seldom suffice to restore renal function. Many patients will require reexploration to control the bleeding point.

Technical Complications   Thrombosis of the renal arterial anastomosis is rare. Partial obstruction due to torsion or kinking of the vessels is more common and should be promptly repaired. When the renogram demonstrates poor concentration of the ^{131}I Hippuran, an arteriogram should be performed to detect correctable technical complications. Thrombosis of the renal vein occurs even more rarely than thrombosis of the renal artery. When it does occur, thrombosis of the artery ensues because the collateral venous circulation of the kidney has been interrupted by the transplant procedure. Partial thrombosis of the renal and iliac veins has occurred. Usually, this is accompanied by swelling of the ipsilateral lower extremity, fever, and evidence of pulmonary embolism.

Formerly, one of the most common, and most frequently fatal, complications following renal transplantation was urinary extravasation due to distal ureteral necrosis. Rejection was seldom at fault. Urinary extravasation is a serious complication that can lead to infection. It demands urgent reexploration with reimplantation of the ureter into the bladder, nephrostomy, or performance of a pyeloureterostomy to the host ureter. Delay in definitive repair frequently will lead to infection, loss of kidney, and death.

Technical errors can become manifest long after the immediate posttransplant period. Arterial stenosis, venous thrombosis, and late ureteral leaks and strictures frequently are confused with rejection. Prior to any antirejection treatment, technical problems should be ruled out by echography, arteriography, renography, or percutaneous nephrostograms.

Hyperacute Rejection Hyperacute rejection of the kidney is almost always mediated by humoral antibody, with the subsequent participation of the complement, coagulation, and kinin cascade systems. Platelets, PMNs, and vasospasm may also play a role. Classical hyperacute rejection is now rare because laboratory techniques can demonstrate cytotoxic antibody directed against donor histocompatibility antigens positive cross match. A rare patient will have a hyperacute rejection in the absence of demonstrable cytotoxic antibody.

Acute Tubular Necrosis If all other causes of renal functional failure in the early posttransplant period have been ruled out, one must assume that the diagnosis is "acute tubular necrosis." ATN occurs most commonly when the donor has undergone long periods of stress and hypotensive insult to the kidney to be transplanted. Another cause of recipient ATN is a long period of warm ischemia preceding transplantation. Cold ischemia is much better tolerated, and preservation up to 48 h is now satisfactory but not preferable.

Almost all transplanted kidneys have undergone some degree of damage secondary to trauma and ischemia. A second trauma (hypovolemia, hypoxemia, renal compression, bacteremia, allergic reactions to ALG) that normally might not result in ATN in normal kidneys may cause oliguria in transplanted kidneys. One must not diagnose rejection and institute massive steroid therapy in the early posttransplantation period without ruling out the possibility that an additional insult to an already damaged kidney has occurred and that the diagnosis is not acute rejection but ATN. Renal biopsy may be necessary to make this differentiation.

Rejection With better immunosuppression, the acute rejection episodes that formerly appeared in the first month following transplantation are seen less frequently. The majority of patients, however, will sustain at least one acute rejection episode during the first 3–4 months following transplantation. Clinical rejection is rarely an all-or-nothing re-action, and the first episode seldom progresses to complete renal destruction. The functional changes induced by rejec-tion appear to be in large part reversible; therefore, the recognition and treatment of the rejection episode prior to the development of severe renal damage is of extreme importance. Usually the rejection reaction responds to in-creased prednisone doses. Even with prompt treatment the creatinine clearance may be permanently impaired, however slightly, following each clinical rejection episode.

Differential Diagnosis The clinical picture of a rejection reaction may be distressingly similar to several other prob-lems: ureter leak or obstruction, hemorrhage with consequent ATN, infection, or stenosis or twist in the renal artery or vein. Classic renal rejection is characterized by oliguria, enlargement and tenderness of the graft, malaise, fever, leukocytosis, hypertension, weight gain, and peripheral edema. Laboratory studies have shown lymphocyturia, red cell casts, proteinuria, immunoglobulin fragments, fibrin fragments in the urine, complementuria, lysozymuria, decreased urine sodium excretion, renal tubular acidosis, and increased lactic dehydrogenase in the urine. The level of the blood urea nitrogen increases, as does serum creatinine. Creatinine clearance is obviously decreased; renograms will show slow uptake of the Hippuran and slow urinary excretion. Echog-raphy can show edema of the renal papillae.

The most important parameter to follow is the serum creatinine level. Unlike the BUN, which is sensitive to a number of changes (steroid administration, fever, and high-protein diet), serum creatinine levels are relatively stable for each patient.

Treatment Most institutions have developed a standard rejection regimen for allografted kidneys utilizing injections of steroids, ALG, and monoclonal antibodies. This standard regimen can be repeated as many as three times within a 2-month period in patients for whom rejection appears to be unremitting. If it is repeated more often than that, infection may appear and be lethal. The decision to stop immuno-suppression and sacrifice the transplant frequently depends on subtle factors and is difficult to make, particularly in patients who have deterioration of renal function over a period of months and years.

Special Topics Certain diseases are known to recur in the transplanted kidney. Transplantation is not necessarily con-traindicated in these diseases, since the recurrence is unpre-dictable. The best example is diabetes, in which the histolgic features of diabetes often recur with only gradual deterioration of function. Graft survivals are > 95% with HLA-identical transplants and 85–90% with cadaveric grafts using ALG, prednisone, cyclosporine, and imuran.

Traditionally, young children have not been considered ideal candidates for renal transplantation, although excellent results have been reported. The small caliber of vessels and active social behavior of children make their management on hemodialysis extremely difficult. Long-term hemodialysis is seldom satisfactory, and a parent is almost always willing to donate a kidney. Several infants have had transplants, and at least one has survived for more than 1 year. Most children with allografts grow slightly more slowly than normal. A number of studies have shown that second and third transplants arè less successful than the first, if the first was rejected soon after transplantation. The rejection of one transplant may sensitize the patient to a number of weaker histocompatibility antigens that cannot be easily detected by sensitive cross-match techniques.

ORGAN PRESERVATION

Only cadaver donors can be used for some organs (heart and liver), and even when the organ is expendable (as in one of a pair of kidneys), the use of cadaver donors avoids the risks inherent in surgical removal of the organ from living persons. Time-consuming procedures, such as tolerance induction, may ultimately become available to pretreat the recipient and make him or her unresponsive to specific histocompatibility antigens.

Methods of Viable Organ Preservation

The main problem associated with preservation of organs in a viable state seems to be hypoxia. When the organ is removed from its physiologic state, it is deprived of its normal oxygenation. Metabolic inhibition seeks to prevent the normal catabolic processes from causing severe or irreversible damage to the tissues, during the period of preservation. It is currently best achieved by hypothermia, which protects the organ by slowing metabolic activity and decreasing oxygen need. Two techniques of cooling are currently available: (1) simple cooling of a kidney by immersing it in or flushing it with a cold solution, and (2) perfusion cooling, which allows longer periods of preservation.

Metabolic maintenance, attempts to sustain a level of

metabolic activity as close to physiologic normalcy as is feasible. Usually it implies perfusion of the organ in vitro with a carefully controlled fluid medium. In practice metabolic maintenance is always best combined with perfusion cooling. There is evidence that an adequate flow rate during perfusion is a good prognostic sign of the viability and transplantability of the organ. Causes of interstitial edema are perfusate osmolarity and excessive perfusion pressure. Even hypothermia alone may cause cellular swelling. When plasma products are used as perfusates, immunologic damage is possible. This may be due to antibodies directed against organ antigens or to the precipitation of circulating antigen-antibody complexes within the organ. Various pharmacologic agents have also been used as metabolic inhibitors. These include such drugs as magnesium sulfate, chlorpromazine, chloroquine, hydrocortisone, and diuretics such as mersalyl. Unfortunately, experiments utilizing such agents in addition to hypothermia show little additive effect.

11 COMPLICATIONS

Surgical care must fully encompass an appreciation and anticipation of postoperative complications from the disease process per se, or from errors of omission or commission.

Wound Complications

Disruption or dehiscence generally refers to a separation of an abdominal wound involving the anterior fascial sheath and deeper layers. The frequency is reported in ranges from 0.5–3% for abdominal wounds. (See Table 11-1.)

CLINICAL MANIFESTATIONS Most dehiscences are concealed in deeper layers of the wound and do not manifest until the fifth postoperative day, although the separation may occur in the operating room or recovery room. The presenting sign that precedes the diagnosis in 85% of cases is serosanguineous drainage from the wounds, and if it occurs more than 24 h postoperatively, is pathognomonic.

TREATMENT Operative closure with through-and-through horizontal mattress sutures placed superficial to the peritoneum or buried figure-of-eight monofilament stainless-steel sutures are preferred to approximate the muscle and fascial layers. In some instances, it is preferable to treat the patient conservatively with occlusive dressing and a binder.

The main morbidity is prolonged hospitalization. The incidence of postoperative hernia is at least 32%.

Wound Infection

Most wounds become infected in the operating room while they are open, but the presence of bacteria in the wound at the end of surgical procedure does not usually result in a wound infection.

The most common infection is *Staphylococcus aureus,* but enteric organisms may be the causative agents when bowel operations have been performed, and hemolytic streptocci account for about 3%. Other common organisms include enterococci, *Pseudomonas, Proteus,* and *Klebsiella.*

Factors that influence wound infection are break in sterile technique, traumatic wounds, age, diabetes, steroids, mal-

TABLE 11-1.   Dehiscence

Local factors	General factors
Hemorrhage	Hypoproteinemia
Infection	Increased interabdominal
Excessive suture material	pressure
Poor technique	Coughing
	Retching
	Hiccuping
	Obesity
	Steroids

nutrition, patients with other infections, duration of surgery, use of drains, prolonged preoperative hospitalization, and multi-antibiotics.

CLINICAL MANIFESTATIONS   Typically infection occurs 3–4 days following operation. Signs and symptoms include fever, edema of wound, redness of wound, pain, and thrombosis of surrounding vessels.

TREATMENT   The treatment consists of surgical drainage. As a general principle antimicrobial drugs are not required unless the organism is *Streptoccus pyogenes* or hemolytic streptococci. Patients with infections around the face or associated systemic bacteremia or spreading cellulitis require antimicrobial therapy. The antibiotic used is determined by culture and sensitivity studies of the wound.

Wound Hemorrhage, Hematoma, and Seroma

Wound hemorrhage is related to an error in technique in which hemostasis was not accomplished. Hemostasis is compromised in patients receiving anticoagulant therapy, polycythemia vera, and myeloproliferative disorders, and in patients with coagulation defects.

POSTOPERATIVE RESPIRATORY COMPLICATIONS

Respiratory Failure

Acute respiratory failure is when the Pa_{O_2} is below the predicted normal for the patient's age or the Pa_{CO_2} is above 50 mmHg in the absence of metabolic alkalosis.

The pathophysiologic components include hypoventilation,

TABLE 11-2.   Indications for Ventilatory Support

Mechanics	Normal	Close monitoring	Intubation
Respiratory rate	12–20	20–30	>30
Vital capacity, mL/kg	70–30	30–15	<15
Inspiratory force, cmH_2	100–50	50–25	<25
Oxygenation, $(A–a)D_{O_2}$, torr*	100–200	200–350	>350
Ventilation, VD/VT	0.3–0.4	0.4–0.6	>0.6
Ventilation, Pa_{CO_2} torr	35–45	45–50	>50

* After 15 min of 100% 0_2.

diffusion defects, abnormalities in the ventilation/perfusion ratio, shunting that is either anatomic or related to atelectasis, reduction in cardiac output with shunt, alteration in the hemoglobin level, and changes in dissociation curve.

Clinical manifestations that should alert the observer to the development of postoperative pulmonary insufficiency include congestive failure, dyspnea, cyanosis, evidence of obstructive lung disease, pulmonary edema, and unexplained deterioration of arterial O_2 tension.

Tachypnea and hypoxemia are the earliest manifestations of respiratory insufficiency.

The diagnosis of adult respiratory distress syndrome (ARDS) is usually assigned when conservative measures such as oxygen by mask, pulmonary toilet, and/or bronchodilators fail to maintain the Pa_{O_2} above 60 torr.

TREATMENT   Control of postoperative pain can effect a significant reduction in the incidence of pulmonary complications following thoracic or upper abdominal operations. Use of epidural local anesthesia, spinal narcotics, and continuous narcotic infusion have all been used to control pain. The treatment of acute respiratory insufficiency is based primarily on ventilatory support.

Atelectasis

Atelectasis comprises 90% of all postoperative pulmonary complications. The two major factors that cause atelectasis are bronchial obstruction with distal gas absorption and hypoventilation or ineffectual respiration.

CLINICAL MANIFESTATIONS   Clinical manifestations usually appear in the first 24 h after an operation and rarely appear after 48 h. These include fever, tachycardia, rales, diminished breath sounds, bronchial breathing, and cyanosis.

TREATMENT Prophylaxis begins preoperatively by insisting that the patient cease smoking and instructing the patient in deep abdominal breathing and productive coughing.

Postoperative prophylaxis includes the minimal use of depressant drugs, the prevention of pain that may limit respiration, frequent changes of body position, deep breathing and coughing exercises, and early ambulation.

Pulmonary Edema

Pulmonary edema occurs during or immediately after an operation. The increased use of massive blood transfusions, plasma expanders, and other fluids during operative procedures has increased the incidence of this complication. Circulatory overload represents the most common cause of pulmonary edema. Other factors include left ventricular failure, shift of blood from the peripheral to pulmonary vascular bed, negative pressure on the airway that increases the gradient between the transmural capillary pressure and the alveolar pressure favoring transudation, and injury to the alveolar membrane by noxious substances. The early disturbances of pulmonary edema are accumulation of fluid in the sheath around small pulmonary arteries and thickening of the capillary and alveolar membranes.

Clinical manifestations are widening $A-a_{O_2}$ gradient, reduction in lung compliance, carbon dioxide retention, bronchospasm, frothy pink-stained fluids, and rales.

TREATMENT Therapy is directed at providing oxygen, allowing oxygen access to alveoli by removing obstructive fluid, and correcting circulatory overload.

Drug therapy includes furosemide or ethacrynic acid for rapid diuresis, and digitalis glycosides for heart failure or arrhythmia. CPAP can reverse the process in the nonintubated patient, whereas PEEP is most effective in the intubated patient.

CARDIAC COMPLICATIONS

Abnormal electrocardiograms are a common finding in the postoperative period. Although every type of EKG pattern may be seen postoperatively, certain arrhythmias occur with greater frequency following certain types of surgery or associated with specific clinical situations.

TABLE 11-3.   Etiology

1. Underlying cardiac disease
   a. Valvular disease
   b. Previous MI
2. Other medical conditions
   a. Chronic obstructive lung disease
   b. Hypertension
   c. Hyperthyroidism
   d. Diabetes mellitus
   e. Malignancy
3. Preoperative medication
   a. Digoxin
   b. Furosemide
   c. Tricyclic antidepressants
4. Electrolyte abnormalities
5. Types of surgery
   a. Head and neck surgery
   b. Involving the thorax
   c. Major vascular

Arrhythmias

Postoperative arrhythmia may be defined as any new disturbance of the cardiac rhythm or conduction abnormality excluding sinus tachycardia. The etiology involves several fractors. (See Table 11-3.)

EVALUATION OF POSTOPERATIVE ARRHYTHMIAS   Postoperative arrhythmias are most commonly paroxysmal supraventricular tachycardia (PAT); usually a routine EKG will provide an accurate diagnosis. The patient, because of obtundation, disorientation, endotracheal intubation, or incisional pain may not be able to accurately express cardiac symptoms. A substantial percentage of arrhythmias will be picked up by the routine EKG monitoring. Comparison of the current tracing with previous recordings is essential.

A systematic approach is the key (see Figs. 11-1 and 11-2).

EXTRASYSTOLE

1. Atrial premature contractions (APC). A premature QRS of normal contour is preceded by a P wave of abnormal morphology and axis.
2. A-V junctional premature contractions (JPC) may arise from any A-V junctional focus, and in most cases will

activate the entire atria by retrograde conduction and the ventricles by antegrade conduction.
3. Ventricular premature contractions (VPC) may originate from a single focus or multiple foci in the ventricles. The diagnostic criteria are: a bizarre and wide QRS (0.12 s or more); not preceded by an ectopic P wave; a constant coupling interval; and a fully compensating postectopic pause.

PARASYSTOLE Parasystole results from the simultaneous activity of two independent pacemakers, one usually in the sinus node and the other located most often in the ventricle.

TACHYARRHYTHMIAS The majority of arrhythmias occurring in the postoperative period have a rapid ventricular response rate. They may be atrial, A-V junctional, or ventricular in origin, but they are conveniently grouped as supraventricular tachyarrhythmias (SVT) or ventricular tachyarrhythmias. As a rule the lower the ectopic pacemaker, the more serious the nature and consequences of the arrhythmia.

Supraventricular Tachyarrhythmias The most common postoperative arrhythmias, SVTs, are often triggered by an ectopic supraventricular premature contraction, usually have a self-limiting and benign course, and are closely interrelated.

SVTs are often differentiated on the basis of the rate of the atrial activity:

60–150/min	=	nonparoxysmal A-V junctional tachycardia
160–250/min	=	paroxysmal atrial on A-V junctional tachycardia
250–300	=	atrial flutter
400–650	=	atrial fibrillation

Paroxysmal Atrial Tachycardia (PAT) Postoperative PAT is often triggered by an APC and has the potential to be converted into atrial flutter or fibrillation.

The diagnostic criteria are: regular ventricular activity, regular ectopic atrial P waves at a rate 160–250/min, isoelectric base line, constant A-V relationship, and narrow QRS.

Digoxin, propranolol, quinidine, and esmolol are all helpful in the treatment of PAT.

ATRIAL FLUTTER The diagnostic criteria are: regular ventricular beats, regular atrial activity rate 250–350, sawtooth pattern, constant A-V relationship, and narrow QRS.

Digoxin, quinidine, propranolol, esmolol, procainamide,

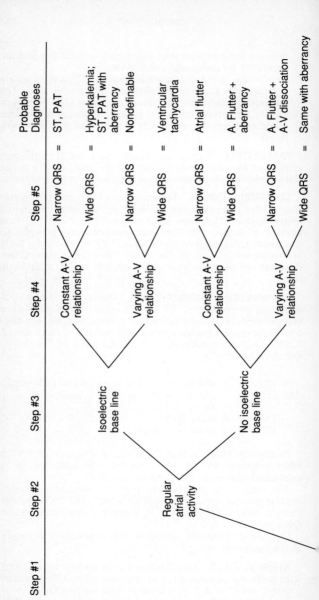

Step #1	Step #2	Step #3	Step #4	Step #5		Probable Diagnoses
	Regular atrial activity	Isoelectric base line	Constant A-V relationship	Narrow QRS	=	ST, PAT
				Wide QRS	=	Hyperkalemia; ST, PAT with aberrancy
			Varying A-V relationship	Narrow QRS	=	Nondefinable
				Wide QRS	=	Ventricular tachycardia
		No isoelectric base line	Constant A-V relationship	Narrow QRS	=	Atrial flutter
				Wide QRS	=	A. Flutter + aberrancy
			Varying A-V relationship	Narrow QRS	=	A. Flutter + A-V dissociation
				Wide QRS	=	Same with aberrancy

186

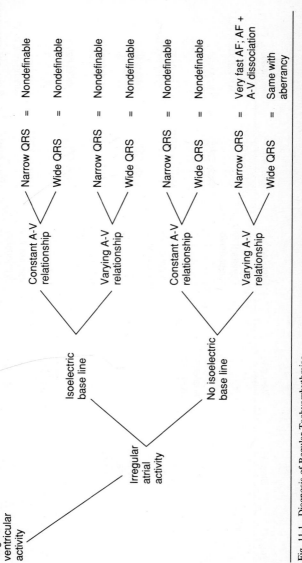

Fig. 11-1 Diagnosis of Regular Tachyarrhythmias

Step #1	Step #2	Step #3	Step #4	Step #5	Probable Diagnoses
	Regular atrial activity	Isoelectric base line	Constant A-V relationship	Narrow QRS =	Parasystole; ST or PAT + JPCs/PVCs
				Wide QRS =	Same with aberrancy
			Varying A-V relationship	Narrow QRS =	ST or PAT + varying A-V block
				Wide QRS =	Same with aberrancy
		No isoelectric base line	Constant A-V relationship	Narrow QRS =	Nondefinable
				Wide QRS =	Nondefinable
			Varying A-V relationship	Narrow QRS =	A. Flutter + varying A-V block
				Wide QRS =	Same with aberrancy

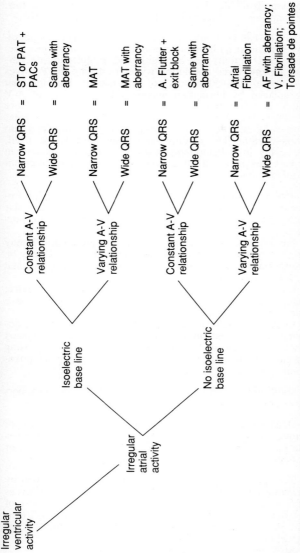

Fig. 11-2   Diagnosis of Irregular Tachyarrhythmias

and verapamil are all useful in the treatment of atrial flutter. DC cardioversion using very low energy is also effective.

ATRIAL FIBRILLATION (AF) The most common postoperative SVT is atrial fibrillation and the diagnostic criteria are: ventricular activity that is chaotic and irregular in rate 120–180; chaotic atrial fibrillation waves replacing the P waves at a rate of 400–650; absence of an isoelectric base line that is replaced by fibrillation waves; varying degree of A-V block; and narrow QRS. Digoxin or carotid sinus pressure increases the A-V block and slows the ventricular rate. Verapamil may do the same, or occasionally convert it into sinus rhythm. DC cardioversion may have to be used, especially in a hemodynamically compromised patient in order to restore an effective atrial systole, which will augment cardiac output.

VENTRICULAR TACHYCARDIA (VT) In spite of the high frequency of PVCs in the postoperative period, ventricular tachyarrhythmias are remarkably uncommon following surgery.

Present when three or more VPCs are grouped, VT may originate from any ectopic focus in the ventricles. It may be paroxysmal with a rate of 160–250/min or nonparoxysmal with a slower rate of 70–130/min.

Diagnostic criteria include regular ventricular activity; independent, mostly regular, atrial activity; isoelectric base line; A-V dissociation; and wide and bizarre QRS.

Ventricular tachycardia frequently compromises the hemodynamics of the patient, especially when the underlying heart disease is advanced. The treatment must be immediate, using an antiarrhythmic agent and/or DC cardioversion. Hypokalemia must be corrected.

BRADYARRHYTHMIAS Unlike tachyarrhythmias postoperative bradyarrhythmias are relatively uncommon events.

Sinus Arrest. In this arrhythmia, there is an absence of impulse generation by the sinus node. In prolonged cases the lower pacemaker usually takes over (A-V junctional or idioventricular).

Sinus Exit (S-A) Block. When the impulse is generated by the sinus node, but fails to activate the atria, various degrees of S-A block are said to be present, although only those of the second degree can be diagnosed with the surface EKG. The second-degree S-A block is classified into Mobitz Type I (Wenckebach), and Mobitz Type II block. Atropine is the drug of choice.

MYOCARDIAL INFARCTION

The majority of patients who died suddenly during the operative and immediate postoperative period demonstrated coronary artery thrombosis or myocardial infarction at autopsy.

Clinical Manifestations   The majority of cases occur on the operative day or during the first 3 postoperative days.

Treatment   Treatment of myocardial infarction consists of relief of pain, relief of hypoxia, and treatment of arrhythmias.

12 PHYSIOLOGIC MONITORING OF THE SURGICAL PATIENT

With all the technical breakthroughs in the last decade, the physician is now overwhelmed with monitors in the critical care and operative areas. But the most sophisticated and advanced electronic systems can never substitute for the close surveillance by an experienced and qualified health professional.

BASIC MONITORING

Monitoring is noninvasive or invasive (listed in Table 12-1). These monitors provide a collection of physiologic variables, shown in Table 12-2. Arterial pressures, heart rate, temperature, and respiratory rate are the most commonly monitored variables because they are the most easily measured. These measurements should be determined routinely in all patients.

Observations of the patient's mental status provide important clues to the presence of hypoxemia, hypercapnia, and acidosis. Restlessness and confusion can be early warning signs of sepsis and low-output states.

ARTERIAL PRESSURE Arterial pressure, the most frequently monitored circulatory variable, reflects the overall circulatory status. Arterial pressure falls after hypovolemia from blood or fluid loss, cardiac failure, and in the terminal stage of most diseases. The pressures do not directly measure reductions of blood flow and volume; rather, they measure the failure of circulatory compensations.

Normal blood pressure taken by sphygmomanometer cuff is approximately 120/80 mmHg for young adults, but this increases with age. A simple guide is that the upper limit of normal systolic pressure is 160 and diastolic pressure is 100; above these parameters is considered hypertensive.

An important measurement is the pulse pressure, which is the difference between systolic and diastolic pressure. Mean arterial pressure (MAP) is the diastolic pressure plus one-third of the pulse pressure.

Intraarterial pressure is commonly measured in critically ill patients and gives a continuous waveform. Indications for this type of continuous monitoring are shock, critical illness, and intraoperative and postoperatirve monitoring in extensive

TABLE 12-1.   Monitoring Procedures

Noninvasive procedures
  Physical examination
  Electrical sensing with surface electrodes. e.g., ECG and EEF
  Impedance phlebography
  Arterial tonometry
  Gas sampling using skin surface probes
  Radiologic examination
  Bedside mass spectrometry
  Expired gas analysis
Invasive procedures
  Intravenous injection and blood sampling from capillaries and peripheral
    veins
  Cutaneous needle electrodes for ECG and EEG
  Rectal probe for temperature
  Bladder catheter for renal function
  Tissue oxygen probe
  Intraarterial and venous gas tension and pH analysis
Highly invasive procedures
  Arterial and central venous catheter
  Intracardiac probes
  Transcardiac probes for pulmonary artery catheter for pressures and
    flows
  Subarachnoid probes for pressure
  Intracranial probes for CSF pressures and flows

TABLE 12-2.   Physiologic Variables (in Order of Increased Specificity)

1. Arterial blood pressure
2. Heart rate, respiratory rate
3. Temperature
4. Hematocrit and hemoglobin concentration
5. Urine output rate
6. Central venous pressure (CVP)
7. Electrocardiogram (ECG), chest x-ray
8. Serum electrolytes: Na^+, Cl^-, HCO_3^-, BUN, creatinine
9. Arterial blood gases—pH
10. Tidal volume (V_T), respiratory rate (f), minute volume (MV)
11. FeNa, RF1, creatinine clearance
12. Plasma and urine osmolalities, osmolar and free water clearances
13. Electroencephalogram (EEG)
14. Intracranial pressure (ICP)
15. Pulmonary arterial and capillary wedge pressure (PAP and PCWP)
16. Cardiac output and hemodynamic variables
17. O_2 transport variables: O_2 delivery, O_2 consumption (V_{O_2}), and O_2 extraction rate
18. End-tidal CO_2 (PET_{CO_2}, V_{CO_2}, V_D/V_T, $P(A\text{-}a)D_{O_2}$)
19. Mass spectrometry
20. Transcutaneous O_2 and CO_2

operations. This type of monitoring also allows for frequent arterial blood gas measurements. Intraarterial catheters may be placed in the radial, femoral, or axillary arteries. Complications are infrequent, but may include hematoma and bleeding at the catheter site; dissection of the intima by needle or the guide wire; arteriovenous fistula and pseudoaneurysm; arterial thrombosis; arterial occlusion, ischemia, or infection.

HEART RATE   This is usually counted by manual palpation of the radial artery. Heart rate is also measured automatically with the EKG or the intraarterial pressure monitor. Tachycardia is a rate above 100. The EKG should be evaluated for rate, irregularities in waveforms, dropped beats, and differences from base line.

Heart rate is very nonspecific, but an increase may suggest infection, anxiety, poor volume status, pain, and discomfort.

TEMPERATURE   Body temperature is taken orally or rectally. In the operating room and the ICU it is determined by thermocouples.

Elevations are associated with infection, tissue necrosis, late-stage carcinomatosis, Hodgkin's disease, leukemias, and hypermetabolic states. Hypothermia is associated with late septic shock, reduced metabolism associated with hypothyroidism, malnutrition, and cold exposure.

RESPIRATORY RATE   One of the earliest responses to a decrease in Pa_{O_2} or a rise in Pa_{CO_2} is an increase in respiratory rate. The normal range is 10–16 breaths per minute. Rates over 30 indicate severe respiratory distress. The health care worker should also observe the respiratory pattern. Rapid, shallow respirations are common with interstitial edema, whereas large tidal volumes are typical of pulmonary vascular disease, metabolic acidosis, and sepsis. Rates of less than 12 suggest central nervous system depression. Irregular patterns may indicate central nervous system disease or cardiovascular disease.

BODY WEIGHT   A daily record of body weight is often an important indicator of fluid balance.

URINE OUTPUT   The hourly rate of urine output (normal output = $\frac{1}{2}$ mL/kg/h) is a reasonable measure of perfusion of the kidney. Renal function can also be monitored by measurement of plasma (P_{osm}) and urine (U_{osm}) osmolality as well as calculation of osmolar and free water clearance. The ratio of U_{osm}/P_{osm} of over 1.7 indicates a good concentrating ability. The osmolar clearance (C_{osm}) formula is

$$C_{osm} = \frac{U_{osm}}{P_{osm}} \times \text{urine output (1 h)} \qquad N: 100\text{--}125 \text{ mL/h}$$

Creatine clearance (C_{cr}) reflects the glomerular function:

$$C_{cr} = \frac{U_{cr} \times \text{urine vol (1 h)} \times 1.73}{P_{cr} \times 60 \times \text{body surface area}} \quad N: 100-125 \text{ mL/h}$$

INVASIVE MONITORING

Arterial Blood-Gas Analysis

These data provide information on pH, efficiency of gas transfer, shunting, O_2-carrying capacity, and O_2 delivery.

Oxygen is carried in combination with hemoglobin; delivery depends on flow and the amount of oxygen available to the hemoglobin. Calculation of alveolar O_2 can be calculated from the equation:

$$Pa_{O_2} = Fi_{O_2}(P_B - 47) - P_{CO_2}/0.8$$

where P_B = barometric pressure;

　　　47 = H_2O, water vapor pressure.

Oxygen consumption = arterial O_2 transport − venous O_2
　　　　　　　　　　　　　transport
　　　　　　　　　　 = (C.I.)(13.9)(Hb) (arterial O_2 SAT
　　　　　　　　　　　　　− venous O_2 SAT)

Oxygen content = bound O_2 + dissolved O_2
　　　　　　　　 = Hb × 1.39 × O_2 + P_{O_2} × 0.003

The frequency for measurement of blood gases depends on the clinical situation. It is important to monitor trends in blood gases in order to predict and treat acute respiratory decompensation.

End-tidal CO_2 monitoring can be an extremely valuable diagnostic tool for detecting many conditions including malignant hyperthermia, pulmonary embolus, and decreased cardiac output.

CARDIOVASCULAR PHYSIOLOGY IN ACUTE ILLNESS

The assessment of oxygen transport (or the delivery of oxygen from the atmosphere to the mitochondria of the body cell mass) can be used as the most important monitor of patient outcome. The period immediately after acute injury is characterized by systemic O_2 consumption ($\dot{V}_{O_2}$) that may be less than normal. The period of initial resuscitation is quickly followed by an increase in $\dot{V}_{O_2}$. An increase in systemic $\dot{V}_{O_2}$ is, therefore, a characteristic response to injury and sepsis.

To ensure cellular survival, microcirculation ($\dot{D}_{O_2}$) must balance systemic $\dot{V}_{O_2}$.

Serum lactate levels.   The clinician can use arterial blood lactate levels to discover areas of impaired tissue perfusion. Tissue hypoxia stimulates anaerobic metabolism, with subsequent overproduction of lactate.

CARDIOVASCULAR MONITORING

Two important points must be made about the physiology of blood flow. Cardiac output alone is not an indicator of myocardial contractility, and arterial blood pressure is not an indicator of blood flow.

Cardiac output, the actual amount of blood ejected by the heart, is related to stroke volume and heart rate and is governed by preload and afterload.

The afterload is the impedance to cardiac ejection during systole imposed by vascular resistance, blood pressure, and blood viscosity. The preload is the degree of muscle fiber stretch imposed by filling of the ventricles during diastole.

The bedside determination of fundamental hemodynamic variables such as cardiac output and wedge pressure is essential for proper management of critically ill surgical patients. Placement of the pulmonary artery catheter (Swan-Ganz) is now common practice.

Pulmonary capillary wedge pressure (PCWP) equated with left atrial pressure assumes an open circuit from the catheter tip to the left atrium. Factors that can influence PCWP include mitral valve disease, pulmonary disease, reduced ventricular compliance, and positive pressure ventilation.

Central venous oximetry is one of the most important data points collected from the pulmonary artery catheter. The mixed venous oxygen ($S_{V_{O_2}}$) level reflects an estimate to

TABLE 12-3.   Hemodynamic and Respiratory Profile

Data to be gathered and used for calculations	Abbreviations
1. Determine body surface area by using height and weight and referring to BSA chart. (BSA is used to index measured and derived values to the size of the patient.)	BSA
2. Determine cardiac output using average of 5 outputs. (10 cc D_5W injected onto prox. port.)	CO
3. Draw arterial blood sample, process in blood-gas machine and in co-oximeter.	Arterial: pH (art.), P_{O_2}, P_{CO_2} Art. O_2 Sat. (CO - OX)
4. Draw mixed venous blood sample (using heparinized syringe) from distal pulm. art. cath. port over 2–3 min. time span. Process in blood-gas machine and in co-oximeter.	Mixed venous: pH, P_{CO_2}, PV_{O_2} MV_{O_2} Sat. (CO − OX)
5. Note heart rate.	HR
6. Note central venous pressure.	CVP
7. Note pulm. cap. wedge pressure. Also known as pulmonary artery occlusion pressure.	PCWP, PAoP
8. Note systemic arterial systolic and diastolic blood pressures or mean arterial pressure [mean = DP + ⅓ (SP − DP)]	SYST/DIAS, MAP
9. Note pulmonary artery systolic and diastolic blood pressures or mean PA pressure.	PA.SYST/PS DIAS, MPAP or PA
10. Note fraction of inspired oxygen.	Fi_{O_2}
11. Note hemoglobin.	Hb
12. Note positive end-expiratory pressure.	PEEP
13. Cardiovascular drugs and lactic acid measurements should also be noted when applicable.	

which the body is using oxygen. In critically ill surgical patients Sv_{O_2} does not correlate with individual tissue determinations of oxygen transport but only reflects the overall balance between oxygen consumption and delivery. A recent development has been pulmonary artery catheters with fiberoptic light bundles to allow for continuous measurements of oxygen saturation of mixed venous blood.

The goal of hemodynamic monitoring is therefore to ensure that oxygen delivery to the tissue meets or exceeds metabolic demands (see Table 12-3).

Noninvasive Techniques

As medical electronics develop more and more, data can be gained by the noninvasive means of pulse oximetry, end-tidal CO_2 monitors, echocardiographic devices, and metabolic charts.

A summary of selected variables is shown in Table 12-4.

TABLE 12-4.   Selected Variables

Calculation	Normal values, units
Hemodynamic Formulas	
1. Cardiac index $= \dfrac{CO}{BSA}$ (Prime determinant of hemodynamic function, volume of blood pumped by ventricle per minute)	$CI = 2.5\text{--}4$ L/min/m^2
2. Stroke index $= \dfrac{CI \times 1000}{HR}$ (Average volume ejected by ventricle with each beat)	$SI = 35\text{--}40$ cc/beat/m^2 BSA
3. Systemic vascular resistance index $=$ MAP $-$ CVP $\times$ 80 (customary measure of resistance in systemic circuit)	SVRI* $= 2180 \pm 210$ dyne/s/cm^5/m^2
4. Pulmonary vascular resistance index $=$ MPAP $-$ PCW $\times$ 80 (measure of resistance in pulmonary vasculature, computation is analogous to SVRI)	PVRI* $= 240 \pm 45$ dyne/s/cm^5/m^2
Oxygen and Respiratory Formulas Oxygen Content $=$ bound O_2 + dissolved O_2 $= $ (Hb $\times$ 1.39 $\times$ O_2 sat. $+$ ($P_{O_2} \times 0.003$) (1.39 mL O_2 can combine with 1 g Hb; however, others use 1.34 or 1.36, as uncertainty exists about this value; 0.003 is the oxygen solubility coefficient)	
5. Art. O_2 content $=$ (Hb $\times$ 1.39 $\times$ Sa_{O_2}) $+$ ($Pa_{O_2} \times 0.003$) $Sa_{O_2} =$ Arterial oxygen saturation $Pa_{O_2} =$ arterial P_{O_2}	Ca_{O_2} (20 vol%)
6. Mixed venous O_2 content $=$ (Hb $\times$ 1.39 $\times$ Sv_{O_2}) $+$ ($Pv_{O_2} \times 0.003$) $Sv_{O_2} =$ Mixed venous oxygen saturation $Pv_{O_2} =$ Mixed venous P_{O_2}	Cv_{O_2} (15 vol%)

* SVRI & PVRI can be expressed as Wood units (toor/L/min) if not multiplied by 80.

TABLE 12-4. (Continued)

Calculation	Normal values, units

7. Arterial − venous O_2 differ: $C(a\text{-}v)O_2$ (3.5–5 vol%)
$(A - VO_2 \text{ diff}) = Ca_{O_2} - Cv_{O_2}$
(Measurement of difference in O_2 content in arterial and venous blood)

8. Oxygen transport = O_2 content D_{O_2} (900–1200 mL/
          × C.O. × 10   min)
   Calculate: (a) Arterial O_2 transport using Ca_{O_2}
           (b) Mixed venous O_2 transport using Cv_{O_2}
           (c) 10 = factor to convert mL O_2/100 mL blood to mL
              O_2/L blood
(D_{O_2} is known at oxygen delivery or transport and represents the
total oxygen delivered to the tissues.

9. Oxygen consumption
   A, indexed V_{O_2} (110–150 mL/min/
                               m²)
      = $(Ca_{O_2} - Cv_{O_2} \times \text{C.I.} \times 10$
      = Art. O_2 transport − venous O_2 transport
      = (C.I.) (13.9) (Hb) (art. O_2 Sat. − ven. O_2 sat.)
   B, not indexed, instead use CO V_{O_2} (250 mL min)
      = $C(a\text{-}v)_{O_2} \times \text{C.O.} \times 10$
(Oxygen extracted by the tissues from arterial blood per unit time)

10. Alveolar O_2 (alv. O_2)
     = $Fi_{O_2} (760\text{-}47) - p_{CO_2}/0.8$
     (760 = barometric pressure, 47 = H_2O vapor pressure, 0.8 =
respiratory quotient)

11. Alveolar − arterial O gradient (A-a gradient)
     = Alv. O_2 − art. O_2
     = $PA_{O_2} = Pa_{O_2}$
(Represents the difference between the partial pressures of alv. and
art. O_2)

12. Pulmonary capillary O_2 content Cc_{O_2} (21 vol%)
     = Bound O_2 + dissolved O_2
     = (Hb × 1.39 × O_2 sat.) + (alv. P_{O_2} × 0.003)
     (a) Assume O_2 sat. = 100% or 1
     (b) Calculate alv. P_{O_2} as above in 10
     (Oxygen content of blood perfusing ventilated alveoli when
Pa_{O_2} is sufficient to fully saturate hemoglobin)

13. Shunt or venous admixture = Q_s/Q_t Q_s/Q_t (<0.05)
                = $\dfrac{(Cc_{O_2} - Ca_{O_2}}{(Cc_{O_2} - Cv_{O_2}}$
     (a) Q = cardiac output; (b) S = shunt; (c) T = total
(Fraction of CO not oxygenated in an idealized lung)

13 SKIN AND SUBCUTANEOUS TISSUE

PHYSICAL PROPERTIES

Tension and elasticity are the primary physical properties of the skin. Tension is the characteristic that accounts for the fact that the skin can resist stretching. Tension is most marked where the skin contains very dense elastic fibers, particularly if the skin is thin. Anatomic lines of tension are called *Langer's lines,* which were described in 1861.

Elasticity refers to the skin's ability to resume its original shape after an external force has been applied. As with tension, elasticity decreases in the elderly.

Tensile strength is the resistance of skin to tearing under tension. The average strength is 1.8 kg/m². Abnormally low values of tensile strength are found in diseases such as Ehlers-Danlos syndrome, in which a defective form of collagen is produced. Also, tensile strength is reduced in patients taking high doses of cortisone for a prolonged period.

FUNCTIONS OF SKIN

Functions of skin include: (1) percutaneous absorption; (2) an important role in the circulatory system; (3) serving as an organ of senses; (4) secretion of sweat; (5) providing an avenue for the insensible loss of water; and (6) contributing to thermal regulation.

Percutaneous Absorption This function of skin permits entry of substances into the bloodstream. The stratum corneum is the major barrier to diffusion. Water and lipid-soluble substances diffuse rapidly across the skin. Most electrolytes, including sodium and calcium, cannot penetrate the skin.

Percutaneous absorption of phenol and carbolic acid is rapid and may cause fatal poisoning. Estrogenic hormones and hydrocortisone also absorb rapidly and can be therapeutically effective with percutaneous application.

Substances in gas form, with the exception of carbon monoxide, penetrate the skin easily. This method has been employed pharmaceutically with the use of dimethylsulfoxide as a vehicle.

Circulation and Vascular Reactions   The cutaneous vascular system is extremely complex. Changes in skin circulation contribute significantly to general vascular and circulatory physiology. Skin blood flow can be directly visualized through the beds of the nail. The color of skin is dependent upon the quantity of blood in the subdermal plexus as much as upon melanin and keratin pigments. In addition, skin temperature is dependent on the rate of blood flow.

Local vascular response may result from direct action on the vessel wall or its contractile elements. A red local reaction can develop after dilatation of small vessels. A "skin wheal" is a circumscribed area of skin edema secondary to dilated blood vessels and leakage of plasma into the extracellular space. Conversely, stimulation of sympathetic nerve fibers causes vasoconstriction of these cutaneous vessels. In addition, the cutaneous vessels respond to various chemical agents such as acetylcholine and nitrites, which cause vasodilatation, while norepinephrine, epinephrine, and vasopressin cause vasoconstriction. Although nitrites cause a sensation of flushing and increased blood flow, smoking paradoxically decreases blood flow through skin.

Sensory Function   Many specific sensory functions are facilitated by the skin. The Krause end bulbs mediate cold sensitivity. Ruffini's endings are the receptors for warmth. Meissner's corpuscles provide tactile sensation and Pacinian corpuscles are involved in the sensation of pressure. Pain is mediated by nonmyelinated nerve endings.

Causalgia is a syndrome of pain and vasodilatation that occurs after injury of major nerves. This syndrome is also called *reflux sympathetic dystrophy*. The most common cause is a prior operation with transection of minor nerve branches. Treatment of this condition is difficult and requires institution of physical and occupational therapeutic resources. Active use of the involved extremity is important. For advanced cases blockade of the contributing sympathetic ganglion with neurolytic agents is used. If ganglion blocks are transiently successful, a surgical sympathectomy might be curative.

Sweat Secretion   Sweat glands in skin are either eccrine glands or apocrine glands. The eccrine glands are distributed all over the body and are primarily responsible for heat regulation. The apocrine glands are similar to sebaceous glands and develop mostly during puberty. Their activity is in response to autonomic nervous stimulation rather than thermal conditions.

Sweating is a response to local application of heat or to nervous impulses. Sympathetic nerve fibers liberate acetylcholine to stimulate sweat glands. Atropine and other anticholinergic drugs can block these receptors and interfere with sweat secretion. Hyperhidrosis, that is, increased sweating, results from an abnormal increase in nerve impulses or emotional states.

The content of sweat is primarily water with small amounts of sodium chloride. Potassium is also lost through sweat. Nitrogen compounds are secreted in sweat as well. The concentration of urea in sweat is twice as high as that in blood. Sweat also contains large amounts of lactic acid and ammonia.

Insensible Water Loss Besides sweat secretion, water is lost through the epidermis by continuous evaporation. In contrast to sweat, water losses through evaporation do not contain electrolytes or other solutes. Approximately 700 mL total water loss occurs through the skin each day. Hypothyroidism decreases the daily amount of water loss, whereas thyrotoxicosis greatly increases this amount.

Thermoregulation Regulation of body temperature is an important function of the skin. Heat escapes through skin under the processes of radiation, convection, conduction, and evaporation. Sweating is a primary process for heat evaporation. Increased humidity markedly decreases the efficiency of sweating for thermoregulation because of the impairment of evaporation.

Thermoregulation is accomplished in skin also by shifting blood flow from the interior to the skin. Cold stimuli result in pallor of the skin by relative vasoconstriction. After the stimulus has ceased there is a reactive arterial vasodilatation. This results in a reddish discoloration of skin. In contrast, prolonged cold stimulus causes paresis of the venous limbs of capillaries. A reddish discoloration also may result from this condition, which is not associated with increased blood flow, and skin temperature does not rise. This condition leads to frostbite. Prolonged exposure of skin to cold temperature should be treated by emersion of the involved portion into water at a temperature of 40°C.

Heat exhaustion is a syndrome of excessive loss of salt and water during exposure to high temperatures. The clinical symptoms are exhaustion, headache, palpitation, dizziness, and confusion. Treatment is immediate cooling by evaporation or application of ice. Simultaneously, intravascular volume replacement of fluids is indicated.

PRESSURE SORES

Pressure on an area of skin for 2 or more h may result in ischemia sufficient to cause a decubitus ulcer. Factors contributing to pressure sores include skin over bony prominence, anemia, malnutrition, and immobilization. Surgical therapy requires sharp debridement to excise the ulcer and underlying fascia and necrotic material. Frequently, a bony prominence must be modified to prevent subsequent pressure. Occasionally, the remaining wound must be covered with a myocutaneous flap.

HIDRADENITIS SUPPURATIVA

Hidradenitis suppurativa is a chronic infection of the cutaneous apocrine glands, subcutaneous tissue, and fascia. This disease occurs in the axilla, areola of the nipple, groin, or perineum. Commonly there is slight induration and subsequent inflammation of the skin. Eventually, suppuration develops and cellulitis surrounds the abscess. Initial treatment is incision and drainage, but frequently this produces only a few drops of purulent material. Then, the chronic stage develops, with multiple painful cutaneous nodules. Culture of these abscesses reveals a preponderance of staphylococci and streptococci.

Definitive treatment requires complete excision of the involved area and improved hygiene to prevent recurrence. Myocutaneous flaps or advancement flaps enhance wound coverage.

CYSTS

Epidermal Inclusion Cysts An epidermal inclusion cyst results from epithelium of skin that is trapped subdermally due to trauma or other reasons and begins to grow and desquamate. The cyst is filled with keratin and desquamated cells. These cysts can occur anywhere on the body. They are generally cured by complete removal. If the cyst is secondarily infected, incision and drainage is indicated first.

Sebaceous Cysts Sebaceous glands are associated with hair follicles and are generally found on the midline of the trunk and on the face. A cyst is formed from a sebaceous gland when the exit of sebum is blocked. True sebaceous cysts are very rare and usually represent epidermal cysts that have been incorrectly diagnosed. The presence of glandular epithelium lining is necessary for the diagnosis.

Dermoid Cysts Dermoid cysts are congenital lesions that arise in early childhood. They generally occur in the midline of the body, the lateral eyebrow, on the scalp, or in the abdominal and sacral regions. There have been no reports of malignant degeneration of these cysts. Dermoid cysts in the nasal region have a remote possibility of communication with the central nervous system. A CT scan should be obtained prior to excising nasal dermoids.

Pilonidal Cysts   Pilonidal cysts are malformations of the neuroenteric canal that occur in the sacrococcygeal region. The ingrowth of hair in the coccygeal region sets the stage for cyst formation and repeated infections. This disease has been referred to as "jeep driver's disease," because long hours of sitting and bumpy driving aggravate the congenital condition. Chronic infection and drainage is the usual presentation. Treatment includes incision and drainage followed by secondary removal of the cyst or sinus when infection has subsided. Excision of the entire sinus is essential for successful treatment. This may be facilitated by injection of methylene blue to determine the extent of arborization of the sinus tract. A skin graft or muscle advancement flap may be necessary to close the defect. Some surgeons prefer to allow closure by secondary intention, particularly if there is residual infection.

Ganglia   Ganglia are the areas of mucoid degeneration of retinacular structures. They are cystic masses frequently found over the dorsum of the wrist and over tendon sheaths of hands or feet. These cysts contain clear fluid similar to joint fluid. Aspiration of the ganglion alone has a 75% recurrence rate. Surgical excision of the entire ganglion is the recommended treatment. This may require excision of a part of the joint capsule in some cases.

BENIGN TUMORS

Warts   Verruca vulgaris, the common wart, is caused by a virus that is contagious. Warts usually occur on the hand or soles of the feet. They are quite tender and painful.

Treatment of verruca vulgaris can be accomplished with liquid nitrogen freezing or electrodesiccation under local anesthesia. Caustic agents have been used also, but with a higher recurrence rate.

Keratosis   Keratosis is a precancerous lesion manifested by hypertrophy of the epidermis. Senile keratoses occur in older individuals with fair complexion. They should be treated by surgical excision if the lesion is large and the suspicion of malignancy is low. Topical treatment with 5-fluorouracil or liquid nitrogen may be done.

Seborrheic keratosis is a thickened area of skin that may

appear brown, gray, or black. Occasionally these lesions are mistaken for melanoma. Electrocoagulation is adequate treatment if biopsy is benign.

Keloids Keloids are dense accumulations of fibrous tissue that extend above the surface of the skin from traumatic wounds or surgical incisions. They are the result of a failure of collagen breakdown and occur most commonly in blacks. Recurrence is common after simple excision.

First line treatment of keloids is steroid injection. This method is effective in relieving the burning and itching, as well as producing actual shrinkage of the lesion. Postoperative radiation therapy is controversial in treating keloids. Subcuticular sutures should be avoided in patients with a history of keloid formation.

Capillary Malformation Capillary malformations are commonly known as "port wine stains" of the skin. They represent dilated abnormal capillaries in the subdermal plexus. They are smooth lesions with reddish or purplish patchy distribution. Excision of small lesions is appropriate. The larger lesions are being treated now with argon laser. This is reserved, however, for patients over 14 years of age.

Hemangioma Hemangiomas appear in infancy and may enlarge over the first year of life but usually regress thereafter. They are bright red, raised, and irregular skin lesions. Episodes of ulceration or superficial infection actually hasten spontaneous resolution of these lesions. Spontaneous resolution usually occurs by age 7.

Arteriovenous Malformation Arteriovenous malformations are also called *cavernous hemangiomas*. These lesions are evident at birth and do not change during growth of the child. Occasionally they involve deep structures such as the central nervous system or muscles. Nonetheless, wide excision is the treatment of choice. Occasionally, preoperative embolization of feeding vessels can assist wide excision.

Glomus Tumor Glomus tumor is a benign, rare neoplasm of the skin that usually occurs in the nail beds of the hands and feet. These lesions are extremely painful because they are derived from the giomic end organ, a nerve apparatus that normally functions to regulate blood flow in the extremity. These lesions are also called *angiomyoneuroma,* and are generally benign. The malignant counterpart to this tumor is called *hemangiopericytoma.*

Neural Tumors Neurofibromas and Schwann cell tumors can occur in the skin. Their treatment is surgical excision. Neurofibromas are associated with von Recklinghausen's disease. Approximately 10% of patients with neurofibromatosis will have sarcomatous degeneration of these tumors.

MALIGNANT TUMORS

Skin cancer is associated with exposure. Ultraviolet light, ionizing radiation, and chemicals are causative factors. Skin cancer usually is manifested by a low-grade malignant tumor that metastasizes late. Therefore, cure rates of carcinoma of the skin are relatively high.

Basal Cell Carcinoma   Basal cell carcinoma is a skin malignancy that grows slowly and accounts for at least three-fourths of cancers in most clinical series. These lesions are waxy and grayish-yellow and often have telangiectasia below the surface. Most basal cell cancers are located on the head and neck. They tend to invade and erode into deep structures including the skull, orbit, or brain if left untreated.

Squamous Cell Carcinoma   Squamous cell carcinoma usually presents as an ulcerated skin lesion that tends to grow more rapidly than basal cell cancer. Biopsy is necessary to differentiate this lesion from other types of skin cancer. Again, most occur on the head and neck. The typical appearance is an ulcer with rolled margins resembling a small volcanic crater. Squamous cell carcinoma is more malignant than basal cell and will metastasize to regional nodes more rapidly.

Squamous cell cancers are found in areas of frequent irritation such as the vermillion border of the lip, or areas of postradiation dermatitis, or ulcerations in old burn scars.

Bowen's disease is a slowly growing squamous cell carcinoma in situ for which excision is recommended.

Sweat Gland Carcinoma   This rare tumor usually occurs in the sixth and seventh decades of life. Therapy consists of wide local excision and consideration of lymphadenectomy. Regional lymph nodes will be involved in approximately 50% of cases.

Treatment   Options for treatment of skin cancer include electrodesiccation, cryosurgery, chemosurgery, radiation therapy, and surgical therapy. Biopsy of the skin lesion and relevant history determine the choice of therapy. Electrodesiccation and curettage are applicable for superficial, nonrecurrent basal cell carcinomas. Chemosurgery is described as the Mohs technique. The lesion is excised under local anesthesia, and frozen sections are taken of the entire surface of the resection. Four or five resections may be necessary to completely excise the lesion. The advantage of this method is the possibility of eradicating small extensions of the central lesion with greater certainty than conventional excision provides. This technique is particularly useful in recurrent basal cell or squamous cell carcinomas. Radiation therapy can be used to cure basal or squamous cell carcinomas. In some instances a better cosmetic result with less effort can be accomplished. Surgical therapy is conventional treatment for most skin cancers. Controversy continues regarding an adequate margin of normal tissue. Most recommendations have been 0.5 cm around basal cell carcinomas and 1 cm around squamous cell carcinomas. In recurrent lesions, frozen section or permanent section determination of tumor-free margins should precede definitive reconstruction. Regional lymph node dissection is performed only for clinical evidence of node involvement.

Approximately one-third of patients with positive margins after resection of basal cell carcinoma will develop recurrence. If the patient is reliable, simple observation may be all that is indicated. Repeat surgical excision is the best treatment for recurrence.

Eighty percent of squamous cell carcinomas are cured by surgical excision. Mohs has reported about a 95% cure rate for recurrent basal cell carcinoma and a 75% cure rate for recurrent squamous cell carcinoma.

Fibrosarcoma This tumor occurs commonly in women in the thigh, buttock, or inguinal region. It is usually a relatively low-grade malignancy and is radioresistant. Wide surgical excision is the treatment of choice. Local recurrence is common.

Hemangiopericytoma This is a malignant tumor of angio-blastic origin and is probably a variant of the glomus tumor. Prognosis is distinctly poor, with only 27% 5-year disease-free survival. Radiation therapy is considered the treatment of choice, especially for larger tumors.

Kaposi's Sarcoma This tumor has a markedly increased incidence in homosexuals. Acquired immunodeficiency syndrome is commonly associated with Kaposi's sarcoma. Usually, the tumor begins in the hands or feet as multiple plaques that are reddish to purple and may be flat, ulcerated, or polypoid. Lymph node involvement is common. Radiation can retard the growth of Kaposi's sarcoma, but surgical excision is also helpful. Actinomycin D has given some responses. Overall, the prognosis is poor.

Dermatofibrosarcoma Protuberans This tumor is a relatively low-grade malignancy that generally occurs on the trunk. It is radioresistant but responds to surgical excision with a 70% 5-year disease-free survival.

PIGMENTED LESIONS

Intradermal nevus, junctional nevus, and compound nevus are examples of benign pigmented lesions; however, they have variable degrees of malignant potential. The intradermal nevus is a nest of melanoblasts confined to the dermis. Frequently, these nevi contain hair. The junctional nevus is a proliferation of melanoblasts that originates in the basal layer of the epidermis and extends down into the dermis. These lesions occur around the genitalia, palms, nail beds, and mucous membranes. The compound nevus has both junctional and intradermal elements. These lesions are benign but have some malignant potential.

Juvenile melanomas are nevi that occur prior to puberty. Most occur in the face and enlarge slowly.

The differential between benign pigmented skin lesions and melanoma can be difficult. Changes in various characteristics of pigmented lesions are indications for excision. These include change in color or pigment distribution; development of erythema; change in size or consistency; and change in the surface characteristic, such as oozing, bleeding, or erosion.

The Hutchinson freckle (lentigo maligna) is a precancerous melanosis of the face that usually occurs in elderly people. Approximately one-third of these lesions will become malignant melanoma. Their prognosis is excellent, however, especially when the lesion is excised from the face. Any suspicious lesions should be completely excised with a margin of normal skin.

MELANOMA Melanoma is a malignant lesion originating in the melanoblast of the skin. Mucous membranes and pigmented regions of the eye can also harbor primary melanoma. The lesion is usually darkly pigmented, smooth, firm, and nonhairy. At some phases of development the melanoma cells do not contain melanin and are referred to as *amelanotic melanoma*.

Staging of melanoma was introduced by Clark. Clark's levels of invasion are: (I) all tumor cells above the basement membrane, (II) has tumor extension into the papillary but not the reticular dermis, (III) has tumor adjacent to the interface between the papillary and reticular dermis, (IV) is characterized by tumor cells in the reticular dermis, (V) has invasion into the subcutaneous fat.

A new system of staging has been introduced by Breslow, which is based on thickness of the primary lesion using an occulomicrometer. In this sytem level I tumors are 0.75 mm or less, level II are 0.76–1.50 mm, level III are 1.51—3.0 mm, and level IV are greater than 3.0 mm. At this time Breslow's classification is usually used for critical decision about therapy.

Staging of melanoma is based on critical examination of regional nodes and thickness of the primary lesion. Stage I refers to thin lesions without node involvement. Stage II refers to thick lesions without node involvement. Stage III refers to any lesions with nodal involvement, and Stage IV includes any lesions with distal metastases.

The incidence of melanoma is increased by exposure to solar radiation in light-skinned races. The presence of melanin in the skin has a protective effect against ultraviolet light acting as a stimulus. Melanoma is much more common in patients with xeroderma pigmentosum, a genetic disorder associated with hypersensitivity to ultraviolet light.

Melanomas usually arise in nevi that have a junctional activity. Nevi of the palm, soles, nail beds, genitalia, and mucous membranes have functional elements that make them more prone to be the source of melanoma than moles at other sites. Malignant melanoma rarely occurs in prepubertal children.

Four types of melanoma are described: superficial spreading melanoma, nodular melanoma, lentigo maligna melanoma, and acral-lentiginous melanoma. Superficial spreading melanoma is characterized by intradermal spreading and accounts for almost 70% of all cutaneous melanoma. Nodular melanoma is less common and is characterized by little radial growth but more invasive growth. The prognosis for nodular melanoma is significantly worse. Lentigo maligna melanoma is the most indolent of all and occurs mostly in older individuals. Acral-lentiginous melanoma occurs in the palms, soles, and subungual regions; its histology is similar to that of lentigo maligna.

Surgical Treatment Surgical excision is the primary therapy for melanoma. For most pigmented lesions an excisional biopsy with a margin of 2–5 mm is indicated. However, extremely large lesions may require an incisional biopsy, which is appropriate prior to planning definitive therapy.

The acceptable margins for definitive excision of melanomas depends on thickness of the lesion. A margin of 0.5 cm is probably adequate for lesions less than 0.75 mm in thickness. Lesions between 0.76 and 1.5 mm in thickness require a 2-cm margin. Thicker lesions require a 4-cm margin.

Amputation of a digit is indicated for acral-lentiginous melanomas.

Removal of regional lymph nodes should be performed when there is clinical evidence of adenopathy and no distant metastases. Prophylactic dissection of regional lymph nodes is more controversial. The choice between a prophylactic lymph node dissection vs. waiting for clinical evidence of node involvement may be based on the probability of occult lymph node metastases with a given stage of primary tumor. Tumors less than 1.5 mm have about a 15% association with positive lymph nodes. Thicker lesions between 1.6 and 3.7 mm have a 35% association with positive lymph nodes. Tumors thicker than 3.7 mm have a 50% chance of positive lymph nodes.

Some retrospective studies show a survival advantage for immediate lymph node dissection of clinical Stage I melanoma. A prospective randomized study by the World Health Organization, however, showed no survival improvement for patients in this category. A prospective, multi-institutional trial is proceeding in North America to confirm or refute these results. Nonetheless, immediate lymph node dissection should be used when the melanoma originates in the skin covering a lymph node basin, since the changes following excision of the primary tumor may complicate the clinical evaluation of lymph nodes.

Adjunctive Treatment   *Regional Chemotherapy and Hyperthermia.*   Isolated regional perfusion has been tested for melanoma. The involved extremity is perfused with a solution approximately 40°C. The chemotherapeutic agent most commonly used in melphalan. This therapy is probably beneficial only in those patients whose primary tumor is thicker than 3.7 mm. Also, patients with numerous satellite and transit metastases may benefit from isolated regional perfusion.

Immunotherapy.   A variety of agents have temporarily controlled cutaneous metastases of melanoma. Local intralesional injections of BCG provide remission to approximately 20% of patients in one study. Systemic treatment with biologic response modifiers has begun to show some impact on disseminated melanoma.

Prognosis for patients with melanoma depends on the staging. The 5-year cure rate for Stage I lesions smaller than 0.76 mm is almost 95%. Lesions between .76 and 1.5 mm have an 85% 5-year cure rate. Stage II lesions are less favorable, with a 60% 5-year survival rate. Patients who are Stage III (positive lymph node involvement) have approximately 35% 5-year survival.

14 BREAST

EMBRYOLOGY

- Mammary ridge or milk line appears in sixth week as ectodermal thickening from axilla to groin. Caudal two-thirds of the line regresses; anomalous persistence often mistaken for nevi. Aberrant breast tissue in axilla or elsewhere off milk line apparent during stimulation of pregnancy. Treatment: excision.
- In the fifth month in utero, 15–20 cords develop, which form lumina in the seventh month.
- Falling maternal estrogen levels after birth stimulate fetal production of prolactin, with secretion of colostrum for several days after birth in boys and girls.

ANATOMY

- Except for mild hypertrophy during neonatal period and puberty, male breast undergoes little change throughout life.
- Prepubertal female "bud" develops from 11–15 years. Lobulation occurs after first ovulation.
- Young adult female breast extends from second to sixth rib, from sternum to anterior axillary line. Glandular tissue circular in outline except for tail of Spence extending to axilla. Cooper's fibrous ligaments help to suspend the glandular tissue to the anterior superficial fascia under the skin. Subareolar area and nipple contain smooth muscle that contracts with tactile stimulation.
- Arterial supply: Perforating branches of internal mammary artery (first through fourth interspace) medially, lateral thoracic artery from the axillary artery lateral to pectoralis major, and pectoral branch of acromiothoracic artery medial to muscle.
- Venous drainage: Superficial subcutaneous veins drain into internal mammary or neck veins; deep veins correspond to arterial supply. Mammary cancer may metastasize to vertebral bodies or pelvis, bypassing lungs because of intercostal drainage to vertebral veins (Batson's plexus).

- Lymphatic: Internal mammary and axillary lymph nodes drain the breast. Axillary levels: I—lateral to pectoralis minor, II—beneath pectoralis minor, III—medial to pectoralis minor. Drainage proceeds inferior to superior, eventually to supraclavicular nodes and then via thoracic duct to the venous system. Average lymph node harvest surgically is 5 internal mammary nodes and 20 axillary nodes (levels I, II, and III).

Histology Breast composed of multiple alveolar glands. Terminal ducts lined by columnar epithelium. Milk sinus in subareolar region lined by squamous epithelium. Multiple alveoli form lobules.

- Cyclic change: Volume increases nearly 50% after eighth day of menstrual cycle. Vascular congestion and lobular proliferation regress with menses.

- Pregnancy and lactation: Alveolar and lobular ducts proliferate with regression after nursing ceases. Nipple and areola darken and Montgomery's glands (of the areola) become prominent. Striae appear.

- Menopause: Lobules involute. Fat replaces parenchyma.

- Aberrations: Asymmetric development or virginal hypertrophy in girls may be corrected surgically after maturity. Gynecomastia in pubertal boys may be corrected if there is no regression or hormonal abnormalities.

EXAMINATION

- Inspection: Asymmetry, skin dimpling, edema, nipple inversion more easily detected with patient seated, hands on hips and then elevated over head.

- Palpation: With patient seated erect, supraclavicular and axillary fossae are examined with tail of Spence and central breast tissue. Entire breast reexamined with patient supine and arm overhead. Women over age 35 who practice monthly breast self-exam detect smaller cancers with fewer lymph nodes.

- Mammography: Absorbed dose of radiation is 0.1 rad at midbreast with negligible risk after age 30. American Cancer Society recommends base-line x-ray between ages 35–40, then every 2 years between ages 40–50, then annually after age 50. If family history present, first mammogram should be obtained at age 35, with annual film after age 40. The mammogram evaluates stromal changes in contrast to fatty areas of the breast, so it is most accurate in postmenopausal fatty breasts as opposed to premenopausal glandular breasts. Patterns suspicious for carcinoma include skin thickening, stromal densities with starburst parenchymal invasion, and microcalcifications (debris extruded into the ducts from rapidly dividing cells, especially common in intraductal cancers). Mammogram is especially useful in exam for nonpalpable lesions, for the contralateral breast in patients with cancer, and for pendulous breasts. False-positive rate 11%, false-negative rate 6%. Prospective trials demonstrated earlier cancer detection and increased survival because of mammographic screening. Xeroradiography is similar to mammography, but images are positive rather than negative and radiation exposure is increased; not recommended.

- Thermography: Tumors or infections generate "hot spots," but method unreliable.

- Ultrasonography: Cysts differentiated from solid lesions on ultrasound, but this method cannot detect microcalcifications. Needle aspiration simpler and less expensive for cyst detection.

- Other methods: Angiography, CT, and MRI still experimental in detection of breast cancer.

BENIGN CONDITIONS

- Fibrocystic mastopathy: Known by many names, including chronic cystic mastitis, this condition increases in incidence with age but tends to be more symptomatic in younger woman, with tenderness and swelling premenstrually. Only those patients with severe hyperplasia or atypia on biopsy are at increased risk for carcinoma. Claims of symptom relief from intake of vitamin E, or abstinence from caffeine or xanthine derivatives have never been proved. Danazol (a synthetic androgen analogue), tamoxifen (an antiestrogen), and even progesterone have been used effectively for treatment.

- Cysts: These firm, round, distinct masses vary from 1 mm to several centimeters in diameter and may increase in size toward the end of the menstrual cycle. Physiologic fluid typically is clear or brownish-green on aspiration. Biopsy is indicated if fluid is bloody, if mass does not completely resolve after aspiration, or if cyst fluid reaccumulates.

- Fibroadenomas: These lobular, firm, rubbery, well-circumscribed masses are most often solitary and present in young women; best treated by excision.

- Ductal papilloma: About one-third of patients with bloody nipple drainage have an intraductal papilloma, although nearly 20% have carcinoma. Diagnosis is established by excision of major duct system and breast tissue in the subareolar area.

- Sclerosing adenosis: Fibrotic irregular areas of breast tissue with microcalcifications require biopsy to distinguish from carcinoma.

- Fat necrosis: Only about half the patients with fat necrosis recall the related trauma, which results in a superficial, firm, irregular area of fibrosis with overlying skin retraction; frequently confused with carcinoma until examined histologically.

- Granular cell myoblastoma of the breast appears similar to an early breast cancer grossly.

- Mondor's disease is thrombophlebitis of a superficial vein of the breast, often with tenderness and skin retraction.

- Acute infections are most common in lactating women who sustain nipple abrasions, and most often present with pain and erythema. Cellulitis may be treated by antibiotics, but abscesses require incision, interruption of loculations, and dependent drainage (usually *Staph aureus* cultured). Nonnursing women require biopsy as well as drainage to distinguish duct ectasia from post-obstructive abscess secondary to ductal carcinoma.

- Chronic infection is rare except in immunosuppressed patients, but histologically is most often caused by tuberculosis, from the lungs, or a mediastinal node erosion of a costal cartilage.

CARCINOMA

- Incidence: Breast carcinoma is the most common malignant neoplasm in females, with an increasing age-adjusted incidence rate since 1940; breast cancer is now diagnosed in 1 of every 10 women in the U.S. during their lifetimes.

- Etiology is probably multifactional. Female sex is a predisposing factor, since only 1 male acquires breast carcinoma for every 100 females diagnosed. Incidence increases with age: It begins after age 20 and plateaus around menopause, then rises steeply thereafter. Genetic factors are important in about 15% of cases and are most marked in patients whose mothers had premenopausal bilateral breast carcinoma. Younger age at diagnosis is associated with blood type O, benign breast disease, and ovarian cysts; older age at diagnosis is associated with blood type A, diabetes, hypertension, and uterine disorders. The Dutch have the highest national breast cancer mortality, while the Japanese have the least. Higher risk is associated with nulliparity and late age at first pregnancy. Although estrogens induce mammary cancer in mice, no theory of induction secondary to hormones or birth control pills has been proved in human beings. Obesity, high consumption of animal fat, viral factors transmitted via breast milk, and even wet ear wax have been associated as risk factors.

- Natural history is cited in studies from the late 1800s at London's Middlesex Hospital, where median survival for 1000 untreated cases was 2.7 years; survival was calculated from the description of onset of the first symptoms. Five-year survival was 18%, and 10-year survival 3.76%. Autopsies showed that 95% of the women died of breast carcinoma, with breast ulceration in 75% at death.

- Biology of breast cancer: A typical scirrhous adenocarcinoma begins in the upper outer quadrant (45%) of the left breast (60%) and takes 30 doublings from the one-cell stage over 5–8 years to reach 1 cm in diameter. Metastasis occurs when the tumor is greater than 0.5 cm in diameter, and prognosis is adversely affected by the number of axillary lymph nodes involved. With enlargement, fibrosis shortens Cooper's ligament with characteristic skin dimpling. Systemic spread is most common to lung (65%), bone (56%), and liver (56%).

- Diagnostic workup proceeds in an orderly progression (Table 14-1). Every suspicious lesion deserves biopsy, and then biopsy incision should be made in the direction of the skin lines (periareolar) or as convenient for possible subsequent segmental resection or mastectomy. Staging should be accomplished prior to definite treatment. The TNM classification proposed by the International Union Against Cancer helps to establish four stages of disease (Table 14-2).

HISTOLOGY

- Ductal carcinomas constitute 80% of the malignant neoplasms of the breast.

TABLE 14-1.   Diagnosis and Evaluation of Breast Cancer

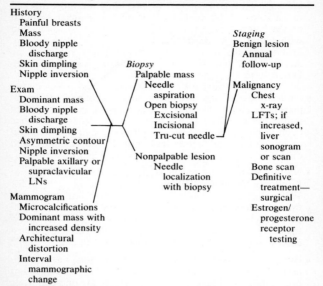

History
  Painful breasts
  Mass
  Bloody nipple
    discharge
  Skin dimpling
  Nipple inversion

Exam
  Dominant mass
  Bloody nipple
    discharge
  Skin dimpling
  Asymmetric contour
  Nipple inversion
  Palpable axillary or
    supraclavicular
    LNs

Mammogram
  Microcalcifications
  Dominant mass with
    increased density
  Architectural
    distortion
  Interval
    mammographic
    change

Biopsy
  Palpable mass
    Needle
      aspiration
    Open biopsy
      Excisional
      Incisional
    Tru-cut needle

  Nonpalpable lesion
    Needle
      localization
      with biopsy

Staging
  Benign lesion
    Annual
      follow-up

  Malignancy
    Chest
      x-ray
    LFTs; if
      increased,
      liver
      sonogram
      or scan
    Bone scan
    Definitive
      treatment—
      surgical
    Estrogen/
      progesterone
      receptor
      testing

- Noninfiltrating ductal carcinomas (ductal carcinoma in situ) constitute 1% of all carcinomas, and excision should be curative; survival at 5 years is only 90%, however, suggesting that this lesion is often multicentric and associated with infiltrating ductal carcinoma and later disease.

- Infiltrating ductal carcinoma is the most common form of breast cancer. Lesion is typically hard, crablike, with infiltrating tentacles, and gritty on cross section.

TABLE 14-2.   Staging of Breast Carcinoma

Stage I	Tumor less than 2 cm, no lymph node (LN) or distant spread
II	Tumor less than 5 cm, with or without LN involvement, no distant spread
IIIa	Tumor greater than 5 cm with or without LN involvement or any tumor with matted LN; no distant spread
IIIb	Any tumor with direct extension to chest wall or skin or any tumor with arm edema or supraclavicular LN involvement
IV	Any tumor, any LN involvement *with* distant metastases

- Comedocarcinoma is typified by ducts lined with abundant necrotic hyperplasia and mitotic debris, which on gross section is extruded, much like a comedo when squeezed.

- Paget's disease is the manifestation of ductal carcinoma that invades the nipple with a scaling eczematoid lesion. Histologically large cells with clear cytoplasm are noted and tend to be associated with a better prognosis than the average ductal carcinoma.

- Papillary carcinoma presents as a softer tumor with larger growth prior to lymph node metastasis, and therefore has a better prognosis.

- Medullary carcinomas are large, soft, bulky lesions, often with areas of central necrosis and lymphoid infiltration. Metastases occur late.

- Colloid carcinomas are soft, ill-defined lesions with large mucinous lakes on cross section and a good prognosis.

- Tubular carcinoma is a well-differentiated tumor with good prognosis.

- Inflammatory carcinoma is generally ductal carcinoma involving the dermal lymphatics, indicative of advanced disease and presenting as "peau-d'orange," or "orange peel" skin (stage IIIb).

- Lobular carcinomas arise in terminal duct epithelium and spread in a sheetlike invasive fashion. They are often multicentric in the same breast and show bilateral invasive lesions about 30% of the time.

- Sarcomas of the breast are rare, but the most common is a giant benign variant of fibroadenoma, cystosarcoma phylloides. Only 1 in 10 tumors is malignant. They are present in patients older than those who have fibroadenoma (forties) and are more cellular. Total mastectomy is recommended for both benign and malignant varieties because axillary lymph node metastases are rare (with mets more common to lung and bone).

TREATMENT

- Halsted initiated the modern era with his first radical mastectomy in 1882. Removal of breast, axillary nodes, and both pectoralis major and minor muscles established reliable local-regional control of advanced breast carcinoma. His "criteria of inoperability" excluded those patients (25%) who would surely develop distant metastases:

fixation of lesion to chest wall (ribs or pleura), fixation of axillary nodes, or presence of supraclavicular lymph nodes, inflammatory breast carcinoma. Halsted's radical mastectomy became the only accepted treatment for operative breast carcinoma until the 1960s.

- Over the ensuing 20 years, alternative operations were debated: sparing the pectoralis major (Patey), sparing both pectoralis muscles (Madden), and extending the radical (Urban harvested the internal mammary lymph nodes and the adjacent chest wall in addition to the radical mastectomy).

- Limited resections were first tried successfully in the last decade. In 1980, Veronesi reported the same survival and local recurrence rates in patients who had tumors 2 cm or smaller with palpable axillary nodes and who underwent radical mastectomy vs. quadrantectomy, axillary dissection, and whole breast radiotherapy. In 1985, Fisher reported the National Surgical Adjuvant Breast Project (NSABP) results, which compared modified radical mastectomy with segmental resection/axillary dissection/radiation therapy in patients with tumors 4 cm or smaller, with or without palpable axillary nodes. Survival and local recurrence rates again were equal. In a third arm of the NSABP, patients underwent segmental resection/axillary dissection without radiation therapy and showed a high local recurrence rate (24% in node-negative and 36% in node-positive patients). This supported local treatment of the entire breast (with either excision or radiotherapy) because of multicentricity of breast cancer, causing local recurrence.

- For stages I and II cancers, either modified radical mastectomy or segmental resection/axillary dissection/radiation therapy is acceptable surgical treatment. Axillary dissection (not sampling) should be performed to adequately stage the disease and to prevent local axillary recurrence (and to avoid radiation to the axilla with potential morbidity of brachial plexopathy and increased lymphedema). Approach may be modified according to patient preference, while not compromising local-regional control. Modified radical mastectomy is recommended for extensive multicentric disease, subareolar lesions, large or medial quadrant lesions that would produce large deformity with segmental resection, and patients whose general health status would be compromised by radiation treatment. Extensive intraductal carcinoma with invasion is associated with 10% increased local recurrence when treated with local excision and radiation therapy, and mastectomy is therefore preferable. Operative mortality for either treatment is less than 1%. Morbidity includes infarction, skin necrosis, seroma, and lymphedema.

- Surgery for stage III or IV breast cancer may be indicated for large or deep tumors to prevent recurrent uncontrollable local disease, although eventual outcome may be death from distant metastases.

- Subcutaneous mastectomy is generally not indicated for any malignant lesion, because recurrence rate is greater than the proportion of breast tissue remaining under the areola. Total mastectomy (removal of the areolar-nipple complex along with all breast tissue) may be indicated for ductal or lobular carcinoma in situ or for patients with strong risk factors for development of carcinoma. Controversy exists about these groups of patients over surgery vs. close surveillance. Approximately 30% of patients with in situ lesions develop invasive carcinoma, although not necessarily in the same quadrant (for lobular CIS, there is equal probability of an invasive lesion developing in the opposite breast, and contralateral biopsy is advised). For those who have had carcinoma in one breast, the risk for development of carcinoma in the opposite breast is about 1% per year.

Adjuvant Therapy

- Standard adjuvant therapy postoperatively for pre- or perimenopausal node-positive patients consists of 6 months of treatment with cytoxan, methotrexate, and 5-fluorouracil (CMF). Variations include addition of vincristine and prednisone or addition of adriamycin.

- Postmenopausal patients who are node-positive and estrogen receptor (ER)–negative also require chemotherapy. Those who are node-positive and ER-positive may be treated with the antiestrogen tamoxifen.

- Subgroups of stage I patients of any age at risk for recurrence—such as those with lymphatic invasion, those with high-grade tumors, or those not having a less aggressive tumor such as colloid, tubular, papillary, or medullary—may also be candidates for adjuvant chemotherapy (preliminary report in *New England Journal of Medicine*, 1988).

- Adjuvant radiotherapy is used postoperatively only in patients at high risk for local recurrence.

TABLE 14-3. Response to Endocrine Therapy by Hormonal Markers

Receptor status	Distribution in patients	Response to tamoxifen
ER$^+$, PgR$^+$	41%	68%
ER$^+$, PgR$^-$	30%	32%
ER$^-$, PgR$^+$	2%	42%
ER$^-$, PgR$^-$	27%	9%

Prognosis

- Early breast cancer: 5-year survival for stage I patients is 95% and for stage II is 80%, with local recurrence rate about 6% using adjuvant therapy as indicated. Patients at high risk have tumors with poor cytologic differentiation, lymphatic and vascular permeation, poor circumscription, high thymidine labeling index (increased number of dividing cells), and estrogen receptor negativity (about 50%).

- Prognosis for stage III disease has risen from 20 to 40% at 5 years, with the advent of adjuvant therapy. Stage IV disease still has a survival of less than 10% at 5 years.

- Inflammatory carcinoma (IIIb), previously considered the most lethal of all breast carcinomas, now has a 5-year survival of nearly 50% using sequential multimodal therapy.

- Patients with discovery of breast cancer during pregnancy or lactation tend to be diagnosed at a later stage of disease than age-matched controls, probably because of the difficulty in assessing their thickly glandular breasts. They should be treated as indicated by stage.

RECURRENT CANCER

- Local recurrence may be treated by excision. Regional recurrence or localized osseous metastases may be helped by radiation therapy.

- Treatment of recurrence is palliative, not curative.

- Most patients with recurrence should receive systemic therapy: hormonal if indicated (Table 14-3), otherwise chemotherapy. No controlled trials have evaluated efficacy of sequential chemotherapy and hormone manipulation. Patients who are either ER- or progesterone receptor (PgR)–positive should be given a trial of hormonal therapy manipulation. All techniques produce the same regression (about 60%): (1) ablation (oophorectomy or adrenalectomy); (2) additive therapy (high-dose estrogen or progesterone to block binding of endogenous estrones and other breakdown products); (3) antiestrogens (tamoxifen or diethylstilbesterol vs. the antiadrenal agent aminoglutethimide). Tamoxifen has the least side effects (hot flashes and mild cytopenia) and is the therapy of choice.

- Patients who are hormone receptor–negative or who fail to respond to hormonal manipulation are candidates for previously described CMF regimen or adriamycin. Partial or complete remission is achieved in 65% of patients.

REHABILITATION

Patients should regain full function of the arm on the side of operation, although physical therapy may be beneficial. Exercise, elevation and sequential compression pumps help to decrease lymphedema. Women who have undergone breast surgery help to provide psychologic support to others through the American Cancer Society's Reach to Recovery program.

Breast reconstruction, if desired, is begun at the time of initial therapeutic surgery or delayed until completion of chemotherapy. Reconstruction is most easily accomplished with submuscular silastic implants or via myocutaneous flaps (latissimus dorsi or transverse rectus).

15 TUMORS OF THE HEAD AND NECK

BACKGROUND

Rational operations for cancer of the head and neck awaited the discovery of the primary origin of cancer in the various organs of this region and the ability to differentiate cancer grossly and microscopically from other confusingly similar diseases. With the advent of anesthesia and microscopic pathology in the mid-1800s, operative attack on cancer in all areas moved swiftly forward. Partial laryngectomy was introduced in 1853, and total laryngectomy was first accomplished by Billroth in 1873. Mortality rates exceeded 50%, however, primarily due to the lack of antibiotics. Theodor Kocher was the first to recommend the excision of the lymphatic contents of both the anterior and posterior triangles of the neck together with the jugular vein and sternocleidomastoid muscle.

During the early 1900s radiation therapy for cancer of the neck was introduced. By 1930 primary therapy for these tumors was radiation. With refinement of this technique cure rates were increasing. However, metastatic deposits in the neck did not respond to radiation as well as to operation.

The improvements of blood transfusions, anesthesia, and antibiotics markedly changed the ability of surgeons to do radical operations for combined excision of primary lesions and cervical metastases. Grant Ward of the Johns Hopkins Hospital and Hays Martin of the Memorial Center for Cancer were pioneers in this sector of surgery.

Today, considerable common ground for radiation therapy and surgery exists for treatment of tumors of the head and neck. Patients frequently benefit from both operation and radiation as a planned course of integrated treatment.

DIAGNOSIS

PHYSICAL EXAMINATION Examination for head and neck cancers begins with close scrutinization of the skin. Basal and squamous cell carcinomas of the skin are the most common of all cancers, with the head and neck area the most common site for these lesions. All lumps of the skin should be palpated to observe their firmness, whether they have a cystic or solid quality, and whether they are fixed to the underlying tissues.

The oral cavity is a rich source of pathologic processes. Proper examination requires the use of a tongue depressor, glove, and good lighting. If the patient has dentures of any sort they should be removed. The openings of Wharton's ducts should be examined. Then, the floor of the mouth is observed and the tonsillar pillar on either side. The undersurface of the anterior and lateral tongue can also be examined.

The buccal mucosa is examined also. In this region the nipple indicating the opening of Stensen's duct is observed. Pressure on the parotid gland should express saliva from the orifice.

The tongue is carefully inspected and palpated for lesions commonly found on the edges or tip. Vitamin deficiencies are frequently reflected by atrophy or "hairiness" of the tongue.

The tonsils and soft palate may contain lesions and should be inspected also. Inappropriate hypertrophy of one tonsil may reflect a lymphoma. Inspection and palpation of the hard palate may reveal a lobular elevation running down the midline called a "torus," a harmless congenital deformity.

Neck Examination of the neck should include the larynx, thyroid, trachea, sternocleidomastoid muscle, and lymph node–bearing areas. Also, salivary glands should be examined.

The angle of the jaw is a common site for enlarged lymph nodes or a tumor of the tail of the parotid gland. On the anterior border of the sternocleidomastoid muscle a cystic mass may appear representing a branchial cleft cyst.

Occasionally, normal structures of the neck may mimic lymphadenopathy. The carotid bulb, the tip of the hyoid bone, and the tips of the transverse processes of the second cervical vertebra are structures that might be mistaken for lymph nodes.

Masses in the thyroid are best felt if the examiner stands behind the patient and palpates the lobes of the gland between the thumb and forefinger. A mass in the midline of the neck may represent an enlarged lymph node, a pyramidal lobe of the thyroid, or a thyroglossal duct cyst.

Indirect Laryngoscopy Indirect laryngoscopy should be part of the armamentarium of any physician and part of the routine general physical examination. By using a mirror in the oropharynx, the posterior third of the tongue, lateral pharyngeal walls, posterior pharyngeal wall, epiglottis, valleculae, and piriform sinuses can be examined thoroughly. Skillful use of the laryngoscopy mirror also can provide examination of the aryepiglottic folds, posterior epiglottis, and vocal cords. Movement of the vocal cords is an important assessment of the neck and mediastinum.

The flexible fiber-optic nasopharyngoscope is a handy office instrument that can give novice examiners a better view of the larynx than is available on indirect laryngoscopy.

Direct laryngoscopy is a more complex procedure, requiring general anesthesia. The chief reason for resorting to direct laryngoscopy is the biopsy of lesions deep in the larynx.

The laryngoscopy mirror can also be used for examination of the nasopharynx. Complete examination of the nasopharynx is done by inserting a soft rubber #10 French catheter through either nasal passage, drawing its tip out through the mouth, and retracting the soft palate forward, revealing the entire nasopharynx. The adenoids, normal lymphatic tissue in this region, lend a granular appearance of the posterior and superior mucosal surfaces. The fiber-optic nasopharyngoscope facilitates examination of this region also.

DIAGNOSTIC STUDIES Plain radiographs of the bones of the face and neck are useful for suspicion of lesions of the paranasal sinuses, nasal cavity, orbit, mandible, or larynx. Arteriography has been used to evaluate tumors within the cranium or rare tumor of the carotid body. Computed tomography (CT) is especially useful in the assessment of head and neck tumors. Enlarged cervical lymph nodes can be detected, as can tumors in the nasopharynx, paranasal sinuses, and larynx. Some studies have demonstrated superior differentiation between abnormal and normal tissue using magnetic resonance imaging (MRI) versus CT.

Biopsy of head and neck lesions is the best diagnostic maneuver. Lesions of the lip, skin, gingiva, floor of the mouth, tongue, and buccal mucosa are easily biopsied with a 4-mm skin punch. Lesions of the soft palate, tonsillar palate, or posterior tongue can be biopsied with a cervical biopsy forceps.

Occasionally enlarged cervical nodes may require biopsy when no primary tumor can be found. In this situation needle biopsy of the cervical node is indicated if an exhaustive search for the primary lesion is unsuccessful. Squamous cell carcinoma can be diagnosed easily with this maneuver. Lymphoma, however, is virtually impossible to diagnose by needle biopsy.

Some cancers of the oral mucosa are quite soft and superficial in their early stages. Application of toluidine blue will aid in making the diagnosis. This technique distinguishes areas of dysplasia and carcinoma in situ.

Tumor Markers Some head and neck tumors secrete a parathormone-like substance associated with an elevated calcium in approximately 10% of Stage III and IV cancers. Also, carcinoembryonic antigen (CEA) is sometimes elevated in head and neck tumors and can be used to follow therapy. Recently, a squamous cell carcinoma–associated antigen has been identified in 60–70% of advanced head and neck cancers.

Cancer Staging. The American Joint Commission for Cancer Staging has implemented TNM staging for head and neck cancer. This system is quite complex and therefore should not be used from memory but only with a good staging reference. Recent studies show that thickness of an oral lesion is more important than the area covered when predicting subsequent involvement of lymph nodes and overall survival.

LIP

Squamous cell carcinoma of the lip constitutes 15% of all cancers of the oral cavity. Benign lesions that occur in the lip include mucous cysts, tumors of the minor salivary glands, hemangiomas, and fibromas.

Tumors of the lip are invariably related to exposure to sunlight. The incidence of carcinoma of the lip increases progressively the farther south the latitude of the patient population being considered. Fishermen, sailors, and farmers are occupational groups with a high incidence.

There is a relationship between cancer and tobacco. The residents of nursing homes and institutions are more prone to have carcinoma of the lip from cigarette smoking, presumably because they tend to smoke their cigarettes down to the smallest possible butt. The heat and moist tobacco are directly applied to the lips.

Benign lesions of the lip mentioned above have some interesting systemic correlations. Multiple pigmented spots may be associated with Puetz-Jeghers syndrome, denoting the presence of multiple small intestinal polyps. Scattered small hemangiomas of the lip may be associated with similar lesions elsewhere in the oral cavity and gastrointestinal tract, those of Rendu-Osler-Weber disease.

Hyperkeratosis is a premalignant condition of the lips, usually associated with sunlight exposure. The normal distinct line marking the mucocutaneous borders becomes indistinct. The lip becomes pale, thin, and more fragile. A white film indicative of early hyperkeratosis gradually grows thicker and more exophytic with time. Ultimately, ulceration may appear and give rise to carcinoma in situ and eventually invasive carcinoma. Thirty to forty percent of all carcinomas of the lip are preceded by this condition. Most cancers of the lip are squamous carcinoma. Over 90% of these cancers occur on the lower lip and are slow but relentless in growth. Metastases increase with increasing size. Only approximately 10% of all patients have cervical lymph node metastases. The usual spread is from the lower lip to the submental nodes on the ipsilateral side. Lesions of the upper lip drain to lymph nodes in the anterior portion of the submaxillary gland.

Treatment of carcinoma of the lip can be radiation therapy or operation. There is no statistical difference between these two methods for cure rate. The choice is usually determined by the size of the primary lesion. Small lesions of the lip can be excised easily. Medium-sized lesions require more complex operations and therefore are usually treated with radiotherapy instead. Very large lesions generally require a combination of radiation and surgical therapy with radical neck dissection.

The prognosis for patients with lip cancer is excellent in those with lesions less than 1 cm. Patients with advanced lesions have a 5-year survival of 50%.

ORAL CAVITY

The oral cavity includes the buccal mucosa, anterior two-thirds of the tongue, floor of the mouth, and hard palate. Again, squamous cell carcinoma is the most common tumor. Factors that contribute are smoking, heavy intake of alcohol, poor oral hygiene, and syphilis. The relative risk for oral cancer is higher in pipe and cigar smokers than in other populations. In India, the habit of smoking a cigar with the burning end inside the mouth is widespread and thought to be related to a very high incidence of cancer of the oral cavity.

Alcoholism has a highly suggestive role in oral cancer. As many as 42% of all patients so afflicted have a history of alcoholism.

There is a direct relationship of syphilis to cancer of the tongue. Syphilitic glossitis often leaves a fibrotic tongue scarred with longitudinal fissures and thick hyperkeratotic plaques. Squamous cell cancer of the tongue develops from this base.

BENIGN LESIONS   Inflammatory Hyperplasia   A number of irritating conditions can produce tumor-like projections of the oral mucosa that are not true neoplasms. Some of these are called *fibroepithelial polyp* or *irritation fibroma*. Diagnosis should be confirmed by biopsy. Treatment is usually correction of the causative factor, either by design of new dentures or by discouraging the patient from traumatizing the area.

Mucous cysts are also common in the oral cavity. They arise from salivary gland–bearing areas of the oral mucosa. They are probably secondary to obstruction of the excretory duct of minor salivary glands. Treatment consists of wide surgical unroofing of the lesion.

Ranula is the special name for large mucoceles that result from obstruction of major excretory ducts in the floor of the mouth. Reparative granulomas are benign tumors of the gingiva. They are slow-growing, sessile tumors that bleed easily. Histologic sampling usually reveals multinucleated giant cells distributed throughout the area of fibroblastic proliferation. These lesions have no propensity for malignant transformation but should be treated by complete excision.

Granuloma Pyogenicum   This is an elevated pedunculated or sessile lesion that can occur on the lips, tongue, buccal mucosa, or gingiva. This lesion can be associated with pregnancy and is sometimes called a "granuloma gravidarium." It is usually advisable to wait until the end of pregnancy to treat these granulomas.

Pleomorphic adenomas can arise from minor salivary glands in the oral cavity. They have the potential of becoming malignant, similar to their counterpart in the parotid glands. Treatment is by wide local excision.

Capillary hemangiomas are sometimes seen in the mucous membranes of infants. They usually regress spontaneously by the end of the fifth year. Extremely large vascular malformations can occur and do not regress spontaneously. These lesions require multiple operations to excise hemangiomatous tissue and reconstruct the oral cavity.

Granular cell myoblastoma is a rare lesion that occurs within the muscle of the tongue and appears as a small, firm, spheroid mass. There is no malignant potential, and treatment is simple excision.

HYPERKERATOSIS AND ERYTHROPLASIA   The mucosa of the oral cavity may contain white patches commonly known as *leukoplakia*. More specifically these lesions represent hyperplasia, keratosis, and dyskeratosis. They are usually a response to inflammation. Leukoplakia carries a connotation of a premalignant lesion, but most pathologists prefer to describe specific microscopic changes rather than use this term. Lichen planus and chronic discoid lupus are diseases of the oral mucosa that can cause keratosis and hyperplasia.

Erythroplasia is the appearance of a reddened area in the mucosa and can be the very earliest indication of dysplasia. This occurs most commonly in the floor of the mouth, lingual border, and tonsillar pillars. Erythroplasia is a more definite sign of premalignant change, and all such lesions should be excised promptly.

Squamous cell carcinomas are the most common malignancy of the oral cavity. Some adenocarcinomas occur as derivations from minor salivary glands. In general, lesions of the oral cavity are better differentiated and less malignant than lesions occurring in the oropharynx.

Tongue Carcinoma of the tongue commonly begins at the tip or along the free borders. A small area of ulceration may be seen with a large tumor mass residing in the parenchyma of the tongue itself. Cancer of the tip of the tongue metastasizes to submental lymph nodes, while lesions along the borders metastasize to ipsilateral submandibular nodes.

Tongue carcinomas are quick to metastasize; nearly 40% of patients have adenopathy on first presentation. Therapy is designed, therefore, to attack not only the primary lesion but also the ipsilateral lymph nodes. Surgical treatment includes wide resection of the oral lesion together with radical neck dissection. Pre- or postoperative radiation therapy is frequently used. The horizontal ramus of the mandible must be resected together with the tumor if there is any contact with the periosteum.

Five-year survival rates for patients with cancer of the tongue are approximately 30–40%. Over 50% survival can be obtained if no palpable lymph nodes are present.

Floor of the Mouth Squamous cell cancer in the floor of the mouth tends to extend anteriorly and posteriorly around the rim of the mandible. This pattern of growth results in common bilateral involvement of the anterior floor of the mouth with frequent bilateral cervical metastases. Metastases occur first to the submaxillary lymph nodes. Sixty percent of patients will have palpable cervical metastases on presentation, and 90% will develop cervical lymph node involvement within 1 year of diagnosis.

Large lesions of the floor of the mouth require wide excision in continuity of a portion of the mandible and radical neck dissection. Neck dissection should be done regardless of palpable adenopathy. The 5-year survival rates for patients with this cancer are comparable to those of patients with cancer of the tongue.

Gingiva Cancer of the gums is better differentiated and slower growing than lesions of the tongue. These neoplasms can involve the mandibular nerve with the presentation of numbness in the mental and submental areas.

Treatment of cancer of the lower gum requires resection of the involved mandible together with a radical neck dissection. As metastases of the cervical nodes are relatively less common, treatment is restricted to local excision of the tumor. Five-year survival rate averages 45%.

Hard Palate The most common malignant lesions of the hard palate are tumors of the minor salivary glands. Squamous cell carcinomas are rare in this region. The usual malignancy is an adenoid cystic carcinoma or adenocarcinoma.

The primary symptom is a mass usually noted first by the patient. The tumor is slow growing, and metastases occur late. Primary treatment is by surgical excision. Adequate excision must include resection of the hard palate together with the tumor mass.

Buccal Mucosa Cancers of the buccal mucosa are usually epidermoid. Their natural evolution varies according to the grade of the tumor. A less aggressive form of buccal cancer is encountered in patients who are tobacco chewers and is called *verrucous carcinoma*. This tumor progresses very slowly and is easily recognized by its exophytic form and shaggy white appearance. These tumors are fairly radiosensitive but have a marked tendency to recur and become a much higher grade of malignancy after being exposed to radiation. Therefore, the initial therapy is wide excision. For high-grade lesions, block dissection of the cheek with radical neck dissection is the operative treatment of choice. Five-year survival rate is approximately 55%.

OROPHARYNX

The oropharynx is the region of the mouth posterior to the tonsillar pillars and the circumvallate papillae of the tongue. The most common site for malignant tumors in this area is the tonsil itself. Other structures in this region are the anterior surface of the epiglottis, the soft palate, and the posterior third of the tongue.

Tonsil Inflammatory swelling, or tonsillitis, is the most common benign lesion of the tonsil. Common malignant lesions are high-grade epidermoid carcinomas and lymphosarcomas. These lesions appear grossly as a swelling of the tonsil with a central ulcer. They may present as a typical sore throat with a slight feeling of tenderness. Trismus and pain in the ear are common complaints. These cancers usually spread to lymph nodes near the angle of the mandible. Lymphosarcomas of the tonsil usually present as more bulky primary masses and can be bilateral.

Treatment of tonsillar cancer depends on the diagnosis. Lymphosarcomas are radiosensitive and should be treated primarily by radiation. Epidermoid carcinomas of the tonsil, however, require integrated therapy with pre- or postoperative radiation and resection of the tonsillar mass in continuity with a radical neck dissection. Five-year survival is approximately 25%.

Posterior Third of the Tongue   Lesions on the posterior third are of much higher grade than in other areas of the tongue. They spread rapidly to the cervical lymph nodes. These lesions may attain considerable size before they cause pain or dysfunction. Operation often results in total loss of the tongue, an overwhelming psychologic and functional deficit. Bilateral neck dissection must be combined with resection of the tongue for adequate extirpation of metastatic disease.

Soft Palate   Malignant tumors of the soft palate are almost always squamous cell carcinomas. In contrast to other areas of the oral pharynx these carcinomas tend to metastasize late. Resection is more likely to produce a cure but often leads to a severe functional defect.

Epiglottis   Carcinoma on the anterior surface of the epiglottis is usually exophytic and well differentiated. Radiation therapy is quite successful in treating these lesions. Resection usually requires hemilaryngectomy or total laryngectomy.

LARYNX

The supraglottic larynx is that portion above the true vocal cords. The glottic portion of the larynx is that area made up to the true cords themselves. The mucosa lining the area underneath the true cords down to the lower border of the cricoid cartilage is the infraglottic portion of the larynx. Lesions involving any portion of the exterior of the larynx are spoken of as hypopharyngeal.

Cancer of the larynx overwhelmingly affects men compared to women. Numerous epidemiologic studies have related smoking to carcinoma of the larynx. The induction of carcinoma of the larynx cannot occur solely as a result of tobacco, however; a further agent, or a co-carcinogen, is required. Alcohol is thought to be a co-carcinogen in this disease because a high percentage of patients are alcoholics.

Fifty-six percent of squamous epidermoid cancers of the larynx occur in the glottic region, 42% occur in the supraglottic region, and only 2% are subglottic. Glottic cancers are usually very well differentiated, slow growing, and late to metastasize. Supraglottic and infraglottic cancers are less well differentiated and more likely to spread to lymph nodes when first seen.

Hoarseness is the first symptom of laryngeal cancer. Respiratory obstruction is a late sign. The finding of a tumor on the vocal cord associated with stridor, retraction, or the use of accessory muscles to breath indicates an immediate tracheostomy. Other late signs of malignant lesions of the larynx are pain on swallowing, weight loss, and hemoptysis.

Any patient who has persistent hoarseness for more than 3 weeks should have a careful inspection of the vocal cords by indirect laryngoscopy. If no pathology is found, direct laryngoscopy should be used to examine the cords even more closely.

Benign tumors of the larynx include simple polyps, vocal cord nodules, and retention cysts. These are usually removed by biopsy forceps.

Hyperkeratosis can affect vocal cords as it does the lips and oral cavity. This lesion is evidence of premalignant change and should be stripped off the cord with biopsy forceps.

Viral papillomas occur on the vocal cords of children generally prior to adolescence. Repeated excision is the only effective treatment.

MALIGNANT LESIONS   Carcinoma of the vocal cords usually presents early through hoarseness. These lesions grow slowly enough that early therapy is rewarded by a 90% or better 5-year survival rate. Late presentations are manifested by perforation of the thyroid cartilage and invasion of the soft tissues of the neck.

Radiotherapy alone is appropriate for early vocal cord lesions. For stage II, III, and IV cancers, partial or total laryngectomy is mandatory. A radical or modified radical neck dissection ipsilateral to the lesion is usually performed. Combined radiation therapy and operation in treatment of advanced lesions of the larynx improves the long-term survival rate. In addition, adding chemotherapy to treatment of stage IV lesions has increased survival to as high as 50%.

Following laryngectomy most patients learn to use effective esophageal speech. For the remaining patients, electric vibrating devices can be used to provide tone in the oral cavity that is modulated by the patient's oral structures. Also, the development of the Blum-Singer prosthesis provides artificial speech for many patients. This prosthesis is a silicone valve placed in a passage connecting the trachea and posterior pharynx. Between 60 and 90% success has been obtained with this device. The major problem has been prevention of aspiration of saliva.

HYPOPHARYNX

The hypopharynx includes the piriform sinuses, exterior portion of the aryepiglottic folds, and the lateral and posterior pharyngeal walls. Tumors in this region are also related to smoking. Another etiologic factor is the Plummer-Vinson syndrome, found most commonly in Scandinavian women.

Most of these tumors are epidermoid carcinomas and tend to be of a higher grade than lesions of the oral cavity or larynx. Metastatic spread generally occurs through the lymphatic channels leading to the midjugular chain of lymph nodes. Distant metastases are more common with involvement of the mediastinal nodes, lung, and liver.

The most common presentation of hypopharyngeal cancer is interference with swallowing, either by choking or aspiration. Aspiration pneumonia may be the illness that first brings the patient to the physician. Not uncommonly the first sign of disease is the appearance of a midjugular lymph node.

Treatment requires a judicious combination of radiation and operation. Five-year survival rates are generally reported at 30%. Reconstruction of this region following operation includes myocutaneous skin flaps, free transfer of segments of small bowel with arterial microanastomosis in the neck, or mobilization of the stomach and anastomosis to the base of the tongue.

NASOPHARYNX

Tumors in the nasopharynx are uncommon but not rare. Nasopharyngeal cancer is frequent in the Near East, among the Filipinos, and especially among the Chinese. Thirty percent of all cancers in Taiwan are nasopharyngeal.

The most common benign lesion of the nasopharynx is hypertrophied adenoids. The adenoids represent a portion of the large circle of lymphatic tissue surrounding the respiratory passageway at the level of the posterior tongue and tonsils. Chronic respiratory tract infections cause persistent hypertrophy of this tissue. Occasionally, children will have disturbed breathing patterns and obstruction of the eustachian tube leading to chronic ear infections secondary to hypertrophy of the adenoids. These symptoms are an indication for operative excision.

Epidermoid carcinoma, lymphosarcoma, and adenoid cystic carcinoma are the most common malignancies of the nasopharynx. Epidermoid carcinoma develops in areas of metaplasia along the respiratory epithelium. These lesions invade the roof of the nasopharynx, and then the cavernous sinus with paralysis of cranial nerves III, IV, V, and VI. Pain in the distribution of the supraorbital and infraorbital nerves is frequent. Metastatic disease along the base of the skull causes difficulty with deglutition from hemiparesis of the superior constrictor muscle. Other symptoms are hypesthesia of the mucous membranes of the soft palate, and Horner's syndrome from compression of the cervical sympathetic chain.

The early signs of nasopharyngeal cancer such as brief periods of epistaxis or nasal obstruction are usually missed. Most often, this disease presents as cervical adenopathy. Generally, metastatic nodes are found high in the neck behind the lower portion of the ear.

Treatment of the primary lesion and metastases is usually by radiation therapy. Five-year survival rates are approximately 30%. With no involvement of cervical nodes, five-year survival may be as high as 55%.

Lymphosarcoma of the nasopharynx tends to occur at the extremes of age. These tumors are usually bulky with a rubbery consistency. They do not frequently invade bone, and therefore paralysis of nerves is much less common. Radiation and chemotherapy are the treatments of choice. Five-year survival is approximately 40%.

NASAL CAVITY AND PARANASAL SINUSES

Four pairs of nasal sinuses are found surrounding the nasal cavity. These are the maxillary, ethmoid, frontal, and sphenoid sinuses. Benign tumors of the sinuses are usually polyps secondary to chronic inflammation or allergy. They should be treated by local excision as well as treatment of the underlying pathologic condition that led to their growth.

Most malignant tumors of the nasal sinuses are epidermoid carcinomas followed by lymphoma and tumors from minor salivary tissue. They generally present with pain, nasal obstruction, and persistent nasal secretion. Repeated epistaxis is very suggestive but occurs in only 10% of patients. Bone destruction may be seen on plain radiographs, but this is a late sign.

Treatment of these tumors depends on the tissue diagnosis. Lymphomas are ordinarily treated by radiation therapy alone. Epidermoid carcinomas require preoperative radiation combined with excision. Radical neck dissection is not done unless palpable nodes are present.

MANDIBLE

Tumors of the mandible arise from either the tooth forming (odontogenic) tissue or from bone (osteogenic) tissue. The lesions derived from odontogenic tissue are usually follicular or radicular cysts. These cysts are remnants of tissues sequestered during development that may undergo proliferation and cystic change. Treatment is by intraoral excision. A radicular cyst is caused by infection of the dental pulp. These cysts may grow to several centimeters in size. They are treated by extraction of the involved tooth and excision of the cyst only.

Ameloblastoma is the most common solid tumor of the mandible. It is a slow-growing, relatively asymptomatic tumor that can attain large size. This tumor is treated by segmental resection of the mandible along with the tumor.

Osteogenic tumors of the mandible are generally the same as tumors of any other bone in the body. Benign lesions include torus mandibularis, Padget disease, and giant cell tumor. The malignant lesions of the mandible include multiple myeloma, Ewing sarcoma, chondrosarcoma, and osteogenic sarcoma.

SALIVARY GLANDS

Salivary tissue is found in the parotid gland, submaxillary gland, lingual gland, and numerous other salivary glands. The parotid gland bends around the posterior portion of the mandible and is divided into a large superficial lobe and a smaller deep lobe. The seventh cranial nerve exits from the skull by way of the stylohyoid foramen and passes through the parotid gland, bifurcating within the substance of the gland. Most parotid tumors lie within the superficial lobe. For this reason, great care must be taken during the excision of these tumors not to cut branches of the facial nerve.

The submaxillary gland is found in the digastric triangle of the neck. It is closely related to the mandibular branch of the facial nerve. Also, the lingual nerve passes deep to the inferior surface of the submaxillary gland and parallels the course of Wharton's duct, which conducts saliva from the submaxillary gland to the mouth.

Approximately 60% of all salivary tumors occur in the parotid gland. Women with malignant tumors of the salivary glands are known to have a higher incidence of cancer of the breast.

The most common lesion of the salivary gland is the mixed tumor (pleomorphic adenoma). These are benign tumors that have a loose, myxoid pattern and structures resembling cartilage. Sometimes well-differentiated squamous epithelium can be found.

Papillary cystadenoma lymphomatosum (Warthin tumor) is another benign lesion of the parotid gland that occurs exclusively in males. Ten percent may be bilateral. These tumors usually have well-developed lymphoid tissue.

Mikulicz disease represents a dense infiltration of lymphocytes occasionally arranged in follicles throughout the salivary tissues. This process may be a phase of the larger disease complex called Sjögren syndrome. Most frequently this disease involves a single parotid gland.

Nutritional deficiencies may produce enlargement of the parotid glands. Also, cirrhosis of the liver, kwashiorkor, and diabetes mellitus can cause an increase in the glandular acini of the salivary glands.

Most malignant salivary tumors are found in the parotid gland. Overall, however, only 25% of all parotid tumors are malignant. One-third of these malignant tumors are adenocarcinomas, another third are epidermoid carcinomas, and the remaining third are anaplastic lesions.

Mucoepidermoid carcinoma is a type of epidermoid carcinoma that contains mucous-secreting cells and is found in the parotid gland. The proportion of mucous-secreting cells is inversely related to the grade of the tumor. In the highly malignant tumors epidermoid and intermediate cells dominate the picture. Regional metastases are more common in this situation.

Adenoid cystic carcinoma is a type of adenocarcinoma found in the salivary glands. Besides the presence of mucin these tumors are marked by an arrangement of small, darkly staining cells with relatively low cytoplasm. Cervical lymph node metastases develop in approximately 30% of the cases.

The distinction of benign versus malignant tumors of the salivary gland is made by detection of fixation of the gland to underlying structures, enlargement of cervical lymph nodes, and paralysis of the seventh nerve. In any case, excision of the mass and histologic examination is indicated. Incisional biopsy should not be done. Tumors of the parotid gland should be excised with preservation of the seventh nerve and diagnosis by frozen section. If a low-grade malignant lesion is identified the remainder of the gland and seventh nerve should be removed. If a high-grade lesion is found a radical neck dissection should accompany the procedure.

Most salivary tumors are poorly sensitive to radiation. An occasional epidermoid or adenocarcinoma may be an exception to this generality.

Benign mixed tumors will recur in 40–50% of patients if improperly excised. Malignant tumors have a 5-year survival of 80–90%. Adenocarcinomas have a similar course, with survival dropping to 60% at 10 years.

TUMORS OF THE NECK

Inflammation   Inflammatory swelling in the adult neck is only rarely a hospital problem. In large series of neck masses only 3–4% were inflammatory, with 84% being neoplastic. Tuberculous adenitis, so-called scrofula, was once a common cause of neck masses but now is quite rare.

Malignant Tumors   Almost 80% of malignant tumors of the neck are metastatic from some other site. Of the primary cervical neoplasms most are lymphomas; another large group are tumors of major salivary glands.

Considering these probabilities, the first responsibility of a clinician faced with a hard cervical node is to perform a thorough exploration of possible sites of origin. Masses below and behind the ear are more likely to come from the nasopharynx. Lymphadenopathy at the angle of the mandible suggests a primary lesion in the submaxillary gland, tonsillar area, or floor of the mouth. Enlarged lymph nodes in the submental area should provoke an examination of the tip of tongue, lower lip, and gingivobuccal gutter. Lymph nodes along the middle third of the neck are suspect for primary lesions in the oropharynx, larynx, or thyroid. Only when lymphadenopathy occurs in the supraclavicular area does metastasis from below the clavicle become a major possibility, i.e., lung, mediastinum, or breast. The left supraclavicular nodes are frequently involved by malignant tumors below the diaphragm and are called Virchow's nodes.

If a thorough search for primary lesions is unfruitful, biopsy of the cervical node is carried out. If this confirms the clinical impression of malignancy, further invasive tests are indicated to find the primary. This may include surgical exploration of the maxillary sinus. If a primary lesion still cannot be identified, a radical neck dissection for treatment of the neck is warranted. Eighty percent of patients in this clinical situation will ultimately manifest the primary lesion within 5 years. The other 20% of patients who survive without any apparent sign of a primary lesion are thought to have either a true branchiogenic carcinoma or possibly spontaneous regression of the primary.

Other primary lesions of the neck include dermoid cysts, which usually occur in the midline, and sebaceous cysts, which are common in men and are probably secondary to trauma of shaving. Carotid body tumors (chemodectomas) are rare tumors of the paraganglionic tissue found at the carotid bifurcation. Although malignant transformation is rare, early removal is indicated to avoid complications with the carotid artery.

Masses of the neck in children are more likely to be inflammatory. The most common malignant lesion is lymphoma, and the second most common is carcinoma of the thyroid.

OPERATIONS OF THE HEAD AND NECK

The most commonly performed major operation for cancer of the head and neck is the radical neck dissection. This procedure was originally designed by Crile to eradicate the cervical lymphatic network. Today, surgeons combine radical neck dissection with a simultaneous resection of the primary lesion. These are frequently called *composite resections* or *commando operations*.

Incisions for radical neck dissection are numerous, but among the most common is a hockey-stick incision with the ascending line along the posterior border of the sternocleidomastoid and the horizontal portion across the neck slightly above the clavicle. Skin flaps are made in a plane underneath the platysma muscle. The fibroareolar node-bearing tissue of the neck is dissected away from the trapezius in a medial direction toward the scalene muscle. The phrenic nerve is preserved. The sternocleidomastoid and internal jugular vein are divided. The vagus nerve is spared. The dissection is then carried upward where the hypoglossal nerve is identified and spared. The sternocleidomastoid is transected at the mastoid process. The submaxillary gland is included with the specimen. The spinal accessory nerve is usually sacrificed. The last step is transection of the jugular vein at the point where it leaves the base of the skull.

A modified or "functional" neck dissection spares the sternocleidomastoid muscle, the spinal accessory nerve, and the jugular vein in order to limit the morbidity of the operation.

The indication for this procedure is a neck dissection without clinically positive nodes in the presence of a primary lesion with a relatively high risk of occult nodal metastases.

The mortality of radical neck dissection alone is less than 1%. If neck dissection is combined with en bloc excision of a primary lesion, mortality rates range from 2 to 5%.

Some lesions are at risk for nodal metastases to both sides of the neck and require bilateral neck dissection. This causes marked facial edema that can persist for several weeks. Some surgeons prefer to spare the jugular vein on one side to decrease the amount of edema, while others stage the dissection, allowing a delay of several weeks before operating on the contralateral side.

Parotidectomy   Most lesions in the parotid gland require a superficial parotidectomy. This dissection is carried out through a Y-shaped incision positioned behind the angle of the mandible with the arms of the incision on either side of the earlobe. The main trunk of the VIIth cranial nerve is identified and traced into the parotid parenchyma. Dissection is continued along the external surface of the nerve. Stensen's duct is identified at the midpoint of the gland and is ligated. Temporary weakness of the VIIth nerve is to be expected.

Total Laryngectomy   Total laryngectomy can be accomplished through a transverse incision in the lower neck, similar to thyroidectomy. The upper limit of dissection is approximately 1 cm above the hyoid. All the anterior strap muscles should be removed. The body of the hyoid bone is cut at the junction of the attachments to the lateral wing on either side. The pharyngeal constrictors are cut at the lateral edge of the thyroid cartilages bilaterally. Upon entry into the pharynx the muscles of the tongue are severed from the hyoid and the larynx is pulled forward. Then, vascular pedicles are ligated bilaterally and the trachea is divided obliquely. A tracheostomy is created by careful anastomosis of the mucosa to the skin. The defect in the pharynx is closed transversely with inverting sutures. Before closure a feeding tube is inserted through the nose and into the esophagus for postoperative nutrition.

POSTOPERATIVE CARE FOLLOWING HEAD AND NECK OPERATIONS

Tracheostomy is performed at the time of operation in any patient in whom a portion of the mandible is removed and there is extensive resection of oral structures. The tracheostomy tube must be aspirated frequently and requires the presence of well-trained nursing personnel. Only diligent suction will prevent accumulation of tracheal secretions, which can cause catastrophic anoxia.

Humidification of air for the patient's trachea is essential. This can be done with a moist 4 by 4 sponge draped over the tracheostomy.

On the first postoperative day nasal feedings of half-strength formula should begin. Soon, the patient can be advanced to a pureed regular diet through the feeding tube.

Appropriate antibiotics should be used perioperatively due to contamination of the tissue planes in head and neck operations.

Most important, patients require adequate counseling in preparation for these large operations. Patients do not panic if they understand and expect the problems that can occur, including mental stress, control of saliva, aspiration, and persistent headaches.

In recent years rehabilitation following head and neck resections has made a positive impact on the quality of life in these patients. Major impairments of appearance, swallowing, and speech are important quality-of-life issues for these patients. Myocutaneous flaps and free flaps have improved reconstruction of soft tissues in the head and neck. The pectoralis major flap has been the most popular. Replacement of the mandible has been accomplished with bone transplantations or metal prostheses. The maximum results of rehabilitation are usually obtained by team efforts utilizing the skills of the head and neck surgeon, plastic surgeon, oral surgeon, speech therapist, and psychotherapist.

16 CHEST WALL, PLEURA, LUNG, AND MEDIASTINUM

ANATOMY

Framework   The thoracic cage, which tapers sharply in the upper chest and is conical in shape, consists of the sternum, 12 thoracic vertebrae, 10 pairs of ribs that end anteriorly in segments of cartilage, and 2 pairs of floating ribs. The cartilages of the first 6 ribs have separate articulations with the sternum; the cartilages of the seventh through the tenth ribs fuse to form the costal margin before attaching to the lower margin of the sternum.

Musculature   The pectoralis major and minor muscles constitute the principal musculature of the anterior thorax. The latissimus dorsi, trapezius, rhomboid, and other shoulder girdle muscles form the muscular coat for the posterior thorax. The lower margin of the pectoralis major forms the anterior axillary fold, and the convergence of the latissimus dorsi and teres major muscles forms the posterior axillary fold.

Pleura   The pleura is an active serous membrane with a vascular and lymphatic network. There is constant movement of fluid, phagocytosis of debris, and sealing of air and capillary leaks. The visceral pleura covers the lung and is insensitive. It is continuous over the hilum and mediastinum with the parietal pleura, which covers the inside of the chest wall and diaphragm. The parietal pleura has nerve endings for pain; only when disease extends to this pleura of the chest wall is pain produced. The pleura extends slightly beyond the lung border in each direction and is completely filled with normal lung expansion; only a potential space exists.

Intercostal Space   The parietal pleura constitutes the innermost layer, followed by three layers of muscles, which elevate the ribs during quiet respiration. The vein, artery, and nerve of each interspace are located behind the lower margin of the rib. Hence, a thoracentesis needle or a clamp used to enter the pleura should be inserted across the top of the lower rib of the selected interspace.

Diaphragm   The peripheral muscular portions arise from the lower six ribs and costal cartilages, from the lumbar vertebrae, and from the lumbocostal arches; the muscular portion converges to form a central tendon. The phrenic nerve supplies the motor innervation, and the lower intercostals supply the sensory innervation. The diaphragm, which rises as high as the nipple, contributes 75% of pulmonary ventilation during quiet respiration.

THORACIC INCISIONS

Lateral Thoracotomy *Anterolateral.*   This incision extends from the sternal border above the fourth interspace to the midaxillary line. It requires division of the pectoralis major and minor muscles and the serratus anterior. The incision allows rapid entry into the chest with the patient in the semidecubitus position. Therefore, it is the preferred incision for trauma and hemodynamically unstable patients. Exposure is adequate for mediastinal operations, for some cardiac procedures, and for resection of the middle and upper lung lobes.

Posterolateral.   This incision is used for the majority of pulmonary resections, for esophageal operations, and for the approach to the posterior mediastinum and vertebral column. The skin incision starts at the anterior axillary line just below the nipple, extends posteriorly below the tip of the scapula, and ascends between the scapula and the vertebral column. Parts of the serratus anterior, latissimus dorsi, and trapezius are divided, and the thoracic cavity entered usually in the fifth interspace.

Midlateral.   No major muscle groups are divided, allowing for quick closure and less patient discomfort. Good exposure is attained with single lung ventilation.

In general, with lateral thoracotomies postoperative respiratory therapy is essential as the patients experience significant pain and avoid using their chest muscles. Patients must also be properly positioned to prevent posterior dislocation of the shoulder and brachial plexus injury.

Median Sternotomy   Median sternotomy is the optimal incision for anterior mediastinal and cardiac surgery. The pleural spaces can be entered or avoided as desired. The skin incision extends from the sternal notch to the xyphoid, and the sternum is split to enter the chest. Since fewer muscles are divided, patients have less postoperative pain and impaired pulmonary function than with a lateral thoracotomy.

Bilateral anterior thoracotomy and thoracoabdominal incisions are avoided, as they cause significant patient discomfort and postoperative complications.

PREOPERATIVE EVALUATION

All operations on the chest result in some short-term respiratory disability, and many effect removal or permanent alterations in function of intrathoracic organs. Hence, the following factors are examined to assess the ability of the patient to undergo surgery.

CARDIAC STATUS Electrocardiogram is essential. If history, examination, or EKG reveal any abnormalities, cardiology consultation is required. Further evaluation may entail echocardiograms, nuclear scans, or coronary angiograms. Goldman and associates have identified nine factors (S_3 gallop, MI <6 months ago, >5 PVCs, age >70, aortic stenosis, emergency operation, poor general medical health, rhythm other than sinus or PACs, intraperitoneal, aortic or intrathoracic operations), which are assigned point values and correlate with incidence of cardiac complications.

NUTRITION Malnutrition increases the morbidity and mortality of any surgical procedure. Particularly important in thoracic surgery patients are the adverse effects of protein depletion on respiratory function. The muscle groups in the thorax, shoulder, and diaphragm that are involved in respiration and coughing share in the unselected loss of strength seen in all muscles. Coupled with the increased tendency for pulmonary edema and the relative immunosuppression of malnutrition, the risk of a thoracic operation rises. Nutritional status should be assessed by history, physical exam, and laboratory tests (i.e., hemoglobin, coagulation, liver enzymes, total lymphocyte count).

PULMONARY FUNCTION Pulmonary function must be adequate to tolerate the operation and the postoperative period. No single test is available that provides an adequate overall evaluation of lung function. Measurements of value include lung volumes, mechanics of breathing, regional lung function, diffusion capacity, and arterial blood gases.

Spirometry. Vital capacity (VC, normal 70 mL/kg), the amount of air that can be forcefully expelled from a maximally inflated lung position, is normal or near-normal in patients with moderately severe obstructive airway disease, and is reduced in individuals with restrictive pulmonary or neuromuscular disease. The forced expiratory volume (FEV_1) is reduced in obstructive airway disease, but the degree of reduction varies in the same individual. The FEV_1 may be the most useful test to monitor patients with marginal pulmonary function who are being prepared for operation by aggressive respiratory therapy. The FEV_1 is reported as an actual volume and as a percentage of the VC (FEV_1/VC). The values obtained with spirometry in patients are compared with those obtained from other normal individuals of the same sex, age, and height, and are reported as a percentage of normal.

Blood-Gas Determination.   The Pa_{CO_2} measurement provides an immediate indication of the patient's alveolar ventilation; any value above 46 torr signifies hypoventilation. Elevation of the Pa_{CO_2} suggests abnormalities in distribution of ventilation and perfusion; patients with chronic lung disease may be treated aggressively to improve pulmonary function and then be considered for operation. Normal Pa_{O_2} is 85 torr at sea level. If it is below 70 torr, an attempt should be made to determine the cause and to improve the patient's respiratory exchange.

Specialized Tests.   Radionuclide perfusion scanning for regional lung function allows determination of the separate contributions of the right and left lungs to overall pulmonary function ("split-function" study) and is helpful for patients with compromised pulmonary reserve determined by spirometry. Postoperative VC and FEV_1 can be predicted for the patient who requires pulmonary resection (predicted postoperative FEV_1 = preoperative FEV_1 × percent perfusion in noninvolved lung segments). Perioperative mortality is increased significantly if the predicted postoperative FEV_1 is less than 800 mL.

Exercise Testing.   This is indicated for patients with reasonable exercise capability despite severe obstructive airway disease. The treadmill speed is increased to 3 m/h and the elevation is raised in 10° increments; patients who complete the test are good risks to tolerate pneumonectomy even with significant impairment on spirometry.

Many patients are smokers, and every effort should be made to stop for 2 or more weeks before operation. Aggressive attention should be given to reduce the amount and tenacity of secretion, as well as to identify and treat any pulmonary infection.

POSTTHORACOTOMY CONSIDERATIONS

Pulmonary Function Changes   Vital capacity is reduced 25–50% in addition to the amount of functioning lung that was removed. This is often accompanied by an increase in the closing volume, thus potentiating the development of atelectasis. The severe pain and the sedative effects of the postoperative analgesia produce reductions in tidal volume and elimination of normal sighs. Coughing is inhibited, as is ciliary function and alveolar macrophage activity; hence, the protection against inhaled particulate matter and microbes is diminished.

Complications   Atelectasis means closure of lung units, and it exists as microatelectasis (not visible on chest x-ray), and macroatelectasis (the collapse of a segment, lobe, or entire lung). It is caused by retained bronchopulmonary secretions, decreased sighing, and decreased expiratory reserve volume, and may lead to fever and ventilation/perfusion mismatch. Postoperative bronchopulmonary infectious complications consist of tracheobronchitis and pneumonitis. They are a consequence of diminished pulmonary function and can hinder postoperative recovery.

Pain   Incisional pain is severe, and unless it is well managed it will cause diminished respiratory mechanics. It is a challenge to give patients enough pain medication so that they are able to cough, without giving them so much that they lose their drive to do so. Analgesia is usually administered IM or IV, but there is reported success with intercostal blocks and epidural anesthesia.

THORACIC INJURIES

The predominant types of injury include high-velocity penetrating wounds (usually military), knife or low-velocity gunshot wounds (civilian), or blunt injury from motor vehicle accidents.

CONDITIONS REQUIRING URGENT CORRECTION Airway Obstruction   The oropharynx should be cleared of debris and the neck positioned by an anterior chin-thrust motion while applying continuous cephalad traction to the head. Nasotracheal or orotracheal intubation or cricothyroidotomy should be performed as indicated.

Tension Pneumothorax   When injury to the lung parenchyma allows air to enter (but not exit) the intrapleural space, the pressure increases, causing a shift of the mediastinum and compression of the contralateral lung as well as a decrease in venous return. Release of tension by a thoracostomy tube or large bore needle is life-saving.

Open Pneumothorax   When a segment of chest wall that is greater than the cross-sectional area of the trachea is destroyed, air is sucked through the wound into the chest rather than through the trachea into the alveoli. A watertight seal should be placed and a tube inserted into the pleural space.

Massive Flail Chest   When severe blunt injury results in a two-point fracture of four or more ribs, the chest wall becomes flail. The patient is unable to develop sufficient negative pressure to maintain ventilation; intubation and positive pressure ventilation is mandatory.

Massive Hemothorax   If a patient has percussion dullness of a hemithorax after trauma, a chest tube should be inserted. If massive hemothorax is found (>1500 mL initially, or >200 mL/h for 4 h), the patient should be explored.

Conditions Requiring Urgent Thoracotomy

1. Massive air leak: This signifies disruption of the trachea or a major bronchus. Greater than 80% of injuries are within 2.5 cm of the carina.
2. Pericardial tamponade in the presence of trauma.
3. Esophageal perforation.

DANGEROUS BUT LESS COMPELLING INJURIES   Diaphragm Rupture   Rupture is most commonly caused by penetrating trauma or crush injuries. The left hemidiaphragm is more prone to rupture (ratio of 9:1 compared to the right side). Repair is required to prevent herniation of abdominal contents, which can strangulate and perforate or prevent adequate ventilation by occupying the thoracic cavity.

Pneumothorax   Pneumothorax is usually the result of injury to the lung or the tracheobronchial tree, and can be associated with a hemothorax. In cases with greater than 50% collapse, in those with hemopneumothorax, and in patients with penetrating chest trauma, an intercostal catheter should be inserted and attached to 10–25 cmH$_2$O suction. If the pneumothorax is stable, it can be observed and will resorb at a rate of ~1.25%/day.

Interstitial Emphysema   This condition is caused by disruption of the respiratory tract or esophagus without air entering the pleural space: The air spreads into the mediastinum, the deep tissue planes, and the subcutaneous space. The patient's appearance is markedly distorted, but there is no reason to "treat" the condition, except to take steps to stop the air leak.

Rib Fractures and Lesser Flail Injuries   The main concerns are pain control and for the patient to maintain adequate ventilation. Intubation and positive pressure ventilation are required if there is any respiratory distress. Associated factors to beware of include: delayed pneumothorax, hemothorax, pulmonary contusion, and subclavian injury from an anterior first rib fracture.

Sternal Fractures   Sternal fractures are usually transverse, occuring at or near the manubrium, and are painful. It is essential to rule out injury to underlying structures, especially the heart (echocardiograms, continuous EKG monitoring for at least 24 h, CPK enzymes).

Hemothorax   Massive or continued intrathoracic bleeding requires a thoracotomy. If the costophrenic angle is merely blunted (implying <300 cc), a hemothorax may be followed. Larger amounts of blood need to be evacuated with a thoracostomy catheter. If the hemothorax persists because of a poorly functioning tube, thoracotomy and removal of the clot is indicated to prevent fibrothorax and empyema.

Pulmonary Injury   The lungs have a remarkable ability to tolerate penetrating and blunt trauma. Any penetrating object causes a degree of pneumothorax and bleeding. With insertion of an intercostal catheter the lung reexpands, tamponades the injury, the eventually heals. Thoracotomy is rarely needed to control bleeding. Contusion is caused by blunt injury and is characterized by capillary disruption and a "fluffy" infiltrate on chest x-ray 24–48 h after the injury. If a significant area is involved, mechanical assistance may be required, but usually not for more than 48–72 h.

CHEST WALL

Congenital Deformities

PECTUS EXCAVATUM   Pectus excavatum is the most common congenital deformity of the chest wall, and is attributed to overgrowth of the lower costal cartilages and ribs. The body of the sternum is displaced posteriorly to produce a funnel-shaped depression. Asymmetry is common and the defect varies widely in expression. The anomaly is three times more common in males and there is a familial tendency. Thirty to 70% of patients report symptoms including exercise intolerance, atypical chest pain, dyspnea, bronchospasm, and arrhythmias. However, there is little solid evidence to support functional cardiopulmonary impairment. Operative correction is recommended between 18 months and 5 years to prevent postural and psychological consequences of the defect, but correction in adolescence is also justifiable in order to allow evolution of the defect. The operative technique involves excising the deformed costal cartilage, separating the intercostal muscle bundles from the sternum, and then correcting the sternal concavity. This is done by combining a forward fracture of the sternum with an insertion of bone posteriorly, inserting a metal strut to elevate the sternum, or inverting the entire sternum.

PECTUS CARINATUM   The protrusion deformities of the sternum are much less common than pectus excavatum. Most patients are asymptomatic, and operative treatment consists of resection of the deformed cartilage and contouring of the sternum with transverse osteotomies.

STERNAL FISSURES   Fissures are caused by failure of the sternal primordia to fuse. The superior sternal cleft is broad and extends to the fourth costal cartilage. Osteotomies of each half and reapproximation can usually be performed. Distal sternal cleft is invariably part of Cantrell's pentology, which consists of other defects in the heart, diaphragm, and ventral abdominal wall. Complete sternal cleft is the rarest form of fissure and should be repaired during infancy.

Thoracic Outlet Syndrome

The thoracic outlet is a tight space with rigid delimiters. Any further confinement (cervical rib, healed clavicular fracture, variation in insertion of the scalene muscles) can cause compression of neurovascular components that traverse the space. Compression usually occurs in the small space between the first thoracic rib and clavicle: other sites are the scalene triangle and the pectoralis minor space. Symptoms are primarily neurogenic (90%) and include: aching in the base of the neck, shoulder, or arm; paresthesias down the medial side of the arm; weakness in grip; and forearm fatigue. The nerve most often affected is the ulnar. Symptoms of arterial compression (<10%) include numbness, pallor, fatigue, coolness, and sensitivity to cold.

Diagnosis is made by careful history (focusing on trauma, or occupation or exercise activities) and physical exam. The tests, which include the Adson maneuver (loss of radial pulse on scalene contraction), pressure over the brachial plexus to reproduce the typical pain, percussion-induced pain, and hyperabduction maneuvers, are positive in a large proportion of normal patients. Objective tests include ulnar nerve conduction velocity and somatosensory evoked potentials.

Initial treatment is conservative and consists of physical

therapy. The basic surgical treatment of refractory symptoms is first rib resection, which requires division of the anterior and middle scalene muscles, along with release of any congenital bands or cervical ribs. Arterial reconstruction is performed as required for subclavian artery abnormalities.

Chest Wall Tumors

Metastatic lesions from the breast or lung primaries are the most common chest wall tumors. About half of primary tumors are malignant, and hence the initial biopsy should provide adequate tissue for proper diagnosis.

BENIGN TUMORS

- Fibrous dysplasia (osteofibroma, bone cyst) presents as a slowly enlarging nonpainful mass.

- Eosinophilic granuloma is a solitary destructive process associated with pain and tenderness and may heal spontaneously.

- Osteochondroma is a slow-growing tumor from the cortex of a rib.

- Chondroma occurs at the costochondral junction in children and young people. It can be confused pathologically with a chondrosarcoma, and therefore initial wide local excision is recommended.

- Desmoid tumors have a tendency to recur and should be resected with a wide margin.

MALIGNANT TUMORS

- Fibrosarcoma usually arises from the soft tissue and commonly metastasize to the lungs. Wide resection and chemotherapy is currently recommended.

- Chondrosarcoma is a slow-growing malignancy that occurs in the anterior chest and requires wide local excision.

- Osteogenic sarcoma grows rapidly and results in both bone destruction and production. Aggressive chemotherapy, radiotherapy, and wide excision are required.

- Ewing's sarcoma occurs in the first two decades of life and presents with fever, malaise, and a rapidly growing painful mass. Onion skin appearance on x-rays is classical, and the treatment is irradiation with radial surgery. The prognosis is poor.

- Myeloma is a disease primarily of the elderly and is usually systemic. Solitary myeloma confined to a rib is rare but has a better prognosis.

Chest Wall Reconstruction

Radial excision of malignant chest wall tumors can be accomplished with respiratory support and adequate reconstruction to provide chest wall stability. Many techniques for reconstruction are employed including synthetic meshes, acrylic plates, and myocutaneous flaps.

DISEASES OF THE PLEURA AND PLEURAL SPACE

Pleural Effusion

A pleural effusion is an accumulation of fluid in the pleural space. A concave meniscus in the costophrenic angle suggests the presence of at least 250 mL fluid. Lateral decubitus views can detect smaller amounts of fluid and can confirm that the fluid is free. A transudate is a protein-poor ultrafiltrate of plasma and is caused by alterations in systemic hydrostatic colloid osmotic pressure. Examples include CHF, cirrhosis, nephrotic syndrome, hypoproteinemia, and peritoneal dialysis. Changes in capillary permeability caused by inflammation or infiltration of the pleura produce a protein-rich effusion classified as an exudate. Examples include malignancy, infection, infarction, trauma, and sympathetic effusion. Characteristics of the fluid that distinguish exudate from transudate are pH <7.2, high protein, foul smell, red cell count >100,000, elevated amylase, and Gram's stain positive for bacteria. Pleural effusions can produce dyspnea. Thoracentesis is the mainstay of diagnosis. Therapeutic drainage of transudative effusions is rarely indicated, since they will reaccumulate unless the underlying condition is improved. Exudative effusions usually warrant a more aggressive approach.

MALIGNANT PLEURAL EFFUSION   Malignant effusions are caused by interference of venous and lymphatic drainage by direct tumor invasion and are frequently massive and symptomatic. The fluid is exudative and often bloody. The presence of a malignant effusion is a poor prognostic sign and treatment is palliative, consisting of tube thoracostomy to evacuate all fluid and pleurodesis (usually with tetracycline).

EMPYEMA   Empyema is a suppurative infection of the pleural space, most often associated with pneumonia (*Staphylococcus, Streptococcus,* and gram-negative organisms), trauma, pulmonary infarction, or extension from an intraabdominal source. Initially the fluid is free but the suppuration leads to a fibrinous "peel" that traps the lung and prevents reexpansion. Thoracentesis with Gram's stain confirms the diagnosis, and a CT scan is useful in delineating abscess, loculations, and lung parenchyma.

The first step of treatment is chest tube insertion and closed suction. If the lung reexpands and the cavity is obliterated, the tube can be simply removed. If the drainage persists and the lung is adherent to the chest wall, the closed drainage can be easily converted to open drainage. If the lung is trapped and does not reexpand with high suction, thoracotomy and decortication are indicated.

CHYLOTHORAX   Chylothorax is a milky, odorless effusion consisting of leaking lymphatic fluid from the thoracic duct. The most common cause is surgical trauma followed by noniatrogenic trauma and malignancy. Chylothorax is frequently massive (average loss >750 mL/day) and can produce dehydration, malnutrition, and loss of circulating lymphocytes. Conservative treatment is usually successful and consists of keeping the lung expanded and decreasing chyle production by eliminating oral intake and starting parenteral nutrition. If conservative treatment fails (persistent drainage after 2 weeks, or >500 mL/day in an adult), surgical treatment is indicated. If it is hard to find the actual site of injury, the thoracic duct is ligated in the right chest close to the diaphragm.

Tumors

MESOTHELIOMA   This neoplasm originates from the mesothelial lining of serosal cavities. Eighty percent of cases present in the pleura, with 20% in the peritoneum. It is associated with asbestos exposure, with smoking as an important cofactor. Mesothelioma exists in a benign (15% of the total) and a malignant form (85% of the total). The benign form is usually asymptomatic and unifocal, and resection is the treatment of choice.

Malignant mesothelioma is locally aggressive, 2:1-male predominant, and multicentric, with multiple pleural-based nodules forming sheets separated by loculated, cystic spaces. Most patients die of the primary tumor, although hematogenous and lymphatic spread occurs in one-third of the cases.

Radical extrapleural pneumonectomy or complete pleurectomy combined with chemotherapy and radiation can extend survival, but long-term survivors are rare.

METASTATIC PLEURAL TUMORS Over 90% of pleural tumors are metastatic, with lung and breast being the most common primaries.

Spontaneous Pneumothorax

Spontaneous pneumothorax most commonly results from rupture of a pulmonary bleb or bullae and occurs in young males without significant pulmonary disease. The incidence of recurrence increases after each episode. An asymptomatic pneumothorax with less than 30% collapse that does not increase in size over 8 h can be observed. Otherwise a thoracostomy tube is inserted to allow lung reexpansion. Operation may be required for a persistent air leak (> 1 week), massive air leak preventing lung expansion, or after the second episode. At thoracotomy, the site of leak is closed and a pleural abrasion is performed.

LUNG

Anatomy

Segmental Anatomy The right lung has three lobes (upper, middle, lower), while the left lung has two lobes (upper and lower). Each lobe contains a segmental blood supply and bronchial network, with the right lung containing 10 segments and the left lung containing 9 segments. Separation of the bronchial and vascular stalks allows subsegmental and segmental resections when lung tissue needs to be preserved.

Lymphatic Drainage Two groups of lymph nodes drain the lungs: the pulmonary or N_1 nodes and the mediastinal or N_2 nodes. In turn, the pulmonary nodes consist of intrapulmonary, lobar, interlobar (referred to as the lymphatic sump of Borrie, as all lobes of the corresponding lung drain into that group of nodes), and hilar nodes. The mediastinal nodes consist of anterior mediastinal, posterior mediastinal, tracheobronchial, and paratracheal nodes.

Diagnostic Modalities

AIRWAY INVESTIGATION Sputum Sputum is needed for culture and cytology, and must be obtained past the level of the larynx. This is done by percutaneous transtracheal or orotracheal aspiration, or by saline-induced coughing.

Bronchoscopy Bronchoscopy allows direct visual examination of the tracheobronchial tree, direct biopsies of bronchial neoplasms, and the ability to assess mobility of surrounding structures, extent of endobronchial involvement, and on occasion the source of bleeding. Therapeutic uses include removal of foreign bodies or inspissated secretions.

IMAGING The standard posteroanterior (PA) chest x-ray remains the most frequently used study and is an adequate screening tool. For better definition, the computed tomography (CT) scan and the magnetic resonance imaging (MRI) scan are used. Nuclear medicine imaging plays an important role in ventilation/perfusion studies (i.e., for diagnosing pulmonary embolus) and split function testing. Bronchography and pulmonary angiography are used rarely.

BIOPSIES Needle Biopsies Percutaneous transthoracic needle biopsy (PTNB) is gaining popularity as the skills of the radiologists and pathologists improve. It is performed under local anesthesia, and is associated with few complications that require further therapy. It can help identify malignancies, infections, sarcoidosis, and other pulmonary diseases. Contraindications include coagulopathy, pulmonary hypertension, bullous lung disease, and positive-pressure ventilation.

Mediastinoscopy This is used to evaluate and biopsy mediastinal masses or identify spread of pulmonary neoplasms. The paratracheal, tracheobronchial, and subcarinal nodes are accessible, while posterior nodes and nodes between the trachea and esophagus are not.

Parasternal Mediastinotomy The second and third costal cartilages are removed and the mediastinum visualized. This is particularly useful for evaluation of nodes left of the aortic arch and in the pulmonary hilum.

Open Lung Biopsy The chief indication for open lung biopsy is failure of other less invasive techniques to make a diagnosis. A formal operation under general anesthesia is required, and there is some morbidity associated with the procedure.

Thoracoscopy This is useful in diagnosing enigmatic pleural effusions, in staging tumors, in removing foreign bodies, in assisting therapeutic pleurodesis for malignant effusions, and for evacuation of hemothorax.

Congenital Lung Lesions

Agenesis   Bilateral pulmonary agenesis is not compatible with life. Isolated unilateral agenesis (usually on the left) allows for normal life.

Hypoplasia   This is most often seen in association with anomalies that compete with the lungs for space, such as diaphragmatic hernia.

Cystic Adenomatoid Malformation   Neonates present with acute respiratory distress in the first few hours of life. Chest x-ray shows a multicystic "swiss cheese" region with over-expansion and mediastinal shift toward the normal lung. Lobectomy is the treatment of choice and prognosis is excellent.

Pulmonary Sequestration   A portion of lung may be isolated during development and receive its blood supply from the aorta instead of the pulmonary artery. Intralobar sequestrations rest within a lobe, do not have a visceral pleural envelope, but communicate with the tracheobronchial tree. They occur in the posteriobasal segments and present as recurrent pneumonias; the treatment is lobectomy. Extralobar sequestration is less common, does not have tracheobronchial communication, is enclosed by its own pleural sheath, and appears as an unexplained triangular mass in the posterior lung field. Treatment is resection.

Congenital Cysts   These cysts can be single or multiple and are confined to a segment or lobe. They invariably present with infection, as the viscous fluid they contain becomes contaminated after communication with the airway. Resection, after preoperative bronchoscopy and arteriography, is indicated.

Arteriovenous Malformation (AVM)   Pulmonary AVM is a fistula between pulmonary arteries and veins. Multiple small lesions associated with the Osler-Weber-Rendu syndrome account for half of all cases. The other half have lesions that are fewer in number and larger in size. When shunt fraction exceeds 25% of total blood flow, patients can present with cyanosis and polycythemia. Pulmonary angiography confirms the diagnosis. Resection is indicated whenever possible.

Lobar Emphysema   Lobar emphysema presents with massive distention of a lobe or segment that shifts the mediastinum and compresses the contralateral lung. Involvement of the upper or middle lobe is the most frequent finding; lower lobe involvement is rare. Resection is straightforward and curative.

Pulmonary Infections

LUNG ABSCESS Lung abscess is a focus of infection with parenchymal necrosis and cavitation. It is most commonly a complication of necrotizing pneumonia secondary to aspiration and is, therefore, located in segments that are dependent in the supine position (i.e., posterior segments of the upper lobes and the superior segments of the lower lobes). Other causes are bronchial obstruction, seeding from systemic sepsis, pulmonary trauma, and direct extension from extraparenchymal infection. The patients present with fever, appear chronically ill, and describe recent onset of copious foul sputum production. Hemoptysis can occur and be massive; dyspnea is not common.

Treatment is primarily high-dose antibiotics and drainage. Spontaneous drainage by expectoration is adequate, but bronchoscopic aspiration may be needed. Conservative treatment is successful in 75% of patients. When internal drainage is inadequate, external drainage is established by tube pneumonostomy or pneumonotomy, which opens the cavity to the outside. Both procedures depend on pleural symphysis; spillage of the abscess material into the free pleural space can be catastrophic. Lobectomy is the definitive treatment. The indications are chronic symptoms, serious hemorrhage, and suspicion of carcinoma.

BRONCHIECTASIS Bronchiectasis is characterized by bronchial dilatation and variable involvement of surrounding parenchyma. The bronchial mucosa usually remains intact but the bronchi are filled with pus, mucus, and an occasional broncholith. Segmental bronchi of the lower lobes, the right middle lobes, and the lingula are most frequently involved. The disease is most commonly idiopathic; it can be associated with cystic fibrosis or obstruction by tumor, foreign body, or bronchostenosis.

The clinical picture is dominated by cough and mucopurulent sputum production (scant to 1000 ml/day), low-grade fever, weight loss, and hemoptysis. Complete bronchography is the definitive test. Postural drainage, chest physical therapy, and antibiotics will obviate operative treatment in a majority of patients. If symptoms persist and the disease is localized, segmentectomy or lobectomy is indicated.

TUBERCULOSIS Pulmonary infection with *Mycobacterium tuberculosis* behaves like a lung abscess: The smoldering central focus of infection communicates with the tracheobronchial tree, providing drainage for bacilli-loaded sputum and allowing ingress of air to cause cavitation. The intense inflammatory process promotes arterial hypertrophy, and erosion into these vessels can cause life-threatening hemoptysis. Chest x-ray showing upper lobe cavitary changes or a positive PPD is suggestive of the diagnosis. Definitive diagnosis rests on growth of the organism in culture.

Treatment is primarily medical with a combination of drugs including isoniazid, streptomycin, and rifampin. Pulmonary destruction with bronchopleural fistula and empyema, persistently active disease, hemorrhage, or inability to rule out cancer are indications for surgical resection. If limited pulmonary reserve precludes resection, thoracoplasty (resection of the ribs) can be used to collapse the pleural space and obviate infection.

FUNGAL AND FUNGAL-LIKE INFECTIONS   Actinomycosis-*Actinomyces israelii* is an anaerobic bacillus (not fungus) that inhabits the oral cavity and tonsilar crypts. Thoracic infection is thought to occur from aspiration and is characterized by suppuration, abscess, and sinus tract formation and relentless invasion. Diagnosis is made by the presence of sulfur granules (yellow-brown clusters of microorganisms) from sputum, sinus tracts, or biopsies. The organism is sensitive to penicillin, and surgery is very rarely required.

Nocardia   *Nocardia asteroides* is a rare pathogen except in immunocompromised hosts and begins as a pneumonic process grossly similar to tuberculosis and carcinoma. It is a bacillus (not fungus), is relatively easy to culture, and is usually successfully treated with sulfonamides.

Histoplasmosis   *Histoplasma capsulatum* is the most common systemic fungal infection in the U.S. The severity of infection is determined by the size of the inoculum and the immune competence of the host. The disease can take many forms and is distinguishable from tuberculosis only by culture. Amphotericin B is effective in the majority of cases and is the treatment of choice for serious illness. Asymptomatic patients with positive skin tests need not receive chemotherapy. Large, thick-walled cavities that fail to improve after a course of amphotericin B are the most common indication for surgery.

Aspergillosis   *Aspergillus* infection presents in three forms—allergic bronchospasm, invasive (invariably fatal), and saprophytic. Saprophytic disease is caused by colonization of a preexisting pulmonary cavity ("fungus ball"). Diagnosis can be made by skin tests and sputum cultures. Amphotericin B is the treatment for disseminated disease, but it does not enter into a cavity. Hence, surgical resection is the treatment of choice for localized lesions.

Tumors

PRIMARY CARCINOMA Lung cancer is the main cancer killer for both sexes. The primary etiology is tobacco addiction; long-term exposure or co-carcinogens are required, and the risk is reduced by cessation of smoking.

Pathologic Classification Most primary bronchogenic carcinomas arise from basal or mucous cells in the surface epithelium of the bronchial tree. Other sites of origin are the neurosecretory cells (Clara cells) and Kultchintsky cells (carcinoid tumors). The simplest division, based on approach and management, is between non-small-cell lung cancer (NSCLC) and small-cell lung cancer (SCLC).

NSCLC.
- Squamous cell carcinomas: Though more common in the upper lobes, bronchogenic carcinomas develop in all parts of the lung. They are very slow growing, late to metastasize, and may present as central bulky masses with bronchial obstruction or as peripheral lesions with cavitation. Peripheral tumors may present with extensive chest wall invasion before metastases occur. The Pancoast syndrome represents a specific example wherein a tumor in the superior sulcus may invade the brachial plexus, the upper two ribs, and the vascular structures at the thoracic apex. Squamous carcinoma was the leading pulmonary neoplasm in the U.S., but it is now being replaced by adenocarcinoma.

- Adenocarcinomas: These tumors arise in the subsegmental bronchi away from the hilum. Growth is more rapid than in squamous tumors, and early metastasis by the vascular route is common, particularly to the brain and adrenal.

- Bronchoalveolar carcinomas: This variant of lung cancer, with one-third of the patients not having a smoking history, has a more encouraging biologic behavior. It can remain localized as a peripheral tumor with a 5-year cure rate after resection of 50–75%. The diffuse form of the disease presents with rapid dissemination in one or both lungs, with no consideration of operative treatment. The typical cell of the neoplasm arises from the alveolus, with some tumors also containing bronchiole Clara cells.

- Scar carcinomas: This term is used for adenocarcinomas, bronchiolar cell carcinomas, or mixed cellular neoplasms arising from sites of previous pulmonary disease, usually tuberculosis. They are located predominantly in the upper lobes.

SCLC. The small-cell anaplastic carcinoma ("oat cell carcinoma") is a highly malignant, rapidly growing neoplasm, often located centrally because of its origin from a proximal bronchus. It spreads by hilar and mediastinal lymph node involvement, local invasion, and hematologic dissemination. Because of its aggressive behavior, surgical resection was thought to be futile, with chemotherapy being the primary treatment modality. However, there are certain subtypes (specifically the polygonal, fusiform cell type) that can be resected if located in the periphery without lymph node spread.

Staging The TNM classification is used with recent modifications by the American Joint Committee on Cancer (AJCC) (Primary tumor = T):

- T_1: <3.0 cm, without invasion.

- T_2 >3.0 cm, invades the visceral pleura or has associated obstructive pneumonitis. The proximal extent of the tumor must be within a lobar bronchus or at least 2.0 cm distal to the carina.

- T_3: Any size with direct extension to the chest wall, diaphragm, pericardium, or mediastinal pleura, or within 2.0 cm of the carina without involving the carina.

- T_4: Invasion of the heart, great vessels, trachea, esophagus, or carina, or presence of a pleural effusion.

(Nodal involvement = N):

- N_1: metastasis to peribronchial or ipsilateral hilar nodes.

- N_2: Metastasis to ipsilateral mediastinal or subcarinal nodes.

- N_3: Metastasis to scalene, supraclavicular, or contralateral mediastinal or hilar nodes.

Distal metastasis = M; M_1: distant metastasis present:
Stage I: T_1 or T_2 with N_0 M_0. Stage II: T_1 or T_2 with N_1 M_0. Stage IIIa: T_3 N_0 M_0; T_3 N_1 M_0; T_{1-3} N_2 M_0. Stage IIIb: any T N_3 M_0; T_4 any N M_0; Stage IV: any T any N M_1.

Clinical Manifestations Bronchogenic carcinoma is seen predominantly in the 45–65 age group, although it is not rare in men less than 45 years of age. The disease may be discovered incidentally in an asymptomatic patient, but symptoms are usually present: cough (75%), blood-streaked sputum (50%), dull chest pain without chest wall involvement, sputum (50%), dull chest pain without chest wall involvement, localized or radicular pain with chest wall involvement, fever and purulent sputum with bronchial obstruction, hoarseness with left recurrent laryngeal nerve invasion, or dyspnea with a pleural effusion. Loss of appetite and weight loss is an ominous sign: Such patients usually have an unresectable tumor or systemic metastases.

A small percentage of patients, not necessarily with systemic spread, present with extrapulmonary nonmetastatic manifestations, which may be relieved by resection of the primary tumor. They include pulmonary hypertrophic osteoarthropathy with clubbing of the digits, secretions of hormone-like substances (ACTH, ADH, serotonin, PTH), or myasthenia-like syndrome.

Diagnosis and Workup Almost any type of pulmonary infiltrate, nodule, mass, or atelectasis should raise the suspicion of carcinoma, particularly if the patient is or lives with a smoker. Diagnostic modalities include cytology (sputum, lavage, or bronchoscopic washings) and biopsy (bronchoscopic or transthoracic fine needle aspiration). Ten to twenty percent of patients undergo thoracotomy without a proven diagnosis. An effort must also be made to determine whether localized or metastatic spread has occurred, since half the patients are beyond consideration for operative treatment on initial presentation. The key elements are (1) history, (2) examination for suggestive lymph nodes and biopsy if indicated, (3) CT scanning to evaluate mediastinal, abdominal (liver, adrenal), and brain involvement, (4) bronchoscopy, (5) mediastinoscopy, and (6) pleural biopsy and cytology if an effusion is present.

Treatment The treatment of lung cancer involves deciding what is best for the given tumor according to its stage and cell type, and the physical capability of the patient to withstand optimal tumor treatment. Surgery is the only therapeutic option with cure potential: Radiotherapy may provide long-term disease-free survival, but it, along with chemotherapy, is adjunctive or palliative treatment at the current time. Historically, the total pneumonectomy was considered the optimal operation for lung cancer. As reports indicated that prognosis was not compromised by lesser resection, lobectomy became the operation of choice whenever it was possible to adequately remove the primary tumor. A similar evolution is taking place with sleeve and segmental resections, with good short- and long-term control of tumor.

- Stage I NSCLC: Five-year survival in patients who undergo resection is up to 80%. In medically inoperable patients, radiotherapy has a 20% 3-year survival. Females and patients under age 70 have a better prognosis, and cell type makes no significant difference in survival.

- Stage II NSCLC: Surgery is the treatment of choice, and patients can expect a 30–50% 5-year survival. Medically inoperable patients have up to 20% 3-year survival. Seventy percent of surgically treated patients develop regional or distant metastatic disease. Therefore, adjuvant therapy, either radiation or chemotherapy, is recommended.

- Stage IIIa NSCLC: Lymph node metastases decrease survival in bronchogenic carcinoma, but some groups advocate aggressive surgical and adjuvant therapy. In patients who have a potentially curative resection of their pulmonary tumor, including all accessible lymph nodes and chest wall if invasion is present, the addition of radiation may provide up to a 50% 3-year survival. Chemotherapeutic agents (cisplatinum, doxorubicin, and cytoxan) can increase survival.

- Stage IIIb and IV NSCLC: Radiation therapy is indicated for decompression (trachea, esophagus, SVC) for growing tumor. Otherwise, none of the reported therapeutic programs offer patients any significant survival benefit.

- SCLC: Median survival without treatment is 2–4 months. Chemotherapy can prolong survival up to 2 years with a small percentage of cure. Stages I and II patients treated by resection and adjuvant therapy have a reported 5-year survival of 30%, but most patients present initially with diffuse disease.

SOLITARY PULMONARY NODULES (SPN) SPN are defined as an abnormal rounded or ovoid density up to 4 cm in diameter, surrounded by a zone of lung tissue and free of cavitation. Because of the favorable outlook if the nodule is a cancer, there is considerable interest in the differential diagnosis of these "coin lesions." The differential diagnosis includes hamartoma, granuloma, AV fistula, infarct, and several benign and malignant tumors. Reports suggest a malignancy rate of 40–65% in SPN, and 80% in the above-50 age group. A logical approach to SPN would include early thoracotomy for lesions in known risk populations: > 50 years old, smoking history, absence of certain knowledge of a similar lesion on chest film more than 2 years old. In nonsmokers under 35 years old with a small chance for malignancy, needle biopsy and bronchial brush biopsy with observation for growth is appropriate.

OTHER LUNG TUMORS   *Bronchopulmonary Neuroendo-
crine tumors.*   Carcinoid tumors are slow-growing tumors
that metastasize late and can produce serotonin leading to
the carcinoid syndrome. The tumors protrude into the lumen
(80% arise in the proximal bronchi), making bronchial obstruction with infection and atelectasis the most common
clinical presentation. Conservative surgical resection, such
as sleeve resection or local bronchial excision with broncho-
plasty, is the preferred treatment.

Tumors of Bronchial Gland Origin.   Cylindroma and mucoepidermoid tumors are the most common neoplasms arising
from the bronchial glands. Their location is predominantly
central, and may show a spectrum of behavior from benign
to malignant, with distant metastases. Treatment is en-bloc
surgical resection, with cure rates higher than those of
primary carcinoma.

Sarcomas.   A variety of mesodermal sarcomas may occur
in the lung (leiomyosarcoma, lymphosarcoma, fibrosarcoma,
and others) with the same symptoms of primary carcinoma.
There is no increased incidence with cigarette smoking.
Treatment is surgical resection, with prognosis depending on
the stage of the neoplasm.

Benign Tumors.   Benign tumors compromise only 1% of
pulmonary neoplasms. Hamartoma, which is comprised of
disorganized adipose, muscular, and fibrous tissue, is the
most common. They are usually asymptomatic and can be
simply enucleated. Other tumors from epithelial, mesenchymal, or lymphoid origin can occur; their significance is related
to the differential diagnosis from malignancy.

METASTATIC TUMORS   Metastases to the lung are common
during the clinical course of many extrathoracic primary
neoplasms, and resection of these nodules can result in a
significantly improved survival rate. Aggressive treatment is
indicated when the tumor doubling time is greater than 40
days and metastases to other sites have been excluded. As
much lung tissue as possible should be preserved; hence,
wedge resection or segmental resections are strongly preferred.

TRACHEA

Anatomy

The trachea is a centrally located unpaired organ that has an
average length in adults of 11 cm segmented by 18–22

cartilaginous rings. The rings are rigid for the anterior two-thirds, with a membranous portion posteriorly. This allows for flexibility without collapse. The blood supply is derived laterally from the inferior thyroid and bronchial arteries.

Congenital Lesions

The most common lesion is the tracheoesophageal fistula, which is discussed in detail elsewhere. Congenital stenosis, which is rare, presents in several variants: weblike diaphragms, tracheomalacia at sites of compression by a vascular ring, or absence of the membranous trachea with fusion of the rings posteriorly. Congenital stenosis should be suspected in infants with noisy breathing, wheezing, and retractions after birth. Operative treatment is indicated if repeated dilatation or tracheostomy fails to allow growth. When possible, the stenotic segment is resected and the trachea reconstructed with an end-to-end anastomosis. Diffuse involvement may require bone or cartilage splints.

Trauma

The most common injury requiring treatment is that occurring as a complication of tracheal intubation. Soft, low-pressure tubes have reduced but not eliminated the problem. Ischemic necrosis at the tube cuff site can produce stricture, tracheomalacia, or erosion and fistula formation. Blunt and penetrating trauma produce a spectrum of injury ranging from laceration to complete transection.

Resection and end-to-end anastomosis is the preferred treatment. Fistulas are repaired by separating the two structures, closing the defects, and interposing muscle.

Neoplasms

Primary tracheal neoplasms are uncommon; more than 80% are malignant, and squamous cell and adenoid cystic carcinomas account for the majority of histologic types. Patients present with dyspnea, cough, wheezing, stridor, or hemoptysis. Laser ablation is used for palliation with excellent results in 60% of treated patients. Operative resection is both a surgical and anesthesia challenge, as obstructing lesions make ventilation difficult. Ventilation is delivered by placing an endotracheal tube through the distal trachea or bronchus or by "jet" ventilation. A surprising amount of trachea can be resected (up to 5 cm or 10 rings) and reconstructed with ane end-to-end anastomosis. Prosthetic material for tracheal reconstruction remains experimental.

MEDIASTINUM

The mediastinum is the central cavity of the thorax bounded laterally by the pleural cavities, inferiorly by the diaphragm, and superiorly by the thoracic inlet. It is divided into three compartments: (1) the anterior mediastinum, which lies above the heart and contains the thymus along with lymphoid and adipose tissue; (2) the posterior mediastinum, which lies behind the heart and contains the esophagus, thoracic duct, descending aorta, and the autonomic nerve trunks; and (3) the middle mediastinum, which contains the heart, pericardium, aorta, trachea, main stem bronchi, and related lymph nodes.

Tumor and Cysts

Neurogenic tumors are the most common mediastinal tumors in adults (about 20%), followed closely by thymoma, congenital cysts, and lymphoma. Recently, the Mayo Clinic reported on a large series of children where lymphoma was present in >50% of patients followed by neurogenic tumors. Approximately 30% of all mediastinal tumors are malignant, with lymphoma being the most common malignant tumor.

Manifestations and Diagnosis   The most common symptoms are nonspecific (chest pain, cough, dyspnea) and are ascribed to compression of the trachea and esophagus. Other symptoms include SVC syndrome, hoarseness from recurrent nerve palsy, and Horner's syndrome. Nerve root compression through the intervertebral foramen (''dumbbell extension'') can produce localized neurologic deficits. More than a third of patients are asymptomatic. CT scans and magnetic resonance imaging (MRI) provide great potential for imaging the mediastinum. Tissue for pathologic examination may be obtained by endoscopy, percutaneous needle biopsy, mediastinoscopy, or mediastinotomy. Operation provides definitive diagnosis and frequently definitive treatment, and remains an important part of combined protocols for chemotherapy and radiation.

NEUROGENIC TUMORS

1. Neurilemmoma. Neurilemmomas account for 40–60% of all neurogenic tumors. They arise from mature Schwann cells in intercostal nerves and are usually benign.
2. Neurofibromas. Neurofibromas contain elements of both nerve sheath and nerve cells and account for 10% of all neurogenic tumors. Advanced age or presence of neurofibromatosis increases the risk of malignancy to 30%, which carries a poor prognosis.
3. Neuroblastomas. They are poorly differentiated tumors arising from the sympathetic nervous system and can be hormonally active. More than 75% occur in children under 4 years of age. Bone, liver, and lymph node metastases are not infrequent and may make the lesion unresectable. Neuroblastomas are radiosensitive, and debulking followed by radiation can have favorable results.
4. Pheochromocytomas. Intrathoracic primary pheochromocytomas are rare and are usually nonsecreting. Thirty percent are malignant.

THYMOMAS   Thymoma is the most common anterior mediastinal mass in adults, is rare in children, and has a peak age incidence between 40 and 50 years. Symptomatic patients present either with mass effects on adjacent organs or with paraneoplastic syndromes such as myasthenia gravis, hypogammaglobulinemia and red cell aplasia. Histology contributes nothing to the distinction between malignant and benign, which is based entirely on invasive gross characteristics. Benign thymomas can be resected for cure, but malignant thymomas have a poor prognosis.

LYMPHOMAS   Mediastinal lymphoma is most frequently located in the anterior compartment and is present in 50% of patients with Hodgkin's and non-Hodgkin's lymphoma. Radiation is the standard treatment, with the addition of chemotherapy in the presence of systemic spread.

TERATODERMOID TUMORS   Teratomas are found in the anterior mediastinum, are often partially cystic, and consist of ectodermal elements including hair, teeth, and sebaceous glands. Surgical excision through a median sternotomy is the preferred treatment. Eighty percent are benign, and resection is curative. The prognosis for malignant tumors is poor because of local recurrence and distant metastasis.

GERM-CELL TUMORS   Five cell types of extragonadal germ-cell tumors are present. Seminoma and embryonal cell carcinoma are the most common, followed by choriocarcinoma, malignant teratoma, and endodermal sinus carcinoma.

The tumors are highly malignant, and 90% of patients present with symptoms of compression of adjacent structures. Most patients deserve median sternotomy and an attempt at resection. However, prognosis is poor, although various chemotherapy regimens can provide palliation. Seminoma needs to be separated from the other cell types because it is very radiosensitive and 5-year survival approaches 75%.

MESENCHYMAL TUMORS   Lipomas are the most common, followed by fibromas. The malignant forms are rare. Other tumors include hamartoma, leiomyoma, and others. Surgical resection is the treatment of choice.

Mediastinal Cysts

Congenital cysts constitute 20% of mediastinal masses and account for a majority of middle mediastinal lesions. A CT scan demonstrating a mass with near water density occurring in a characteristic location is diagnostic.

Pericardial Cysts   These are the most common cysts occurring in the mediastinum, appear at the right costophrenic angle as a smooth walled cystic mass, and can communicate with the pericardium. If diagnosis is certain, they may be observed.

Bronchogenic Cysts   Bronchogenic cysts are most frequently located posterior to the carina or main stem bronchi. They can communicate with the tracheobronchial tree, producing an air-fluid level, allowing for confusion with lung or mediastinal abscess. All bronchogenic cysts should be resected to remove a site for potential chronic inflammation.

Enteric Cysts   Enteric cysts are located in the posterior mediastinum adjacent to the esophagus. When lined with aberrant gastric mucosa, peptic ulceration can lead to perforation and abscess formation. Resection is always indicated.

Mediastinitis

ACUTE MEDIASTINITIS   Acute mediastinitis is a fulminant infectious process with high morbidity and mortality. It is initiated most frequently by esophageal perforation and less often by tracheal rupture and direct spread from oropharyngeal infections. Chest pain, dysphagia, respiratory distress, and crepitus are the chief findings with florid sepsis and hemodynamic instability supervening rapidly in untreated cases.

Antibiotics and fluid resuscitation are begun immediately. The primary problem, such as esophageal rupture, is treated according to accepted principles. Drainage through the chest and neck is created as required.

CHRONIC MEDIASTINITIS   Chronic inflammation and fibrosis in the mediastinum are thought to result from granulomatous infections, although identification of an organism is rare. The process remains silent until it progresses to produce obstruction. Operative exploration is frequently required to establish a diagnosis and to relieve obstruction.

17 CONGENITAL HEART DISEASE

INTRODUCTION

Incidence of congenital heart disease (CHD) is 3–4/1000 live births, and is 10 times more frequent within family members. Sibling risk is about 2%. In the majority, an etiology cannot be established, though rubella in the first trimester is known to cause CHD (usually PDA).

EMBRYOLOGY

Fetal heart develops between 3 and 8 weeks' gestation. Of the six branchial aortic arches, only the left fourth and left sixth remain. They become the transverse aortic arch and PDA, respectively. Abnormalities of the bulbus cordis septation lead to transposition of the great vessels, truncus arteriosus, and other aortic abnormalities. Septal malformation leads to the varieties of atrial septal defect (ASD), ventricular septal defect (VSD), atrio-ventricular canal, and others.

Fetal circulation is primarily a right-to-left shunted system as oxygenated blood is shunted through ductus arteriosus (DA) and foramen ovale (FO) and bypasses the pulmonary circuit. With expansion of the lungs and decreased pulmonary vascular resistance, the flap valve of the FO is closed [as left atrial (LA) pressures exceed right atrial (RA) pressures] and the DA closes.

Of the large number of CHDs, seven malformations comprise the majority: VSD (20%); and ASD, PDA, coarctation, aortic stenosis, pulmonary stenosis, and transposition of the great arteries (TGA), (each 10–15%).

CLASSIFICATION

Three major physiologic disturbances result from CHD, and therefore three general classifications of CHD exist.

I. Ventricular outflow obstruction (e.g., aortic stenosis, pulmonary valve stenosis, and coarctation of the aorta).
   A. Impede ventricular emptying.

    B. Result in systolic overload with secondary ventricular hypertrophy.

II. Left-to-right shunts (acyanotic group) (e.g., uncomplicated septal defects and PDA).

    A. Result in overload of pulmonary system and CHF is manifest (usually when shunt >1.5–2.0).

    B. Increased pulmonary vascular resistance is the late result of increased pulmonary blood flow.

    C. Considerations:

        1. Pulmonary HTN is more damaging than simply increased pulmonary blood flow. Therefore, ASDs cause less injury to the pulmonary bed than VSDs (provided equal shunt fractions).

        2. It is the pulmonary vascular resistance, not the systolic BP, that is of concern. Once increased resistance has occurred, it usually represents irreversible pulmonary vascular disease and precludes successful surgical correction of their underlying CHD.

        3. Histologic changes in the pulmonary bed are medial hypertrophy (early), intimal thickening (later), and fibrosis (end-stage and irreversible).

    D. Reduction in systemic blood flow may lead to growth and developmental delay.

III. Right-to-left shunts (cyanotic group) (e.g., tetralogy, TGA, truncus arteriosus, tricuspid atresia, and total anomalous pulmonary venous connection).

    A. These result from intracardiac septal defects combined with obstruction to pulmonary blood flow, and are characterized by arterial hypoxemia and cyanosis.

    B. Features

        1. Cyanosis: depends on degree of anoxia and hemoglobin concentration (more easily seen in polycythemic states).

        2. Polycythemia: physiologic response to chronic anoxia, and will result in increased viscosity of blood with thrombotic complications (Hct's >80% associated with cerebral venous thrombosis).

        3. Clubbing of digits: hypertrophic osteoarthropathy, which usually occurs after 2 years of age and will subside after correction of anoxia.

        4. Decreased exercise tolerance with dyspnea on exertion (DOE).

        5. Neurologic damage: three scenarios

            a. Anoxic injury: "cyanotic spells" are periods of unconsciousness secondary to cerebral anoxia and have grave implications.

  b. Brain abscesses: bacteria have direct access to left-sided circulation.
  c. Paradoxical venous thromboembolism: DVTs can migrate through intracardiac defect and be expelled out aorta

EVALUATION OF THE PATIENT

  I. History
    A. Prenatal exposures/diseases
    B. Family diseases
    C. Age when murmur or symptoms (e.g., cyanosis, poor feeding, increasing fatigue) appeared
 II. Physical examination
    A. Assess growth and development
    B. Cyanosis (clubbing)
    C. Heart (murmur, thrill, size, lift)
    D. Lungs (CHF)
    E. Liver enlargement is hallmark of CHF in children
    F. Extremities (pulses, clubbing)
III. Laboratory
    A. CXR (heart size and contour, lung vascularity, rib notching)
    B. EKG (ventricular hypertrophy, axis deviation, conduction defects)
    C. Echocardiography: noninvasive but quite precise and sensitive modality; except for few complex abnormalities, it is the diagnostic method of choice
    D. Cardiac catheterization: advantages of pressure measurements, abnormal shunts detected, flow ratios and valve areas calculated

PRINCIPLES OF CARE

  I. Operative management: four keys for safe surgery
    A. Temperature of patient
    B. Precise fluid management
    C. Prevention of air embolus (especially those with right-to-left shunts)
    D. Serial arterial blood gas (ABGs)
 II. Postoperative: four important principles
    A. Constant observation
    B. Telemetry
    C. Serial ABGs
    D. Attentive respiratory physiotherapy

SPECIFIC ABNORMALITIES

I. Obstructive lesions
   A. Pulmonary stenosis
      1. Incidence
         a. 10% of all CHD
         b. No known etiologic factors
      2. Pathology
         a. Spectrum of valvular, annular, and RV and PA disorders
         b. Most commonly 2° to fused valve cusps
         c. Atresia (true) is rare
         d. Annular hypoplasia is important to recognize, as it affects the approach to the repair
         e. Foramen ovale is always patent 2° to increased RA pressures
      3. Pathophysiology
         a. Increased RV systolic pressures with 2° right ventricular hypertrophy (RVH)
         b. Severity is graded by RV systolic–PA systolic gradient
            Mild: < 50 mmHg
            Moderate: 50–80 mmHg
            Severe: 80 . . . may reach 100–200 mmHg
         c. Progressive RVH with RV failure usually occurs late
      4. Clinical
         a. Symptoms: frequently none, but mild dyspnea and easy fatigability are most common
         b. Examination: weak S2, harsh systolic ejection murmur at 2d intercostal space; RV lift, palpable
         c. Laboratory: CXR—increased RV size and decreased vascularity
            EKG: RVH
            Echocardiography is diagnostic
            Catheterization: essential to outline RV outflow
      5. Treatment
         a. Critically ill neonates
            i. PGE₁—to keep PDA open
            ii. Balloon valvuloplasty
         b. Operative repair
            i. Longitudinal arteriotomy (in PA) dividing fused commisures
            ii. Calibrate annular size using Hegar dilators
            iii. May require ventriculotomy with patch if infundibular stenosis is present

    iv. Close foramen ovale, measure pressures after procedure to check gradient

    v. 1% operative mortality after neonatal period

B. Congenital aortic stenosis

  1. Incidence: about 10% of all CHD

    a. 3–4 times more common in males

    b. No etiologic factors identified

  2. Pathology: four types identified

    a. Bicuspid valve: common (about 2% of general population) and usually results from undeveloped commisures

    b. Tricuspid valve with fused commisures

    c. Subvalvular stenosis: ranges from a discrete ring to a complete fibromuscular tunnel

    d. Supravalvular stenosis: most rare (described later)

  3. Associated anomalies occur in up to 20% (PDA, coarctation, VSD, pulmonary stenosis)

  4. Pathophysiology: directly related to degree of obstruction

    a. Cardiac catheter quantifies obstruction by measuring peak LV systolic and peak aortic root pressures (gradient)

    b. Valve cross-sectional area may be calculated using pressure gradients and cardiac output; severe lesions have valve area < 0.5 cm^2

    c. Using pressure gradients alone
      Mild stenosis: <40 mmHg
      Moderate stenosis: 40–75 mmHg
      Severe stenosis: >80 mmHg

    d. LVH develops to a varying degree

    e. Pressure gradient may fall as the ventricle fails

    f. Calcification of fused cusps universal by third or fourth decade

    g. LV impairment is rarely manifest in childhood, but when signs/symptoms appear, there is a 4–9% risk of sudden death

    h. Endocarditis is rare (1–3%)

  5. Clinical

    a. Children frequently asymptomatic, but symptoms of fatigue, dyspnea, angina, and syncope are usually seen when gradient > 50 mmHg

    b. Examination features

      i. Basal systolic ejection murmur with wide transmission to neck and arms

      ii. LV heave

      iii. Palpable thrill in >80%

      iv. Decreased pulse pressure in 30–40%

  6. Laboratory

    a. EKG: LVH & LV strain

    b. CXR: normal to slightly increased heart size

    c. Echocardiography: concentric LVH

    d. Catheterization: establishes diagnosis and quantifies severity

  7. Treatment: usually on an elective basis
Techniques

    a. Commissurotomy (care to cause no aortic insufficiency)

    b. Resect the ring in subvalvular stenosis (care to bundle and mitral valve, safe area is between right and left coronary cusps)

    c. If LV outflow tract obstruction is severe, Konno procedure is preferred

C. Supravalvular aortic stenosis, special type of AS

  1. Rarest form

  2. Pathologic anatomy ranges from hourglass > diffuse hypoplastic > membranous forms

  3. Frequent associated anomalies

     i. $\frac{1}{3}$ have abnormal AV cusps

     ii. $>\frac{1}{2}$ have abnormal coronary arteries (dilated and tortuous)

    iii. Focal stenotic lesions of arch and PA found

    iv. Associated with "elfin facies" and mental retardation

  4. Symptoms are angina and syncope

  5. Sudden death more comon, and rarely reach adulthood

  6. Treatment

     i. Patch angioplasty for hourglass and hypoplastic

     ii. Konno when annular hypoplasia present

D. Idiopathic hypertrophic subaortic stenosis

  1. Pathology: hypertrophic myopathy of LV muscle with LV outflow tract obstruction in 20% secondary to septal hypertrophy

  2. Genetic predisposition

  3. Symptoms increase with age and are those of aortic stenosis; atrial fibrillation, systemic emboli, and sudden death common (presumed from arrhythmias)

  4. Diagnosis easily made by echocardiography

  5. Treatment

    a. Medical: decrease contractility (β blockade)

b. Surgical: septal myomectomy; indications for surgery include pressure gradient >50 mmHG and/or persistent symptoms despite adequate medical trial

E. Coarctation of the aorta
   1. Incidence: 10–15% of all CHD; 3 times more common in males
   2. Etiology: cause unknown, but probably an extension of the fibrotic process that obliterates the PDA
   3. Pathology
      a. Localized stenosis of aorta 2–4 cm distal to left subclavian artery (⅓ atretic, ⅓ pinhole, ⅓ moderate narrowing)
      b. Layers of wall are infolded media with intimal hyperplasia
      c. Aorta is dilated distal to the coarctation
      d. Aorta is always in continuity
      e. Associated with aortic valve disease and other varieties of LV outflow tract obstruction
      f. Rarely, the coarct is preductal, and severe symptoms occur in infancy when ductus closes
   4. Pathophysiology
      a. 5–10% of affected infants will have severe LV failure requiring surgical intervention; most, however, will be asymptomatic until fourth decade
      b. Large collaterals develop—typically with inflow from a subclavian trunk (IMA, thyrocervical, etc.) and outflow via large intercostals (with reversed flow) into the thoracic aorta
      c. Cause of death if untreated: ruptured aorta> LV failure> intracranial aneurysm rupture> endocarditis
   5. Symptoms
      a. Children: usually have none and are discovered on routine exam to have elevated systemic blood pressure (SBP)
      b. Adults: headache, epistaxis, and leg fatigue are common complaints
   6. Examination
      a. Hypertension (HTN) with decreased or absent femoral pulses
      b. Systolic murmur over left chest
      c. Collateral pulsations
   7. Laboratory
      a. CXR is diagnostic, with rib notching a constant

feature over age 14 (unusual < 6 yrs); rib notching most prominent in ribs 3–6
  b. EKG shows LVH
  c. Echocardiography and catheterization will rule out other abnormalities
8. Treatment is surgical, and ideally done when 3–4 years old unless infant is severely ill (these usually have associated anomalies such as VSD)
  a. Technique is simple end-to-end anastomosis except in those <1 year old, when subclavian flap technique probably gives better results by reducing incidence of late stenosis
  b. Postoperative care involves attention to rebound HTN and frequent incidence of abdominal pain and ileus (presumed secondary to increased SBP in mesenteric vessels)
  c. Postoperative paraplegia is rare (0.5%)
F. Vascular rings
  1. Incidence: uncommon
  2. Etiology: failure of regression or malformation of the six embryonic aortic arches; normally:
  1 & 2: disappear
  Right 3: right common carotid artery
  Right 4: innominate artery
  Left 4: transverse aortic arch
  5: never fully develops
  Left 6: ductus arteriosus
  3. Pathology: five significant abnormalities
    a. Double aortic arch (DAA): usually has one limb behind and one in front of the trachea with right descending thoracic aorta; most frequent and severe, with symptoms usually presenting during infancy
    b. Right aortic arch with left ligamentum arteriosus (retroesophageal); next in frequency
    c. Retroesophageal right subclavian artery: has origin distal to left subclavian, and courses posterior to the esophagus; relatively common, though usually asymptomatic
    d. Anomalous origin of innominate; compresses trachea
    e. Anomalous origin of left common carotid; compresses trachea
  4. Clinical: nearly always related to tracheal, not esophageal, compression
    a. Symptoms
      i. Infants with DAA develop stridor early ("crowing")

        ii. Recurrent pneumonia seen
        iii. Dysphagia
     b. Diagnosis
        i. Barium swallow (will outline esophageal compression at 3d and 4th thoracic vertebrae)
        ii. Tracheogram
        iii. Angiogram
  5. Treatment: *only for symptoms*
     i. DAA: divide smaller of arches
     ii. Others: divide, mobilize, and reimplant vessels as indicated
  6. Postoperative: watch for increased tracheal compression secondary to early edema formation
  7. Excellent surgical results with low mortality and morbidity

LEFT-TO-RIGHT SHUNTS (ACYANOTIC GROUP)

I. Atrial septal defects (ASDs)
  A. Types
    1. Foramen ovale (FO): present (probe patent) in 15–25% of all adults
    2. Ostium primum: partial atrioventricular (AV) canal; discussed later in separate section
    3. Ostium secundum: most common and focus of this section; incidence of secundum ASDs: 10–15% of all CHD
  B. Pathology
    1. Size: wide variance, but most 2–3 cm
    2. Location: majority in midatrial septum; however,
     a. High: near SVC orifice ("sinus venosus type"), and usually have associated anomalous entrance of superior pulmonary vein into the SVC
     b. Low: near IVC, and can see right-to-left shunting
    3. Associations
     a. 10–15% have anomalous pulmonary veins
       i. Right veins drain to SVC, left veins drain to coronary sinus or innominate vein
       ii. Note: it is unusual to have anomalous pulmonary drainage with intact atrial septum
     b. Lutembacher syndrome: secundum ASD plus mitral valve stenosis; leads to huge left-to-right shunt with massive PA dilatation
    4. Pathophysiology

    a. Left-to-right shunt occurs because of decreased compliance of LV compared to RV

    b. Shunt is less in infants because the ventricular compliances are similar

    c. Volume of the shunt is dependant upon ventricular compliance and pulmonary vascular resistance

       i. Size of defect matters little

       ii. Significant shunts have pulmonary flow 2–4 times systemic flow

    d. Effects of increased pulmonary blood flow

       i. CHF with DOE

       ii. Late pulmonary HTN

       iii. Increased susceptibility to pneumonia

       iv. No increased risk of subacute bacterial endocarditis (SBE)

    e. Effects of decreased systemic flow is "gracile habitus" (see below)

    f. Pulmonary HTN in children rare (<15%), but will eventually develop in about 15% of adults

    g. Arrhythmias become more common in adults

5. Clinical

    a. Symptoms

       i. Usually asymptomatic, especially in early years

       ii. When present, fatigue, palpitations, and DOE are most frequent

       iii. Overt CHF appears in adults, and may be first seen during pregnancy

    b. Signs

       i. Soft systolic murmur (pulmonary flow murmur)

       ii. Fixed and widely split S2

       iii. "Gracile habitus" (thin, decreased muscular tone, narrow bones)

    c. Lab

       i. CXR: mild cardiomegaly, mild CHF

       ii. EKG: RVH, RBBB

       iii. Echocardiography is diagnostic

       iv. Catheterization angiography: only if associated anomalies suspected

6. Indication for repair is shunt fraction > 1.5–2.0, or symptoms; only contraindication is Eisenmenger syndrome

7. Repair is done with full cardiopulmonary bypass, and defect closed using either pericardium or dacron if too large for primary closure; if there

are anomalous pulmonary veins, close the septum using patch, and include the pulmonary vein orifice (to direct it to the LA)

II. Total anomalous drainage of the pulmonary veins
  A. Anatomy; in all variations, ASD and PDA invariably present
    1. Supracardiac (45%): pulmonary veins drain into innominate vein
    2. Cardiac (25%): pulmonary veins drain into RA or coronary sinus
    3. Infradiaphragmatic (25%): pulmonary veins drain to portal vein or adjacent structures
  B. Pathophysiology
    1. Venous outflow obstruction is the major problem and produces severe pulmonary HTN
    2. It produces severe disability, with 50% 3-month and 80% 1-year mortality if untreated
  C. Clinical
    1. Symptoms are those of CHF
    2. Laboratory echocardiography makes the diagnosis, but angiogram mandatory for anatomy definition
  D. Surgical repair
    1. Must be performed early, and carries 15–20% mortality
    2. Done using hypothermic arrest
      a. Create a large connection between common venous trunk and the LA, ligate the anomalous vein, and close the ASD
      b. If connected to the coronary sinus, simply open this widely so it drains to the LA freely

III. Partial AV canal defect (ostium primum ASD, or partial endocardial cushion defect)
  A. Embryology: defect in the formation of the septum primum and its confluence with the ventricular septum
  B. Anatomy
    1. Two defects
      a. Cleft in anterior leaflet of mitral valve (may be partial or complete)
      b. Crescent-shaped defect low in atrial septum
    2. Usually the chordae are attached to both margins of the cleft leaflet, so it functions as a "trileaflet valve" without insufficiency
    3. Associated cleft in the tricuspid valve is frequent
    4. Conduction system is displaced inferiorly
    5. Distinguish from complete AV canal by presence

of intact ventricular septum and separate, intact tricuspid and mitral rings

C. Pathophysiology is of left-to-right shunt +/− mitral insufficiency

D. Clinical
   1. Symptoms: degree of mitral regurgitation (MR) determines symptoms
      a. When MR small, symptoms similar to simple ASD
      b. With large MR, symptoms of CHF present early
   2. Signs
      a. Cardiomegaly with apical thrill
      b. Harsh systolic murmur of MR
      c. Retarded growth
   3. Laboratory
      a. CXR: cardiomegaly and CHF
      b. EKG: left axis deviation
      c. Echocardiography is diagnostic

E. Surgical repair
   1. Timing: usually between 1–4 years of age unless CHF and/or pulmonary HTN present
   2. Technique
      a. Correct the MR (interrupted sutures)
      b. Close the ASD (pericardial patch)
      c. Avoid heart block (note proximity to conduction bundle)
   3. Postoperative
      a. Mortality: 5%
      b. Morbidity: heart block <5%, arrhythmias 18%, and residual MR 18%

IV. Complete atrioventricular canal
   A. Embryology: extensive failure of endocardial cushion development
   B. Pathology
      1. Large atrioventricular defect involving both atrial and ventricular septums
      2. Mitral and tricuspid valve abnormalities
      3. Rastelli classification of valve defects
   C. Pathophysiology
      1. Left-to-right shunt at both atrial and ventricular levels
      2. CHF and pulmonary HTN occur early
      3. Severity most influenced by size of VSD and degree of MR
   D. Diagnosis best made by echocardiography and cardiac catheterization

E. Surgical repair
   1. Timing: within first year
   2. Patch repair of septal defects with reconstruction of valves
   3. Mortality 75% in earlier series, now 5–15%
V. Ventricular septal defect
   A. Etiology: no identified etiologic factors
   B. Incidence: common (20–30% of all CHD)
   C. Pathology
      1. Four major anatomic types
         a. Perimembranous (80%): in membranous septum, just below aortic cusps, with the conduction system at the posterior-superior rim
         b. Outflow (infundibular or supracristal): anterior to crista supraventricularis, near pulmonary valve, and away from conduction system
         c. Inflow: posterior to papillary muscle beneath tricuspid valve
         d. Muscular: in inferior muscular portion of septum, and are frequently multiple ("swiss cheese")
         e. LV to RA defects: these are most rare, and occur in the membranous septum above the tricuspid annulus; small defects, but large shunts because of pressure gradient
      2. Size of VSD: varies 3 mm to 3 cm
         a. "Restrictive": VSD is smaller than the aortic valve area
            i. RV pressure up, but still < LV pressure
            ii. Shunt flow dependent on size of VSD
         b. "Nonrestrictive": VSD larger than aortic valve area
            i. RV pressure = LV pressure
            ii. Shunt flow is dependant on pulmonary vascular resistance
            iii. Causes early pulmonary HTN and vascular changes
      3. Pulmonary arteriolar disease develops early in those with nonrestrictive VSDs
      4. Associated anomalies are common (e.g., PDA, coarctation, ASD, pulmonary valve stenosis, and aortic insufficiency)
   D. Pathophysiology: two major consequences
      1. Cardiac failure: shunts > 2.0 may produce failure, and can be up to 4.0–5.0 with severe CHF in infancy; chronic congestion may lead to recurrent pneumonia
      2. Increased pulmonary vascular resistance

        i. As pulmonary vascular resistance increases, left-to-right shunt decreases

        ii. Eventually, shunt will reverse (Eisenmenger) with resulting cyanosis of right-to-left shunt

    3. Small VSDs have increased risk of SBE

E. Clinical

    1. Symptoms: usually asymptomatic with smaller VSDs, but develop symptoms of CHF with larger defects, and may develop cyanosis following shunt reversal

    2. Signs: loud, harsh pansystolic murmur and growth retardation

    3. Laboratory

        a. CXR: CHF and cardiomegaly

        b. EKG: biventricular hypertrophy

        c. Echocardiography is diagnostic

F. Treatment

    1. Timing: delay repair of small defects, as 60–70% will close spontaneously (spontaneous closure common in membranous and muscular, but rare in outflow and inflow types)

    2. Surgical Rx

        a. Severe CHF in infancy may be treated with either PA banding or direct repair

        b. Large VSDs should be repaired in first year

    3. Technique

        a. Approach is either via right atrium or through a transverse ventriculotomy

        b. Dacron or pericardial patch

        c. Avoid conduction system, avoid air embolus, and identify multiple VSDs

VI. Patent ductus arteriosus

A. Incidence: 10% of all CHD with 3:1 male preponderance

B. Etiology: ductus arteriosus is a remnant of the left 6th aortic arch, which functions in utero to bypass the pulmonary circuit

    1. Normally closes within few days of birth because of decreasing pulmonary vascular resistance

    2. Failure to close is related to fetal rubella, but majority of cases have unknown etiology

C. Anatomy

    1. Located just beyond left subclavian artery

    2. Diameter 2 mm to 1 cm (usually 7–8 mm)

    3. Length 5–10 mm

    4. 15% incidence of associated anomalies (VSD and coarctation are most common)

D. Pathophysiology: left-to-right shunt

1. Pulmonary blood flow may reach 10–15 L/min with large shunts and may lead to early and severe CHF
2. Pulmonary vascular resistance rises as in VSD, but will usually decrease following ligation
3. Fixed increased pulmonary vascular resistance may develop and result in reversed shunt (Eisenmenger)
4. Susceptible to *Streptococcus viridans* SBE

E. Clinical
1. Symptoms: infants range from asymptomatic to severe CHF (after 1 year, patients usually asymptomatic)
2. Signs: hallmark is continuous murmur at left 2d interspace with wide transmission
    a. Wide pulse pressure
    b. Cyanosis indicates associated anomaly or Eisenmenger syndrome
3. Laboratory: echocardiography is accurate, but angiography is best study

F. Surgical treatment
1. Ligation via left posterolateral thoracotomy in infants
2. Adults have friable PDA with surrounding calcification and require patch closure using cardiopulmonary bypass and hypothermia

G. Special: PDA in premature infants usually can be closed using indomethacin (79% success), however operation may still be indicated and is safely done

RIGHT-TO-LEFT SHUNTS (CYANOTIC GROUP)

I. Tetralogy of Fallot
A. Incidence: 50% of all cyanotic heart disease
B. Anatomy
1. Classic description of four abnormalities
    a. Right ventricular outflow tract obstruction (RVOTO)
    b. VSD
    c. Dextroposition of the aorta (''overriding aorta'')
    d. Right ventricular hypertrophy (RVH)
2. All anatomic defects are secondary to single developmental defect—malalignment of the infundibular septum
3. The infundibular septum is deviated anteriorly and cephalad and results in

a. Large (2–3 cm) VSD at point of nonunion in the membranous septum
b. RVOTO: most have combination of valvular stenosis and infundibular obstruction
   i. 20% have pulmonary atresia
   ii. Can have diffuse hypoplasia of the entire RV outflow tract
c. "Overriding aorta"
   i. 5–10% have abnormal coronary artery anatomy
   ii. 25% have right aortic arch
4. RVH develops secondary to the above defects
5. PDA is often present, and when closes there is increased cyanosis
C. Pathophysiology
1. VSD + RVOTO
  a. RV pressures = LV pressures
  b. pulmonary blood flow is decreased with right-to-left shunting and leads to cyanosis
  c. CHF and cardiomegaly are rare
2. Anoxia varies with pulmonary blood flow, and is exacerbated with exercise
3. Polycythemia with Hct's 60–75% common after 2 years, and may reach 85–90%
4. Cyanosis is more easily seen with increased Hct
5. Clubbing of digits develops over first few years
D. Symptoms (most are symptomatic)
1. Dyspnea and cyanosis, which are aggravated by exertion
2. Cyanotic "spells": episodes of deep cyanosis followed by periods of unconsciousness
   i. Ominous sign, which results from cerebral anoxia
   ii. Death or hemiplegia may result
   iii. Indicates need for emergency operation
3. Squatting: characteristic position, which will lessen dyspnea presumably by increasing peripheral vascular resistance and resulting in increased pulmonary blood flow
4. Brain abscesses are commonly seen
E. Examination
1. Cyanosis and clubbing of digits
2. Systolic murmur and weak S2
3. 50% have palpable thrill
F. Laboratory
1. CXR: "Sabot"-shaped heart
2. EKG: RVH and right axis deviation
3. Echocardiography is diagnostic

       4. Catheterization and angiography are mandatory to delineate RVOTO anatomy, VSD location, and coronary anatomy

  G. Operative treatment
    1. Indications
      a. Cyanotic spells—immediate Rx
      b. For emergency operations < 6 months, palliative shunt probably best
      c. When older than 6 months, corrective repair indicated
    2. Palliative shunt—will direct systemic blood flow to pulmonary system
      a. Blalock-Taussig: right subclavian artery to pulmonary artery shunt (direct connection) or left subclavian to pulmonary artery shunt using interposition graft
      b. Potts and Waterston shunts no longer used
    3. Corrective operation
      a. RVOTO: Rx depends upon anatomy (may require annuloplasty, valve commissurotomy, or outflow patch if hypoplasia present)
      b. VSD: close using pericardium or dacron patch
      c. When completed, RV systolic should be < 65% of LV systolic

II. Transposition of the great arteries (TGA)
  A. Incidence: 5–8% of all CHD (25% of all neonatal deaths due to CHD)
  B. Etiology: abnormal division of bulbar trunk
    1. 4:1 male predominance
    2. No known risk factors
  C. Anatomy
    1. Ventriculo-arterial discordant connection with atrio-ventricular concordant connection
      a. Aorta arises from RV
      b. Pulmonary artery arises from LV
      c. Basically, two parallel circuits—there must be an area of blood mixing for survival
    2. Three areas of blood mixing
      a. ASD (frequent)
      b. VSD (50–70%)
      c. PDA (50%)
    3. Associated anomalies are common (e.g., pulmonary stenosis or atresia, coarctation, dextrocardia)
  D. Pathophysiology
    1. Systemic anoxia and progressive CHF are the two basic problems
    2. Three basic groups of patients

      a. No VSD: "poor mixing"; early anoxia, cerebral damage, and death

      b. Large VSD: "good mixing"; early CHF and pulmonary HTN

      c. Large VSD + LVOTO (i.e., pulmonary valve stenosis)

        i. Better course (similar to tetralogy patients)

        ii. Later symptoms of anoxia, but rarely CHF

E. Clinical

  1. Symptoms depend upon anatomy, either CHF or cyanosis

  2. Systolic murmur is usually present

  3. Echocardiography is diagnostic

F. Treatment

  1. Palliative: create or enlarge ASD to improve mixing

    a. Operative atrial septectomy

    b. Balloon atrial septostomy (BAS)—current palliative procedure of choice

  2. Operative repair

    a. Atrial "switch": use atrial baffle to direct systemic venous blood to the LV (via mitral valve) and oxygenated pulmonary venous blood to RV (via tricuspid valve)

      i. Senning: uses atrial septum for baffle

      ii. Mustard: uses pericardium for baffle

    b. Arterial "switch": transposes PA and aorta

      i. Requires concomitant transposition of the coronaries

      ii. Potential advantage over atrial switch is that RV is not required to handle systemic pressures

  3. Timing

    a. Those with large VSDs should be repaired early to prevent development of pulmonary HTN

    b. Those with no VSD may be palliated for months with BAS and repaired later

    c. Those with VSD + LVOTO may be palliated with a Blalock shunt for years and later (5–7 years) have Rastelli procedure

III. Tricuspid atresia

A. Incidence 3–8% of cyanotic heart disease

B. Anatomy

  1. Four basic abnormalities present: tricuspid valve atresia, ASD, RV hypoplasia, and VSD; blood usually enters RV via VSD

2. 30% have associated TGA
C. Pathophysiology is of severe hypoxemia
   1. 90% die in 1 year without repair
   2. Those with TGA will usually have CHF instead of anoxia
D. Clinical
   1. Usually present with cyanosis and anoxic spells
   2. Echocardiography is diagnostic, but catheterization required to outline anatomy
E. Treatment
   1. Emergency systemic to PA shunt usually required early
   2. Occasionally, BAS may temporize if ASD is small and gradient present
   3. Definitive repair deferred until 6–12 months
      a. Fontan procedure—three variations:
         i. RA to PA anastomosis
         ii. RV to PA using conduit
         iii. RA to RV conduit
      b. Operative success depends on systemic venous pressure to perfuse the pulmonary bed. Increased pulmonary vascular resistance is contraindication to this procedure
   4. In those few who have CHF, PA banding early followed later by debanding and Fontan (must protect pulmonary vascular bed)

RARE MALFORMATIONS

I. Cor triatriatum
   A. Anatomy: variant of TAPVC with common venous chamber draining to LA through restricted opening; chamber is above and in back of the normal LA, and is separated by a thick muscular diaphragm; 70% have ASD with right-to-left shunt
   B. Pathophysiology is of pulmonary HTN (as in mitral stenosis)
   C. Clinical: patients present with severe pulmonary congestion, pulmonary HTN, and heart failure
      1. 75% will die in first year without treatment
      2. Diagnosis best made by echocardiography
   D. Treatment: prompt operation indicated; excise abnormal septum and close the ASD (good results)
II. Congenital mitral valve disease
   A. Rare, and usually associated with multiple abnormalities

B. Symptoms of CHF appear early

C. Treatment is valve repair, preferably when child is older

III. Aortic-pulmonary window

A. Rare, and results from incomplete development of spiral septum that divides truncus arteriosus, and leaves an opening (or window) between the aorta and PA (5–30 mm size); results in large left-to-right shunt (similar to PDA or VSD), with malignant course

B. Clinical findings similar to PDA except that murmur is only systolic

C. Echocardiography can be diagnostic, but aortography should be performed

D. Repair is transaortic closure using patch if necessary

IV. Ruptured sinus of Valsalva

A. Anatomy: primary abnormality is thinning of aortic media in wall of sinus secondary to failure of aortic wall to extend to the aortic valve annulus; usually, right coronary sinus is involved

B. Pathophysiology: sinus wall ruptures into the RA, and produces large left-to-right shunt with relentless CHF

C. Diagnosis is by echocardiography

D. Surgical repair indicated promptly, and technique is transaortic excision and patch closure

V. Truncus arteriosus

A. Rare, and results from failure of aortic/PA division; entire outflow circulation (aorta, PA, coronaries) arises from common trunk

B. Pathophysiology: severe pulmonary overload with early CHF and development of increased pulmonary vascular resistance (< 6 months); severe disability with 50% dead in 1 month and 90% dead in 1 year if untreated

C. Treatment: conduit from RV to PA after closure of VSD and detachment of PA from truncus, PA banding is attendant with high mortality

VI. Single ventricle

A. Anatomy: both atrioventricular valves empty into common chamber (may be morphologically right or left); varieties of outflow arrangements are seen

B. Pathophysiology: depending on outflow anatomy, either CHF of hypoxemia is seen

C. Treatment

1. Early palliation may require PA banding (those with CHF) or Blalock shunt (those with decreased pulmonary blood flow)

2. Definitive treatment options include Fontan or ventricular septation

VII. Ebstein anomaly
  A. Anatomy: malformation of tricuspid valve with downward displacement of septal and posterior leaflets creating a third heart chamber; leaves "atrialized" portion of RV wall and hypoplasia of distal functioning RV chamber
  B. Pathophysiology: major problem is decreased output from RV (secondary to tricuspid insufficiency and RV dysfunction)
    1. Massive RA dilatation
    2. Arrhythmias commonly seen
    3. Right-to-left shunt via ASD is commonly seen
  C. Symptoms
    1. Early, infants have tachypnea and cyanosis, which decreases later
    2. Average age at diagnosis is midteens, but only 5% will live > 50 years
  D. Diagnosis can usually be made by auscultatory findings and CXR, but echocardiography is diagnostic
  E. Treatment is recommended for symptoms or increasing cardiomegaly, and is usually valve repair or (less commonly) valve replacement

ANOMALIES OF CORONARY ARTERIES

I. Anomalous left coronary origin from PA
  A. Rare 1/300,000 births
  B. Described as clinically similar to adult myocardial infarction, and retrograde flow in left coronary has been demonstrated
  C. Severe disability with MI and LV failure presenting usually within 3 months of age; EKG will show Q-wave infarction, and catheterization is diagnostic
  D. Treatment involves (1) transplanting the origin of the left coronary artery to the aorta, (2) performing bypass graft (vein or subclavian artery), or (3) simply ligating the origin to prevent retrograde flow; 50% mortality

II. Coronary arteriovenous fistula
  A. Anatomy
    1. Usually a single, small (2–5 mm) fistula, and involved coronary artery is tortuous and dilated
    2. $\frac{2}{3}$ arise from right coronary artery, $\frac{1}{3}$ from left coronary

    3. 90% drain into a right heart chamber or its connecting vessel

  B. Clinical
    1. Most patients asymptomatic, and are evaluated because of characteristic continuous murmur
    2. Adults may develop mild CHF from left-to-right shunt or, more rarely, develop angina from coronary steal
    3. Catheterization establishes diagnosis

  C. Treatment ligation (on bypass for larger fistulas)

III. Corrected transposition

  A. Anatomy
    1. "Double discordance": TGA is present and there is atrioventricular discordant connection
    2. Morphologic RV receives pulmonary venous blood from mitral valve, and outflow is to the aorta; while morphologic LV receives systemic venous blood from tricuspid valve, and outflow is the PA
    3. High incidence of associated anomalies (98%)
      a. Conduction defect (>50% have AV block)
      b. VSD (80%)
      c. Pulmonary stenosis
      d. Mitral insufficiency

  B. Treatment
    1. Echocardiography makes diagnosis
    2. Closure of VSD must be done to prevent pulmonary HTN

IV. Double outlet right ventricle (DORV)

  A. Anatomy
    1. Both great arteries arise from the morphologic RV
    2. Wide variation in anatomy
      a. Four described relationships of the great arteries
      b. Four described VSDs
        i. Subaortic
        ii. Subpulmonic
        iii. Beneath both ("doubly committed")
        iv. Beneath neither "uncommitted")
    3. Therefore, there are 16 possible anatomic varieties, and range from classic TGA at one extreme to tetralogy at the other
    4. Taussig-Bing syndrome is a form of DORV, which is a DORV with subpulmonic VSD

  B. Clinically, three types of disabilities seen
    1. With simply a large VSD, symptoms of large VSD develop early

     2. With pulmonic stenosis and subaortic VSD, symptoms of tetralogy develop

     3. With Taussig-Bing variant, symptoms of TGA develop

  C. Surgical repair: in general involves creation of intra cardiac tunnel to direct LV outflow to aorta

V. Pulmonary artery sling

  A. Anatomy: left PA arises from right PA, and courses between trachea and esophagus—this forms a sling around the trachea

  B. Clinical

     1. Symptoms develop early (first months), and are stridor, wheezing, and choking

     2. Esophagram and bronchoscopy establish diagnosis

  C. Repair: divide the left PA at its origin, and reinsert on the main PA

18 ACQUIRED HEART DISEASE

DETERMINATION OF CARDIAC FUNCTION

Evaluation of cardiac function, both preoperative and post-operative, requires an understanding of the heart as a pump. Cardiac output (CO) measures the ability of the heart to supply metabolic substrates and remove waste. CO is proportional to heart rate (HR) multiplied by stroke volume (SV). CO divided by the patient's body surface area equals cardiac index (CI). This allows a normal value for all patients. SV has three major determinates.

Preload This is measured as the end-diastolic pressure within the ventricle. A normal value is 8 mmHg. Within limits the ventricle can be volume loaded to increase preload. This results in increased force of contraction. Sarcomere length of 2.2 nanomeres results in maximal force of contraction. In a normal heart, this occurs with end-diastolic pressure of 14. A Swan-Ganz catheter is often used to measure left ventricular end-diastolic pressure. When there are no obstructions between the pulmonary vascular bed and left ventricle, the wedge pressure reflects left ventricular end-diastolic pressure.

Afterload This is the impedance to left ventricular emptying. The greater the afterload, the lower the SV. The mean systolic pressure approximates afterload.

Contractility This represents the intrinsic ability of cardiac muscle to contract. It is measured as a maximal velocity of fiber shortening.

Each of these factors may be manipulated postoperatively to alter CI. Hazard function curves show increased mortality postoperatively with CI less than 2. It is important to realize that blood pressure, urine output, temperature, and cerebral function are all unreliable determinates of cardiac function in the postoperative state. If CI falls below 2, the first intervention is usually to increase preload to 14–18 mmHg. Occasionally in stiff ventricles, left ventricular end-diastolic pressure has to be pushed to 20 mmHg. Afterload is reduced by decreasing MAP with nitroglycerin or nitroprusside. In severe cases, intraaortic balloon pump may be required. Contractility may be increased with the use of inotropes; dopamine, dobutamine, and epinephrine are frequently used.

EXTRACORPOREAL CIRCULATION

Gibbon accomplished the first open heart operation in 1953 using cardiopulmonary bypass. Currently, most centers use a roller pump, originally designed by DeBakey. The nonpulsatile flow provided by this pump appears to be well tolerated for up to 4 h. Since 1970 most centers have used either membrane or bubble oxygenators. Priming solutions are usually crystalloid with albumin added to keep oncotic pressure 10–20 mmHg. Hemodilution is allowed to a hematocrit of 25. Starting heparin doses are usually 4 mg/kg and are checked with activated clotting times. Perfusion rates are usually 2.5 mm/m²/min, and core body temperature is lowered to about 30°C. Mean systemic pressure of about 50–60 mmHg is sought. In most cases, myocardial preservation is obtained using cold crystalloid or blood cardioplegia in combination with body hypothermia (28–30°C) and topical cooling. With this, myocardial temperatures below 15°C can be obtained and a cross clamp time up to 4 h is possible.

Postoperative Complications

Bleeding Blood coagulation mechanics are abnormal for at least 18–24 h after coronary artery bypass. Unless bleeding is excessive, transfusion of platelets or FFP is seldom required. Brisk bleeding requires urgent return to the operating room.

Cardiac Tamponade Classic findings include elevated central venous pressure, hypotension, low CO, and mediastinal widening. Findings may be subtle. If a low CO is present and does not respond rapidly to specific treatments, reexploration for cardiac tamponade needs to be considered.

Inadequate Cardiac Index CI of 2–2.5 L/min early postoperative is adequate. CI below 2 requires rapid diagnosis and treatment, since death from inadequate perfusion may occur rapidly.

Preload, afterload, and contractility may be manipulated as noted above. The combination of fluid resuscitation and afterload reduction often restores cardiac index. Inotropes may be required. An intraaortic balloon pump (IABP) may be required if the above efforts fail. IABP can raise CO by 700 mL/min.

Early postoperative cardiac rhythm disturbances require close attention. Temporary pacing wires are placed in the right ventricle and right atrium before leaving the operating room. Cardiac pacing with atrial or AV sequential pacing may be useful. Premature ventricular contractions may deteriorate into ventricular fibrillation or ventricular tachycardia. Potassium levels should be checked and kept well above 4 meq/L. Lidocaine at 1–3 mg/L is useful.

Renal Failure Intravenous infusion of 1500 mL/m^2 for the first 24 h is customary. Renal failure is uncommon with postoperative cardiac indexes above 2, unless there is preexisting disease. Renal failure may be treated with hemodialysis or peritoneal dialysis.

Respiratory Insufficiency With curent pump oxygenators, respiratory insufficiency is uncommon. The simplest numerical expression of this failure is elevation of A-a gradient.

Low-Grade Fever Low-grade fevers are common in the first 24–48 h postoperation. After this time, postpericardiotomy syndrome is usually the cause. This is treated with anti-inflammatory medication. Obvious specific causes need to be sought. The most serious of these is a mediastinal wound infection. If this is present, a prompt return to the operating room is mandatory. This occurs in approximately 1% of open heart patients.

Central Nervous System Dysfunction Stroke occurs in approximately 1–2% of open heart patients. Specific cause is often not found. Every effort should be made to remove air and debris from cardiac chambers before unclamping the aorta. Mean pressures during the pump run should be kept at 60 mmHg, especially in the elderly.

GI Disturbance Acute abdomen occurs in approximately 1% of pump cases. Specific causes need be sought.

SPECIFIC DISEASES

MITRAL STENOSIS All evidence indicates that mitral stenosis is almost always due to rheumatic fever, even though a definitive history of this can be obtained in only 50% of patients. Symptoms of mitral stenosis develop as early as 3 years following rheumatic fever, but may take as long as 25 years. Rheumatic fever produces a pancarditis, but it is the endocardial changes that predominate. Rheumatic fever results in scarring of the valve tissue. This results in turbulent flow, and hemodynamic changes result in commissural fusion, valve fibrosis, and calcification. This decreases leaflet mobility. The subvalvular apparatus (chordae tendineae) and papillary muscles become thickened, fibrotic, and contracted.

It is important to emphasize that the pathologic changes of mitral stenosis do not develop from multiple episodes of rheumatic fever, but rather from the turbulent flow resulting from the initial episode. Therefore, repair of the mitral valve and decreasing leaflet turbulence may result in a good long-term result.

Normal mitral valve cross-sectional area is 4–6 cm^2. Reduction to 2–2.5 cm^2 constitutes mild mitral stenosis (class I). Patients with cross-sectional area less than 1 cm^2 are severely disabled (class IV). Mitral stenosis results in very significant physiologic derangement:

1. Increased left atrial pressure. When left atrial pressure rises to exceed oncotic pressure of plasma (25–30 mmHg) transudation of fluid across the pulmonary capillaries occurs. When this fluid load exceeds lymphatic capacity, pulmonary edema occurs. This will vary with the cross-sectional area of the orifice (the degree of mitral stenosis), total flow (CO), and duration of flow (HR).
2. A decrease in CO. The CO is fixed at a low level by the stenotic orifice.
3. Increase in pulmonary vascular resistance. The degree to which pulmonary vascular resistance increases with mitral stenosis varies greatly among patients. This increase is primarily a result of vasoconstriction in the pulmonary arterioles; ultimately it intensifies by hypertrophy of the media and intima. In the vast majority of patients, pulmonary hypertension abates following surgical repair.

A few other serious problems include atrial fibrillation and systemic emboli. Atrial fibrillation produces decrease in CO. In addition, thrombus develops in the enlarged left atrial appendage in 15–20% of the patients. Systemic emboli can occur.

The symptoms in mitral stenosis relate to pulmonary congestion (dyspnea, and pulmonary edema) and decreased CO (fatigue). Systemic emboli occur with increase in left atrial size and atrial fibrillation. Hemoptysis may occur but is usually not severe. Angina pectoris occurs in 10% of patients. Right-sided failure eventually occurs. Physical exam usually shows cardiac cachexia. Pulmonary congestion is frequent. Auscultatory findings include a sharply localized apical diastolic rumble. The intensity does not correlate with the severity of mitral stenosis. In addition, the first heart sound is increased and an opening snap classically follows the second heart sound.

Imaging techniques help make the diagnosis of mitral stenosis. Barium swallow shows a characteristic displacement of its middle third due to left atrial enlargement. Chest x-ray demonstrates a left atrium as a double shadow behind the heart. The usual concavity between the aorta and left ventricle appears as a "straight" left heart border. Mitral valve calcification may also be seen. Pulmonary hypertension produces the large pulmonary arteries, and Kerley lines may be present.

Echocardiography can determine the degree of atrial enlargement. It can also estimate the degree of mitral stenosis and also provide information about leaflet mobility. Cardiac catheterization provides additional information in uncomplicated cases; in patients under age 40 it may not be required if good echocardiography data are available. Characteristic findings show left atrial pressure increased to 20–30 mmHg from the usual 5–10 mmHg. Severe stenosis produces a diastolic gradient of 10–20 mmHg across the mitral valve. Coronary arteriography may be desired in certain patients.

Operation should be routinely considered with hemodynamically significant mitral stenosis even if symptoms are minimal. The risk is approximately 1%, and chance of cerebral emboli is always possible. In early mitral stenosis, reconstruction rather than replacement is often possible (90%). Systemic emboli are indications for surgery because recurrent emboli almost always occur. It is also important to remember that mitral stenosis may be successfully operated on, no matter how advanced or how severe the pulmonary hypertension. The left ventricle in pure mitral stenosis is protected and the pulmonary hypertension postop abates or disappears in most cases.

Reconstruction technique (commissurotomy, repair of subvalvular apparatus) is always preferable to replacement. This preserves left ventricular function and avoids the complications of a prosthetic device. Open precise repair on cardiopulmonary bypass is preferred to closed commissurotomy. Standard median sternotomy incision is used. The incision is made into the left atrium at the intraatrial groove and extended beneath the superior and inferior vena cava. A self-retaining retractor is used. Thrombus is removed and the left atrial appendage may be excluded. The mitral valve is evaluated. The repair may be performed if pliable leaflets and an adequate opening can be obtained. Clearly this may be possible more often on mitral stenosis operated early in its natural history. Commissurotomy is accomplished by applying traction sutures to the leaflets. Valvular and subvalvular apparatus is freed and mobilized according to Carpentier's techniques. Careful attention is given to avoid creation of mitral regurgitation. After discontinuing cardiopulmonary bypass, the repair is evaluated. Intraoperative echocardiogram is often used. In addition the transvalvular gradient is evaluated with direct needle puncture. Significant residual gradient (5–7 mm) requires additional procedures.

If reconstruction cannot be accomplished, replacement with bioprosthesis or metal valve is done. Removal of the valve must preserve the chordae to the posterior leaflet. This has been found to preserve left ventricular function. In addition, there is some evidence that it protects against left ventricular rupture in the early postoperative period. Individual sutures should be placed to avoid the circumflex artery and the conduction system. As with repair, great care is taken to remove air from the ventricle prior to left ventricular ejection.

Antibiotics are given perioperatively and continued until all intracardiac lines are removed. Anticoagulation is started within the first 3 days. With bioprosthesis, coumadin is stopped after 3 months if there is normal sinus rhythm and the left atrium is not too large. Mechanical valves require anticoagulation for life. There is no ideal cardiac prosthesis. Mechanical valves are durable and will probably last the life of the patient. They are, however, thrombogenic. One study of frequency of thromboembolism was 4% per patient year. The frequency of thrombosis of the prosthetic was 1% per year. To prevent valve thrombosis and/or thromboembolism, life-long anticoagulation, with its attendant risk, is required. A bioprosthesis requires anticoagulation for 3 months and then may be stopped if the left atrium is not too large and the patient is in normal sinus rhythm. These valves, however, degrade with time, so that in 10 years, 20% of the bioprosthesis fails, requiring a second operation. In general, for patients under 60 years old who can reliably take coumadin, a metal valve is recommended. Older patients often receive the bioprosthesis.

Prognosis following valve repair is very good. Clearly the freedom from reoperation is dependent on residual turbulence following repair. One can expect greater than 80% freedom from the operation for 10 years, with an operative mortality under 2%. Prognosis for mitral valve replacement is poorer, probably due to selection, and to severity of left ventricular function preoperatively. With either metal or bioprosthetic valve there is a mortality rate of 1–2% per patient year.

MITRAL INSUFFICIENCY   Mitral insufficiency in the United States due to rheumatic fever has steadily decreased in frequency, and now represents less than half the patients seen. In most cases, the most common cause is mitral valve prolapse, often complicated by rupture of chordae tendineae. Ischemic papillary muscle disease has become more frequent.

Bacterial endocarditis can result in mitral insufficiency. Mitral insufficiency may occur from prolapse of the anterior or posterior leaflet, lack of coaptation of both leaflets, or structural abnormality of the leaflet itself. In each instance, the annulus may deform so that the AP diameter enlarges, creating a more circular structure.

The physiologic derangement of this condition is regurgitation of blood from the left ventricle to the left atrium during systole. The "V" wave in the left atrium is commonly 30–40 mmHg; however, it could get as high as 80–90 mmHg. In diastole, the left atrial pressure falls rapidly to approach left ventricular pressure. Mean left atrial pressure is 15–25 mmHg. Pulmonary vascular changes appear late, and left atrial size could be very large. Stasis of blood does not occur and therefore emboli are rare. The left ventricle may function adequately for long periods of time before failure. Systolic murmur radiating to the axilla is characteristic of mitral regurgitation. In more severe cases, it may become pansystolic. Symptoms are mostly respiratory and are mild until late in the course.

Diagnosis and quantitation can be made with echocardiography, but cardiac catheterization is usually done. Timing of the operation is difficult, especially since the symptoms are mild until late in the course. An operation should be done before onset of irreversible left ventricular failure. A fall in the ejection fraction with exercise measured with radionuclide is one way to time surgery. As with mitral stenosis, an attempt is always made to repair rather than replace the valve. Chordi shortening, chordi transplantation, and quadrangular resection with annuloplasty have been used by Carpentier and others with good results. Thromboembolism is less than 1%. Recurrent insufficiency has occurred in only a small number of patients. If valve replacement is required, valve selection is as in mitral stenosis.

AORTIC STENOSIS A normal aortic valve has a cross-sectional area of 2.5–3.0 cm². Moderate aortic stenosis is present at about 1.0 cm. Valve areas as low as 0.4–0.6 cm² may be found with severe aortic stenosis. A gradient of at least 50 mmHg is found with significant aortic stenosis. This results in progressive concentric hypertrophy of the left ventricle. Pathologic features of 377 diseased aortic valves were reviewed at the operation. A calcified congenital bicuspid valve represents 46%. Here there is heavy infiltration with calcium on the leaflets as well as the aorta above and the ventricle below. Rheumatic aortic stenosis with commissural fusion and calcification accounts for 35%. Approximately 10% of the patients had acquired aortic stenosis. Here the leaflets are normal size and there is no commissural fusion. The bases of the cusps are heavily infiltrated with calcium. In older patients (greater than 40 years old) coronary atherosclerosis occurs in at least 30–50% of the patients. Characteristically, there is a long asymptomatic period, up to 20–30 years. The classic symptoms include angina pectoris, syncope, and failure. Once symptoms develop, life expectancy is about 3 years. Sudden death accounts for 15–20% of fatalities. Syncope develops in one-third of patients and may be related to cerebral blood flow or arrhythmia. Angina occurs in 30–40%. There may or may not be associated coronary artery disease. Apparently, left ventricular hypertrophy and decreased cardiac output can result in ischemia. This is obviously made worse with coronary artery disease.

Congestive heart failure is more ominous, with life expectancy approximately 1 year. This, as well as atrial fibrillation represents a failing ventricle. Physical exam shows a prolonged heave at the apical impulse instead of a forceful thrust found in mitral regurgitation or aortic insufficiency. Peripheral pulses have slow upstroke. Heart size is usually normal. Cardiac catheterization with coronary angiography is usually used. Surgery has been recommended with valve areas of 0.8–1.0 cm². Currently, exercise radionuclide studies seem to indicate when a decreased ejection fraction is present. Operative replacement of the aortic valve is the only real option. Valve debridement with balloon angioplasty is possible, but is reserved for special cases. Choice of either bioprosthetic or metal valve is made as in mitral valve surgery. It is imperative that in the aortic position, a large enough valve is chosen so that the residual gradient will be acceptable (10–20 mmHg). Some institutions are using homograft aortic valves with good long-term follow-up.

Postoperative care includes anticoagulation and observation for arrhythmias. Operative mortality is low (1–2%). Five-year survival is 80–90% for good ventricles.

AORTIC INSUFFICIENCY   Aortic insufficiency causes volume overload of a left ventricle. The regurgitant volume may be up to 2 to 3 times the normal stroke volume, 60–70 mL. The cardiac response is to increase SV by dilation of the heart. This causes some of the largest hearts seen in clinical cardiology. The response is quite different from aortic stenosis where concentric muscular hypertrophy occurs. Due to this compensation mechanism, LVEDP and LA pressures remain normal until late in the course when left ventricular failure occurs. Mitral regurgitation may become manifest at this point due to annular dilation.

A variety of diseases can produce aortic insufficiency.

Quite common today is bacterial endocarditis. Rheumatic fever is occurring with decreasing frequency. Syphilis is a rarity. Annular ectasia is a collagen disease seen with increasing frequency as the population ages. Cystic medial necrosis is the pathologic substrate and is seen in its most severe form with Marfan syndrome. The aortic root gradually increases starting at the sinus of Valsalva and progresses to a discrete aneurysm in the ascending aorta.

Aortic insufficiency occurs due to annular dilation. Atherosclerotic aneurysms may also cause aortic insufficiency from annular dilation; however, the underlying pathology is different. Aortic insufficiency may also occur from aortic dissection with valve cusps detached from the aortic wall. The clinical course is highly variable depending on the degree and rate of increased aortic insufficiency. Symptom-free intervals of 8–10 years are common. Symptoms usually develop once left ventricular failure begins in the chronic form. Death will usually occur within 4–5 years due to progressive left ventricular failure.

Anginal symptoms may also be present with severe disease. On physical exam, the murmur is a high-pitched decrescendo diastolic murmur along the left sternal border starting immediately after the second heart sound. The peripheral pulses increase and can often be visualized. This is due to a large pulse pressure.

Timing an operation is difficult. Once symptoms develop, some degree of left ventricular failure is usually present. Means of detecting the left ventricular failure have been attempted. Echocardiogram, showing end-systolic dimension greater than 55 mm, has been recommended. A decreased ejection fraction with exercise has also been used. Even with moderate or severe left ventricular dysfunction, operation is recommended, since death is almost always a certainty otherwise. In this subset of patients, degree of improvement postoperation is difficult to predict.

TRICUSPID INSUFFICIENCY   Distinction needs to be made between organic and functional tricuspid valve disease. Organic tricuspid valve disease is almost always due to rheumatic fever; 10–30% of patients with left-sided disease will also have tricuspid valve involvement. In this situation, the pathology is similar to the more familiar mitral valve disease. Organic tricuspid stenosis is more frequent than insufficiency. Endocarditis and trauma are also causes of tricuspid valve disease. Functional tricuspid valve disease occurs when normal leaflets do not coapt due to annular dilation. This is due to left-sided heart disease with subsequent pulmonary hypertension and right-sided failure.

Normal right atrial pressure is 4–5 mmHg. When the tricuspid orifice becomes smaller than 1.5 cm² the pressure rises with a mean gradient of at least 5–15 mmHg and this results in symptoms similar to right heart failure with edema, ascites, and hepatomegaly. A characteristic murmur of tricuspid stenosis is a diastolic murmur at the lower sternum. Inspiration will increase its intensity. A mild degree of tricuspid insufficiency may be tolerated with a little adverse influence. Tricuspid insufficiency produces a systolic murmur at the lower sternum.

Laboratory diagnosis can be accomplished with ultrasound and right heart catheterization. A gradient of 4–5 mm is significant. At the time of operation palpation may not be a reliable indicator of tricuspid insufficiency. Surgical decision about tricuspid insufficiency is difficult. With more minor disease, the tricuspid valve should be left alone. If right atrial hypertrophy is present and the annulus mildly dilated, repair should almost always be done. This could be done by posterior leaflet annuloplasty, DeVega annuloplasty, or the techniques of Carpentier. Tricuspid stenosis usually can be handled with a commissurotomy. When leaflet destruction precludes, repair or replacement needs to be carried out. Mechanical valves have a high incidence of thrombotic complication. Bioprosthesis should be used. When the prosthetic is placed, care must be taken to preserve the septal leaflet. This will avoid complications with the heart block. The conduction bundle lies between the coronary sinus and ventricular septum. With bacterial endocarditis, there is controversy over whether the prosthetic device should be placed at the initial operation. Operative mortality is low (1–2%). Long-term prognosis is dependent on underlying myocardial dysfunction.

MULTIVALVULAR DISEASE   With rheumatic heart disease, more than the cardiac valve may be involved. Prominent signs of disease in one valve can readily be masked by disease in other valves. Echocardiography is a valuable tool to determine the contribution of each valve.

CARDIAC TRAUMA

Penetrating the life-threatening problems are tamponade and hemorrhage. Tamponade develops rapidly because a normal pericardium can accommodate only 100–250 mL blood. Small stab wounds often produce tamponade because the laceration in the pericardium is small, thus holding the clot within the pericardium itself. Large wounds threaten exsanguination due to expulsion of blood into the pleural space. The right ventricle and its chamber are most frequently injured. Rapid transfusion of fluids, intubation, and immediate transfer to the operating room are key principles for treatment. Emergency room thoracotomy is done at some institutions with variable results. This may be accomplished by placing the patient in a slight left anterolateral position; a curvilinear incision is made between the left nipple to parallel the intercostal spaces. The fourth or fifth intercostal space should be entered, as the pectoralis major arises from the third to fifth rib and causes troublesome bleeding with a higher incision. Once the pleural space is entered, the intercostal incision can be quickly completed with scissors or the fingers, separating the ribs, carrying the incision anteriorly on the angle of the rib, almost to the sternum. Unless the incision is long enough, exposure is seriously hampered. Subsequent wound infection following an unsterile thoracotomy is surprisingly rare, less than 5%.

The key to treating cardiac tamponade is considering the diagnosis. Beck's triad (hypotension, elevated venous pressure, and a still quiet heart) is helpful. When the diagnosis is first suspected, pericardial aspiration should be done. As little as 10–15 mL blood may be removed with dramatic improvement. Elevation of intrapericardial pressure to 15–17 mmHg may stop cardiac function unless full resuscitation has been accomplished.

In the operating room, a mediasternotomy is used. Direct suture can usually be accomplished without cardiopulmonary bypass.

Blunt trauma usually results from automobile accidents. Most of these are immediately fatal. Such severe injury can result in cardiac concussion (elevated cardiac enzymes but echocardiogram showing no wall motion abnormalities), or cardiac contusion (positive echocardiogram). Patients with contusions need to be observed in the same manner as those with subendocardial myocardial infarction.

CARDIAC TUMORS

Metastases are the most common cardiac tumors, occurring in 4–12% of autopsies performed in patients with neoplastic disease. The most frequent primary cardiac tumor is myxoma, comprising 50–60% of all primary cardiac tumors. Sarcoma and rhabdomyoma are less common. Benign but extremely rare neoplasms include fibromas, angiomas, lymphomas, and teratomas. 2-D echocardiography is now the keystone of diagnostic studies.

Sixty to sixty-five percent of cardiac myxomas develop in the left atrium, almost always from the atrial septum near the fossa ovalis. Most other myxomas develop in the right atrium. Less than 20 have been found in either the right or left ventricle. Myxomas are true neoplasms. They are usually polypoid, arising from superficial layers of the septum, and invasion does not occur. Metastases are rare. The tumor is friable, so emboli can occur. Myxomas cause symptoms by growing large enough to restrict flow through the mitral or tricuspid valve. Peripheral emboli appear in 40–50% of patients. Myxomas intermittently obstruct flow from the mitral valve by prolapsing through. And some myxomas produce generalized symptoms resembling an autoimmune disorder, including fever, weight loss, arthralgias, and myalgias.

Treatment is operative removal as soon as possible. A biatrial incision is used with good exposure and good exploration. The tumor with the septum is removed. The atrial septum is closed with a patch. Cardiac rhabdomyomas are probably hamartomas. It is said to be the most common cardiac tumor in children, but is rare. About 50% of the patients have tuberous sclerosis of the brain. The tumor is usually fatal.

CORONARY ARTERY DISEASE

Atherosclerosis is the fundamental cause, with the basic lesion being a segmental atherosclerotic plaque often localized within the first 5 cm of the origin of the coronary vessel. Clinical manifestations include angina pectoris, sudden death, myocardial infarction, and congestive heart failure. Angina pectoris is most common, and the differential diagnosis includes the anxiety states, musculoskeletal disease, and esophageal reflux. In 25% of the patients, symptoms are atypical. Laboratory investigations include a stress test, both with EKG monitoring and using radionuclide. Coronary angiography is the cornerstone. A stenosis is considered significant when the diameter is reduced by more than 70%, corresponding to a reduction in the cross-sectional area of 90%. Ventriculography is used to measure ejection fraction. Normal is 0.5–0.7, moderately depressed is 0.3–0.5, and <0.3 is considered severe myocardial dysfunction. In addition, regional wall motion can be described as normal, hypokinetic (impaired), akinetic (little or no visible contraction), and dyskinetic (paradoxical contraction).

Coronary artery disease can be treated both medically and surgically. Surgical treatment includes coronary artery bypass grafting (CABG). Indications for CABG are still evolving. The more severe the proximal atherosclerotic disease and the more depressed the ejection, the greater the likelihood that coronary revascularization will result in an improved survival. Unstable situations such as postinfarction angina and structural defects require more urgent intervention. The place of angioplasty in revascularization is still being evaluated; it has benefits in some settings.

Surgical techniques include the use of cold cardioplegia with systemic hypothermia and topical cooling. Internal mammary arteries are almost always used, and currently the use of sequential and bilateral mammaries has increased. Hospital stay is usually 7–10 days, and full return to activity usually occurs within 3 months. In patients with no complications, mortality risk is approximately 1% and the morbidity rate is approximately 5%. The frequency of stroke is 1–2%. Common carotid surgery is not used unless acute cerebral symptoms emanating from the carotids are present.

Relief of angina is immediate and complete in 90–95% of the patients. This correlates with improvement in wall motion abnormalities. Vein graft patency at 1 month is 90–95%. After that there is an attrition rate of approximately 2–3% per year up to 5 years. Subsequently there is often rapid progression of atherosclerotic disease such that at 10 years, patency rate is about 50%. Progression of native disease is a factor; this may be reduced by decreasing serum cholesterol. Recurrent angina occurs at a rate of 3–5% per patient year. If scar is present, arrhythmia is usually not improved post-CABG. Longevity in patients with coronary artery disease seems to favor operation vs. medical treatment unless there is good ventricular function, little angina, mild degrees of coronary artery disease, or diffuse coronary artery disease.

LEFT VENTRICULAR ANEURYSM

A left ventricular aneurysm develops over a period of 4–8 weeks in 10–15% of patients following a transmural myocardial infarction. Mural thrombus is present in 50% of the patients; however, emboli are rare. Rupture is also rare. Greater than 80% are anterolateral. In 30–40% of cases, single-vessel disease is present. Large aneurysms interfere with ventricular function. Natural history is difficult to determine, but longevity is probably related to underlying ventricular function. Distinction must be made at operation between akinetic scar and true aneurysm. Surgical technique includes (1) not disturbing the aneurysm until the aorta is cross-clamped (this avoids emboli); (2) subtotal resection of scar so that eventual closure does not impinge on viable muscle; (3) possible endocardial resection to treat arrhythmia; and (4) (usually) grafting the LAD to improve septal perfusion.

PERICARDITIS

Acute pyogenic pericarditis is most common in children, with the organism being *Haemophilus influenzae* and *Staphylococcus*. Treatment is drainage either by aspiration or by operation.

Chronic constrictive pericarditis is usually idiopathic. Physiologic derangement is limitation of diastolic filling of ventricles. This results in decreased SV and increased systemic venous pressure. This disease rarely develops after open heart operation.

Findings at cardiac catheterization are characteristic, showing the "square root" sign and equalization of pressures. Treatment is surgical. The approach is through median sternotomy. Pericardium is removed as completely as possible from both ventricles. The atria and cavae are also freed as much as possible; however, this is optional. The plane of resection is usually between the epicardium and pericardium. If thickened, the epicardium may also require removal. Often this can be difficult, and therefore the epicardium may be cut in a gridlike fashion.

HEART BLOCK AND PACEMAKERS

Technology in this field is changing rapidly. The two most common methods of pacing today are R wave-inhibited–demand ventricular and atrioventricular synchronous. Both require an electrode in the right ventricle, and the second requires an additional wire in the right atrium. These are usually placed transvenous to the endocardial surface. Both methods of pacing prevent syncope by pacing the heart during periods of bradycardia. The latter technique allows AV synchrony. The pacemakers of today are programmable such that rate, pulse amplitude, duration, AV delay, and other variables may be changed. Recently a code has been agreed on to describe any pacemaker. Three letters are used, representing chamber pace, chamber sensed, and the mode of generator function. Operative techniques usually involve cut down on a cephalic vein. Optional techniques include external jugular, internal jugular, and subclavian percutaneous introduction. In placing a pacemaker, thresholds need to be checked. They should be between 0.4 and 0.8 mA and

0.2–0.4 V. The most common indicator for pacemaker insertion today is heart block in the elderly (Lev disease). It is uncommon to require a pacemaker following heart block from myocardial infarction. Telephone electrocardiographic surveillance is used, and this has also decreased the morbidity from heart block. Another use of cardiac electrodes is automatic implantable defibrillators. These have been used successfully to terminate malignant ventricular arrhythmias.

ASSISTED CIRCULATION IN ARTIFICIAL HEART

Temporary assisted circulation is a valuable clinical modality when transient cardiac injury is present. It is seldom effective if required for more than 2–3 days. Intraaortic balloon pumping (IABP) is an effective method with electrocardiographic synchronization; the IABP is alternately inflated during diastole and deflated during systole. CI is usually increased 0.5–0.7 L/min. Ischemia of the extremity is the most common complication. The left-heart bypass or assist may also be used. Blood is removed from the left atrium and returned to the systemic circulation, thus assisting in bypassing the left ventricle. This can be used for prolonged periods of time. Work is being done on a total artificial heart. The major obstacle is the lack of an artificial substance that resembles a normal intima in the bloodstream. Thromboembolism is a major obstacle.

19 DISEASES OF THE GREAT VESSELS

ANEURYSMS OF THE THORACIC AORTA

I. General considerations of thoracic aneurysms
   A. Five main groups: Ascending aorta, transverse arch, traumatic, descending thoracic, and thoracoabdominal aneurysms
   B. Most frequent causes
      1. Atherosclerosis
      2. Aortic dissection (considered separately)
      3. Collagen degenerative disease (e.g., Marfan's)
      4. Idiopathic aortic annular dilatation
      5. Trauma (specific, localized areas)
      6. Syphilis (now rare)
      7. Granulomatous disease
   C. Natural history is of progressive enlargement with eventual rupture
      1. Posttraumatic aneurysms tend to grow more slowly.
      2. Overall survival if untreated is 60% and 20% at 1 and 5 years, respectively
   D. Clinical manifestations
      1. Usually asymptomatic until quite large
      2. Majority are discovered on routine CXR
      3. Of those who develop symptoms, pain and symptoms of adjacent structure compression (SVC, trachea, recurrent nerve) are most common
   E. Diagnosis: Echocardiography, CT scan, and aortography (gold standard)
   F. Treatment: In general involves opening the aneurysm, removing thrombus, inserting dacron graft, and wrapping the graft with native aneurysm wall

II. Specific aneurysms
   A. Ascending aortic aneurysms
      1. Etiology: usually secondary to medial degeneration as in Marfan's
      2. Pathology
         a. Develops in proximal aorta and causes dilatation of aortic annulus with resultant aortic insufficiency (AI)
         b. CHF is frequently presenting clinical problem,

and progression is usually rapid once AI develops

3. Clinical: symptoms range from none to those of acute AI, and the murmur of AI is frequently the only abnormal physical finding of exam
4. Diagnosis is made by CT or aortography
5. Treatment
   a. Indicated when AI present or if size >6 cm
   b. Technique is graft replacement with either aortic valve suspension or (less commonly) valve replacement when AI present; if AVR required, valve conduit is used with reimplantation of the coronary arteries

B. Transverse aortic arch aneurysms
1. Etiology: almost always due to atherosclerosis; usually seen >60 years and associated with coronary artery disease and cerebrovascular disease
2. Diagnosis is made by CT or aortography
3. Operative repair
   a. Most difficult, and formerly associated with 75–80% mortality
   b. Currently, utilizing cardiopulmonary bypass, mortality is about 10–20%

C. Traumatic thoracic aneurysms
1. Etiology: nearly all from closed-chest trauma; majority from horizontal deceleration leading to transection of the descending thoracic aorta
2. Anatomy
   a. Most arise just distal to the left subclavian artery origin, opposite the ligamentum arteriosum; involvement of the arch or ascending aorta is rare
   b. Traumatic rupture is fatal at the scene of the accident, but a few will develop a false aneurysm and survive
3. Natural course and clinical signs
   a. Enlarge slowly and may remain asymptomatic for many years
   b. Compression of adjacent structures occurs over time (recurrent nerve, left mainstem, esophagus)
   c. Usually no murmur is heard on exam
4. Diagnosis
   a. CXR: widened mediastinum with loss of aorto-pulmonary window; density near left subclavian; hemothorax
   b. Aortogram is mandatory to outline anatomy
5. Treatment is resection of aneurysm with graft

replacement; use of partial bypass during resection remains controversial

D. Descending thoracic aneurysms
  1. Etiology
     a. Most due to atherosclerosis
     b. Syphilitic are now rare; dissections discussed later
  2. Anatomy
     a. Usually located in proximal descending thoracic aorta, beginning just distal to the left subclavian and extending a variable length down the thorax
     b. Fusiform >> saccular
  3. Natural history
     a. Enlarge and rupture at rate higher than for abdominal aortic aneurysms
     b. 13% 5-year survival if untreated
  4. Clinical
     a. Most are asymptomatic and found on routine CXR; may have symptoms of compression of adjacent structures (recurrent nerve, left mainstem bronchus, esophagus) or erosion into bronchus of lung with hemorrhage
     b. Exam is usually normal
     c. Diagnosis
        i. CXR: mass in region of aorta (some with Ca^{2+})
        ii. CT: accurate and good for follow-up
        iii. Aortogram: precise outline of anatomy
  5. Treatment
     a. Resection indicated when diagnosed
     b. Technique is graft replacement via left posterolateral thoracotomy ($\pm$ partial bypass)
     c. Principal risks are paraplegia and renal failure
        i. Data suggest that maintaining distal aortic perfusion pressure >60 mmHg will guard against paraplegia
        ii. Risk of paraplegia increases quickly as aortic clamp time exceeds 30 min without bypass

E. Thoracoabdominal aneurysms
  1. Etiology and incidence
     a. Due to atherosclerosis
     b. Rare, and occur primarily in elderly patients with extensive atherosclerosis
  2. Anatomy
     a. Begins in descending thoracic aorta and extends to abdominal aorta

        b. Usually involves upper visceral vascular trunks
   3. Natural history
        a. 75% mortality in 2 years without treatment
        b. Of those operated on (Crawford's series), 60% alive at 5 years
   4. Technique
        a. "Intraluminal technique": graft inserted within aneurysm with side-to-side anastomosis made to ostia of important arteries
        b. Reimplantation of large lumbar arteries to graft can decrease incidence of paraplegia; incidence of postoperative paraplegia is still 15–40%

DISSECTING ANEURYSMS

A. Etiology and incidence
   1. HTN and unknown disease or aortic media; not a disease of intima, and is not due to atherosclerosis
   2. Occurs predominantly in older ages (> fifth decade), but may be seen in all age groups
   3. 3–4:1 male preponderance
B. Pathology
   1. Two abnormalities
        a. Transverse tear of intima and media, which permits blood entry (location: 70% ascending, 10% arch, 20% upper thoracic, and 2% abdominal aorta)
        b. Progressive separation ("dissection") of media, which creates inner (true) lumen and outer (false) lumen; extension distally usually occurs rapidly
   2. Four classes proposed by DeBakey
        a. Type A: begins in ascending aorta near AV and extends distally to external iliacs (most common)
        b. Type B: limited to ascending aorta (Marfan's)
        c. Type C1: begins distal to left subclavian and ends in thorax
        d. Type C2: begins distal to left subclavian and extends to abdominal aorta
   3. As dissection proceeds, branches are obliterated or communicate with false channel
        a. Coronaries may be involved by proximal dissection
        b. Aortic insufficiency may develop from proximal dissection

        c. Any artery distal to point of origin of dissection is at risk (carotid, subclavian, spinals, renals, visceral, etc.)

    4. Rupture of false lumen with exsanguination may occur; pericardial tamponade may occur from rupture into pericardium

    5. Untreated, these have a 90% mortality in 1–3 months

C. Clinical

    1. Symptoms: abrupt onset of tearing, excruciating chest pain, frequently radiating to the back; pain is migratory and may radiate widely

    2. Syncope in 20% and neurologic status changes in 30–40%

    3. Other signs: HTN (85%), murmur of AI (25%), unequal pulses

D. Diagnosis

    1. CXR shows widened mediastinum and occasionally left pleural effusion

    2. Echocardiography and CT: fast and fairly accurate

    3. Aortogram remains the gold standard

E. Treatment

    1. Immediate medical control of HTN and myocardial contractility is essential (β blockade and nipride)

    2. Dissections of the ascending aorta are operated upon immediately

        a. Principal objective is excision of ascending aorta

        b. AV suspension is usually required, but AVR rarely necessary

    3. Dissections of the descending aorta treated initially medically (risk of rupture is less) and repaired later unless evidence of continued dissection is present

    4. Operative mortality is 22% for ascending and 14% for descending types; main cause of death is bleeding

F. Long term

    1. HTN needs continued control

    2. Remaining false lumen may enlarge and rupture

    3. Require frequent and continued long-term follow-up

WOUNDS OF THE GREAT VESSELS

I. Penetrating injuries

A. Two immediate threats: Exsanguination and cardiac tamponade

B. Treatment
1. In moribund patient with shock and signs/symptoms of intrathoracic hemorrahage or tamponade, emergency thoracotomy in ER with control of bleeding and or release of tamponade may be lifesaving
2. When relatively stable, aortogram is best to diagnose injury, direct approach, and plan repair
3. Median sternotomy provides best general exposure
   a. May require "T" extension laterally for added exposure (e.g., (left subclavian)
   b. If left subclavian or descending aorta is only injury, left anterior or left posterolateral thoracotomy are best approaches, respectively

II. Nonpenetrating injuries
A. Types
1. Traumatic laceration of thoracic aorta is most common (discussed earlier); laceration with fatal hemorrhage or laceration with contained hematoma and formation of false aneurysm
2. Injuries of other great vessels rare
B. Diagnosis
1. CXR: widened mediastinum (>8 cm)
2. Aortography is best; high index of suspicion (external evidence of severe chest trauma or history suggesting significant deceleration injury) should warrant aortogram
3. Clinically usually silent and hidden by other chest wall complaints
C. Treatment
1. Immediate resection with interposition graft
2. Partial bypass may be used
3. Do not disturb hematoma until proximial and distal control has been achieved
4. Overall mortality is 15–25%, with about 16% paraplegia rate

OBSTRUCTION OF THE SUPERIOR VENA CAVA

A. Etiology
1. 90% are from malignant process (bronchogenic carcinoma >> thymoma > lymphoma)
2. 10% nonmalignant (expanding thoracic aneurysm, chronic fibrosing mediastinitis)

B. Pathophysiology
  1. Increased cerebral venous pressure (20–50 mmHg)
     a. Acute obstruction can produce fatal cerebral edema in minutes
     b. Chronic, slowly developing obstruction may result in only mild symptoms
  2. Obstruction between azygos vein and right atrium is less disabling than when above azygos
C. Clinical
  1. Signs and symptoms
     a. Mild and early: headache, eyelid swelling, neck enlargement, or facial swelling
     b. Severe: symptoms of cerebral anoxia and edema
     c. Chronic: dilated collateral veins, edema, cyanosis
     d. Symptoms increase when recumbent or stooping
  2. Diagnosis
     a. Measure CVP
     b. Venogram to outline anatomy
     c. Must diagnose the primary disease process
D. Treatment
  1. Malignant
     a. SVC involvement usually precludes surgery
     b. Chemo- and radiotherapy are treatments of choice, and most patients will have a rapid, temporary improvement, but death is inevitable
  2. Benign
     a. No treatment if symptoms are mild, as they usually improve as collaterals develop
     b. Only indication for reconstruction is in those with benign disease who fail to develop adequate collaterals and remain symptomatic
     c. Technique for reconstruction is creating a composite "spiral" autogenous saphenous vein graft for interposition

20 PERIPHERAL ARTERIAL DISEASE

ARTERIOVENOUS FISTULAS

Arteriovenous fistulas represent abnormal communications between arteries and veins. The congential variety is frequently associated with numerous communicating vessels. For this reason, complete excision is frequently impossible. Treatment may comprise transcatheter embolization or surgical excision. Recurrence is common with either form of therapy.

ARTERIAL TRAUMA

Arterial trauma is best handled by understanding a set of caveats relating to the problem:

1. It is safest to approach arterial injuries only after adequate proximal and distal control has been achieved. By contrast, proximal and distal control is not helpful in venous injuries, and control must be achieved using direct compression with the digits or a sponge stick.
2. Early restoration of perfusion is important, and if orthopedic instability precludes an effective arterial repair, a shunt should be used while stabilization is being accomplished.
3. Proximity of an injury to an arterial structure should make one suspicious of a vascular injury, even if distal pulses are intact. Traumatic AV fistulas, false aneurysms, and intimal defects may all occur in the presence of normal distal pulsations. Maintaining a high index of suspicion is important, with liberal indications for arteriography.
4. Preoperative arrteriography is undertaken unless (a) the patient is actively bleeding, (b) there is an unstable hematoma, or (c) the limb is severely ischemic.
5. Suspected carotid arterial injury should be managed with preoperative arteriography if the process is above the angle of the mandible or below the level of the clavicle. Midcervical injuries may be explored without arteriography, but should not be seen if the injury traverses the plethysma muscle.

6. Neither autogenous nor prosthetic grafts have been shown to be clearly superior in reconstruction of traumatic arterial injuries.
7. It is important to repair the vein as well as the artery in combined arterial and venous injuries of the lower extremity.
8. If saphenous vein is used for the arterial reconstruction, it should be taken from the contralateral extremity because the ipsilateral saphenous vein may provide an important route for venous return in the presence of combined arterial and venous injury.
9. Right subclavian injuries are best approached via a median sternotomy, while left subclavian injuries are best managed with a left antilateral thoracotomy or "open book" incision.

THORACIC OUTLET SYNDROME

The thoracic outlet syndrome is an ill-defined, controversial entity that is thought to result from compression of the neurovascular structures between (1) the first rib, (2) the clavicle, and (3) the scalenus anticus muscle. Neurologic symptoms are most frequent, and generally comprise pain and sensory deficits in a lower root (arm and hand, principally ulnar distribution) or upper root (occiput, neck, shoulder, and radial distribution).

Venous symptoms occur less frequently than neurologic symptoms, and usually comprise acute or chronic venous obstruction. Acute axillary vein thrombosis may occur with vigorous activity and has been labeled "effort thombosis." Arterial symptoms are the rarest. Subclavian aneurysms may occur and are prone to produce embolization.

Diagnosis of thoracic outlet syndrome is difficult. Diagnoses to be excluded are carpal tunnel syndrome, cervical degenerative osteoarthritis, and cervical disc disease. Disappearance of the radial pulse with arm abduction is not useful because this occurs in a significant number of normal individuals. The Adson maneuver has been disappointing. The "elevated arm stress test" may be helpful, with the reproduction of symptoms by repeated hand grasps with the arms at the 90° abducted position. The most useful maneuver has been the reproduction of symptoms with arm abduction alone, and the most severely symptomatic patients will frequently complain of symptoms after only 30° abduction. Nerve conduction studies have been helpful in some instances, usually to rule out the diagnosis of carpal tunnel syndrome.

Treatment of thoracic outlet syndrome is primarily conservative for neurologic and venous symptoms, and operative for arterial pathology. Conservative management entails (1) limitation of activities that produce the symptoms, and (2) shoulder-girdle strengthening exercises. Operative therapy is indicated when conservative measures fail, and comprises:

1. First rib resection: probably the best form of therapy, generally through a transaxillary approach
2. Anterior scalenectomy: applicable when upper root neurologic symptoms exist alone
3. Medial claviculectomy: useful when concurrent venous thrombectomy is planned

ACUTE ARTERIAL OCCLUSION

Acute arterial occlusion of the extremity is manifest by the sudden onset of ischemic symptoms. These usually comprise the "6 Ps": (1) pain, (2) pallor, (3) paresthesia, (4) poikilothermia, (5) pulselessness, (6) paralysis.

The cause of ischemia is either embolus or in situ thrombosis. It is difficult to differentiate between these two etiologies. However, embolus frequently occurs in the setting of cardiac arrhythmias, while thrombosis occurs in the presence of preexisting peripheral arterial occlusive disease with contralateral pulse deficits and chronic symptoms.

The vast majority of emboli originate from the heart, and the remainder comprise arterioarterial emboli originating from aneurysms or ulcerated plaques. The most common site of embolus is the common femoral bifurcation. These patients present with "water hammer" femoral pulses initially, with disappearance of the femoral pulse as the thrombus propagates proximally. The next most frequent site of embolus is the popliteal trifurcation. These patients usually present with a palpable popliteal pulse and absent pulses distally.

Patients with presumed common femoral emboli are usually taken to the operating room without arteriography. The common femoral artery is then explored under local anesthesia. The embolus and propagated thrombus are then removed with balloon catheters. Interarterial thrombolytic agents may be infused to clear residual thrombus. Coumadin is begun during the early postoperative period, with duration of therapy dependent on the etiology of the process.

Arteriography is important in the management of acute arterial thrombosis. Patients are treated early if the ischemic process is severe. Interarterial thrombolytic agents have been useful in this group of patients, lysing the clot and allowing operative revascularization or percutaneous angioplasty of more localized lesions to proceed on an elective basis.

CHRONIC ARTERIAL OCCLUSION

Chronic peripheral arterial occlusion is usually secondary to atherosclerosis. Other less common causes include inflammatory arterititis, Buerger disease, giant cell arteritis, Takayasu arteritis, popliteal entrapment syndrome, adventitial cystic disease, and drug-induced spasm.

Peripheral occlusive disease is subdivided on the basis of anatomic location:

1. Aortoiliac occlusive disease: inflow disease; Leriche syndrome—infrarenal aorta and iliac vessels: impotence, buttock, thigh, and calf claudication; not limb threatening in the absence of distal disease
2. Infrainguinal occlusive disease: outlow disease; involves the femoropopliteal/tibial vessels below the inguinal ligament; adductor canal is the most common site of disease; calf claudication, rest pain in the foot; less than 10% of untreated claudicants will progress to amputation within 5 years

Treatment The indications for operative intervention in *aortoiliac occlusive disease* include severe claudication, threatened limb loss (rest pain, ulceration, gangrene), and distal embolization. This disease may be treated with one of three techniques:

1. Operative bypass: generally involves placing a bifurcated tube from the infrarenal aorta to both common femoral vessels. Unilateral aortic femoral or iliofemoral bypasses may be used for unilateral disease. Dacron or polytetrafluorethylene (PTFE) prosthetic material may be used. Patency rates are high (80–90% at 5 years), despite the use of prosthetic material.
2. Aortoiliac endarterectomy: appropriate when disease is limited to the aorta and common iliac vessels. Patency rates are high when the external iliac vessels are disease-free.
3. Percutaneous transluminal angioplasty: most appropriate in patients with short lesions localized to the common iliac artery or occasionally the aorta; long-term patency decreases distal to the common iliac bifurcation.

The indications for operative intervention in *infrainguinal occlusive disease* have been limited to threatened limb loss and lifestyle-limiting claudication. Although open endarterectomy may be appropriate for short lesions of the superficial femoral artery, operative bypass remains the mainstay of treatment. Percutaneous angioplasty has been disappointing in patients with infrainguinal occlusive disease. Prosthetic materials have been avoided when the bypass must traverse the knee joint, as patency falls dramatically with nonautogenous tissue below this point. Vein may be used in a reversed or nonreversed fashion. A variety of instruments have been used to lyse the valves if the vein is not reversed, and in situ bypass is accomplished when the vein is left in its own bed.

The patency rate for vein bypasses to the lower extremity is 60% or greater at 5 years. The patency rate for PTFE above the knee approximates that of vein grafts. The patency of PTFE below the knee is dismal, with a minority of the grafts patent at 2 years of follow-up.

EXTRACRANIAL CEREBRAL OCCLUSIVE DISEASE

Atherosclertoic occlusive disease in the brachiocephalic vessels occurs in remarkably discrete areas. Disease in the subclavian vessels is almost always localized at their origin, while disease in the carotid arteries begins and ends within a few centimeters of the common carotid bifurcation. Subclavian disease is frequently asymptomatic. When symptoms occur, they usually comprise arm claudication. A "subclavian steal" occurs in the presence of a subclavian stenosis proximal to the vertebral takeoff, with retrograde flow in that vertebral artery that may, in effect, steal the blood from the brain. This entity is frequently asymptomatic, and less severe concurrent carotid stenoses exist. Cerebral symptoms may be divided into two groups:

1. *Hemispheric symptoms:* occur as a result of carotid arterial emboli; localized to one side of the body; amaurosis fugax occurs after emboli travel through the ophthalmic artery
2. *Nonhemispheric symptoms:* comprise ataxia, dizziness, diplopia, dysarthria; pathophysiology may be (a) low flow to the hind brain, usually from concurrent carotid and vertebral basilar disease, (b) secondary to emboli originating from the proximal subclavian or vertebral vessels.

Various noninvasive tests have been used in the initial workup of patients with suspected extracranial cerebral vascular disease. Auscultation of bruits is inaccurate, because moderate stenosis may exist without an audible bruit, and a high-grade stenosis may lose its bruit as the flow across the stenosis begins to decrease. Duplex scanning employs B-mode ultrasound for anatomic information and Doppler ultrasound for velocity information. The oculoplethysmogram has been used to provide an index of ophthalmic arterial blood pressure, and is positive only when the stenosis exceeds 60% diameter reduction.

The indications for operative intervention in subclavian occlusive disease include: significant lifestyle-limiting arm claudication, emboli to the hand, emboli to the hind brain, and nonhemispheric cerebral symptoms secondary to low flow, in the absence of significant carotid disease (implying inadequate collateralization through the circle of Willis).

The choice of operative procedure must be tailored to the individual patient, but may include: (1) bypass from the carotid to the subclavian artery, usually with a prosthetic graft; (2) subclavian/vertebral endarterectomy; (3) transposition of the subclavian artery into the carotid artery; and (4) prosthetic bypass from the aorta.

The operative indications for carotid arterial occlusive disease are controversial, but may include a carotid stenosis in the setting of (1) transient ischemic attacks (>24 h), (2) resolved ischemic neurologic deficit (>24h, <3 weeks), (3) completed stroke with good residual function, (4) amaurosis fugax or retinal stroke, and (5) asymptomatic high-grade stenosis.

Carotid endarterectomy is the operation of choice for carotid disease. An intraluminal shunt may be used during the carotid cross clamp, and its use may be selectively based on carotid stump pressures or interoperative electroencephalographic findings.

ARTERIAL ANEURYSMS

The most common location of arterial aneurysms is the infrarenal abdominal aorta. Less frequent sites include the popliteal arteries, the renal and visceral vessels, and the thoracic aorta.

Arterial aneurysms may be differentiated into various types on the basis of their pathophysiology:

1. Atherosclerotic: most common
2. Mycotic: secondary to infectious agents
3. Secondary to vasculitis: tend to involve smaller arteries
4. False: usually secondary to arterial trauma or breakdown

of an arterial anastomosis; do not include the normal layers of the arterial wall
5. Dissecting: not aneurysms at all; rather, they represent bleeding into the medial layers of the artery

Abdominal aortic aneurysms and popliteal aneurysms are most commonly discovered by palpation. Ultrasound and CT may be used to define the extent and size of the aneurysm. Arteriography is not helpful in defining the size or extent of an aneurysm, because the lumen is frequently filled with thrombus, and arteriography delineates only the lumen.

The complications of aneurysms depend on their location. The most important complication of abdominal aortic aneurysms is rupture, while the most common complication associated with popliteal aneurysm is thrombosis.

The operative indications for abdominal aortic aneurysm relate to its size. In general, aneurysms smaller than 4 cm are followed with serial imaging tests. Aneurysms greater than 4 cm are treated operatively if the patient is medically fit, whereas aneurysms greater than 6 cm in diameter are managed operatively in almost all individuals.

Ruptured abdominal aortic aneurysms are grave surgical emergencies with onset of hypotension, abdominal or flank pain, and anemia. Operation should be formed as quickly as possible, and the aorta is clamped at the level of the diaphragm or, if the hematoma is not massive, below the renal vessels. Death results in 30–50% of patients. The unheralded rupture of asymptomatic aneurysms with high fatality rates is the most urgent reason for recommending routine operation of significant aortic abdominal aneurysms.

Popliteal aneurysms are treated when they approach 2.0 cm in diameter or when symptoms result from the aneurysms. The high rate of limb loss with popliteal artery thrombosis makes repair advisable, even in asymptomatic patients, provided a vein is available as a conduit. Patients with acutely thrombosed popliteal arteries can sometimes be managed successfully with thrombolytic therapy, and with definitive repair thereafter.

BUERGER DISEASE

Buerger disease, also known as *thromboangiitis obliterans,* is a vasculitic disease of the vessels that occurs most frequently in middle-aged male smokers. It is a rare problem that involves both the arteries and the veins. The distribution of arterial involvement is different from that of atherosclerosis, with Buerger disease involving the smaller, more peripheral arteries. Involvement of the upper extremities is present in 30% of patients. Recurrent superficial phlebitis is common, while the deeper veins are rarely affected. The most important aspect of treatment is restraint from tobacco in any form. Direct surgical approach is usually not possible. Sympathectomy has been performed, but its benefit is unproved.

21 VENOUS AND LYMPHATIC DISEASE

ANATOMY OF THE VENOUS SYSTEM

The veins of the extremities are divided into three systems. There is a deep system, below the level of the fascia of the muscles. The valves in the deep system serve to direct blood flow toward the heart. There is a superficial system residing in the subcutaneous tissue of the extremities. The valves in the superficial system are also oriented so that the direction of blood flow is toward the heart. Finally, there is a system of communicating veins connecting the superficial system with the deep system. The communicating veins have valves oriented so that the flow of blood is from the superficial to the deep system. The communicating veins are most prominent along the medial aspect of the calf, where they are known as "perforating veins."

The flow of blood in veins is phasic with respiration. During inspiration, abdominal pressure increases, and venous flow in the lower extremities transiently decreases. During expiration, abdominal pressure decreases and lower extremity venous flow increases.

DEEP VENOUS THROMBOSIS (DVT)

Virchow postulated three mechanisms for the development of venous thrombosis: endothelial damage, hypercoagulability, and stasis. These factors account for the high incidence of deep venous thrombosis following an operation.

Thrombi occurring in areas of rapid blood flow (arteries) are generally gray in color and primarily composed of platelets. By contrast, thrombi occurring in relatively slow flowing systems (veins) are red in color and primarily composed of fibrin and red blood cells.

CONDITIONS ASSOCIATED WITH A THROMBOTIC DIATHESIS

I. Endothelial cell damage
  A. Immune vasculitis
    1. Systemic lupus erythematosus

  2. Buerger's disease
  3. Giant cell arteritis
  4. Takayasu's disease
  5. Vasculitis with anticardiolipin factor

II. Hypercoagulability (inappropriate fibrin deposition)
  A. Disseminated intravascular coagulation
  B. Antithrombin III deficiency
  C. Protein C deficiency
  D. Dysfibrinogenemia

III. Stasis
  A. Congestive heart failure
  B. Hyperviscosity
  C. Prolonged bed rest
  D. Neurologic disorders with loss of muscle pump

DIAGNOSIS OF DEEP VENOUS THROMBOSIS The clinical diagnosis of DVT is notoriously inaccurate, and objective tests have become the cornerstone of diagnosis. Contrast phlebography still remains the gold standard test. (See following for Table 21–1.)

TABLE 21-1.

| | Accuracy | | |
Test	Calf veins	Proximal veins	Ability to localize thrombus
Doppler ultrasound	−	+/−	+/−
Radiolabelled fibrinogen	+	−	+/−
Impedance plethysmography	−	+	−
Duplex scanning	+/−	+	+

PROPHYLAXIS OF DEEP VENOUS THROMBOSIS

TABLE 21-2.

Method	Efficacy	Safety
Early ambulation	?	+
Warfarin therapy	+	−(Bleeding)
Dextran	+	
		−(Allergic reactions congestive heart failure)
Full heparinization	+	−(Bleeding)
Minidose heparin	?	+
Intermittent compression devices	+/−	+

TREATMENT OF DEEP VENOUS THROMBOSIS   There are presently three options in the treatment of DVT (Table 21-3). Therapy must be individualized for each patient, and is based on the setting in which the process develops.

The patient is placed at bed rest for a period of several days until the thrombus is adherent to the wall of the vein. The patient is anticoagulated, the duration of therapy is at least 3 months after an episode of acute DVT, and frequently 6 months for the treatment of large venous thrombi. Therapy is begun with intravenous heparin, in an initial dose of approximately 100 units/kg followed by continous intravenous infusion to maintain the partial thromboplastin time at least twice the normal time. Oral warfarin therapy may be begun concurrent with heparin therapy, and adequate anticoagulant effect has been observed with only modest increases in the promthrombin time above the control level. Heparin therapy may be rapidly reversed with protamine sulfate, while coumadin therapy requires infusion of fresh frozen plasma or cryoprecipitate for rapid correction, or administration of vitamin K for less rapid normalization.

TABLE 21-3.

Mode of therapy	Safety	Efficacy	Preservation of venous valves
Anticoagulation	−	+	−
Thrombolytic therapy	−	+	+
Operative thrombectomy	+/−	+/−	+/−

INFERIOR VENA CAVAL INTERRUPTION   Vena caval interruption has been used in an effort to prevent pulmonary emboli (Table 21-4). The indications for vena caval interruption include pulmonary embolus with a contraindication for anticoagulation, recurrent pulmonary embolism on adequate anticoagulation, and as prophylaxis against recurrent embolism after pulmonary embolectomy. A relative indication for caval interruption occurs in the pateint with a large iliofemoral DVT with a contraindication to anticoagulation.

TABLE 21-4.

Method of interruption	Safety	Efficacy	Caval thrombosis
Caval ligation	−	+	100%
Adams-De Weese clip	−	+	26%
Mobin-Uddin umbrella	+/−	+	70%
Hunter balloon	+	+	100%
Greenfield filter	+	+	5%

Other Types of Deep Venous Thrombosis

Superficial Thrombophlebitis   This process is characterized by aseptic thrombosis of the superficial veins. In lower extremities, it is usually associated with varicose veins and is dangerous only when it propagates to the common femoral vein. Therapy is usually supportive, including bed rest, warm packs, and anti-inflammatory agents. Superficial thrombophlebitis in the upper limbs is usually secondary to intravenous infusions. Excision of the vein is indicated when the process is infectious.

Subclavian Vein Thrombosis   Thrombosis of the subclavian vein occurs in two settings. The first is in the setting of an indwelling catheter. Removal of the catheter is indicated. It may also occur as an "effort thrombosis," usually in the setting of thoracic outlet syndrome. Thrombolytic therapy has been helpful when an effort thrombosis occurs, and subsequent first rib resection is frequently necessary.

PULMONARY EMBOLISM

A patient with a pulmonary embolism classically presents with chest pain, cough, dyspnea, and tachypnea. Hemoptysis occurs late and is associated with pulmonary infarction. The EKG and chest x-ray are primarily utilized to exclude other diagnoses. Arterial blood gases generally reveal a P_{O_2} below 60 mmHg as well as decreased P_{CO_2}. If a Swan-Ganz catheter is placed, the pulmonary arterial pressures are frequently elevated and the wedge pressure is either normal or decreased (Table 21-5).

TABLE 21-5.

Diagnostic tests	Safety	Accuracy
Ventilation perfusion scan	+	+/−
Pulmonary angiography	−	+

Management   There are three methods of managing pulmonary embolus. The first is anticoagulation, which has been used in the majority of patients. Heparinization prevents propagation of the thrombus and allows the intrinsic thrombolytic mechanisms to clear the thrombus slowly. Thrombolytic therapy is effective in rapid clot lysis, but is associated with significant bleeding complications. Pulmonary embolectomy is indicated in the patient with severe hemodynamic decompensation. The procedure carries a mortality of 50% when done through an open technique. A transvenous technique has been recently developed, but its efficacy has not been well documented.

VARICOSE VEINS

Diagnosis The prevalence of varicose veins increases with age, and is generally greater in women. It is important to distinguish between primary varicose veins and varicosity secondary to underlying deep venous disease. Primary varicose veins may be inherited and are associated with incompetent valves within the superficial system alone. Secondary varicose veins occur as a result of incompetence in the communicating and deep veins of the leg. This results in high pressures within the superficial veins and subsequent dilatation and superficial venous incompetence. Complications are unlikely with primary varicose veins, but secondary varicosities are frequently accompanied by stasis dermatitis and ulceration.

Patients with varicose veins are treated initially with conservative care, employing compression stockings and limitation of prolonged standing. Injection sclerotherapy may be used if the veins are small or localized. Surgical excision is indicated when conservative measures fail. This frequently entails stripping of the greater saphenous vein in its entirety, including ligation of the adjoining branches in the groin. Accessory varicosities are generally excised through multiple small incisions.

CHRONIC VENOUS INSUFFICIENCY

Chronic venous insufficiency develops in the majority of patients who have sustained a DVT. The underlying pathophysiology consists of recanalization of the deep system with subsequent incompetence of the valves. The high venous pressure then promotes fluid and protein loss into the subcutaneous tissues, resulting in subcutaneous fibrosis probably secondary to inadequate tissue oxygenation and metabolism. This "liposclerosis" produces the brawny edema characteristic of the postphlebitic syndrome. Chronic microscopic hemorrhage into these tissues produces deposition of hemosiderin and the characteristic brown pigmentation. Ulceration frequently occurs, and is generally located above the medial malleolus. The chronic edema predisposes the patient to recurrent bouts of cellulitis. The therapy of chronic venous insufficiency is initially supportive. Compression stockings are generally used, as is bed rest with leg elevation and the use of paste boots. Operative therapy is reserved for patients with persistent ulceration despite adequate conservative measures. The perforating veins may be ligated, usually via a subfascial approach; however, this procedure is frequently accompanied by wound infection and recurrent ulceration. Venous reconstruction is indicated in a minority of patients with nonhealing venous ulceration. Ascending and descending phlebography are mandatory in determining whether patients are candidates for venous reconstructive procedures. These patients may be managed using the following algorithm:

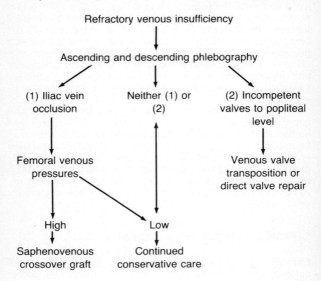

LYMPHEDEMA

Lower extremity edema generally occurs in three clinical settings: cardiac or renal insufficiency is unilateral and clears with elevation; lymphedema is unilateral or bilateral, and is very slow to clear with elevation. The diagnosis of lymphedema is frequently based on clinical grounds. Management is supportive, with compression stockings and care taken to avoid factors that predispose the patient to cellulitis.

Lymphedema may be classified into primary and secondary varieties. The primary lymphedemas are classified as follows:

1. Congenital: present at birth
2. Praecox: onset in childhood
3. Tarda: onset in adulthood

Lymphography has been useful in clarifying the primary lymphedemas into hyperplastic and hypoplastic varieties. Secondary lymphedema is frequently secondary to lymphnode metastases and may also occur after radiation, trauma, or surgical excision, or parasitic invasion.

Operative treatment is only rarely used in patients with lymphedema. The results have been directed at removing the subcutaneous tissues of the extremity. The original procedure of Charles consisted of wide excision of the lymphedemous tissue followed by skin grafting of the extremity. Direct lymphovenous anastomoses have been undertaken at a few centers, but have yet to be proved effective.

22 SURGICALLY CORRECTABLE HYPERTENSION

One in six Americans has hypertension; only one-third of these patients receive treatment, and fewer than one-half are adequately treated. Palliation is the rule with medical management, and opportunities for cure exist in only 5–10% of the total hypertensive population.

There are six basic forms of hypertension that are surgically correctable. These include:

1. Renovascular hypertension
2. Aortic coarctation
3. Pheochromocytoma
4. Hyperadrenocorticism
5. Primary hyperaldosteronism
6. Unilateral renal parenchymal disease

Each condition involves a circulating substance that produces hypertension. The disease entities differ only in the site of origin, and whether the release of the substance is secondary to a parenchymal disorder (e.g., pheochromocytoma) or secondary to reduced perfusion pressure (e.g., renal vascular hypertension). Operative therapy is indicated in each of these conditions, as it offers an opportunity for complete cure rather than palliation.

PATHOPHYSIOLOGY

Pheochromocytoma These tumors produce catecholamines; 15% are malignant, 15% are bilateral (usually associated with multiple endocrine adenomatosis type II syndrome), and 15% are extra-adrenal. The adrenal tumors are localized to the medulla and produce both epinephrine and norepinephrine; the extra-adrenal tumors usually produce only norepinephrine.

Primary hyperaldosteronism These tumors secrete aldosterone and are localized to the zona glomerulosa of the adrenal cortex. Hypokalemia, hypernatremia, and hypervolemia result. Most patients are women between the ages of 30 and 50. The process may be secondary to an adenoma or diffuse cortical hyperplasia.

Hyperadrenocorticism These tumors result in an increase in cortical secretion. The cause may originate in the adrenal gland itself, in the pituitary, or in tumors (ectopic ACTH syndrome). Women between the ages of 30 and 50 are most commonly affected, and hypertension, truncal obesity, amenorrhea, and hirsutism result.

Coarctation of the aorta This is a frequent cause of hypertension in children, and the aortic narrowing usually occurs at the ligamentum arteriosus. The lesion produces decreased renal artery perfusion pressure with secondary hyperreninemia and angiotensin II formation.

Renovascular hypertension Atherosclerosis accounts for 80% of occluded lesions of the renal artery, with fibrodysplasia accounting for the remaining 20%. Fibrodysplasia is the most common cause of renal vascular hypertension in children and young women. The disease may be classified into three types: intimal (5%), medial (85%), or paramedial (10%). The right renal artery is affected 85% of the time, presumably because this is the most mobile kidney and is stretched repeatedly during pregnancy. Renin is produced as perfusion pressure to the kidney is decreased. This activates the juxtaglomerular cells to produce excessive amounts of renin, which then catalyzes the production of angiotensin.

DIAGNOSIS

Surgically correctable hypertension should be suspected in patients who manifest sudden onset of severe hypertension or signs of a hormonal disorder. Hypertension in children or premenopausal women may be surgically correctable.

A basic endocrine and renal screening workup should be undertaken. Examples of appropriate diagnostic techniques are as follows:

PHEOCHROMOCYTOMA Plasma catecholamine levels are more accurate than urinary levels.

PRIMARY HYPERALDOSTERONISM

1. Urinary electrolytes: increased potassium excretion
2. Serum electrolytes: hypokalemia, increased sodium and bicarbonate
3. Plasma renin and aldosterone levels: low plasma renin and high serum aldosterone

HYPERADRENOCORTICISM

1. Urinary 17-hydroxy steroid levels: increased
2. Serum cortisol levels: increased, with loss of diurnal variation
3. ACTH levels: pituitary or adrenal diseases can be differentiated by the ACTH level and the response to dexamethasone suppression

AORTIC COARCTATION   Extremity blood pressures: a difference of more than 20 mmHg is seen between the upper and lower extremities.

RENOVASCULAR HYPERTENSION

1. Physical examination: abdominal bruits
2. Split renal function studies: the ischemic kidney conserves sodium and water, producing a concentration of solutes such as creatinine
3. Howard test: 50% reduction in urine volume, 15% reduction in sodium concentration, 15% increase in creatinine concentration
4. Stamey test: 66% reduction in urine volume, 100% increase in PAH concentration
5. Adrenal vein renin level: ratio (one kidney will have a renin excretion of 1.5 times that of the other kidney) renal systemic renin index (RSRI)

$$\frac{\text{Individual renin activity} - \text{systemic renin activity}}{\text{Systemic renin activity}}$$

(The value of the affected kidney should be greater than 0.48, and the contralateral kidney less than 0.31.)
6. Captopril test: Captopril produces an excess of renin in patients with renovascular hypertension. This increases the sensitivity of both systemic and renal vein renin tests. Administration of 25 mg of captopril produces a marked rise in renin levels at 1 h.

LOCALIZATION OF TUMORS PRODUCING HYPERTENSION

COMPUTERIZED TOMOGRAPHY   Abdominal CT scan or head CT scan, in the case of hyperadrenocorticism, is currently the most useful test in localizing a tumor.

INTRAVENOUS PYELOGRAPHY   This is inaccurate and has been supplanted by newer methods.

ARTERIOGRAPHY This is useful when the tumor is not found with CT scanning.

VENOGRAPHY WITH SELECTIVE SAMPLING This is reserved for ambiguous cases; it is time-consuming but occasionally very helpful.

Treatment

PHEOCHROMOCYTOMA Treatment of pheochromocytoma is operative. Transabdominal adrenalectomy is indicated, with examiniation of both adrenal glands, the organ of Zuckerkandl, and the bladder. Perioperative management requires volume replacement, as all patients are relatively hypervolemic. Phenoxybenzamine and nitroprusside are useful in controlling blood pressure during operation. Vasodilatation and secondary hypotension are common following removal of the tumor.

PRIMARY HYPERALDOSTERONISM The results of treatment for hyperaldosteronism may be predicted with spironolactone. The response to operation is generally good if the blood pressure is decreased preoperatively with this medication. Medical management may be indicated in the absence of a spironolactone response. Operation is generally performed through an anterior abdominal approach. Excision of aldosterone-producing adenomas provides cure rates of 60–90%; however, patients with diffuse cordial hyperplasia do not respond well to adrenalectomy.

HYPERADRENOCORTICISM The treatment of hyperadrenocorticism is dependent on the type of lesion. Extra-adrenal lesions are best treated by excision of the tumor. Bilateral adrenal hyperplasia is associated with pituitary tumors and is effectively managed with pituitary irradiation or transsphenoidal hypophysectomy. In the case of adenoma, unilateral adrenalectomy affords excellent cure rates, though both glands should be examined. Adrenal carcinoma requires wide excision of the tumor, and cure rates are poor.

COARCTATION OF THE AORTA Treatment of aortic coarctation has but one goal: to restore normal arterial pressures to the distal aorta. Therapy is always operative, and the choice of the procedure depends on the anatomy of the lesion. When the problem presents early, the lesion should be treated between the ages of 6 and 16 unless cardiac decompensation develops prior to that time. These lesions are usually located at the ligamentun arteriosum. Excision of the lesion with primary aortic end-to-end anastomosis is desirable, though a short bypass is frequently necessary. As an alternate form of therapy, use of the left subclavian artery as a patch graft is feasible, incising the artery longitudinally and swinging it down onto the aorta over the area of coarctation.

More diffuse aortic coarctation is a rarer problem. Treatment requires bypass grafting, and extra anatomic procedures such as axillofemoral bypass are frequently necessary.

RENOVASCULAR HYPERTENSION There are four modes of therapy for renovascular hypertension: medical management, renal vascular revascularization, percutaneous transluminal dilatation, and nephrectomy. Medical management has been shown to be fraught wth long-term complications and is therefore reserved for only the most frail patients. The choice between revascularization and nephrectomy is dependent on the functional potential of the involved kidney. There are two clinical situations where nephrectomy is indicated: (1) The kidney is small, under 9 cm in length, or (2) the ischemic insult was total and acute, occurring in the absence of collateralization to the kidney.

Renal biopsy has been utilized to predict the potential for function after revascularization, looking for viable cortical glomeruli. In addition, the presence of a nephrogram on arteriography and measurable perfusion on a renal scan indicates a potential for renal function.

The choice of the specific operative procedure depends on the anatomy of the problem and the experience of the surgeon.

Aortorenal Bypass This is applicable only when the aorta is minimally diseased; there are no clear differences between autogenous and prosthetic grafts. Veins should not be utilized in children, however, because aneurysm formation is frequent. Autogenous hypogastric artery provides a suitable alternative in young patients. If an aortic graft is to be placed, it is feasible to run separate graft limbs up the involved renal arteries.

Bypass from Branches of the Celiac Trunk The hepatorenal bypass is on the right, utilizing vein or prosthetic; the splenorenal bypass is on the left, transsecting the splenic artery, leaving the spleen intact and anastomosing the splenic artery to the left renal artery. Hepatorenal and splenorenal bypasses are useful in the setting of a heavily diseased aorta or a fragile patient, as they avoid the necessity for an aortic cross clamp. They do require adequate views of the celiac system on preoperative arteriography.

Renal Endarterectomy This may be accomplished with a longitudinal incision from the aorta to one or both renal arteries. Alternatively, the orifices may be endarectomized through the transsected aorta if an aortofemoral bypass is to be undertaken concurrently. A transaortic renal endarterectomy is useful in the setting of multiple renal arterial stenoses, especially where multiple renal arteries are present.

Percutaneous Transluminal Dilatation This procedure is contraindicated in the presence of lesions at the most proximal portions of the renal arteries and lesions distally at branch points in the renal vessels. The procedure is most appropriate for patients with fibromuscular dysplasia of the renal arteries.

23 MANIFESTATIONS OF GASTROINTESTINAL DISEASE

COMMON SYMPTOMS OF GASTROINTESTINAL (GI) DISEASE

Abdominal pain, dysphagia, anorexia, nausea and vomiting, bloating or distention, and constipation and diarrhea.

COMMON SIGNS

Tenderness, rigidity, palpable masses, altered bowel sounds, GI bleeding, nutritional deficits, jaundice, and stigmata of hepatic dysfunction.

Abdominal Pain

Pain Pathways Pain perception from the abdominal cavity is mediated by one of three routes: (1) visceral sympathetic afferents; (2) visceral parasympathetic afferents; (3) somatic afferents of the parietal peritoneum, root of the mesentery, body wall, and diaphragm.

Variability Abdominal pain can have a marked variability in its perception. With a given pathologic process, the patient may experience somatic, visceral, or referred pain, or any combination thereof.

Visceral Pain Pain impulses originate in the wall of a viscus and travel to the spinal cord via visceral afferents in the splanchnic nerves. Stimuli that cause intense somatic pain, such as cutting and crushing, produce little, if any, visceral sensation. Important stimuli for visceral pain are increased wall tension of a hollow viscus (distention, spasticity, obstruction), capsule stretching (subcapsular liver hematoma), ischemia, and certain chemicals (potassium, bradykinin). Inflammation and ischemia exacerbate visceral pain perception. Visceral pain is poorly localized. *Autonomic reflexes* may accompany severe abdominal pain. These are nausea, vomiting, changes in heart rate, hypotension, and muscular contractions.

Somatic Pain Somatic afferents mediate pain arising in the abdominal wall, parietal peritoneum, root of the mesentery, and diaphragm. The character is usually sharp, well localized, and lateralized. Abdominal wall muscular rigidity is commonly seen with inflammation of the parietal peritoneum.

Referred Pain Visceral disease may present as pain localized to superficial body areas often at a distance from their pathologic origin. The pattern is usually dermatomal.

Etiology Both intraperitoneal and extraperitoneal disorders may be manifest as abdominal pain. See Tables 23-1 and 23-2.

Clinical Evaluation *History.* Accurately define the character, severity, location, timing, radiation, and exacerbating or alleviating factors. Include relationship to meals, sleep patterns, and the effects of position, movement, and respiration. Obtain a chronological report of all changes in character from onset. Record the frequency of vomiting and its nature (clear, bilious, feculent) and the bowel movement and flatus history, and document the menstrual cycle.

Physical Exam. *Observe* the patient for general appearance, muscle spasm, autonomic responses to pain, position in bed, level of activity (writhing accompanies colicky pain, restricted motion accompanies peritonitis), tissue turgor, and vital signs. *Abdominal exam* includes inspection, auscultation (bowel sounds), and palpation (masses, peritonitis, hernias, tenderness, guarding, rigidity). *Pelvic* and *rectal* exams are essential.

Laboratory Procedures. Hemoglobin, white blood count, differential, amylase, bilirubin, SMA7. *X-ray* supine and upright abdomen (decubitus if patient can't stand) and chest. EKG. Fecal occult blood. Culdocentesis.

Intractable Pain This is pain associated with chronic diseases that cannot be definitively treated (pancreatic carcinoma, chronic pancreatitis). Treatment options include opiates, neurosurgical intervention (rarely helpful), splanchnicectomy, and celiac ganglionectomy or ablative block. Recently, dorsal column stimulation with a TENS unit has shown some promise.

Dysphagia

Dysphagia refers to difficulty in swallowing. *Odynophagia* is the term used for painful swallowing. Swallowing occurs in

TABLE 23-1. Gastrointestinal and Intraperitoneal Causes of Abdominal Pain

I. Inflammation
  A. Peritoneum
    1. Chemical and nonbacterial peritonitis—perforated peptic ulcer, gallbladder, ruptured ovarian cyst, mittelschmerz
    2. Bacterial peritonitis
      a. Primary peritonitis—pneumococcal, streptococcal, tuberculous
      b. Perforated hollow viscus—stomach, intestine, biliary tract
  B. Hollow intestinal organs
    1. Appendicitis
    2. Cholecystitis
    3. Peptic ulceration
    4. Gastroenteritis
    5. Regional enteritis
    6. Meckel's diverticulitis
    7. Colitis—ulcerative, bacterial, amebic
    8. Diverticulitis
  C. Solid viscera
    1. Pancreatitis
    2. Hepatitis
    3. Hepatic abscess
    4. Splenic abscess
  D. Mesentery
    1. Lymphadenitis
  E. Pelvic organs
    1. Pelvic inflammatory disease
    2. Tuboovarian abscess
    3. Endometritis

II. Mechanical (obstruction, acute distention)
  A. Hollow intestinal organs
    1. Intestinal obstruction—adhesions, hernia, tumor, volvulus, intussusception
    2. Biliary obstruction—calculi, tumor, choledochal cyst, hematobilia
  B. Solid viscera
    1. Acute splenomegaly
    2. Acute hepatomegaly—cardiac failure, Budd-Chiari syndrome
  C. Mesentery
    1. Omental torsion
  D. Pelvic organs
    1. Ovarian cyst
    2. Torsion or degeneration of fibroid
    3. Ectopic pregnancy

III. Vascular
  A. Intraperitoneal bleeding
    1. Ruptured liver
    2. Ruptured spleen
    3. Ruptured mesentery
    4. Ruptured ectopic pregnancy
    5. Ruptured aortic, splenic, or hepatic aneurysm
  B. Ischemia
    1. Mesenteric thrombosis
    2. Hepatic infarction—toxemia, purpura
    3. Splenic infarction
    4. Omental ischemia

IV. Miscellaneous
  A. Endometriosis

TABLE 23-2.   Extraperitoneal Causes of Abdominal Pain

Cardiopulmonary	*Vascular*
Pneumonia	Dissection, rupture, or
Empyema	expansion of aortic aneurysm
Myocardial ischemia	Periarteritis
Active rheumatic heart disease	*Metabolic*
Blood	Uremia
Leukemia	Diabetic acidosis
Sickle cell crisis	Porphyria
Neurogenic	Addisonian crisis
Spinal cord tumors	*Toxins*
Osteomyelitis of spine	Bacterial (tetanus)
Tabes dorsalis	Insect bites
Herpes zoster	Venoms
Abdominal epilepsy	Drugs
Genitourinary	Lead poisoning
Nephritis	*Abdominal wall*
Pyelitis	Intramuscular hematoma
Perinephric abscesses	*Psychogenic*
Ureteral obstruction (calculi,	
tumors)	
Prostatitis	
Seminal vesiculitis	
Epidydimitis	

three stages: (1) voluntary movement of food bolus into pharynx, (2) reflex (involuntary) propulsion of food through pharynx by waves of contraction, and (3) transportation of bolus through esophagus into stomach via positive-pressure waves (primary peristalsis), followed by reflex lower esophageal sphincter relaxation.

Etiology   *Oropharyngeal causes* are disorders of the mouth, upper respiratory tract, or pharynx, including anatomic, neoplastic, infectious, and neurologic entities. *Esophageal causes* are carcinoma, esophagitis, achalasia, contractile ring, diffuse spasm, Zenker's diverticulum, scleroderma, extrinsic masses, paraesophageal hernias, esophageal webs, strictures, vascular anomalies, and emotional disorders.

Clinical Evaluation   *History* must include duration, location, and timing in relation to ingestion. Determine the amount of weight loss and the presence of associated vomiting. *Examine* for cervical nodes, stigmata of scleroderma and oral lesions. *Diagnostic studies* include barium cine-esophagograms, manometry, and esophagoscopy with biopsy.

Anorexia

Anorexia is the absence of the desire to eat. Appetite is a central phenomenon and anorexia is thus dependent upon central effects. Feeding and satiety centers are in lateral and medial hypothalamus. *Organic causes* include intestinal inflammatory processes; carcinoma of the pancreas, stomach, and liver; hepatitis; alcoholism; ESRD; CHF; panhypopituitarism; adrenal cortical insufficiency and hyperparathyroidism.

Nausea and Vomiting

Pathophysiology The two centers in the reticular core of the medulla oblongata are the chemoreceptive trigger zone (uremia, drug-induced, and radiation emesis), and the integrated center. Afferent pathways emanate from almost all body sites. The vagal pathways are very important, but vagotomy does not abolish vomiting. Sympathetic afferent pathways mediate vomiting associated with intestinal distention. Vomiting occurs when both somatic and visceral efferent pathways cause closure of the glottis, contraction of the diaphragm, pyloric closure, and gastric relaxation followed by peristaltic contractions passing from midstomach to the incisura ending with abdominal, diaphragmatic, and intercostal contractions. Vomiting is associated with signs and symptoms of autonomic discharge.

Etiology Associations exist with all alimentary tract disorders, especially obstructions, with a high acute obstruction causing early vomiting. Autonomic derangements, drugs, psychogenic disorders, and ingestion of noxious substances are other frequent causes. Factors that reduce blood supply and oxygen delivery to the medulla (shock, vascular occlusion, increased ICP) may induce emesis. Emetic drugs produce their effects either by direct central stimulation or by gastric mucosal irritation. Metabolic abnormalities such as acidosis, uremia, and hyperkalemia can affect the emesis center.

Patterns Sudden, often projectile vomiting without antecedent nausea strongly suggests a central cause. Hypertrophic pyloric stenosis also causes projectile emesis. Feculent emesis suggests small bowel obstruction or gastrocolic fistula. Vomiting immediately postprandially occurs with uremia, gastritis, high intestinal obstruction, and gastric neoplasms.

Consequences of Vomiting *Metabolic:* With protracted vomiting, hypovolemia, hypokalemia, and metabolic alkalosis and total body sodium depletion occur. Potassium is excreted by the kidney in exchange for sodium, since there is an unavailability of H^+ to exchange. Further volume contraction can result in a paradoxical aciduria in an attempt to conserve sodium. *Other:* Repeated, forceful retching may cause a Mallory-Weiss tear or rupture the distal esophagus (Boerhaave syndrome).

Constipation and Diarrhea

Intestinal Transit   The stomach empties in 3–4 h, with digested food reaching the ileocecal valve by 2–3 h and completing passage by 9 h. Absorption of water occurs in the cecum and ascending colon. Mass peristaltic waves (gastrocolic reflex) occur after meals and propel the bolus from the hepatic flexure onward. Defecation occurs when peristaltic waves accompanied by relaxation at the rectosigmoid junction propel the contents of the left colon and sigmoid into the rectum. The major portion of ingested material requires several days for evacuation. The vagi, splanchnic, and pelvic nerves play a significant role in ordered intestinal motility. Motility is augmented by parasympathetic stimulation and inhibited by sympathetic stimulation. Finally, receptive relaxation of the internal anal sphincter is dependent upon a lower cord reflex, while the external sphincter is under voluntary control. Pharmacologic influences on transit include increased activity by cholinergic drugs, serotonin, vasopressin, and others. Potassium deficiency, morphine, codeine, and atropine may decrease motility.

CONSTIPATION   Constipation is an abnormal retention of feces or undue delay in discharge compared to usual bowel habits. *Psychogenic causes* include improper training resulting in functional megacolon. *Dietary factors* include lack of bulk and overuse of laxatives. (Concerning *drugs,* see "Intestinal Transit," above.) *Decreased muscular power* in abdominal wall, diaphragm, or pelvic musculature may cause constipation. *Neurogenic causes* include tabes dorsalis, MS, cord tumors, trauma, and Hirschsprung disease. *Intrinsic factors* include tumors, fecal impaction, volvulus, intussusception, and anal spasm (fissures, proctitis, hemorrhoids). *Extrinsic causes* include large intraabdominal masses, and obstructing adhesions.

Associated Symptoms and Effects   *Obstipation* (no feces and flatus) suggests mechanical obstruction. Back pain, hip pain, headache, and tachycardia may accompany constipation. Secondary anal ulcers, fissures, and hemorrhoids may form. Colonic diverticula and sigmoid volvulus may develop.

Clinical Evaluation   A complete bowel and dietary history is necessary. Pay attention to stool size and caliber, presence of melena, mucus, blood, undigested foods, and history of tenesmus. Thorough rectal, BE, and proctosigmoidoscopy are helpful.

DIARRHEA   This is excessive rapid evacuation of excessively fluid stool.

Etiology   Causes are countless and broadly include: functional disease, organic colonic disease (colitis, neoplasms), small intestinal disorders (IBD, malabsorption, fistulas, short gut), gastric factors (ZE syndrome, dumping, postvagotomy), pancreatic and biliary disease, enteric infections (bacteria, parasites), metabolic disorders (thyroid, uremia, parathyroid), and drugs.

Pathophysiology   Primary abnormality is of intestinal water and electrolyte transport. Distention then stimulates propulsive contractions. Principal mechanisms include: (1) *excessive intestinal secretion,* or secretory diarrhea. This involves active ion secretion, for which cholera is a classical model. (2) *Osmotic diarrhea* comes from intraluminal poorly absorbed or osmotically active solutes. These are a result of incomplete digestion, failure to absorb, or ingestion. (3) *Malabsorption of normal ions* occurs infrequently, most notably in congenital chloridorrhea. (4) *Deranged bowel motility* is poorly understood and may occur with diabetes, scleroderma, or irritable colon.

Consequences   Severe, prolonged diarrhea may result in dehydration, acidosis, and electrolyte loss (hypokalemia).

Clinical Evaluation   *History.*   Include duration, time of day, description of stool, presence of blood, mucus or fats, pain or urgency, and other GI disease manifestations. Look for epidemiologic factors.

Physical Examination.   Assess for fever and arthritis (IBD). Examine abdominal region thoroughly for masses and tenderness. Rectal and proctoscopic examinations are helpful.

Stool Analysis.   Check for blood (carcinoma, IBD), mucus, and excessive fats (pancreatic insufficiency).

Radiologic Studies.   Abdominal films, barium enema, and UGI series are essential.

Other Diagnostic Studies.   Occasionally laparotomy and small bowel biopsy are indicated.

INTESTINAL OBSTRUCTION

This is an interference with normal aboral progression of intestinal contents, classified as either mechanical or functional (ileus). Table 23-3 lists common etiologies.

Mechanical Obstruction

This may occur from (1) luminal obturation, (2) luminal obstruction by bowel wall pathology, or (3) lesions extrinsic to the bowel. *Simple obstruction* implies obstruction without ischemia, while *strangulated obstruction* implies blockage with occlusion of the mesenteric vessels. *Closed-loop obstruction* refers to blockage of both limbs of the involved bowel. Mechanical obstruction is most frequently caused by *adhesive bands,* followed by strangulated inguinal hernia, and neoplasm. Carcinoma is the most common cause of large bowel obstruction.

Pathophysiology *Fluid and Electrolyte Losses.* Large quantities of fluid and gas accumulate above the obstruction. Net intestinal secretion is the primary cause of fluid loss and distention. Loss of the bowel's ability to handle fluid progresses from adjacent to the obstruction to proximal bowel. As bowel becomes progressively distended, its circulation is impaired, resulting in wall edema and even necrosis. This edema and accompanying fluid exudation from bowel wall exacerbates losses. Finally, vomiting further adds to dehydration.

Intestinal Gas. This is mostly swallowed air, 70% nitrogen, which diffuses poorly and contributes to distention.

Bowel Motility. Initially, motility increases in an effort to overcome the obstruction, but eventually peristalsis occurs in bursts with quiescent periods. Distal bowel becomes hypoactive.

Strangulated Bowel Obstruction. This is mechanical obstruction with occlusion of the mesenteric blood supply. Venous outflow blockage leads to bloody fluid accumulation within the bowel and bowel wall. Gangrenous bowel leaks bacterial toxins into peritoneal cavity, leading to septic shock. Perforation ultimately ensues.

Closed-Loop Obstruction. Both afferent and efferent loops are blocked, which progresses rapidly to strangulation from mechanics or intraluminal pressure.

TABLE 23-3. Mechanisms of Intestinal Obstructions

Mechanical obstruction of the lumen
  Obturation of the lumen
    Meconium
    Intussusception
    Gallstones
    Impactions—fecal, barium, bezoar, worms
  Lesions of bowel
    Congenital
      Atresia and stenosis
      Imperforate anus
      Duplications
      Meckel's diverticulum
    Traumatic
    Inflammatory
      Regional enteritis
      Diverticulitis
      Chronic ulcerative colitis
    Neoplastic
    Miscellaneous
      K^+-induced stricture
      Radiation stricture
      Endometriosis
  Lesions extrinsic to bowel
    Adhesive band constriction or angulation by adhesion
    Hernia and wound dehiscence
    Extrinsic masses
      Annular pancreas
      Anomalous vessels
      Abscesses and hematomas
      Neoplasms
  Volvulus
Inadequate propulsive motility
  Neuromuscular defects
    Megacolon
    Paralytic ileus
      Abdominal causes
        Intestinal distention
        Peritonitis
        Retroperitoneal lesions
      Systemic causes
        Electrolyte imbalance
        Toxemias
    Spastic ileus
  Vascular occlusion
    Arterial
    Venous

Colonic Obstruction.   Strangulation is rare except with volvulus. Fluid and electrolyte sequestration progresses more slowly. Progressive distention against a competent ileocecal valve is essentailly a closed-loop obstruction and will lead to cecal perforation following the law of Laplace (tension = presssure × diameter × π).

Clinical Manifestations   Initial symptoms are abdominal pain, vomiting, and obstipation followed by abdominal distention, severe colicky pain with hyperperistalsis, quiescent periods, then diffuse pain. Eventually there is a steady generalized discomfort. *Vomiting* occurs immediately (reflex) and at a variable time later depending on the level of obstruction. Feculent material implies low obstruction.

Physical Examination.   Initially there are few findings except for the reported colic. Auscultation early shows loud, high-pitched metallic sounds with rushes and periods of complete silence. With time, dehydration, distention, and acute abdominal findings (strangulated) will develop.

Laboratory Findings.   These include dehydration with increased HCT and BUN and oliguria, metabolic acidosis, and CO_2 retention from abdominal distention. Marked leukocytosis suggests strangulation or ischemia. Amylase elevation can occur.

Radiologic Findings.   Plain supine and upright films are the most important diagnostic study. See Table 23-4. BE is useful in suspected colonic obstruction. Small bowel series helps to differentiate mechanical obstruction from ileus.

Management   Fluid and electrolyte therapy corrects losses followed by surgical operation. Replete potassium. Use urine output, CVP, and initial elevation in HCT to gauge the severity of dehydration. Replace losses with isosmotic fluids. Surgery may not be necessary in immediate postoperative obstruction. Mortality is minimal when operation is undertaken within the first 24 h. Strangulated obstructions are surgical emergencies.

Gastrointestinal Intubation.   A double-lumen nasogastric tube should *always* be used in patient preparation. Long intestinal tubes are of questionable value and may delay treatment of a strangulated obstruction. Prolonged suction therapy should be reserved for immediate postoperative patients, partial obstruction, or cautiously with obstruction secondary to treatable inflammation (i.e., Crohn).

Operation.   Obstructions that are of the closed-loop type, strangulated, colonic, or early complete should be treated as

TABLE 23-4. Radiologic Signs in Intestinal Obstruction

Sign	Simple mechanical obstruction	Adynamic ileus
Gas in intestine	Large bow-shaped loops in ladder pattern	Copious gas diffusely through intestine
Gas in colon	Less than normal	Increased, scattered through colon
Fluid levels in intestine	Definite	Often very large throughout
Tumor	None	None
Peritoneal exudate	None	Present with peritonitis; otherwise absent
Diaphragm	Somewhat elevated: free motion	Elevated; diminished motion

Source: From Eisenberg RL: *Gastrointestinal Radiology.* Philadelphia, Lippincott, 1983, with permission.

surgical emergencies. The five general types of surgical procedures are: (1) lysis, manipulation-reduction procedures; (2) enterotomy for removal of obturation; (3) resection of obstructing lesions or strangulated segments with primary reanastomosis; (4) bypass procedures; and (5) proximal ostomy creation. The *character of the peritoneal fluid* is usually straw-colored, but bloody fluid denotes strangulation. Adhesions should be lysed and loops reduced before resecting loops of questionable viability. *Intraoperative decompression* facilitates closure and improves blood supply. This may be accomplished with a long tube passed orally, nasally, or via a gastrostomy.

Postoperative Care. This includes fluid and electrolyte maintenance, antibiotics, and decompression. There is a continued third-space loss of isotonic fluid in the immediate postoperative period eventually followed by autoinfusion of the sequestered fluid as the bowel recovers. Decompression may be required for up to 5 days.

Ileus

Adynamic ileus is characterized by absent motility due to neuromuscular inhibition with sympathetic overactivity. Extremely common, it occurs after all abdominal procedures. Motility returns at: small bowel 24 h, stomach 48 h, colon 3–5 days. Other causes are intraperitoneal inflammatory processes, retroperitoneal conditions, pneumonia, hypokalemia, hypomagnesemia, sepsis, opiates, and others. *Spastic ileus* caused by uncoordinated hyperactivity is rare. It is seen in uremia and heavy-metal poisoning. *Vascular occlusion ileus* occurs when the bowel is incapable of motility from ischemia.

Clinical Manifestations   These include anorexia, occasional hypoactive bowel sounds, and possibly distention and tympany. Laboratory studies should include SMA7, Ca^{2+} and Mg^{2+}, CBC, and amylase. X-rays may aid in diagnosis, showing gas diffusely throughout intestines. Small bowel barium studies are very useful. Rarely, massive colonic ileus (Ogilvie's syndrome) may lead to cecal perforation.

Treatment   *Treat the primary lesion!* Severe distention may need a short or long nasogastric tube. Metaclopramide may or may not work.

Pseudoobstruction

This is a clinical bowel obstruction with no organic lesion. It may be due to visceral myopathy, diabetes, hypothyroidism, MS, amyloidosis, and others. Treatment of the underlying disorder usually does not work.

GASTROINTESTINAL BLEEDING

This may be the initial symptom of GI disease in 33% of patients. *Hematemesis* is the vomiting of blood. Bleeding is usually proximal to the ligament of Treitz, possibly with concurrent melena. Coffee-ground vomitus suggests a slower bleed. *Melena* is the passage of dark, tarry stool. 50 mL may produce it, and it may last 5 days after bleeding ends. Usually results from upper tract GI bleeding.

Consequences of Gastrointestinal Bleeding   Acutely, the hematocrit is usually an unreliable indicator of the amount lost. Initially there are vasovagal signs, then signs of hypovolemia followed by shock, including oliguria and anuria. Laboratory studies may show azotemia, especially with bleeding varices, *not with colonic bleeding*.

Upper Gastrointestinal Bleeding

Etiology   The majority is due to peptic ulceration, gastritis, esophageal varices, espophagitis, or gastric neoplasms. *Peptic ulceration* accounts for 50–67%. Duodenal: gastric is 4:1. 16% have bleeding as the first symptom. Marginal ulceration occurs after some gastric resections. *Acute mucosal lesions* are erosions confined to mucosa, distinct from ulcers. *Stress ulceration* occurs with shock, sepsis, burns (Curling ulcers), trauma, craniotomy (Cushing ulcers), and major operations, and may be due to decreased splanchnic flow and ischemic damage. *Drugs* such as steroids, alcohol, and aspirin can produce erosive hemorrhagic gastritis. *Esophageal varices* account for 10% of all UGI bleeding and 95% of massive hematemesis in the child. They are secondary to cirrhosis and portal hypertension and are more severe than alcoholic gastritis. *Other lesions* include hiatial hernia, gastric carcinoma, leiomyomas, vascular lesions, Mallory-Weiss tears, hematobilia, and duodenal diverticula.

Diagnosis   *History and Physical.*   History must include previous medical conditions, especially ulcer disease, and intensity and frequency of vomiting (Mallory-Weiss tear). Ingestion of drugs, bleeding tendencies, previous gastric surgery, reflux symptoms, and recent trauma should all be queried. Examination should uncover the stigmata of the etiologic diseases (e.g., cirrhosis, vascular lesions).

Diagnostic Procedures. Hematocrit will not show the extent of loss with acute bleeds. SMA7 (elevated BUN from GI absorption of blood products and from dehydration), blood ammonia. Clotting studies and platelets. *Endoscopy* is mandatory for upper tract bleeding. ^{99m}Tc-labeled erythrocytes can be helpful for intermittent bleeding. Angiography of the celiac and SMA is useful for bleeding in excess of 1–2 mL/min. Selective embolization may be used at this time. Arterial vasopressin via these catheters is no more efficacious than venous administration. UGI series may be done if endoscopy and arteriography are not revealing. Finally, laparotomy should be considered for diagnosis, especially with massive bleeding. A long gastrotomy is used to inspect the duodenum, stomach, and hiatus.

Lower Gastrointestinal Bleeding

This is bleeding distal to the ligament of Treitz; it may be black tarry, *melena,* or bright red, *hematochezia.*

Etiology Causes may vary greatly by age group. See Table 23-5. By anatomic site: *jejunum and ileum*: Meckel's, intussusception, regional enteritis. *Colon:* carcinoma, diverticulosis (massive), vascular ectasias (right colon), colitis, and polyps. *Rectum and anus:* Unaltered blood in stool. Hemorrhoids, fissures, and proctitis.

Diagnosis Include a precise history, familial conditions (polyposis), and drugs. *Examine* for mucosal lesions (OWR, Peutz-Jeghers). Abdominal exam detects masses. Rectal exam is necessary for masses and anal lesions. *Proctosigmoidoscopy must be done early.* Colonoscopy if not massively bleeding. Radioisotope studies for slower bleeding (1 mL/min), and angiography (most accurate) for fast bleeding (2–3 mL/min). Barium studies for nonacute bleeds (carcinomas, polyps).

JAUNDICE

NORMAL BILE PIGMENT METABOLISM Bilirubin is formed from hemoglobin, myoglobin breakdown, and hepatic synthesis. Bilirubin + albumin, (indirect bilirubin, water insoluble, ≤ 0.3 mg/dL), transported to liver, albumin removed and conjugated with glucuronic adid, excreted into bile (direct bilirubin, water soluble, ≤ 1.3 mg/dL). In the intestines, bacteria reduce to urobilinogens (colorless) and urobilin.

TABLE 23-5. Causes of Lower Gastrointestinal Bleeding by Age Group, in Order of Frequency*

Infants and children	Adolescents and young adults	Adults to 60 years	Adults over 60 years
Meckel's diverticulum	Meckel's diverticulum	Diverticulosis	Vascular ectasias
Polyps	Inflammatory bowel disease	Inflammatory bowel disease	Diverticulosis
Ulcerative colitis	Polyps	Polyps	Malignancy
Duplications		Malignancy	Polyps
		Congenital arteriovenous malformations	

* Less frequent causes not specific for any age group.
Infectious diarrheas (amebiasis, shigellosis), ischemic colitis, drug-induced cecal ulceration (e.g., vincristine), vascular lesions, vascular tumors, varices, coagulopathies.
Source: From Boley SJ, Brandt LS, Frank MS: 1981, with permission.

Fecal excretion is 100–200 mg/day. Some unrobilinogen is reabsorbed into the portal system.

ABNORMAL BILE PIGMENT METABOLISM With Normal Bile Excretion Overproduction from hemolysis overloads the liver (elevated indirect and urobilinogen), "shunt" hyperbilirubinemia, liver defects (Gilbert disease, Crigler-Najjar syndrome). All have jaundice but clear urine.

With Impaired Bile Excretion Elevated conjugated bilirubin, excreted into urine.

Intrahepatic Causes. Dubin-Johnson syndrome (normal LFTs, impaired excretion), drugs (phenothiazines, methyltestosterone), primary biliary cirrhosis. Hepatitis and cirrhosis (abnormal LFTs) have both conjugation and excretion deficits. Biliary atresia. Stools may be clay colored.

Extrahepatic Cholestasis. Anatomic obstacle to bile flow out of liver. Atresia, sticture, stones, tumors, cysts, parasites. Increased direct fraction and indirect.

EVALUATION AND MANAGEMENT OF JAUNDICE Clinically apparent with bilirubin $\geq$ 2mg/dL. Sclerae appear earlier.

History Time course is important (extrahepatic obstruction insidious in onset), painless jaundice (carcinoma), presence of RUQ pain (stones, cholangitis), family history, drug ingestion. Decreased appetite, fever (hepatitis), infectious contact, ETOH history.

Physical Examination Rash (drug reactions), spider angiomas (cirrhosis), hepatomegaly and tenderness (hepatitis), palpable gallbladder (malignancy with extrahepatic obstruction, *Courvoisier's law*), ascites.

Laboratory Studies Anemia, increased reticulocyte (hemolysis), sickle cells, spherocytes, WBC elevations (cholangitis), color of stools and occult blood (⅓ pancreatic carcinoma heme-positive). Bilirubin (direct, indirect). Bilirubinuria (not with unconjugated jaundice). Alkaline phosphatase (obstructive jaundice), increased SGOT/SGPT (hepatitis). Increased PT and poor response to aquamenphyton implies hepatocellular disease.

Radiologic Studies Plain films (20% gallstones opaque), OCG ineffective with bili $\geq$ 1.8, ultrasonography, ERCP (with bx), PTC, CT scan, radioisotopic biliary scan, even with bili of 20 mg/dL.

Other Studies *Liver biopsy* may delineate hepatocellular disease. Check coags first! Laparotomy for extrahepatic obstruction.

Algorithm for Obstructive Jaundice With suspicion of extra-hepatic obstruction, start with ultrasound, proceed as per Fig. 23-1.

Figure 23-1 Extrahepatic Ductal Obstruction

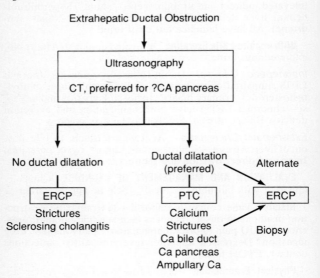

24 ESOPHAGUS AND DIAPHRAGMATIC HERNIAS

ANATOMY

The esophagus is a muscular tube extending from the pharynx at the C_6 vertebra to the junction with the stomach. In the neck it is immediately behind the trachea; in the thorax it curves slightly to the left behind the left main bronchus and then runs anterior to the thoracic aorta crossing it to the left of the midline. It reaches the abdomen through a hiatus created by the right crus of the diaphragm. A segment of variable length has an intraabdominal location.

The blood supply in its cervical portion comes from the inferior thyroid arteries; in the thoracic portion, from the aorta itself and esophageal branches of the bronchial arteries. Lymphatic vessels run longitudinally in the wall of the esophagus before penetrating the muscle layers to reach regional nodes. Malignant lesions of the middle or upper esophagus may metastasize first to the cervical nodes. The esophagus receives vagal and sympathetic nerves as branches from the IXth, Xth, and XIth cranial nerves and also receives sympathetic nerves.

The esophageal wall is composed of an inner circular layer of muscle and an outer longitudinal layer without serosal covering. The mucosal lining is made of squamous epithelium, but the distal 1–2 cm is lined by columnar epithelium.

PHYSIOLOGY

At the upper end of the esophagus there is an upper esophageal sphincter. Peristaltic waves extend down the esophagus. There is a lower esophageal sphincter located in the region of the hiatus. In response to swallowing effort there is relaxation of this zone. The response of the lower esophageal sphincter (LES) to increases in intragastric pressure is dependent on a vagal innervation and parasympathetic activity.

The most sensitive objective test of gastroesophageal reflux is the acid (pH) reflux test performed by placing hydrochloric acid in the stomach and a pH electrode 5 cm proximal to the manometrically defined LES. The acid-clearing test measures the efficiency of the esophagus to clear instilled hydrochloric acid by dry swallowing. The acid perfusion test is a means of reproducing esophageal pain to differentiate the pain from other causes. Radiography and endoscopy provide no direct assessment of esophageal function. Both relaxation and contraction of the LES are due to vagal transmission. Stimulation of alpha-adrenergic nerve receptors causes the LES to contract, and stimulation of beta-adrenergic nerve receptors causes it to relax. Many hormones including gastrin, vasopressin, and glucagon increase LES, while secretin and cholecystokinin decrease the LES.

FUNCTIONAL DISTURBANCES

ACHALASIA This is a condition in which peristalsis is absent from the body of the esophagus and the inferior esophageal sphincter fails to relax in response to swallowing. There is absence or degeneration of the ganglion cells, or Auerbach's plexus, in the esophagus of many patients with this disease.

Clinical Manifestations It occurs with equal frequency in men and women, most frequently between the ages of 30 and 50. The most constant symptom is the obstruction to swallowing, which at first may be intermittent but later becomes persistent. Regurgitation of ingested food and liquid is a common symptom; pain is rare. Carcinoma of the esophagus occurs 7 times more often in these patients than in the general population. The classic radiographic signs are dilatation of the esophagus, with the lower portion projecting into a distal narrow segment. Manometry demonstrates that pressure in the body of the esophagus is higher than normal and the LES fails to relax after swallowing.

Treatment Mechanical pneumatic and hydrostatic dilatation have been said to be successful in about 60% of cases. Operative intervention is generally more popular. The procedure involves an incision through the muscle layers of the distal esophagus. Mucosa is exposed to completely free the distal esophageal segment of its circular musculature, but the incision is extended onto the stomach for only a short distance. 85% of patients have excellent results. Some surgeons have routinely included an antireflux procedure. Rarely is it necessary to perform an esophagogastrectomy.

DIFFUSE SPASM   Clinical Manifestations Pain may be provoked by eating or occur spontaneously. Radiographic abnormalities are uncommon, but a small diaphragmatic hernia may be present. Manometric studies may demonstrate hypertension or hypercontraction of the LES.

Treatment If a hypertensive LES is demonstrated, myotomy should be carried out as for achalasia. Surgical repair of the associated diaphragmatic hernia should be performed. Approximately 75% of patients benefit from operation.

Gastroesophageal Reflux

This is caused by loss of gastroesophageal competence. The majority of patients have associated sliding esophageal hiatal hernia. Scleroderma is the most common systemic disease that causes associated motor failure of the distal esophagus. Other causes include poorly executed myotomies and resections of the esophagogastric junction.

Heartburn is a classic symptom and is described as a substernal distress occurring more commonly during the night. Symptoms may be controlled with topical antacids, weight reduction, and sleeping with the head of the bed elevated. If medical therapy fails, fundoplication is indicated.

ESOPHAGITIS AND BLEEDING Endoscopy is required for the diagnosis of esophagitis. When esophagitis becomes severe, patients complain of painful swallowing. Severe esophagitis usually requires an antireflux operation.

STENOSIS OF THE ESOPHAGUS This is caused by chronic recurrent inflammation and occurs in the lower few centimeters of the esophagus. Most stenotic lesions are amenable to dilatation. If symptoms recur or reflux persists, an antireflux operation is indicated.

SHORTENED ESOPHAGUS This is the result of linear contraction of the esophagus due to repeated inflammation. In most instances, operation is indicated and surgical mobilization usually permits the esophagogastric junction to be reduced below the diaphragm and allows an antireflux procedure. If the esophagus is permanently shortened, a Collis gastroplasty to effectively lengthen the esophagus will allow the antireflux procedure.

BARRETT ESOPHAGUS This is where the lower esophagus is lined with columnar epithelium, a consequence of destruction of the normal squamous epithelium by the corrosive effect of gastroesophageal reflux. This abnormal lining may extend to the level of the aortic arch or higher. The risk of adenocarcinoma developing in these patients is greater than in the general population. Operation is recommended to control the reflux, and a standard antireflux procedure usually suffices; there is a difference of opinion, however, and most surgeons do not feel that a prophylactic resection is indicated.

DIAPHRAGMATIC HERNIAS

Developmental Anatomy

Because the diaphragm is formed from the fusion of several components, a number of developmental defects can occur. There are two major types: (1) a complete or partial absence of the diaphragm, in which case there is no hernial sac, and (2) the failure of muscularization, in which case there is a hernial sac. Classification of general diaphragmatic defects would include: (1) absent diaphragm; (2) diaphragmatic hernia, which includes posterolateral (Bochdalek), anterior (Morgagni), and paraesophageal hernias; and (3) eventration.

The two types of esophageal hiatal hernias are the sliding type and the paraesophageal hernia, and occasionally the two are combined. The sliding type is the more common and is caused by axial displacement of the esophagogastric junction through the esophageal hiatus into the chest. In the paraesophageal type, the esophagogastric junction remains in its normal position below the diaphragm but the fundus and other portions of the stomach become translocated into the chest.

SLIDING ESOPHAGEAL HERNIA This accounts for 90% of the esophageal hiatal hernias. It is of clinical significance because of the related gastroesophageal reflux. Current operations for control of this reflux depend on the anatomic repair of the sliding hernia and reduction by 2 cm or more of the tubular distal esophagus below the diaphragm, as well as an anatomic valvuloplasty. The primary goal is the reestablishment of gastroesophageal competence. The names associated with the operation include Nissen, Hill, and Belsey. All are variations of a basic "wrap-around" procedure. The Belsey operation is a transthoracic procedure that creates a segment of intraabdominal esophagus held in place by a buttress of plicated stomach that surrounds approximately 280° of the distal esophagus. It is successful in relieving symptoms in about 85% of cases. The Nissen fundoplication can be performed transabdominally or transthoracically. This operation totally surrounds the distal esophagus with the adjacent gastric fundus. A success rate of 96% results. The Hill operation is a posterior gastropexy performed transabdominally, and it too is associated with a 96% improvement rate. Other surgeons have encouraged the use of Collis gastroplasty with either a Nissen or Belsey fundoplication to ensure positioning of the gastroesophageal junction below the diaphragm. Collis gastroplasty is particularly effective in the case of a shortened esophagus.

PARAESOPHAGEAL HIATAL HERNIAS The pure paraesophageal hiatal hernia is rare, and usually there is a combined sliding and paraesophageal hernia. The most common complication is the chronic recurrent occult gastrointestinal blood loss. The second most common loss is gastric volvulus, which is seen almost exclusively with massive paraesophageal hernias with most or all of the stomach residing in the chest behind the heart. Because of the high incidence of bleeding in the volvulus, surgical repair is generally indicated even in the absence of symptoms or complications in patients with paraesophageal hernias. In the repair, the lower esophageal sphincter function is normal and the esophagogastric junction is not disturbed. The herniated stomach is reduced; the hernial sac is excised and the widened hiatus is narrowed by placing sutures in the crura. In most instances, an antireflux procedure is added.

Posterolateral (Foramen of Bochdalek) Hernia

(See Chapter 39)

Foramen of Morgagni Hernias

These are also called *anterior diaphragmatic, parasternal,* or *retrosternal hernias* and are seen almost exclusively in adults. 70% of the patients are females. 90% of the hernias occur through the diaphragmatic defect in the right peristernal area. Most patients are asymptomatic. Serious complications are rarely encountered, but the patients may have respiratory distress.

Surgical repair is mandatory for most hernias of the foramen of Morgagni. The hernia is reduced, the sac excised, and the defect is closed, usually through a transabdominal approach.

Eventration of the Diaphragm

Complete or partial unilateral elevation of the diaphragm is referred to as *eventration*. There is no localized diaphragmatic defect but rather diffuse localized bulging of the diaphragm itself. Congenital eventration implies an anomalous development of the diaphragm; acquired eventration may be related to paralysis of the phrenic nerve subsequent to disease or injury. Eventration usually occurs on the left side with a male to female ratio of 2:1. Most patients are asymptomatic but in the newborn, serious respiratory difficulties are frequently encountered.

Prompt emergency surgical repair is indicated in the newborn who is dyspneic and cyanotic. In older children and adults in whom symptoms are disabling, elective surgical repair is indicated and is directed toward restoration of the diaphragm to its normal position. The procedure most frequently used is plication of the diaphragm.

RUPTURE OF THE DIAPHRAGM

This may be caused by either blunt or penetrating injury. Rupture of the left side is 8 times more common.

The diagnosis of traumatic rupture of the diaphragm may be difficult during the early period. Physical findings are nonspecific. Herniation of viscera into the thorax can result in compression of lung parenchyma with interference of alveolar ventilation. With extensive herniation, mediastinal displacement of the contralateral side may interfere with venous return to the heart, and cardiac function may be suppressed by visceral herniation into the pericardial sac.

Any injury involving the area from the fourth intercostal space to the level of the umbilicus should be considered as potentially involving the diaphragm. Careful evaluation of the chest x-ray is crucial. Even in the absence of other operative indications, acute diaphragmatic disruption should be promptly repaired. Abdominal exploration is mandatory in these patients. Upper gastrointestinal contrast studies should be done before discharge. Results of repair of diaphragmatic disruptions are almost universally favorable. Late repair of diaphragmatic hernias is preferably performed through a thoracotomy to permit lysis of adhesions.

DIVERTICULA

Diverticula of the esophagus are acquired lesions resulting from protrusion of the mucosa through a defect in the esophageal musculature (known as *pulsion diverticula*) or from the traction effect of adjacent chronically inflamed granulomatous parabronchial lymph nodes (known as *traction diverticula*).

Pharyngoesophageal Diverticulum

This is the most common diverticulum of the esophagus and arises at the pharyngoesophageal junction. It is located posteriorly in the midline, protruding between the oblique fibers of the inferior pharyngeal constrictors just above the transverse fibers of the cricopharyngeus. It is known as a *Zenker's diverticulum*. It usually occurs after the age of 50.

A sensation of high cervical obstruction to swallowing is the most common symptom. The patients complain of a gurgling sound in their throats when drinking and of the regurgitation of undigested portions of recent meals, often associated with an offensive odor. In extreme cases, malnutrition, hoarseness, and suppurative lung disease may occur. Carcinoma may develop in a chronically neglected diverticulum. The diagnosis is established by radiographic examination of the esophagus. Esophagoscopy is not necessary.

Symptomatic diverticula should be repaired. This is accomplished by a one-stage diverticulectomy through a cervical incision. Some have advised the routine performance of a myotomy in association with the repair, but this has not brought significant improvement in the overall results. Myotomy alone can provide an effective means of dealing with smaller diverticula.

Epiphrenic Diverticula

This usually occurs within 10 cm of the cardia, but may be at higher levels in the thorax. The majority are asymptomatic and do not pose a surgical problem. Symptoms, when present, are those of esophageal obstruction, retention, and regurgitation. Diagnosis is established radiographically. Esophagoscopy is not required. Studies of esophageal motility are essential in planning surgical management of epiphrenic diverticula.

The procedure is performed transthoracically and consists of excision of the diverticulum accompanied by extramucosal esophagomyotomy. If there is an associated diaphragmatic hernia, an antireflux procedure is performed.

Parabronchial or Midesophageal Diverticulum

These are caused by granulomatous infections of mediastinal lymph nodes and are traction diverticula. Generally, they produce no esophageal symptoms and require no treatment. Rarely, obstruction esophagitis, hemorrhage, perforation, or empyema will occur, and in that circumstance treatment is mandated.

BENIGN CYSTS AND TUMORS

These account for less than 10% of esophageal neoplasms. Leiomyomas are the most common benign tumors. Most occur in the lower half of the esophagus, are extramucosal, and can be treated by simple enucleation. Cysts are the second most common benign tumors and in children cause symptoms by compression of the adjacent esophagus or tracheobronchial tree. Most can be removed successfully by enucleation. Some pedunculated benign tumors have produced esophageal defects.

MALIGNANT TUMORS

Carcinoma of the esophagus is predominately a disease of males between the ages of 50 and 70. There is a notably high incidence in Japan, Scotland, and Russia, and among the South African Bantu. Dietary and alcoholic habits, as well as tobacco use, have been implicated. A particularly high incidence has been noted in patients with achalasia and corrosive esophagitis. Other conditions associated with a high incidence include lye burns, diverticula, and the Barrett's esophagus.

Pathology   Nearly all malignant tumors arising in the body of the esophagus are squamous cell carcinomas; most of those involving the esophagogastric junction are adenocarcinomas of gastric origin. Almost as many tumors affect the cardia as affect the entire cervical and thoracic zones. Other malignant tumors are rare and include sarcomas and melanomas.

The tumors spread via lymphatic channels, direct extension, and vascular invasion. Tumors of the cervical esophagus disseminate to the cervical nodes, particularly the anterior jugular and supraclavicular regions. Those arising in the thoracic esophagus spread to peritracheal and esophageal glands as well as supraclavicular and subdiaphragmatic nodes. Lesions of the gastroesophageal junctions spread most frequently to the celiac axis. Neoplasms of the esophagus can metastasize to the liver, lung, or bone. Several Oriental studies have clearly defined a premalignant epithelial change

TABLE 24-1. Postsurgical TNM Classification for Esophageal Carcinoma

T Classification
    T0 = no evidence of tumor
    T1 = tumor invasion of the mucosa or
           submucosa but not the muscle wall
    T2 = tumor invasion of the muscle wall
    T3 = tumor invasion beyond the muscle wall

N Classification
    N0 = no lymph-node metastasis
    N1 = unilateral regional lymph-node metastasis
    N2 = bilateral regional lymph-node metastasis
    N3 = extensive multiple regional lymph-node metastasis

M Classification
    M0 = no evidence of distant metastasis
    M1 = distant metastasis present

with atypia progressing into in situ carcinoma. This evolution takes about 3 years. Routine screening tests with esophageal brushing have led to earlier diagnosis, excision, and improved survival rate.

Clinical Manifestations The earliest and most constant symptom is progressive dysphagia. As obstruction progresses, aspiration pneumonitis may occur. Occult anemia is common. Radiographic studies are highly suggestive. Esophagoscopy is required in all cases to establish a tissue diagnosis by biopsy. Cytologic study of smears is a valuable diagnostic adjunct. A postsurgical staging for esophageal carcinoma has been established (see Table 24-1). Surgical excision is associated with the highest survival rate that is clearly stage-dependent. Most patients present with advanced (stage III) disease. The 5-year survival following surgical excision with stage I neoplasm is about 85%, stage II neoplasm 35%, and stage III 15%. The overall survival rate in one series is approximately 23%, but the more frequently reported figure is 10%. Recently, a combination of chemotherapy and pre- and postoperative radiation therapy with resection has increased the survival of patients with stages II and III disease.

In most cases, the operation consists of resection of almost all the esophagus with anastomosis of the stomach and the thoracic esophagus. This is carried out by a combined abdominal and right thoracic approach freeing the stomach so that its vasculature is based on the right gastric and right gastroepiploic vessel. Since vagotomy necessarily accompanies resection, a pyloroplasty is generally performed, but some surgeons have indicated that with cervical or high thoracic anastomosis and the stomach acting as a conduit rather than a reservoir, pyloroplasty may increase the incidence of reflux. If the stomach does not reach for a proximal anastomosis, interposition can be performed.

There are two additional approaches. In one, the resection is extended widely to include all paraesophageal nodes. The second approach is to perform the esophagectomy blindly using incisions only in the neck and the abdomen and bringing the gastric pedicle up in a substernal position without entering the chest through a separate incision.

In the case of advanced lesions, resection or bypass has provided optimal palliation; over 85% the patients are able to eat, and aspiration is minimized.

Squamous carcinoma of the esophagus is radiosensitive, while adenocarcinoma of the gastroesophagel junction is less sensitive. The overall 5-year survival following therapy with 5000–6000 rad is approximately 6%. Palliative low-dose radiotherapy may alleviate pain and dysphagia. Advanced nonresectable lesions have been treated by laser therapy to provide a conduit for liquids and allow the patient to swallow saliva.

Chemotherapy itself has little demonstrable effect.

ESOPHAGEAL PERFORATION

Most esophageal perforations are caused by instrumentation. Others are caused by accidental ingestion of foreign bodies or the strain of emesis. Infrequently the esophagus may be perforated as a result of either penetrating or nonpenetrating trauma. The most common site of perforation associated with instrumentation is at the esophageal introitus. The second most common site for instrumental perforation is the lower esophagus immediately above the area that it enters through the diaphragmatic hiatus. Postemetic perforation (Boerhaave syndrome) usually occurs in the distal portion of the esophagus. Perforations of the cervical or upper thoracic esophagus enter the pretracheal space and communicate with the mediastinum. Perforations of the lower third of the esophagus are generally into the left pleural space.

Clinical Manifestations　　Perforations of the upper esophagus may be suggested by temperature elevation, pain, and cervical crepitus. There is usually no tenderness. Perforation of the lower esophagus and subphrenic esophageal perforation are associated with cardiorespiratory embarrassment, shock, cyanosis, and abdominal pain.

Radiographic studies are of great assistance in demonstrating mediastinal air associated with cervical perforation or air fluid levels in the pleural space. Studies with opaque medium are indicated to localize the site of perforation. Endoscopic procedures are rarely indicated.

Treatment   Most perforations of the esophagus are best treated by immediate surgical exploration, repair, and drainage. Esophageal leaks that are confined to the upper mediastinum without pleural contamination will resolve with antibiotics and parenteral alimentation. Cervical esophageal perforations that are diagnosed earlier are best treated by repair and drainage. Instrumental and other perforations of the thoracic and subphrenic parts of the esophagus require surgical exploration, repair, and drainage.

CORROSIVE ESOPHAGITIS   (See also Chapter 39)

The ingestion of strong acids or alkalis causes a severe inflammatory reaction of the mucosa, known as *corrosive esophagitis*. Edema and congestion of the submucosal layer are associated with inflammation of the thrombosis of the vessels. This is followed by sloughing of the superficial layers with varying degrees of liquefaction and necrosis of the muscularis followed by fibrosis and delayed reepithelialization. In severe cases the entire mucous membrane may slough and esophageal stricture develops. Full-thickness esophageal and gastric necrosis may occur.

Clinical Manifestations   During the acute phase, pain associated with the burn is noted, as is hoarseness, stridor, and evidence of laryngeal edema. Painful dysphagia is prominent.

Treatment   Early esophagoscopy to define the extent of injury is indicated. The immediate treatment is directed toward management of airway obstruction, administration of intravenous fluids and antibiotics, and discontinuance of oral intake. As soon as the patients can swallow their saliva they are instructed to swallow a thread as a guide for subsequent endoscopy and dilatation. Dilatation is not carried out until the acute inflammation has subsided. Once there is evidence of stricture, dilation by Bouginage over the swallowed thread can be started. If repeat dilatation cannot maintain a satisfactory lumen, a reconstructive operative procedure is indicated. This can be accomplished with colon bypass or by a free transfer of autogenous jejunum with microvascular anastomosis.

MALLORY-WEISS SYNDROME

This consists of a tear of the esophageal mucosa at the esophagogastric junction, usually related to the retching and vomiting associated with alcoholism. A patient presents with upper gastrointestinal bleeding. It will usually cease with conservative management or endoscopic cauterization; rarely does the bleeding require surgical control.

25 STOMACH

ANATOMY

Functional Relationships The *fundus* is located in the upper abdomen, is thin walled and freely distensible, and stores and partially digests food. The *antrum* is thick-walled, distal portion of the stomach; it mixes and grinds food, then releases it slowly through the pyloric sphincter. The *pancreas* is dorsal (inflammation delays gastric emptying, masses cause satiety). The *liver* is right and ventral, while the *spleen* is directly left lateral. Enlargement of either also interferes with gastric capacity. Likewise, gastric disease (peptic ulceration) may affect adjacent organs. The *biliary tree* runs posterior to the duodenum.

Blood Supply and Lymphatics There are four major nutrient arteries (right/left gastric, right/left gastroepiploic) and extensive submocosal arteriole plexus. See Fig. 25-1 for complete details. The stomach can survive on only one major artery. Lymphatic drainage follows the vascular supply.

Innervation Major autonomic supply is vagal. The hepatic branch arises from the left anterior vagus, the celiac branch from the right posterior vagus. Each main vagus terminates in a *nerve of Laterjet,* which gives off small branches to the lesser curvature (secretory innervation to parietal cells).The distal-most branches are the "crow's foot," innervating the motor activity of the antrum. Splanchnic (sympathetic) branches follow arteries and modulate blood flow and muscular function.

Morphology External serosa, outer longitudinal, middle circular, inner oblique smooth muscle, then submucosa, muscularis mucosa and mucosa. Small submucosal arterioles feed rich mucosal capillary network.

Fundic Mucosa. (Proximal two-thirds), comprised of deep glands that open into pits. Glands have surface epithelial (protect surface with mucous, alkaline secretions), mucous neck (line glands), progenitor, chief (secrete pepsinogen), parietal (secrete HCl) and endocrine cells (serotonin).

Antral Mucosa. (Distal one-third), surface epithelial, mucous neck and G cells (produce gastrin).

Sphincters. Lower esophageal sphincter (LES), distal 5 cm

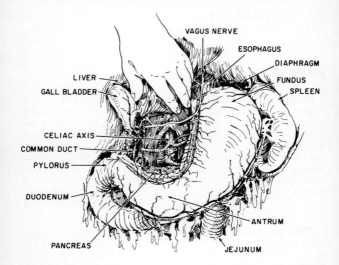

Fig. 25-1   Position of the stomach relative to the other principal organs of the upper abdomen.

of esophagus/stomach junction. Relaxes with swallowing, then contracts to prevent reflux of gastric contents. *Pyloric sphincter*, minimizes duodenogastric reflux, meters movement of food into duodenum, rejects particles > 2 mm.

PHYSIOLOGY

Storage   Stores food for up to 4 h. *Receptive relaxation*, muscular relaxation with ingestion. Solid food settles on greater curvature, liquids pass freely along lesser curvature. The antrum grinds and recirculates food. Pylorus regulates emptying.

Digestion   Salivary amylase acts on starches, only in center of gastric bolus (remains alkaline). Peptic digestion reduces size of meat particles. Gastric lipase assists with early fat digestion.

Gastric Acid Secretion   Interdigestive acid production 2–3 meq/h (BAO = basal acid output). Sight and smell of food stimulate acid, pepsinogen secretion (cephalic phase). Response is vagally mediated, also enhances action of gastrin.

Gastrin, elaborated by G cells in response to gastric distention and vagal stimulation. Gastrin in turn stimulates acid secretion from parietal cells. Luminal acid then suppresses gastrin secretion (negative feedback). Acidification of duodenum causes *secretin* release, which inhibits gastrin and acid production and stimulates pancreatic bicarbonate release. Duodenum and upper jejunum also secrete small amounts of gastrin.

Parietal Cell Function Secretes HCl. Occurs via H^+/K^+ exchange pump, which requires ATP. Acetylcholine (vagal release), gastrin and histamine stimulate. Cimetidine (H_2 blocker), omeprazole (H^+/K^+-ATPase inhibitor), prostaglandins inhibit acid secretion. Vagotomy profoundly diminishes response to gastrin and histamine; however, anticholinergics only partially inhibit.

Surface Cell Function Impervious to H^+. Secrete protective layer of mucus and bicarbonate.

Gastric Analysis Saline lavages before/after histalogue or pentagastrin. Maximal acid output (MAO), 10 to 15 meq/h, BAO, 2–3 meq/h. Duodenal ulcer patients may have higher values; gastric ulcer patients may have lower values. However, significant overlap exists. Zollinger-Ellison (ZE) syndrome shows high BAO with BAO/MAO ≥ 0.6.

Gastric Emptying Meal anticipation causes vagal gastrin release, acid secretion and together with ingestion, receptive relaxation, antral contractions and relaxation of pylorus. Liquids empty continuously, rate dependent on osmolarity. Solids reduced into millimeter-size particles, then traverse pylorus. Osmolality of chyme is diluted by recirculation, prevents dumping. Fats empty slowest. The *gastric pacemaker* is on the greater curvature, action potentials travel toward pylorus. Gastric emptying may be assessed with saline instillation, barium radiographs, bimodal radiolabeled meals. With 750 mL saline instillation, < 200 mL should be left by 30 min.

Other Gastric Function *Instrinsic factor* produced by parietal cell, essential for ileal B_{12} absorption. Gastric acid helps maintain foregut sterility. Gastric mucosa may participate in immunosurveillance and disposal of toxic substances. The stomach also rapidly warms (or cools) ingested contents.

GASTRIC DYSFUNCTION

SYMPTOMS Anorexia Lack of appetite, frequently associated with physiologic stress. Common cause of weight loss with GI neoplasms.

Nausea and vomiting   See Chapter 23.

Pain   Gastric mucosa devoid of pain endings. Gastritis, neoplasms, distention, and even gastric ulcers are relatively painless. Duodenal disease (i.e., ulceration), has characteristic pain patterns: gnawing, midepigastric pain, relieved when acid is buffered (meals, antacids), worse with unopposed acid (early morning). Gastric ulcers have subtle, diffuse pain during or after meals.

Reflux   Gastric contents into esophagus. May cause (1) heartburn, (2) expectoration of chyme, and (3) cough from aspiration. Caused by loss of LES pressure zone. Vagal tone, intraabdominal pressure, drugs, and GI hormones may influence LES pressure.

SIGNS   Bleeding   *Hematemesis* is the vomiting of blood. *Coffee-ground emesis* reflects slow bleeding (acid-hematin), bright-red emesis implies rapid bleeding (varix, ulcer, tears). Stools are usually black (melena) but may be red with rapid bleeds.

Weight Loss   Neoplasia, gastric ulcer usually cause weight loss. Duodenal ulcer is associated with weight *gain*, food neutralizes acid, relieving DU pain.

Gastric Distention   Produces autonomic mediated pallor, tachypnea, bradycardia, and hypotension. Diagnosed by inspection/percussion.

Tenderness   Duodenal ulcers may have associated deep midepigastric tenderness. Gastric ulcers and neoplasms are usually nontender. Perforated ulcers cause generalized peritonitis.

Masses   Distal gastric neoplasms may show anterior, moveable masses. Pancreatic masses are fixed, liver masses descend with inspiration.

DIAGNOSTIC STUDIES   Radiography   Barium studies miss some duodenal lesions and superficial gastric erosions.

Endoscopy   Essential for hemorrhage, gastric ulceration, most duodenal ulceration. Lesions may be biopsied.

POSTGASTRECTOMY SYNDROMES   Procedures that destroy or bypass the pylorus may cause a wide range of disturbances. 20% of patients have transient symptoms; 5% have permanent, nondisabling symptoms; but 1% may become "gastric cripples." Therefore, lesser, pyloric sparing procedures (i.e, parietal cell vagotomy) are being used more frequently.

Dumping Syndrome   Related to ingestion of carbohydrates after pyloric ablation. Characterized by light-headedness, palpitations, cramps, and diarrhea.

Small-Capacity Syndrome Associated with extensive resections.

Postvagotomy Syndrome May cause explosive diarrhea unrelated to meals and gallstones. Mostly with truncal vagotomy, least with parietal cell vagotomy.

Bile Gastritis Erosive gastritis with reflux of bile through incompetent or bypassed pylorus. Low-grade pain, nausea, bilious vomiting. Roux en Y diversion may relieve.

Afferent Loop Syndrome Severe postprandial pain relieved by massive bilious vomiting. From obstruction at junction of afferent limb and gastric remnant.

Other Conditions Acid-reducing procedures may lead to anemia, and there is a question of gastric remnant cancer due to the resulting achlorhydria. Diarrhea may be due to dumping, postvagotomy syndrome.

ULCER DISEASE

Duodenal Peptic Ulceration

Pathophysiology *"No acid, no ulcer"*; however, hypersecretion of acid may not necessarily accompany peptic ulcer disease. Etiology includes gastric acid, pepsin, and duodenal factors (reduction in alkaline secretions, bile, pancreatic juice, hydrogen exchange in duodenal epithelium). Excess, unbalanced acid or prolonged duodenal acidification (pH < 2) may be causative. Severe hyperchlorhydria (ZE syndrome/gastrinoma) has severe ulcer disease, while standard ulcers usually heal with acid neutralization. Surgical therapy thus aims to maximally reduce acid production.

Clinical Manifestations Usually midadult life, male-to-female ratio is 4:1, type A personalities may be high risk, especially with EtOH and tobacco abuse. Genetic factors [multiple endocrine neoplasia (MEN) syndrome] also play a role. *Abdominal pain*, most common feature, gnawing or sharp midepigastric pain, relieved by foods or antacids. May be episodic. Associated back pain may imply posterior penetration into pancreas. Generalized pain implies perforation. *Bleeding* commonly occurs. Massive hemorrhage from posterior bulb ulcerations with erosion into gastroduodenal artery. Most, however, present with minor bleeding and heme-positive or melenic stools. *Obstruction* occurs with pylorospasm or stricture from chronic inflammation. Causes protracted nonbilious vomiting of undigested food, malnutrition, metabolic alkalosis. Treatment is almost always surgical. *Perforation* is usually seen with anterior bulbar ulcers and usually seals with omentum or viscera. 5% have free perforation with generalized periotonitis, fever, dehydration, and free air. This is a true surgical emergency.

Zollinger-Ellison Syndrome Hypergastrinemia and severe peptic ulceration from a gastrinoma. BAO is markedly elevated, gastrin may be > 1000 pg/mL. Equivocal gastrin levels may be stimulated with intravenous calcium or secretin. Gastrinomas are neoplasms, overwhelmingly malignant (≥90%), but slow growing.

Diagnosis Careful history and physical. Relationship to meals, sleeping, antacids. Quality and location of pain. Bleeding, stool heme. Upper GI series, endoscopy, upright chest x-ray for perforation (free air under diaphragm).

Treatment *Nonoperative Therapy.* Typically a 6-week course of the H_2 blocker (cimetidine, ranitidine) and frequent antacids. Reexamine upper GI tract at end of period to document healing.

Operative Therapy. Two main tenants: (1) Correct or prevent life-threatening complications—obstruction, perforation, massive hemorrhage, and (2) cure chronic ulcer disease refractory to nonoperative therapy and prevent recurrence. *Perforation* requires closure of the duodenal opening with an omental patch (Graham patch). This may be accompanied by a definitive acid-reducing procedure [parietal cell vagotomy (PCV)] or by truncal vagotomy, ulcer excision, and pyloroplasty. *Obstruction* is usually treated by resection and gastroenterostomy. *Hemorrhage* requires urgent intervention if massive or unremitting. Technically, the bleeding posterior bulbar duodenal ulcer is undersewn with heavy silk and ulcer diathesis is treated with pyloroplasty or antrectomy and truncal vagotomy. Slower chronic bleeding is treated as recalcitrant ulcer disease. *Chronic persistent disease,* especially with failure or noncompliance with nonoperative therapy, is treated with an acid-reducing procedure with or without drainage/resection. Most recently, *parietal cell vagotomy (PCV)* has shown promise in acceptable recurrence rates with very low morbidity (spares antral pump and thus drainage procedure not required). See Table 25-1. If performed, truncal vagotomy must always be accompanied by a drainage procedure because of denervation of the antral pump and gastric stasis. Resective therapy should be reserved

TABLE 25-1. Results of Operations for Duodenal Ulcer

	Mortality	Morbidity	Recurrence
Partial gastrectomy	3%	10%	5%
Vagotomy and antrectomy	3%	12%	1%
Vagotomy and drainage	1%	15%	10%
Proximal gastric vagotomy	0.5%	5%	15%

for high-risk patients and those with hypergastrinemia. *Zollinger-Ellison syndrome* requires special considerations. If medically uncontrollable on massive doses of H_2 blockers, PCV may be a useful adjunct. A careful search for the gastrinoma must also be made. With unresectable disease, strictures, or unremitting disease, total gastrectomy (not partial) and esophagojejunostomy is the operation of choice.

Stomach Peptic Ulceration

ACUTE EROSIVE GASTRITIS   Most common cause of upper GI bleeding. Accompanies severe, stressful illnesses.

Pathogenesis   Includes acid secretion, back-diffuse of H^+ ions, and submucosal buffers. May be initiated by a disruption in the H^+ barrier. Aspirin, EtOH, or bile salts may contribute.

Diagnosis   Painless UGI bleeding implies acute erosive gastritis. Endoscopy is critical; barium studies are not useful.

Therapy   Directed at (1) repletion of losses from bleeding, (2) gastric rest with lavage of retained blood and clots, 80% will stop bleeding spontaneously, and (3) neutralizing gastric acid with H_2 blockers and antacid pH titration to > 5. Other adjuncts include transendoscopic cautery, pitressin, or intraarterial embolization. Persistent bleeding (> 4–6 units, massive exsanguination), requires operation with gastrotomy and oversewing of bleeding sites accompanied by vagotomy and pyloroplasty. Gastrectomy may be needed if all other therapies fail.

Prevention   Inhibition of acid secretion with acid neutralization by titration in stressed patients is critical. Prostaglandins may be useful.

CHRONIC GASTRIC ULCERATION   Shares common clinical features with malignant disease. *All chronic gastric ulcers require biopsy* via endoscopy.

Pathogenesis   Unclear. Age > 40, F:M ratio, 2:1, drug ingestion (ASA, NSAIDs), and malnutrition have been implicated. Breakdown of mucosal cation barrier. Ulceration occurs within gastric cancer.

Symptoms Anorexia, vague postprandial epigastric discomfort, weight loss. (Exception: pyloric channel ulcers behave like duodenal ulcers.) Massive hemorrhage unusual, chronic slow blood loss with melena or heme-positive stools is common.

Diagnosis Upper GI radiography very useful; this complements endoscopy. Endoscopy with biopsy is essential. Benign lesions appear "punched out," while malignant ulcers have irregular "heaped-up" margins.

Therapy Initially, nonoperative trial of antacids and H_2 blockers. Dietary manipulation, drug avoidance (EtOH, ASA, NSAIDs). Other agents such as sucralfate may be helpful. Operative therapy is for malignant or nonhealing ulcer disease, bleeding, perforation, or obstruction (rare). Resective procedures (vagotomy and antrectomy) are frequently used. Local excision with an acid-reducing/drainage procedure may also be efficacious. Prepyloric and pyloric channel ulcers should be treated as duodenal ulcers.

Gastric Neoplasia

MALIGNANT TUMORS Most gastric neoplasms are malignant. Adenocarcinoma is 95%, lymphoma 4%, and leiomyosarcoma 1%. Highest incidence is in Chile, Japan, Iceland. USA has rapid decline in rate. High-risk groups include family history, pernicious anemia, and, questionably, postgastrectomy remnants. Early detection is critical.

Signs and Symptoms Anorexia, weight loss (> 95%). Symptoms usually occur late. Slow bleeding → hemorrhage. Nausea, vomiting, dysphagia. Pain infrequent and late. Exam reveals a mass (50%), but tenderness is rare. Hepatomegaly (liver metastasis), ovarian involvement (Krukenberg tumor), and pelvic seeding (Bloomer's shelf) may be detected. Advanced malignancy may show an involved left supraclavicular node (Virchow's node).

Pathologic Features Types: (1) superficial spreading, most favorable prognosis, does not penetrate through muscularis mucosa, no ulceration. Early detection has 75% 10-year survival. Detected only by endoscopy/screening. Infiltrating carcinoma may be (2) polypoid, (3) a bulky, ulcerated mass, or (4) *linitis plastica,* extensive wall infiltration without ulceration giving a "leather-bottle" appearance to UGI series. Spread may be via lymphatics, hematogenous, peritoneal seeding or by direct extension. ≥50% have tumor spread at time of diagnosis.

Therapy Primarily surgical. Subtotal gastrectomy, even if palliative, is useful except in most severe circumstances. Include gastrocolic omentum, proximal duodenum. Reestablish continuity via gastrojejunostomy. Adjuvant therapy, especially for recurrence, is poor. Overall 5-year survival is < 10%.

Other Gastric Malignancies

LYMPHOMA/LYMPHOSARCOMA May be isolated or from widespread disease. Thickened rugal folds. Anorexia, weight loss, early satiety common. Diagnosis made by biopsy. May be treated by radiation therapy alone. Survival may approach 85% 5-year.

LEIOMYOSARCOMA Least common. Smooth muscle malignancy. Hemorrhage common. Resection is preferred treatment.

BENIGN GASTRIC NEOPLASMS **Polyps** Most common benign tumors of stomach. (1) Adenomatous polyps occur with pernicious anemia, Peutz-Jeghers, and Gardner. These do have a malignant potential and should be biopsied via endoscopy with snare. Malignant polyps are treated as gastric adenocarcinoma. (2) Inflammatory polyps are sessile and asymptomatic, and may be seen with hypertrophic gastritis (Menetrier's disease) or multiple inflammatory gastric polyps. They must be biopsied but do not require formal resection.

Leiomyomas Common smooth muscle benign neoplasms. At ≥ 4 cm they ulcerate and may have massive hemorrhage, requiring emergent operative with formal resection. Small lesions may be wedged or shelled out.

Miscellaneous Lesions Submucosal lipomas are detected radiographically and are of little consequence. Ectopic pancreas may present as a mucosal dimple.

Other Gastric Pathology

HYPERTROPHIC GASTRITIS (MENETRIER'S DISEASE) Rare gastric epithelial inflammation with massive gastric folds and eventually multiple polyps. There is submucosal edema with inflammatory cells and glandular hypertrophy. Plasma proteins may be lost through this epithelium. Rarely, kwashior-kor may develop. Initially managed nutritionally.

MALLORY-WEISS TEAR   Gastric mucosal disruption at EG junction following violent retching. Massive bleeding in only 10%. Confirm by endoscopy. Operation uncommonly indicated. Massive hemorrhage may require operation with high gastrotomy and deep oversewing without acid reduction.

MISCELLANEOUS CONDITIONS   *Acute gastric dilatation* is followed by vasovagal symptoms. Usually occurs intra- or postoperatively. *Gastric volvulus* is uncommon and associated with paraesophageal hiatal hernia. Gangrene and perforation will develop. *Foreign bodies* occur in children, and sharp objects should be endoscopically retrieved. *Bezoars* are nondigestible conglomerates that occur in postgastrectomy patients. Treatment is with papain or endoscopic fragmentation. *Atrophic gastritis,* or *pernicious anemia,* shows parietal cell loss, achlorhydria, and loss of intrinsic factor, and subsequently B_{12} depletion. There is high risk for malignancy. Last, *corrosive gastritis* may be caused by caustic ingestion (alkali cause esophageal strictures), and strong acid may lead to gastric perforation.

TREATMENT OF MORBID OBESITY

Weight twice or more than ideal. Ultimately hypertension, NIDDM, arthritis, gallstones, and cardiopulmonary dysfunction develop. Almost always refractory to medical therapy. Previously, jejunoileal bypass was successful, but complications (malabsorption, liver disease, renal calculi) have led to its abandonment. Currently, operations aim to limit daily intake to $\leq$ 800 kcal. Gastric bypass with a Roux en Y jejunal limb to a 60-mL gastric pouch has been successful. Alternatively, gastric partitioning (vertical banded gastroplasty) is also used. Results show 50% loss of excess weight in 75% of patients.

ANATOMY

Duodenum 20 cm, jejunum 100–110 cm, ileum 150–160 cm. Jejunoileum extends from *ligament of Treitz* (peritoneal fold at duodenojejunal junction) to ileocecal valve. Jejunum is larger, thicker than ileum and has only one to two vascular arcades versus four to five in the ileum. Small bowel is tethered by the *mesentery*, which carries vascular and lymphatic supply. Mesentery travels obliquely from left of L2 to right S1 joint; it is usually very mobile. Blood supply to jejunum, ileum is via superior mesenteric artery, which also continues supply until proximal transverse colon. Vascular arcades in mesentery provide collateral supply. Venous drainage parallels arterial supply, leading to superior mesenteric vein, joins splenic vein behind pancreas to form portal vein. Lymphatic drainage from bowel wall (lacteals), through mesenteric nodes, to superior mesenteric nodes, into cisterna chyli, and finally to thoracic duct. Mucosal folds form circumferential transverse *plicae circulares*. Innervation is parasympathetic (vagus, celiac ganglia) and affects secretion and motility. Sympathetics come from splanchnic nerves via celiac plexus, affect secretion and bowel and vascular motility, and carry pain afferents.

Histology

Serosa Outermost, visceral peritoneum, encircles jejunum, ileum, only anterior duodenum.

Muscularis Thin outer longitudinal, thick inner circular smooth muscle. *Auerbach's plexus* lies between layers.

Submucosa Fibroelastic connective tissue with vessels, nerves (*Meissner's plexus*), and lymphatics. *Strongest component of bowel wall*.

Mucosa Transvere folds with finger-like villi. Cells of villi have microvilli (brush border) and glycocalyx fuzz, which increase surface area. Villi largest in duodenum. Mucosa is comprised of three distinct layers.

Muscularis Mucosae. Deepest layer, thin sheet of muscle.

Lamina Propria. Continuous connective tissue layer between muscularis mucosae and epithelium. Contains plasma cells, lymphocytes, eosinophils, macrophages, fibroblasts, and smooth muscle. Serves to support epithelium and act as immunogenic barrier.

Epithelium. One layer of cells covering villi and lining crypts of Lieberkuhn. Crypts contain goblet cells (mucous), enterochromaffin cells (endocrine), Paneth cells (zymogen granules), and basal undifferentiated cells. New cells march up crypt onto villus, takes 3–7 days. Villi have endocrine, goblet, and absorptive cells covered by microvilli, which are covered by glycocalyx fuzz. Absorptive cells contain digestive enzymes and some specific absorption receptors. See Fig. 26-1.

PHYSIOLOGY

Motility

Pace-setter potentials originate in duodenum, initiate contractions, propel food through small bowel via *segmentation* (short segment contraction with to and fro mixing) and *peristalsis* (aboral migration of contraction wave and food bolus). The *MMC* (migrating myoelectric complex) sweeps the entire bowel during fasting. Under neurohumoral control, stimulated by *motilin.* Vagal cholinergics are excitatory, vagal peptidergics are inhibitory. Gastrin, CCK, motilin stimulate muscular activity; secretin, glucagon inhibits.

Digestion and Absorption

Fat Pancreatic lipase hydrolyzes triglycerides, components combine with bile salts to form micelles. Micelle then traverses cell membrane passively by diffusion, then it disaggregates, releasing bile salts back into lumen and fatty acids and monoglycerides into cells. Cell then reforms triglyceride and combines these with cholesterol and phospholipids to form chylomicrons, which exit cells and enter the lacteals. Small fatty acids can enter portal vein directly. Bile salts resorbed into enterohepatic circulation in distal bowel. Of 5-g bile salts, 0.5 g is lost daily.

Protein Gastric acid denatures, pepsin begins proteolysis. Pancreatic proteases (trypsinogen, activated by enterokinase to trypsin, and endopeptidases, exopeptidases), further digest

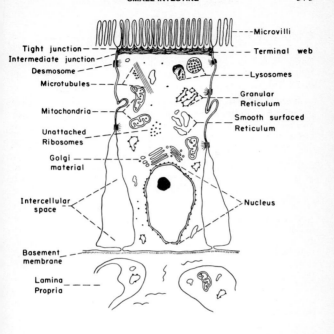

Fig. 26-1 Schematic diagram of an intestinal absorptive cell. [From: Trier JS et al, in Sleisenger MH, Fordtran JS (eds): Gastrointestinal Disease. Pathophysiology, Diagnosis, Management. Philadelphia, Saunders, 1983, chap 48, with permission.]

proteins. Yields amino acids and 2–6 residue peptides. Active transport brings di- and tripeptides into absorptive cells.

Carbohydrate Pancreatic amylase rapidly digests carbohydrates in duodenum. Brush border enzymes complete digestion into hexoses, which are specifically transported into epithelial cells.

Water and Electrolytes Water, bile, gastric, salivary, intestinal fluids are $\approx$ 10 L/day, most of which is absorbed. Water is osmotically and hydrostatically absorbed or may passively diffuse. Sodium, chloride are absorbed by coupling to organic solutes or by active transport. Bicarbonate is absorbed by Na^+/H^+ exchange. Ca^{2+} absorbed via active transport in duodenum, jejunum, facilitated by PTH and vitamin D. K^+ is passive.

Endocrine Function

Small bowel mucosa releases a wealth of hormones into blood (endocrine), via local discharge (paracrine) or as neurotransmitters.

Secretin 27–Amino acid peptide released from small bowel mucosa by acidification or fat. Stimulates pancreatic water and bicarbonate release, which neutralizes gastric acid. Also stimulates bile flow and inhibits gastrin release, gastric acid, and motility.

Cholecystokinin Released by mucosa in response to amino acids and fatty acids. Causes gallbladder contraction with relaxation of sphincter of Oddi and pancreatic enzyme secretion. Also trophic for bowel mucosa and pancreas.

Other Peptides **GIP** released by glucose and fat, stimulates insulin release. Enhances oral vs. intravenous response to glucose load. Others released by small bowel include: VIP, enteroglucagon, motilin (intestinal smooth muscle contraction), bombesin, somatostatin (paracrine inhibitory peptide), PYY.

Immune Function

Mucosa prevents pathogen entrance. Major source of IgA, plasma cells in lamina propria. Lymphocytes in Peyer's patches exposed to antigens migrate to nodes, to bloodstream, then return to redistribute in lamina propria to elaborate specific antibody.

INFLAMMATORY DISEASES

Crohn's Disease

Chronic inflammatory disease of small or large intestine with spontaneous remissions and acute exacerbations. True etiologic agent is unknown. Symptoms included intermittent, sometimes explosive diarrhea associated with meals, weight loss, and abdominal pain. Most common surgical disease of the small intestine. Risk is increased 30 times in siblings and 13 times in first-degree relatives.

Pathology Mucosal and submucosal edema with aphthous ulcers. Progresses to transmural inflammation with intense mononuclear cell infiltration and linear ulcers which may coalesce to form clefts and sinuses, resulting in *cobblestone mucosa*. Wall thickens, becomes edematous. Noncaseating granulomas appear late in bowel wall and nodes. Mesentery becomes thick and short. Fat wraps from mesenteric to antimesenteric border. Scarring and fibrosis occur, narrowing lumen. Typically, involved areas are not contiguous (skip lesions).

Clinical Manifestations   Young adults, abdominal pain (intermittent, crampy), diarrhea (85% of patients), weight loss. Small bowel alone 30%, ileocolitis 55%, colon only 15%. *May involve any enteric mucosa, from mouth to anus.* Anal fissures, fistulas, and perianal abscesses common. Extraabdominal manifestations are arthritis, uveitis, iritis, hepatitis, erythema nodosum, and pyoderma gangrenosum. Stools rarely contain pus, mucus, or blood. Fever in one-third. Patients may present with intestinal obstruction, abscess, enteroenteric or enterocutaneous fistula. Free perforation is rare.

Diagnosis   Enteroclysis (small bowel barium enema) shows nodular contour, luminal narrowing, linear ulcers, sinuses and clefts, cobblestoning. BE may be useful but need to see terminal ileum. *Acute ileitis* is inflammation of the terminal ileum, which can mimic appendicitis but is self-limited and does not lead to Crohn's disease.

Treatment   Patients with obstructive symptoms treated with bowel rest, hyperalimentation, nasogastric decompression, and pulsed steroids. Surgery for complete obstruction (rare) or for chronic high-grade partial obstruction (more common). Nonsurgical treatment for symptoms includes sulfasalazine *(Azulfidine)*, steroids (for acute exacerbations), azathioprine, and 6-mercaptopurine. Surgical therapy is controversial. Appendectomy should be avoided with active appendiceal or cecal disease but is safe in other circumstances. Operation is indicated for complications: obstruction, abscess, fistula, perforation, bleeding, perianal disease, growth retardation. Intraoperatively, only grossly involved intestine should be removed; *wide resections are to be avoided*. Intestinal continuity should be restored whenever possible. Bypass with exclusion is *not* utilized.

Prognosis   Ileal Crohn's increases risk of adenocarcinoma. Surgical therapy is *not* curative. Recurrence at 5, 10, 15, and 25 years is 29, 52, 64, and 84% after surgery. Disease burns out with advancing age, especially > 50.

**TABLE 26-1. Types and Relative Frequency of Small Bowel
Benign Neoplasms**

Neoplasms	Percent
Leiomyomas	17
Lipomas	16
Adenomas	14
Polyps	14
Polyposis, Peutz-Jeghers	3
Hemangiomas	10
Fibromas	10
Neurogenic tumors	5
Fibromyomas	5
Myxomas	2
Lymphangiomas	2
Fibroadenomas	1
Others	1

Tuberculous Enteritis

Rare in Western countries. Mostly secondary infection in
pulmonary TB patients. Ileocecal region involved most often.
May produce: hypertrophic reaction with luminal stenosis,
ulceration, or both. Ulceration produces diarrhea and pain
alternating with constipation. Treatment is with combination
chemotherapy. Surgery reserved for perforation, obstruction,
or hemorrhage.

NEOPLASMS

Primary small bowel neoplasms very rare. Colon is 40 times
small intestine. 75–80% are malignant. Symptoms often
vague: epigastric pain, nausea, vomiting, colic, diarrhea,
bleeding (usually occult). Most common reasons for operation
are obstruction, bleeding, and pain. Benign tumors cause
intussusception in adults; malignant tumors directly obstruct
or kink bowel. Diagnosis is difficult. Endoscopy is useful for
duodenum; rest of bowel requires enteroclysis (small bowel
intubation with barium radiographs).

Benign Neoplasms

Either epithelial or connective tissue origin. Most often
adenomas, leiomyomas, or lipomas. See Table 26-1. Often,
these cause no symptoms unless they cause obstruction by
intussusception; they may also bleed (one-third occult).

Surgery is indicated if the diagnosis is made or suspected. Most often simple segmental resection is employed.

ADENOMA True adenomas, villous adenomas, or Brunner's gland adenomas (hyperplastic duodenal glandular proliferation without malignant potential). 20% in duodenum. Majority asymptomatic. Villous adenomas have 35–55% malignant potential.

LEIOMYOMA Benign, single, smooth muscle lesion. Most commonly present with bleeding.

Peutz-Jeghers Syndrome

Mucocutaneous melanotic pigmentation (circumoral, buccal, palms, soles, perianal) and GI polyps. Simple dominant inheritance. Polyps are multiple jejunal, ileal, and rectal, and are hamartomas. May cause colicky pain from intermittent intussusception. Bleeding may occur. Curative resection usually not possible.

Malignant Neoplasms

Adenocarcinoma (most common), carcinoids, sarcomas, lymphomas. Patients have diarrhea with mucus/tenesmus, obstruction, and chronic blood loss. Usually insidious presentation. Treatment is wide resection, including nodes. Duodenal lesions require pancreaticoduodenectomy. Palliative resections for relief of symptoms/obstruction. Overall survival poor (average 20% 5-year survival). Periampullary carcinoma may have up to 40% 5-year survival.

ADENOCARCINOMA Approximately 50% of small bowel malignancies. Mostly in duodenum and proximal jejunum. 50% of duodenal carcinoma involve the ampulla and are associated with intermittent jaundice. Jejunal lesions are associated with obstruction.

SARCOMAS 20% of small bowel malignancies; leiomyosarcomas most common. May bleed or obstruct.

LYMPHOMA 10–15% of small bowel malignancies. Most common in ileum. May be primary small bowel or part of systemic disease.

CARCINOIDS Arise from enterochromaffin (Kulchitsky) cells. Occur as often as adenocarcinomas of small bowel. Malignant potential is variable. Secrete serotonin and substance P. Carcinoid syndrome (flushing, bronchospasm, diarrhea, vasomotor collapse, hepatomegaly, right heart valvular disease) occurs in <5%. (Some feel that hepatic metastasis must be present before the syndrome will occur.) Most frequently, carcinoids arise in the appendix (46%), ileum (28%), and rectum (17%). Appendiceal tumors metastasize 3% of the time as compared to ileal carcinoids (35% metastatic rate). Of those < 1 cm diameter (75% of GI carcinoids), only 2% metastasize. Gross appearance is yellow or tan round, hard nodule covered with normal mucosa. Symptoms are the carcinoid syndrome (rare) or abdominal pain, obstruction, diarrhea, and weight loss.

Diagnosis Small bowel series, mesenteric arteriorgrams, CT scan are useful. Urine for 5-HIAA with/without penta-gastrin stimulation is used for diagnosis of syndrome.

Treatment Primary carcinoids <1 cm are treated by seg-mental small bowel resection. Larger lesions or lesions with involved nodes require wide bowel excision with inclusion of mesentery. Appendiceal carcinoids <2 cm require only simple appendectomy, ≥ 2 cm should have right hemicolec-tomy. Carcinoid syndrome may be treated by curative or palliative resection, or with long-acting somatostatin.

Prognosis Overall 54%, 75% for local disease, 59% for regional, and 19% for distal spread. Because of indolent nature, debulking and palliative resections are used.

DIVERTICULAR DISEASE

Congenital diverticula are *true*, composed of all layers; acquired ones are *false*, because only mucosa and submucosa protrude through a muscular defect. *Meckel's* and duodenal diverticula are the most common diverticula of the small bowel.

Duodenal Diverticula

10–20% incidence in autopsy series, 90% asymptomatic, <5% require operative intervention. 67–75% found in peri-ampullary region on medial wall. Manifestations may be obstruction, perforation, bleeding. Those associated with the ampulla may produce cholangitis, pancreatitis, and recurrent choledocholithiasis from partial obstruction and stasis or choledochal sphincter dysfunction. Surgical therapy is di-verticulectomy or extended sphincteroplasty for those in-volving the ampulla.

Jejunal and Ileal Diverticula

Less common than in duodenum. Multiple, false diverticula may occur and lead to jejunal pseudoobstruction and dyskinesia. *Meckel's diverticulum* is the most common *true* diverticulum of the GI tract. Congenital, from incomplete closure of omphalomesenteric or vitelline duct. Usually 2–3 ft from ileocecal valve and 1–12 cm long. May have heterotropic gastric mucosa or pancreatic tissue. Overall 2% of population. Complications include intestinal obstruction (via volvulus), bleeding (gastric mucosa produces acid), or acute diverticulitis. Meckel's in a hernia is a *Littre hernia*. Diagnosis is via enteroclysis or ^{99m}Tc-pertechnetate scan. Complications of Meckel's are often confused with acute appendicitis. Asymptomatic Meckel's found incidentally at surgery should *not* be removed.

SMALL BOWEL ULCERATIONS

Most due to drugs (enteric-coated potassium or corticosteroids), vascular disorders, Crohn's disease, syphillis, typhoid fever, TB, lymphoma, gastrinoma, or Meckel's diverticulum. Nonspecific ulcers may be found in the terminal ileum. Treatment is for complications, most often obstruction and bleeding.

FISTULAS

Most often due to surgical trauma. <2% associated with Crohn's disease. Complications include sepsis, fluid and electrolyte imbalances, skin breakdown, and malnutrition. Overall, intestinal fistulas have ≈ 20% mortality, even with TPN. Key to successful management is fluid, electrolyte, and nutritional maintenance with control of sepsis. More proximal fistulas generally have higher output (>500 mL/day) and more severe complications. GI series is essential to identify the anatomical location of the fistula. Treatment includes drainage of fistula or cavity, TPN, bowel rest, skin protection. Somatostatin may be helpful. Factors that prevent spontaneous closure are: high output, distal obstruction, severe disruption in intestinal continuity, inflammation (undrained abscess, active granulomatous disease), foreign body in tract, short tract (<2.5 cm), or epithelialization of the tract. <30% close spontaneously, and most that do close, do so in about 3 weeks.

PNEUMATOSIS CYSTOIDES INTESTINALIS

Uncommon, multiple gas-filled cysts (submucosal, subserosal) in the GI tract. Most often associated with other conditions. Usually does not require surgical therapy.

BLIND LOOP SYNDROME

Bacterial overgrowth in stagnant area of small bowel produces diarrhea, steatorrhea, anemia, weight loss, abdominal pain, vitamin deficiencies (especially B_{12}), and neurologic disorders. Usually secondary to strictures, stenoses, fistulas, blind pouches (postoperative), or diverticula.

SHORT BOWEL SYNDROME

Following emergent massive small bowel resection (volvulus, mesenteric vascular occlusion), short bowel syndrome may arise. Hallmarks are diarrhea, fluid and electrolyte deficiency, and malnutrition. Usually, up to 70% resection can be tolerated if the terminal ileum and ileocecal valve are preserved. Loss of terminal ileum leads to abnormalities of B_{12} and bile salt absorption. Jejunal resection is better tolerated than ileal resection. Following resection, adaptation occurs: villi lengthen, cell number and renewal increase, thus increasing the absorptive surface. Luminal feeding and certain hormones (CCK, secretin, enteroglucagon) appear to be trophic and necessary for adaptation. Adaptation does not occur with TPN alone.

Treatment   Includes: prevention with conservative resection of marginally viable bowel and "second-look" operations to reassess such intestine; early on, treatment is corrective for fluid and electrolyte losses and TPN. Early enteral nutrition is essential. Elemental diets (Vivonex) or polymeric diets (Isocal, Ensure) are useful. Milk products should be avoided. Fat-soluble vitamin supplementation is often needed. B_{12} injections may be used. H_2 blockers may diminish diarrhea from rapid transit. Certain amino acids (glutamine) may specifically aid in adaptation.

INTESTINAL BYPASS

Jejunoileostomy for the treatment of morbid obesity has been completely abandoned. Complications include liver failure, death, cirrhosis, hyperoxaluria, renal calculi, avitaminoses, blind loop syndrome, pancreatitis, and gallstones, among many others. Morbid obesity is now treated with gastric partitioning or gastric bypass. Previously constructed jejunoileal bypass should be taken down and intestinal continuity should be restored if significant metabolic imbalances or hepatic failure exists. There is some early evidence that partial ileal bypass (200 cm) may be useful in refractory hyperlipidemia.

ANATOMY

Structure 3–5 ft long, marked by *tenia coli*—3 strips of longitudinal muscle 120° apart. *Haustrations*—outpouchings.

Arterial Supply Superior mesenteric—right colon to midtransverse colon: (1) ileocolic; (2) right colic; (3) middle colic. Inferior mesenteric—midtransverse colon to superior rectum: (1) left colic; (2) sigmoid branches; (3) superior rectal. Internal iliac—middle and lower rectum: (1) middle rectal; (2) inferior rectal via pudendal.

Venous Drainage Generally follow arteries; superior and inferior veins go to *portal* vein. Middle and inferior veins go to *systemic* system.

Lymphatics From middle rectal up—mesenteric chain. Inferior rectal—internal iliac chain. Anal—inguinal chain.

Innervation Sympathetic and parasympathetic. Major operative concern is in low rectal dissections where injury to pelvis plexus can lead to impotence.

PHYSIOLOGY

Fluid Average uptake 1500 mL/day, but can absorb up to 5000 mL.

Electrolytes *Sodium.* Active transport against a gradient.

Chloride. Active transport with exchange for bicarbonate.

Potassium. Passive absorption and secretion.

Fuels Primarily short-chain fatty acids.

Ammonia and Urea Mostly by-product of protein metabolism. Absorption of ammonia is decreased by acid environment (this is why lactulose is used in hepatic encephalopathy).

Motility Opiates increase muscle tone but decrease propulsion.

Flatus Normally 1000 mL/day is expelled. Hydrogen and methane are primary explosive gases and may be an issue in electrosurgery of unprepared bowel.

Continence Complex series of events. Key points: (1) preservation of puborectalis muscle; (2) maintance of 90° angle of rectum; (3) tonic activity of internal sphincter.

DISEASE STATES

Ulcerative Colitis

Mucosal involvement of large bowel

Clinical Manifestations Bloody stools, diarrhea, crampy abdominal pain—can progress suddenly to toxic megacolon.

Diagnosis Endoscopy—granular, edematous, can have frank ulcerations. *Rectum invariably involved.* Barium enema should *not* be done during acute phase due to risk of perforation. If chronic, barium enema will show foreshortening, "iron-pipe," or fine ulcers. Differential diagnosis—Crohn's infection.

Extraintestinal Manifestations *This disease is a causative factor in colon cancer,* especially after 10 years of activity. Patients must be monitored. Extraintestinal manifestations include primary sclerosing cholangitis, hepatic steatosis progressing to cirrhosis, polyarthritis, erythema nodosum, ocular lesions.

Therapy *Medical Therapy.* Sulfasalazine—broken down to 5-ASA, which is a topical anti-inflammatory. *Steroids* may be useful in acute exacerbations but may be deleterious if toxic megacolon or infection develop.

Surgical Therapy. Should be offered to all patients who would tolerate an anesthetic. *Total proctocolectomy and ileostomy*—"gold standard" removes all disease. Disadvantage—ileostomy may be difficult to maintain. *Colectomy and ileocolorectal anastomosis* preserves continence. *Disadvantage*—frequent bowel movements, leaves mucosa in rectum, which may develop cancer. Ileoanal "pull-through"—advantages of both. Strip the rectal mucosa, but maintain musculature. Pouch of ileum pulled down, and a neorectum created.

Crohn's Colitis

Transmural involvement. Tendency to "skip" areas. Clinical manifestations—similar to ulcerative colitis, however more cramping, fistula drainage.

Perianal involvement is Crohn's disease until proven otherwise.

Diagnosis   Colonoscopy is key although biopsies may be difficult to differentiate from U.C. X-ray studies can show strictures, fistula, and terminal ileal involvement.

Medical Therapy   Brief periods of bowel rest, with parenteral nutrition may be helpful. Steroids give symptomatic relief in acute exacerbations. Full immunosuppression is an option, but secondary malignancies can develop.

Surgical Therapy   Should be limited to complications of the disease—stricture, fistula, hemorrhage. Because this disease recurs, limited resections are in order. For large areas of involvement, total proctocolectomy and ileostomy is appropriate.

The ileoanal pull-through procedure must not be done for Crohn's disease; fistula will form, since the disease is not limited to mucosa.

Diverticular Disease

Actually these are pseudodiverticula, as only mucosa and muscularis layers herniate through the bowel wall at the entry of the nourishing vessels. It is very common in the Western population, increasing in frequency with age. (One-third of patients over 60 have diverticula on barium enema.)

Etiology   Increased intraluminal pressure. Possible bowel dysmotility as evidenced by thickened circular muscle layers. Lack of dietary fiber can lead to a decreased diameter with locally high pressures.

Clinical Manifestations   Majority are asymptomatic. Less commonly present with inflammation, perforation, bleeding, or fistula.

Therapy   *Acute Nonperforated.*   Bowel rest, antibiotics, contrast study after acute phase resolves. Segmental resection if recurrent attacks or stricture. *Exception:* If the first attack is prior to age 50, this signals a virulent form of the disease and should be resected.

Therapeutic Algorithm for Diverticulitis.

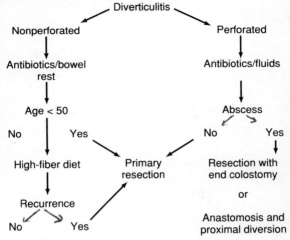

Perforation. Key in therapy is the resection of the disease segment. With limited involvement, primary anastomosis may be done; however, if there is any question, an end colostomy or diverting proximal ostomy is mandatory.

Hemorrhage. Because this is arterial, volume of bleeding can be life-threatening. After initial stabilization, labeled RBC scan can help localize bleeding area. Angiography is less sensitive but more specific. If no site is identified and life-threatening bleeding continues, subtotal colectomy is indicated. *An upper GI tract source or rectal source must be eliminated as the cause of bleeding prior to colectomy.*

Fistula. Usually to bladder. Manifest as pneumaturia "champagne urine." Therapy is one-stage resection in well-prepared colon.

Volvulus

Twisting of colon on itself creates a closed-loop obstruction.

Sigmoid Most common, seen mostly in elderly, debilitated population. Acute distention and pain. X-ray shows "bent inner tube" (Fig. 27-1). These can be decompressed via sigmoidoscope with memorable results. A long rectal tube is left for several days followed by elective resection.

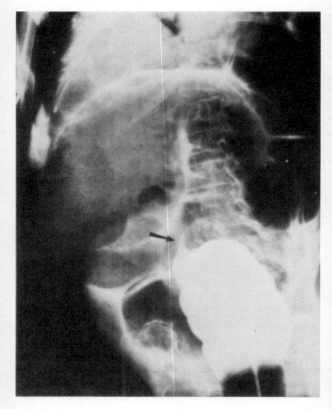

Fig. 27-1 ''Bird-beak'' sign (arrow) on Gastrografin enema in sigmoid volvulus. (From: *Nivatvongs S, Becker ER, 1987, with permission.*)

Cecal Volvulus Rotates about ileocolic pedicle. X-ray shows ''coffee bean'' in LUQ. Rapid gangrene mandates operative intervention with cecopexy or resection.

Angiodysplasia

Second leading cause of lower GI bleeding after diverticulosis. Primarily right-sided. Diagnosis by angiography and scan. Treat by resection if it is localized.

Polyps

Four Categories   Neoplastic, hamartomatous, inflammatory, and unclassified.

Neoplastic   Tubular adenoma, villous adenomous, tubulovillous. Malignant potential increases with size greater than 1 cm. Should be removed by colonoscopy. If pedunculated and tumor is limited to mucosa, no other therapy if stalk is normal. If sessile, colon resection due to malignant potential.

Hamartomatous   Juvenile polyp, Peutz-Jeghers syndrome. Not neoplastic. Local excision adequate.

Inflammatory   Due to previous colitis. Also hyperplastic, no malignant potential. Tend to be small.

Unclassified   Familial adenomatous polyposis coli. Autosomal dominant, multiple adenomatous polyps. Very high cancer risk.

Therapy   Total colectomy with ileal reservoir is most well accepted by young people. (See section on "Ulcerative Colitis".)

Colon Cancer

140,000 new cases; 60,000 deaths yearly.

Etiology   Multifactorial: diet, especially Western low fiber, high meat; genetic predisposition in familial polyposis. Bile salts are carcinogenic. Slight increase postcholecystectomy.

Staging   Classic (and easiest to remember) is Dukes' (see Fig. 27-2):

Stage	Depth	5-Year survival, %
A	Limited to muscularis mucosa	98
B	Full thickness, negative nodes	78
C	Regional nodes positive	32
D	Distant disease	6

Presentation   Varies with location; right-sided lesions tend to be bulky and nonobstructive. These patients present with microcytic anemia and weakness. Left-sided lesions are more likely to obstruct due to the thicker stool and concentric nature. Bleeding per rectum tends to be slower than with

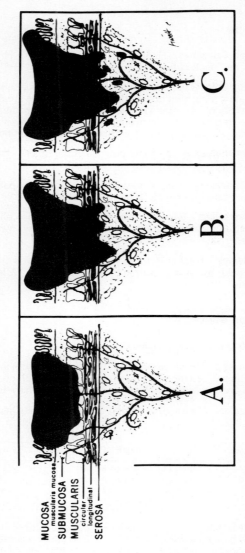

MUCOSA
muscularis mucosa
SUBMUCOSA
MUSCULARIS
circular
longitudinal
SEROSA

A.

B.

C.

Fig. 27-2 The Dukes' staging system (A, B, and C). (From: Goldberg SM, Gordon PH, Nivatvongs S, 1980, with permission.)

diverticular disease. Occult stool testing is vital in early detection of colorectal disease.

Diagnosis   Rectal exam is obligatory in any surgical patient. Flexible colonoscopy allows examination of the entire colonic mucosa, but is operator dependent. Air contrast barium enema can detect lesions as small as 1 cm and will evaluate the cecum in situations where colonoscopy could not reach.

Bowel Preparation   Improvement in perioperative infection rates is dependent on several factors: (1) mechanical cleansing to limit the volume of feces; (2) intraluminal antibiotics to reduce bacterial count of residual feces; (3) parenteral antibiotics given in such a way that adequate tissue levels are available at incision. A suggested regimen follows:

Preoperative Day 1.

- Clear liquid diet
- Reglan 10 mg PO at 3 P.M.
- Golytely or Colyte 4 L over 4–6 h; start at 4 P.M.
- Neomycin 1 g
- Erythromycin base 1 g } orally at 1 P.M., 2 P.M., 11 P.M.
- Wash abdomen with Hibiclens or Betadine
- Do not shave the abdomen

Operation Day   Cefoxitin or cefotetan or cephalothin/metronidazole on call. Clip, not shave, abdominal hair. Use iodine-impregnated plastic drapes or wound towels.

Postoperative Care   24 h of antibiotics postoperatively in uncomplicated cases.

Operative Approach   In emergent surgery primary anastomosis can be carried out for right-colon lesions. Colostomy is most appropriate in unprepared left colon. Elective resections are outlined in Fig. 27-3. Rectal lesions can be treated by low anterior resection if they are 7 cm above the anal verge, below which point abdominoperineal resection (APR) is mandatory.

ANAL NEOPLASMS   One must differentiate squamous cell carcinomas of the anus, treated by radiation and chemotherapy, from adenocarcinomas extending from the rectum which require APR. Moral: Biopsy all anal lesions.

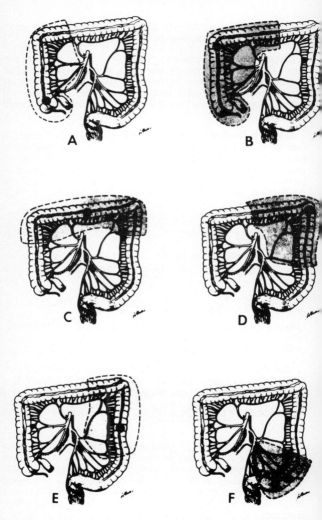

Fig. 27-3 Extent of resection in carcinoma of the colon. *A*. Carcinoma of cecum. *B*. Carcinoma of hepatic flexure. *C*. Carcinoma of transverse colon. *D*. Carcinoma of splenic flexure. *E*. Carcinoma of descending colon. *F*. Carcinoma of sigmoid colon. (From: *Nivatvongs S, Becker ER, 1987, with permission.*)

Benign Disease

Rectal Prolapse   Uncommon, but seen in the elderly with laxity of the pelvic floor. Intussusception to the outside. Repair by proctopexy or rectosigmoidectomy.

Infection   Cadre of sexually transmitted diseases can cause proctitis and discharge; a good history and appropriate cultures are mandatory.

Perirectal Disease   The diagnosis and prompt therapy of perirectal infections is vital to minimize surrounding tissue involvement and incontinence.

Perianal Abscess   This superficial collection does not communicate with the anal canal and can be drained in an outpatient setting.

Perirectal (Intersphincteric) Abscess   There is no obvious external drainage, but severe pain on rectal exam. The patient should be investigated in the operating room under anesthesia. A connection to the anal crypt can usually be identified. Goodsall's rule holds: If the external opening is in the posterior anus, the tract curves to the posterior midline. If the opening is anterior, it tracts straight back (see Fig. 27-4). Fistulas are one of four types (Fig. 27-5): intersphincteric, transsphincteric, suprasphincteric, and extrasphincteric. Therapy is incisional and drainage. The abscess cavity must be laid wide open; however, primary fistulectomy is not necessary at that time.

Necrotizing Perineal Infection   Synergistic, aggressive, fascilitis, and soft tissue infection. Very rapid spread once it has begun. Usually due to neglected perirectal or periurethral infections. Must be widely debrided and proximal diversion performed.

Hemorrhoids   Due to dilated submucosal venous plexus.

Internal.   Above dentate line. Painless bleeding and prolapse. Treat by rubber band ligation or excision if permanently prolapsed.

External.   Tend to thrombose and be fairly painful. Should be excised.

Fissure   Painful tear in posterior midline. Worsened by chronic spasm of internal sphincter. Can be treated with lateral internal sphincterotomy.

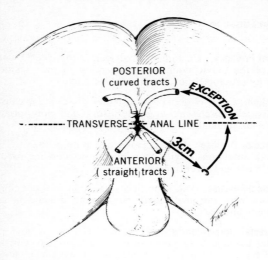

Fig. 27-4 Goodsall's rule.

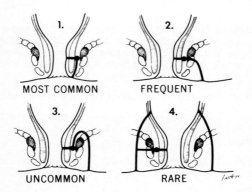

Fig. 27-5 The four main anatomic types of fistula: (1) intersphincteric, (2) transsphincteric, (3) suprasphincteric, and (4) extrasphincteric.

Incontinence Serious social problem. Multiple causes including: birth trauma, destruction of tissues from previous infections, neuromuscular disease, previous operative interventions. Therapy is aimed at reconstructing at least the external sphincter and puborectalis mechanisms.

28 APPENDIX

FUNCTION AND ANATOMY

Lymphoid tissue appears in the appendix 2 weeks after birth. Number of follicles peaks at 200, between ages 12 and 20. Secretory immunoglobins are produced as part of gut-associated lymphoid tissues to protect the milieu interior. Appendectomy does not predispose to bowel cancer or alter immune system. Appendix is useful but not indispensable. The base arises from posteromedial aspect of the cecum where three taeniae coli meet. Length and location of free end is variable: pelvic, retrocecal, or either lower quadrant. Congenital defects are rare and clinically insignificant, supplied by appendiceal artery.

INFLAMMATION—ACUTE APPENDICITIS

Incidence   Most common acute surgical condition of the abdomen. Most frequent in second and third decades, parallels amount of lymphoid tissues in appendix. Male-to-female ratio is 2:1 between ages 15 and 25, but otherwise, 1:1. Incidence has been declining in the last several decades.

Etiology and Pathogenesis   Obstruction of lumen caused by fecalith, lymphoid hypertrophy, inspissated barium, seeds, intestinal worms. Symptomatic closed-loop obstruction develops because of continued mucosal secretion into 0.1-mL capacity lumen and because of rapid multiplication of resident bacteria of the appendix. Distention stimulates visceral afferent pain fibers, producing vague, dull, diffuse mid- and lower abdominal pain. Sudden distention may cause peristalsis with cramping. Venous pressure is exceeded and arteriolar inflow causes vascular congestion of the appendix, with reflex nausea. Serosal engorgement inflames the parietal peritoneum with shift or more severe pain to right lower quadrant. Mucosal compromise allows bacterial invasion, with consequent fever, tachycardia, leukocytosis. With progressive distention, antimesenteric infarction and perforation occur. Occasionally episodes of acute appendicitis resolve if obstruction is relieved; subsequent pathologic exam reveals thickened scarred appendiceal wall.

Clinical Manifestations *Symptoms.* Classic progression of symptoms includes anorexia, followed by constant moderate periumbilical pain with shift in 4–6 h to sharp right lower quadrant pain. Variable position of tip of appendix or malrotation allows variabilty in pain location. Subsequent episodes of emesis may occur, along with obstipation or diarrhea, particularly in children.

Signs. Determined by position of appendix and whether ruptured. Vital signs show mild tachycardia or temperature elevation 1°C. Position of comfort is fetal or supine with legs drawn up, especially right. Positional movement causes pain. Anterior appendix gives maximal tenderness, guarding and rebound, at McBurney's point (one-third of the distance from the anterior superior iliac spine to the umbilicus). Cutaneous hyperaesthesia may be present early in the area supplied by the right spinal nerves T_{10}, T_{11}, T_{12}. Rovsing's sign (pain in the right lower quadrant with palpation in the left lower quadrant) indicates peritoneal irritation. Psoas sign (slowly extending the patient's right thigh when lying on the left side) demonstrates nearby inflammation when stretching the iliopsoas muscle. Obturator sign (passive internal rotation of the flexed right thigh with patient supine) indicates irritation near the obturator internus. A retrocecal appendicitis may present with flank pain. A pelvic appendicitis may give pain on rectal exam, with pressure on the cul-de-sac of Douglas.

Laboratory Findings Moderate leukocytosis of 10,000–18,000/mm³ with moderate polymorphonuclear predominance. Pyuria present when inflamed appendix lies near ureter or bladder. Bacilluria indicates urinary tract infection.

Radiography. X-rays helpful but not diagnostic. Plain abdominal films may show distended cecum, one or two distended small bowel loops, or a fecalith in the right lower quadrant suggestive of appendicitis. Gentle barium enema in acute appendicitis shows nonfilling of the appendix and mass effect on the medial and inferior borders of the cecum; complete filling of the appendix rules out appendicitis. Ultrasonography may be diagnostic. Chest x-ray rules out right lower lung field disease, which may simulate right lower quadrant pain by irritating T_{10}, T_{11}, T_{12} nerves.

Complications—Rupture Rupture occurs after unrelenting obstruction of the lumen leads to gangrene distal to the occlusion. Spillage is contained locally in 95% of patients. A phlegmon of inflamed matted loops of intestine and momentum may resolve or may expand in contained fashion to form a periappendiceal abscess or to cause intestinal obstruction. Spreading peritonitis allow contamination in the pelvic cul-de-sac or the right subhepatic space via the right gutter. Suppurative pyelophlebitis (ascending septic thrombophlebitis of the portal venous system) presents with spiking fever, chills, hepatic pain, jaundice. Septic emboli lead to multiple pyogenic abscesses.

Incidence.   Rupture is present in 15–25% of patients at presentation, with a higher incidence in pediatric and geriatric age groups.

Diagnosis.   Abdominal pain occasionally (only 4%) lessens temporarily after rupture because of sudden relief of distention; in most patients pain continues unabated. A tender, boggy mass may be palpable on rectal or in the right lower quadrant. Degree of distention, ileus, fever, tachycardia, leukocytosis, toxic appearance parallel the severity of peritonitis.

Differential Diagnosis   That of the acute abdomen. Preoperative diagnosis of acute appendicitis should be 85% accurate depending upon the location of the appendix, the length of the symptoms, and the age and sex of the patient.

Acute Mesenteric Adenitis.   Most often in childhood, recent upper respiratory infection, generalized lymphadenopathy.

Acute Gastroenteritis.   Generally viral etiology, associated diarrhea, cramping, and relaxation between hyperperistaltic waves. Salmonella gastroenteritis results from ingestion of contaminated food; historically disables groups of patients. *Salmonella typhosa* infection rare, characterized by rash, inappropriate bradycardia, leukopenia, positive stool cultures.

Diseases of the Male.   The diseases that mimic abdominal pain are testicular torsion, epididymitis, seminal vesiculitis.

Meckel's Diverticulitis.   Same preoperative picture as appendicitis. Requires diverticulectomy, occasionally bowel resection.

Intussusception.   Most under 2 years of age, currant jelly stool, intermittent crampy attacks of pain, RLQ sausage-shaped mass. Initial attempt at reduction by barium enema.

Acute Ileitis or Regional Enteritis.   Associated with diarrhea and often chronic history, but infrequency of anorexia, nausea, emesis. If found at laparotomy, incidental appendectomy indicated to decrease subsequent confusing symptoms (not done if cecum involved because of greater risk of postoperative fistula).

Perforated Peptic Ulcer. Right gutter spillage of UGI contents with rapid sealing of perforation causes prominence of RLQ symptoms.

Diverticulitis or Perforating Carcinoma of Colon. Requires exploration.

Epiploic Appendagitis. Infarction secondary to torsion. Pain present but no peritonitis or obstruction.

Urinary Tract Infection. Right costovertebral angle tenderness and bacteriuria present.

Ureteral Stone. Hematuria and referred pain to scrotum or labia present. Pyelography confirms diagnosis.

Primary Peritonitis. Treated with antibiotics after paracentesis shows simple gram-positive flora.

Henoch-Schönlein Purpura. Occurs several weeks following streptococcal infection, associated with purpura, joint pains, nephritis.

Yersiniosis. Transmitted via contaminated food, mimics appendicitis. *Campylobacter jejuni* causes diarrhea and pain with positive stool cultures.

Gynecologic Disorders. Pelvic inflammatory disease usually bilateral, associated with lower pelvic pain and cervical motion tenderness, occurs perimenstrual; Gram stain of vaginal discharge often shows gram-negative diplococci. Ruptured graafian follicle mimics appendicitis with spillage of sufficient blood and fluid into pelvis; occurs at ovulation (Mittelschmerz). Ruptured ectopic pregnancy: tuboovarian mass and hypovolemia present; culdocentesis yields non-clotting blood.

Others. Foreign body bowel perforations, mesenteric vascular occlusion, right lower chest pleuritis, acute pancreatitis, hematoma of abdominal wall.

Select Groups

The Young Faster progression of disease with high fever and emesis with more frequent rupture at diagnosis (15–50%).

The Elderly Deceptively mild clinical course with increased morbidity because of higher incidence of concomitant disease and because greater than 50% are ruptured at diagnosis.

The Pregnant Expected frequency for age group. Diagnosis more difficult because appendix displaced cephalad and lateral by gravid uterus; pain, nausea, leukocytosis common in normal pregnancy but left shift indicates acute process. Maternal mortality negligible. Fetal mortality overall 2–8.5%; as high as 35% with appendiceal perforation and peritonitis.

Treatment Treatment is always operative because the obstructed lumen will not resolve with antibiotics alone. Acute appendicitis without rupture is treated with immediate appendectomy after medical evaluation complete. Ruptured appendicitis with local peritonitis or phlegmon operated upon early after resuscitation for fluid and electrolyte losses. Ruptured appendicitis with spreading peritonitis requires more extensive fluid resuscitation but patient should undergo operation normally within 4 h to prevent continued peritoneal contamination.

Ruptured appendicitis with periappendiceal abscess formation may be treated acutely with operation but is associated with increased morbidity. If symptoms are of several days' duration, subsiding, and associated with right lower quadrant mass, initial nonoperative therapy with fluid resuscitation, bowel rest, and large doses of antibiotics is appropriate. If vital signs, leukocytosis, and abdominal signs progress, drainage of abscess may be indicated, followed by conservative therapy. Interval appendectomy in 6 weeks to 3 months is advised because of high recurrence rate.

Preoperative antibiotics lower infectious complications, but the regimen is controversial: (1) preoperative antibiotics only for presumed perforation; (2) preoperative antibiotics for all, continued as indicated if perforation or gangrene found; (3) preoperative antibiotics for all, continued for 3–5 days if any stage appendicitis found. Pathogens in acute appendicitis are mixed colonic flora, both aerobic and anaerobic; *Bacteroides fragilis* needs coverage. Clindamycin plus an aminoglycoside or second-generation cephalosporin regimen are popular.

Procedure Incision should be in the right lower quadrant for patients with suspected appendicitis. McBurney incision gives best exposure but necessitates second incision if alternative procedure necessary. Rocky-Davis incision with muscle splitting can be extended medially as needed. Right paramedian or lower midline incision is used for general exploration, but is contraindicated with abscess, since infected material brought through uncontaminated peritoneal cavity.

Appendiceal stump is traditionally ligated and inverted; small risk of intramural cecal abscess from inversion of infected stump. Inversion without ligation risks bleeding from appendiceal artery. Ligation without inversion secures hemostasis but allows peritoneal contamination from the exposed stump mucosa or slipped ligatures.

If appendicitis is not found, the pelvic organs and remaining abdominal viscera are explored. Mesentery is examined for lymphadenitis. Ileum is "run" for terminal ileitis or Meckel's diverticulitis.

Drainage of localized pus accomplished with lateral drains. Peritoneal cavity cannot be drained. If appendix ruptured, subcutaneous fat and skin left open to heal by granulation or secondary closure.

Prognosis Mortality is 0.1% if unruptured acute appendicitis, 3% if ruptured, and 15% if ruptured in the elderly. Death usually from uncontrolled sepsis, pulmonary embolism, or aspiration; improving rates with earlier diagnosis prior to rupture and better antibiotics.

Morbidity is increased with rupture and older age. Early complications are septic. Wound infection requires reopening of the skin incision and it predisposes to dehiscence (less common with muscle-splitting incision). Intraabdominal abscesses may occur from peritoneal contamination after gangrene and perforation. Fecal fistula results from necrosis of a portion of the cecum by abscess or constricting purse string or from a slipped ligature. Intestinal obstruction may occur with loculated abscesses and adhesion formation. Late complications include adhesion formation with mechanical obstruction and hernia.

TUMORS

Neoplasms are uncommon. Benign lesions may cause obstruction with acute appendicitis. Malignant tumors total less than 1% of all appendices.

Carcinoid tumors of the GI tract are found most commonly in the appendix (45–75%). Only 3% of these metastasize, and even fewer produce malignant carcinoid syndrome. Three-fourths present in distal third of appendix as small, firm, circumscribed, yellowish-brown tumors. Treatment: if confined to appendix, appendectomy and wide resection of mesoappendix; if invasion past resection line or nodal metastases present, right hemicolectomy.

Adenocarcinoma usually discovered incidentally at appendectomy and behaves like colon carcinoma. Treatment: right hemicolectomy.

Mucocele is a cystic dilatation of the appendix containing mucoid material. Appendectomy is treatment for benign (noninflammatory proximal appendiceal obstruction) or malignant (mucous papillary adenocarcinoma) lesions. Rupture or iatrogenic spillage results in pseudomyxoma peritonei.

29 LIVER

ANATOMY

Approximately $\frac{1}{50}$ of body weight. See Fig. 29-1 for segmental anatomy. True main interlobar fissure from gallbladder fossa anteroinferiorly to inferior vena cava posteriorly. Biliary drainage through right and left hepatic ducts, which form common hepatic duct anterior in porta hepatis. Hepatic artery is 25% of hepatic blood flow, portal vein is 75%. Celiac→common hepatic→(gastroduodenal, right gastric)→ proper hepatic→(right, left) hepatic. Cystic from right hepatic. In 17%, right hepatic from SMA.

Portal Venous System Formed behind pancreas from superior mesenteric and splenic veins (inferior mesenteric drains into splenic). System is valveless. Travels posterior to bile duct and hepatic artery in porta hepatis, gives off right, left portal branches.

Hepatic Venous System Central veins in liver lobules, sublobular veins, and collecting veins coalesce to form right, left, and middle hepatic veins, which drain into inferior vena cava. System is also valveless. Average blood flow is 1500 mL/min per 1.73 m^2 of BSA.

FUNCTION

Four interrelated physiologic-anatomic units: circulatory, biliary, reticuloendothelial, and functioning hepatocytes.

Function Tests *Proteins.* Proteins synthesized are albumin, fibrinogen, prothrombin, and other clotting factors. Serum albumin will fall with disease but has a half-life of 8–10 days.

Carbohydrates and Lipids. Hypoglycemia rarely seen in liver disease; more often, glycogenesis is impaired. Galactose conversion to glucose may decrease in cirrhosis, hepatitis. Liver synthesizes, esterifies, and excretes cholesterol. Biliary obstruction and primary biliary cirrhosis can show rise in cholesterol. Parenchymal disease may show decreased cholesterol.

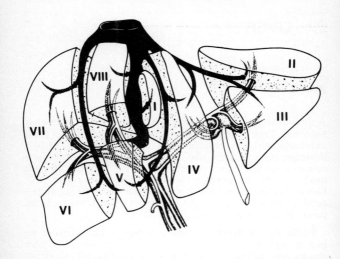

Fig. 29-1 The functional division of the liver and the segments according to Couinaud's nomenclature. (From: *Bismuth H: Surgical anatomy and anatomical surgery of the liver. World J Surg 6:6, 1982, with permission.*)

Enzymes. Most commonly abnormal are alkaline phosphatase, SGOT (AST), and SGPT (ALT). SGOT will rise with liver, cardiac, skeletal muscle, kidney, and pancreatic cellular damage. SGPT is more liver-specific. LDH may also rise. *Alkaline phosphatase* is elevated with biliary obstruction, cholestasis, and space-occupying hepatic lesions. Very sensitive for metastatic carcinoma. 5'-Nucleotidase also elevated in hepatobiliary disease.

Dye Excretion. Certain dyes, especially indocyanine green, can provide an estimate of hepatic blood flow by the Fick principle.

Coagulation Defects. Commonly accompany liver disease. In obstructive jaundice, vitamin K decreases from decreased bile to solubilize it. In hepatocellular disease, prothrombin synthesis falls. Additionally, factors V, VII, IX, and fibrinogen may decrease. Cirrhotics may have increased fibrinolysis.

SPECIAL STUDIES

Needle biopsy obtains tissue with minimal mortality (0.08%) and is useful in diagnosing posthepatitic and postnecrotic cirrhosis and cellular and focal lesions. *Ultrasound, CT, and MRI* define parenchymal disease and provide localization for therapy. Vascular lesions and patency may also be assessed. *Scintillation scanning* with ^{99m}Tc-sulfur colloid has a >65% accuracy in diagnosing hepatic lesions. *Angiography* is useful for demonstrating tumor vascular patterns and for preoperative evaluations.

TRAUMA

Second most commonly injured intraabdominal organ (spleen is first), most commonly from vehicular trauma. Injuries are classified as *transcapsular, subcapsular,* or *central.* Hiatal injuries are frequently fatal. With capsular rupture, intraabdominal blood loss commonly leads to shock. Pain, spasm, and rigidity may also be seen.

Diagnosis   Liver injury should be suspect in blunt abdominal injuries with clinical symptoms (above) or right costal margin rib fractures. Lavage may be negative with subcapsular and central lesions. CT scan is most accurate.

Treatment   As with any major trauma, airway, breathing, and circulation must be restored prior to other definitive therapy. Stable patients with CT scan–documented minor liver injuries may be observed, providing their vital signs remain stable. Prolonged bed rest may be required with expectant therapy. Liver hemorrhage is usually controlled by prompt celiotomy with debridement of devitalized tissue, ligature of major vessels, and packing of hepatic injuries. Deep parenchymal sutures should be avoided. The *Pringle maneuver* (vascular inflow occlusion) may be helpful. External drainage usually accompanies these procedures.

Complications   Hemorrhage accounts for most deaths and infection. *Hematobilia,* blood in the bile, occasionally follows major liver injury or deep parenchymal sutures. Usually episodic GI bleeding weeks after injury. Treatment is via embolization or operation.

Trauma with Major Vascular Injury   Ligation of common or proper hepatic artery is usually followed by good collateral flow. 15% of blunt injuries have hepatic venous disruption with significant mortality. Control may be obtained via inflow occlusion at porta hepatis and vascular isolation from the vena cava with a liver shunt. *Portal vein injury* is rare and should be repaired when feasible. Ligation can be tolerated if necessary.

HEPATIC ABSCESS

Pyogenic Abscesses

Result from (1) ascending biliary infection (*cholangitis from calculi is most common cause*), (2) hematogenous spread via portal system, (3) generalized septicemia with arterial spread (second most common), (4) direct extension, and (5) hepatic trauma. *Pylephlebitis* (portal septicemia) occurs in 3% of perforated appendicitis and acute diverticulitis and may lead to abscess. Cultures show *E. coli* in 33% related to biliary origin: staph and strep predominate with systemic infectious origins.

Clinical Manifestations Symptoms of primary cause. "Spiking" fevers with rigors, diaphoresis, nausea, vomiting, and anorexia. Pain is late, jaundice uncommon, tenderness in 50%.

Diagnosis Leukocytosis, anemia frequent. Blood cultures positive in 30%. LFTs show alkaline phosphatase elevation. Radiographic signs include restricted right diaphragm movement, right cardiophrenic angle blunting, rare air fluid levels. CT is very useful.

Treatment Drainage and antibiotics. Solitary abscesses may be drained percutaneously using CT or ultrasound. Multiple abscesses carry higher mortality, require operative drainage, rarely resection.

Amebic Abscesses

10% of population infected with <u>*Entameba histolytica*</u>. Liver abscesses in middle-aged adults, <u>M:F 9:1</u>. Organisms reach liver via portal system. Usually <u>solitary right lobe abscess with "anchovy paste" fluid</u>.

Clinical Manifestations Fever, liver pain (88%), occasionally right shoulder pain. Fever with diaphoresis and rigors in 75%. 50% antecedent diarrhea, bloody mucous stools in children. Liver tender and enlarged on exam. Jaundice rare.

Diagnostic Studies/Complications Leukocytosis, anemia with prolonged disease. Only 15.4% ameba recover rate in stool. LFTs not helpful. Specific amebic complement fixation test most useful. Scans also useful. Aspiration of cavity shows characteristic material, trophozoites in $<\frac{1}{3}$. Secondary bacterial infection in 22%. Abscesses may rupture (6–9%) or extend into adjacent organs.

Treatment Amebicidal drugs first, metronidazole drug of choice. May require aspiration/drainage if symptoms persist, abscess remains radiographically, or is secondarily infected.

CYSTS

Nonparasitic Cysts

Includes degenerative, dermoid, lymphatic, retention, and proliferative cysts. Solitary cysts usually in right lobe, clear content. Liver may be honeycombed, *polycystic,* which is associated with polycystic kidneys. Rarely, polycystic livers may cause portal hypertension. *Traumatic cysts* usually single and bile-filled. *Cystadenomas* filled with mucoid material. Cysts usually grow slowly with few symptoms, present as painless RUQ mass. Symptoms from pressure on adjacent organs. Jaundice is rare, LFTs of little use. CT/ultrasound are very useful. Pain occurs with rupture, torsion, or hemorrhage.

Treatment For asymptomatic cysts observation only. Surgical treatment should be complete extirpation. Large, deep, sterile cysts may simply be widely unroofed. Purulent contents demand external drainage. Polycystic livers should not be resected. Prognosis follows that of the associated, if any, renal disease.

Hydatid Cysts

Usually unilocular and caused by *Echinococcus granulosus.* Alveolar type caused by *Echinococcus multilocularis.* 70% located in liver, $\frac{1}{3}$ multiple. Right lobe affected 85%. Cyst is two-layer encapsulated with contents under pressure and is colorless, opalescent. Daughter cysts inside main cysts. *Alveolar* disease has no capsule with multiple metastasis, blood, and lymphatic invasion.

Complications Include intrabiliary rupture (5–10%), suppuration with biliary bacteria, intraperitoneal or intrapleural rupture.

Clinical Manifestations Usually asymptomatic. Early symptoms from pressure on adjacent organs. Pain, tenderness, palpable mass common. If secondarily infected, symptoms of pyogenic abscess. May present with anaphylaxis if intraperitoneal rupture. Biliary rupture shows colic, jaundice, and urticaria.

Diagnostic Studies   Round, calcified shadows on plain films. CT scan very useful. Indirect agglutination positive in 85%, Casoni's skin test positive in 90%.

Treatment   Treatment is surgical. Must remove cysts without contaminating peritoneal cavity. Cysts may be intraoperatively drained and flushed with hypertonic saline or alcohol prior to excision. Large cysts may require partial hepatectomy. Cavity may be managed by omentoplasty, simple closure. External drainage has high complication rate.

Benign Tumors

Hamartomas   Composed of normal tissues arranged in disorderly fashion. Firm, nodular, encapsulated, cystic. Usually of no clinical significance.

Adenomas   May be related to oral contraceptives but not definitively proved. Should be resected if enlarging or bleeding. Contraceptives *should* be stopped and asymptomatic lesions followed.

Focal Nodular Hyperplasia   Solitary, tan, unencapsulated tumors near liver edge. Usually asymptomatic, rarely rupture. Resect only if symptomatic. May be response to injury.

Hemangioma   Most common liver nodule. F:M is 5:1. No malignant potential. Majority asymptomatic, rare bruit. Symptoms related to size. May rupture and hemorrhage, especially in children and pregnant women. Diagnosis by angiography, CT, ultrasound. *Avoid needle biopsy*. Infants may have high-output CHF and may respond to steroids, hepatic artery ligation. Resect adults only for symptoms and when size > 4–5 cm; rupture is rare.

MALIGNANT TUMORS

Primary Carcinoma

Primary liver carcinoma is common in Asia, and aborigines. In children, hepatoblastoma is common before age 2. Aflatoxins and low-protein diets have been implicated etiologically. *Postnecrotic cirrhosis* frequently precedes.

Pathology   *Hepatocellular carcinoma* (most common), *cholangiocarcinoma* (bile duct cancer), and *hepatoblastoma*, an immature variant in children. *Fibrolamellar carcinoma* is a hepatocellular variant occurring in young adults. Frequent invasion of portal and hepatic veins. Extension via (1) centrifugal growth, (2) parasinusoidal extension, (3) venous spread, and (4) distal metastasis via lymphatic and vascular systems, most often to nodes and lungs. Metastases occur in 48–73%.

Clinical Manifestations   Weight loss, fatigue in 80%, pain in 50%. Hepatomegaly very common, splenomegaly and portal hypertension in ⅓. Jaundice, ascites common. Children usually present with a mass.

Diagnostic Evaluation   Alkaline phosphatase, 5′ nucleotidase usually elevated, bilirubin often normal. AFP present in 30–75%. Arteriography, CT/MRI useful. Preoperative needle biopsy. Intraoperative ultrasound to define resection limits.

Treatment   Only chance is surgical excision. Cirrhosis compromises resection possibilities. Radiation therapy and chemotherapy are of little use in adults, may help in children. Hepatic arterial chemotherapy may reduce tumor size.

Prognosis   Extremely poor for adults. Resectable children under age 2 have better survivals.

Other Primary Neoplasms   These include angiosarcomas (vinyl choloride, thorotrast), mesenchymomas, and infantile hemangioendotheliomas.

Metastatic Neoplasms

Most common malignant liver tumor by 20:1. Metastasis in liver in 25–50% of all cancer deaths. Routes to liver are (1) portal vein, (2) lymphatics, (3) hepatic artery, and (4) direct extension. Often grow more rapidly than original lesion.

Clinical Manifestations   Symptoms in 67%, pain, ascites, jaundice, anorexia, weight loss. Mass in 50%. Flushing in hepatic carcinoid.

Diagnosis   Alkaline phosphatase elevated in over 80%, SGOT in 67%, AFP normal. CEA may be elevated in colon metastases. CT/MRI, angiography, and intraoperative ultrasound useful.

Treatment   Consider if (1) primary controlled, (2) no other metastases, (3) patient will tolerate procedure, and (4) total extirpation is possible. Resection of metastases has survival benefit for colorectal carcinoma and Wilms tumor. 20% of colon carcinomas have metastases, of which 25% are resectable, of which 50% have other negating factors. Of all colon carcinomas that have metastases, 25% are resectable, of which 50% have other negating factors. Overall, there may be a 30% 5-year survival for resections for colorectal carcinoma. Resection for carcinoid metastases may provide symptomatic relief. Intraarterial FUDR and mitomycin C may provide symptomatic relief and size reduction.

HEPATIC RESECTION

Indications: (1) trauma with necrosis, (2) cysts, (3) granulomas, (4) primary neoplasms, (5) secondary neoplasms. Up to 80% resection may be tolerated in noncirrhotics. Regeneration from marked hypertrophy of remaining tissue. Insulin is an anabolic factor. Preoperative management includes optimization of nutrition, liver function, and coagulation parameters.

Operative Procedures Major aim is to prevent/control hemorrhage. Porta hepatis may be safely clamped for 60 min. Resection follows anatomic planes of segmental anatomy based upon portal distribution. Liver is mobilized by dividing triangular ligament, coronary ligament, and ligamentum teres. Porta hepatis dissection defines artery, vein, and duct to be removed, which are temporarily occluded. Glisson's capsule is incised and hepatic parenchyma is cleaved bluntly, ligating ducts and vessels, heading toward the hepatic veins, which are then doubly ligated at the cava, followed by division of porta hepatis structures.

PORTAL HYPERTENSION

Etiology See Table 29-1. Broad classes include (1) increased inflow (rare), (2) extrahepatic outflow obstruction, (3) extrahepatic portal obstruction, and (4) intrahepatic obstruction. Overwhelming majority ($\geq$ 90%) of cases due to *intrahepatic obstruction*. Factors contributing include (1) fibrosis with portal venule compression, (2) compression by regenerative nodules, (3) increased arterial flow, (4) fatty infiltration and inflammation, and (5) intrahepatic vascular obstruction. *Nutritional cirrhosis* remains the most common etiology worldwide. Related to EtOH in Western civilization. Resistance to flow is postsinusoidal (on the hepatic venous side of the sinusoid). *Postnecrotic cirrhosis* accounts for up to 12%.

TABLE 29-1. Etiology of Portal Hypertension

A. Increased hepatopetal flow without obstruction
  1. Hepatic arterial-portal venous fistula
  2. Splenic arteriovenous fistula
  3. Intrasplenic origin
B. Extrahepatic outflow obstruction
  1. Budd-Chiari syndrome
  2. Failure of right side of heart
C. Obstruction of extrahepatic portal venous system
  1. Congenital obstruction
  2. Cavernomatous transformation of portal vein
  3. Infection
  4. Trauma
  5. Extrinsic compression
D. Intrahepatic obstruction
  1. Nutritional cirrhosis
  2. Postnecrotic cirrhosis
  3. Biliary cirrhosis
  4. Other diseases with hepatic fibrosis
     a. Hemochromatosis
     b. Wilson disease
     c. Congenital hepatic fibrosis
  5. Infiltrative lesions
  6. Venoocclusive diseases
     a. *Senecio* poisoning
     b. Schistosomiasis

Pathophysiology Elevated pressure in portal venous system leads to collateral venous flow. Normally < 25 cm H_2O, mean 21.5 cm. Pressure may be measured intraoperatively, by direct splenic puncture or by occlusive hepatic venous pressure (OHVP), which is analogous to the pulmonary wedge pressure. Anatomy may be defined by *splenoportography* or the venous phase of mesenteric arteriography. Normally, no collaterals should be seen. Collaterals that become functional are: (1) *hepatopetal collaterals,* which shunt blood from an obstructed extrahepatic portal system to normal intrahepatic vasculature; these are the veins of Sappey, cystic, epiploic, hepatocolic, hepatorenal, diaphragmatic, and suspensory ligament veins. (2) *Hepatofugal* are the most common collaterals and include the *coronary and esophageal veins,* the *superior hemorrhoidal veins, umbilical vein,* and the *veins of Retzius.* These vessels shunt blood away from the liver to the systemic venous system.

Esophagogastric Varices

Initially, submucosal veins enlarge; later, submucosa disappears and veins line inside of esophagus and erode from esophagitis and hemorrhage. Gastric varices predominate in the cardia. 30% of cirrhotics with varices will bleed within 2 years of diagnosis. 70% of these patients die within 1 year of the first hemorrhage. 60% rebleed within 1 year.

Acute Bleeding Usually first sign of portal hypertension in children. In adults, varices account for 25–33% of massive UGI bleeds. Cirrhotic bleeding is varices in 50%, gastritis in 30%, and ulcers in 9%. Therefore, a specific diagnosis must be made prior to treatment. Physical shows stigmata for cirrhosis. Esophagoscopy is the most accurate tool in this diagnosis. Arteriography may be useful in ulcer disease.

Treatment *Nonoperative techniques:* (1) Balloon tamponade is risky and has a failure rate of 25–55%. (2) Endoscopic variceal sclerosis may control bleeding in up to 93% of patients with similar mortality to emergency shunts. (3) Vasopressin reduces portal flow by 40%. Peripheral venous is route of choice. Avoid in patients with coronary disease. (4) Inderal may be used as prophylaxis. *Operative therapy:* ligation, esophageal devascularization, and shunting procedures. Effective shunting will stop bleeding and may yield a 50–71% immediate hospitalization survival. Pediatric variceal bleeding, however, often stops spontaneously with bed rest and sedation. Important tenets in treatment include correction of coagulation deficits with component therapy. Additionally, acute bleeding in cirrhotics exacerbates or will induce encephalopathy.

Prevention of Recurrent Hemorrhage Shunting procedures in adults who have bled and stopped are much safer if performed electively. Prognosis is correlated with hepatic function as per Child's criteria. Overall, patients with nutritional, alcoholic, or cryptogenic cirrhosis have a worse prognosis than do patients with biliary cirrhosis or extrahepatic portal vein obstruction.

Ascites

Mechanisms poorly understood. Portal hypertension is a contributory but not solely etiologic factor. Hypoalbuminemia and reduced serum osmotic pressure contribute to ascites. Impairment of hepatic venous outflow appears to be most important. Accompanying ascites is the retention of sodium and water. **Treatment** includes rest, nutritional supplementation, low sodium intake, potassium repletion. Diuretics include furosemide, chlorothiazide (first line), and aldosterone antagonists (spironolactone). Paracentesis is contraindicated. Intractable ascites may require peritoneal venous shunts (complications include DIC).

Hypersplenism

Splenomegaly accompanies portal hypertension. Subsequent hypersplenism may follow (WBC < 4000, PLT < 100,000). Splenectomy is *rarely* indicated and negates future selective shunting.

Hepatic Coma

Portal-systemic encephalopathy rarely occurs in portal hypertension without coexistent hepatocellular dysfunction. Portacaval shunts may show up to 38% incidence. Physiologically, there is hyperammonemia secondary to portal systemic collaterals and impairment of the ornithine-citrulline-arginine cycle. Dietary protein and intraluminal intestinal blood (variceal bleed) are major contributors. Endogenous intestinal urea production also contributes. Clinical manifestations include altered consciousness, reflexes, and motor activity. This may progress from confusion to frank coma. **Treatment** should reduce nitrogen within the gut, reduce ammonia production, and enhance ammonia metabolism. This includes (1) restriction of protein intake, (2) control of bleeding, (3) gastrointestinal catharsis (lactulose), (4) intestinal bacterial reduction (neomycin), and (5) intraluminal ammonia trapping (lactulose).

Surgery for Portal Hypertension

Esophageal Procedures directly attack bleeding varices. These include transesopohageal ligation of varices and esophageal transection. Control, however, is only temporary, with 50% of cirrhotic survivors rebleeding. The *Sugiura* procedure includes esophageal transection, paraesophageal devascularization, splenectomy, and vagotomy with/without drainage. It carries a high mortality and rebleed rate in most hands.

Procedures that Reduce Portal Pressure Classified as totally or partially diverting. Most basic is the *end-to-side portacaval shunt,* which completely diverts all portal inflow from the liver to the vena cava. The *side-to-side portacaval shunt* diverts portal flow but additionally allows reversed portal outflow from the liver. Other functional side-to-side shunts include the mesocaval, central splenorenal, and H-graft procedures. In decompressing the portal vein, all of these do not preserve hepatic portal inflow. The *distal splenorenal*, or *Warren, shunt* is truly selective in decompressing varices while maintaining portal perfusion via a continued hepatic portal hypertension. This procedure is associated with less encephalopathy, but statistical differences in true survival, long-term selectivity, and ascites are unproved.

Shunt Selection.   Should include preoperative portograms to assess portal vein patency. Budd-Chiari syndrome mandates a side-to-side shunt. Ascites may or may not alter shunt preference, with side-to-side shunts having the lowest incidence.

Patient Selection.   Includes evaluation of ascites, coagulation deficits, liver function (bilirubin, BSP retention). Child's classification is associated with operative morbidity/mortality. Overall, group A patients have nearly no elective mortality, whereas group C patients have up to 53% operative mortality.

Intraoperative Technique.   Should always include pre- and postshunt portal pressure.

Complications of Portal-Systemic Shunts.   Include intraoperative bleeding or shunt failure, postoperative rebleeding, hepatic failure, hepatorenal syndrome, cardiorespiratory failure, and delayed complications such as encephalopathy, hemosiderosis, and ulcer disease.

FULMINANT HEPATIC FAILURE

Sudden, severe hepatic failure secondary to massive cellular necrosis. Usual origin in acute viral hepatitis. Also seen with Reye syndrome and with chemical toxins (carbon tetrachloride). Therapy is supportive and includes hemo- and peritoneal dialysis, exchange transfusions, and plasmapheresis. Mortality is 85–90%. Spontaneous recovery occurs in 10–20%.

30 GALLBLADDER AND EXTRAHEPATIC BILIARY SYSTEM

ANATOMY

Duct System Extrahepatic biliary system starts with hepatic ducts; ends at the stoma of the common bile duct in the duodenum. Right hepatic duct enters the confluence with a sharp curve, which accounts for the lesser number of calculi in this segment. Left duct is longer than the right; the two join to form a common hepatic duct 3–4 cm in length. Cystic duct joins to form the common bile duct.

Common bile duct measures 8–11.5 cm in length and 6–10 mm in diameter. Portal vein is posterior to the duct; hepatic artery is to the left. Lower third enters duodenum at the ampulla of Vater, where it is frequently joined by the pancreatic duct. Various portions of the duct have been named according to their other relationships, such as suprapancreatic, intrapancreatic, and intraduodenal.

Bile duct and pancreatic duct join in one of three ways: May join outside of the duodenum and traverse the duodenal wall as a single duct; may join within the duodenal wall and have a common channel; or may exit separately into the duodenum. Sphincter of Oddi surrounds the common bile duct at the papilla of Vater, controlling flow of bile, and sometimes pancreatic juice.

Gallbladder Pear-shaped organ located in bed of liver in line with the anatomic division of that organ into right and left lobes. Divided into fundus, corpus or body, infundibulum, and neck. Fundus extends beyond liver margin and contains smooth muscle; if kinked, has been referred to as a "phyrigian cap." Corpus or body is major storage area and contains primarily elastic tissue. Body tapers into a neck which has a dilatation called the *infundibulum,* or *Hartmann's pouch.*

Wall is composed of smooth muscle and fibrous tissue. A columnar epithelium containing fat and cholesterol crystals also secretes mucus.

Supplied by cystic artery, a branch of the right hepatic artery. Venous return consists of small veins that directly enter the liver bed, and a cystic vein that enters the right portal vein. Lymph flows directly into liver and also to nodes along surface of the portal vein. Nerves arise from the celiac axis and lie along the hepatic artery.

Empties into the cystic duct, which enters common hepatic duct to form common bile duct. Variations of cystic duct union with the common hepatic duct are surgically important. It may run parallel with the hepatic duct and unite in the duodenum; may be very short or even absent; may enter the right hepatic duct; and may rarely spiral around the common hepatic duct and enter on the left side. Mucosal folds in the cystic duct are called the "valves of Heister."

Anomalies

Classic anatomic description of the extrahepatic biliary tree and its vascular supply occurs in only one-third of patients. Isolated congenital absence of the gallbladder is rare, occurring in 0.03% of autopsy cases. Duplication of gallbladder with two separate cavities and cystic ducts occurs in 1 in 4000.

Gallbladder may assume many abnormal positions. "Floating gallbladder" occurs when there is an increase in the peritoneal investment. Gallbladder may even be suspended by a complete mesentery; occurring only 5% of the time, may predispose to torsion and gangrene. Left-sided gallbladder is extremely rare and is referred to as "retrodisplacement." Totally intrahepatic gallbladder can occur and is associated with an increased incidence of gallstones.

Accessory hepatic ducts present in 15% of cases. Small ducts (Luschka) may drain directly from the liver into the gallbladder.

Anomalies of the hepatic artery and cystic artery occur in 50% of cases. An accessory left hepatic artery arises from the left gastric artery in 5% of cases. In 20%, the right hepatic artery arises from the superior mesenteric artery. Right hepatic artery is vulnerable to injury especially when a "caterpillar hump" artery is mistaken for the cystic artery. Cystic artery may arise from left hepatic artery or junction of both right and left arteries. Double cystic arteries occur in 25% of cases. In 15%, cystic artery arises in front of the common hepatic duct.

CYSTIC DISEASE OF THE EXTRAHEPATIC BILIARY TRACT (CHOLEDOCHAL CYST)   See Chap. 38.

CONGENITAL BILIARY ATRESIA   See Chap. 38.

PHYSIOLOGY

Bile Secretion   Normal adult secretes 250–1000 mL bile per day. Bile secretion is responsive to neurogenic, humoral, and chemical control. Vagal stimulation increases secretion; splanchnic stimulation decreases bile flow. Bile flow also stimulated by secretin release from duodenum, which itself is stimulated by hydrochloric acid, protein breakdown products, and fatty acids.

Composition of Bile   Main constituents of bile are electrolytes in the same concentration as the plasma, bile salts, proteins, cholesterol, fats, and bile pigments.

Bile salts act as anions that are balanced by sodium. Major bile salts are cholic, deoxycholic, and chenodeoxycholic acids. These conjugate with taurine or glycine. Liver bile contains unesterified cholesterol, lecithin, and neutral fat.

The color of bile secreted by the liver is due to the pigment bilirubin diglucuronide, which is the breakdown product of hemoglobin. In the intestine, this is acted on by bacteria and converted to urobilinogen, a small fraction of which is absorbed.

Gallbladder Function   Gallbladder stores and concentrates bile. Sodium, chloride, and water are selectively absorbed, resulting in a 10-fold increase in concentration of bile salts, bile pigments, and cholesterol.

Mucus secretion protects mucosa from the lytic action of bile and facilitates passage of bile through the cystic duct. This mucus comprises the "white bile" of a hydrops of the gallbladder arising from obstruction of the cystic duct. Calcium is also secreted in the presence of inflammation or cystic duct obstruction.

Motor activity is complex. Depends on coordinated contraction of gallbladder and relaxation of sphincter of Oddi. Gallbladder can generate pressures up to 300 mm water. Since hepatic secretory pressure is 375 mm water, passage of bile depends upon relaxation of the sphincter of Oddi. Gallbladder emptying is mediated by both humoral and nervous stimulation. Cholecystokinin is main stimulus and is released from intestinal mucosa in response to food. Intravenous cholecystokinin relaxes terminal bile duct, sphincter of Oddi, and duodenal musculature; it also causes the gallbladder to evacuate 70% within 30 min. Vagal innervation stimulates contraction, whereas sympathetic stimulation inhibits motor activity. Parasympathomimetic drugs contract the gallbladder, while atropine relaxes the organ.

The gallbladder evacuates in $\frac{1}{2}$ h following a fatty meal.

Patients receiving total parenteral nutrition have an increased risk of gallbladder disease due to stasis. Incidence of cholecystitis in this group approaches 45%.

Oral Cholecystography   Graham and Cole introduced the use of contrast media for the gallbladder in 1924. Visualization of gallbladder is dependent on absorption of the radiopaque iodine-containing compound across the GI mucosa, blood flow to the liver, uptake and excretion by hepatocytes, patency of hepatic and cystic ducts, and water absorption by gallbladder.

An abnormal oral cholecystogram consists of a poorly visualizing or nonvisualizing gallbladder. The so-called Telepaque exam is 98% reliable. Nonvisualization of the gallbladder may be due to failure to retain the oral medication, faulty absorption, hepatic dysfunction, hepatic or cystic duct obstruction, a nonabsorbing gallbladder mucosa, or faulty x-ray technique. If the serum bilirubin is greater than 1.8 mg/dL, this test will be ineffective.

Calculi can be demonstrated either as filling defects or as a nonopacifying gallbladder. Tumors and polyps may be visualized in a similar manner.

Cholecystokinin (CCK) cholecystography may be used in those patients with a history suggestive of biliary calculous disease, but with a normal oral cholecystogram and a normal ultrasound (see next section). Normal gallbladder will demonstrate a volume reduction of greater than 50% in 20 min with this test. Duodenal aspiration of bile is usually done in conjunction with this test. A finding of cholesterol monohydrate or calcium bilirubinate crystals constitutes an abnormal or positive test.

Sphincter of Oddi maintains a resting pressure of 300 mm water during starvation, approximately that of the maximal expulsive force of the gallbladder. Following a meal, this is reduced to 100 mm water. Bile secretion, on the other hand, stops at a pressure of 360 mm water. The appearance of jaundice with a totally obstructed common bile duct depends on the presence and function of the gallbladder. In the presence of a functioning gallbladder, jaundice occurs 46–48 h following obstruction, whereas in its absence, jaundice may occur within 6 h.

Motor Dysfunction   Biliary dyskinesia, originally referring to all functional disturbances of biliary tract motility, now refers to a motor disorder of the sphincter of Oddi. Experimentally induced pain has been shown to occur when the gallbladder is stimulated to contract with cholecystokinin or a fatty meal against a closed sphincter of Oddi. With distention of the bile duct by a balloon catheter, a similar colicky pain results.

DIAGNOSIS OF BILIARY TRACT DISEASE

(See also ''Jaundice'' in Chap. 23.)

Radiologic Studies

Routine Abdominal X-Rays   Demonstrate radiopaque stones in up to 15% of cases. Generally, bile pigment calculi are nonradiopaque unless they contain sufficient amounts of calcium. Pure cholesterol and mixed calculi are nonradiopaque, whereas calcium carbonate stones are all radiopaque.

PERCUTANEOUS TRANSHEPATIC CHOLANGIOGRAPHY (PTC), ENDOSCOPIC RETROGRADE CHOLANGIOPANCREATOGRAPHY (ERCP)   (See ''Jaundice'' in Chap. 23.)

Operative Cholangiography   This test has become routine for many surgeons and even mandatory for others; performed in the operating room at the time of cholecystectomy to demonstrate common bile duct stones. Others adopt a policy of selective cholangiography, employing this modality only in certain instances such as ultrasound documentation of common duct stones, biochemical or clinical evidence of obstructive jaundice, dilatation of the common bile duct, cholangitis, or the presence of preoperative pancreatitis.

This technique is used to avoid unnecessary common bile duct exploration and also to identify common duct calculi that have escaped detection by palpation.

Cholangiogram can be obtained through the cystic duct or through a T tube placed at the time of common bile duct exploration. A complete study demonstrates filling of the duodenum, absence of filling defects (calculi) in the common bile and hepatic ducts, and a smooth taper of the distal common bile duct.

Ultrasonography and Computed Tomography

Gray-scale B-mode ultrasonography has a diagnostic accuracy over 90% and in most institutions has essentially replaced oral cholecystography as the diagnostic modality of choice for uncomplicated cholelithiasis. Especially useful in the pregnant patient, the patient who is vomiting, in the emergency setting, and in the jaundiced patient. Computed tomography (CT) has little role in the diagnosis of calculous disease of the gallbladder.

Isotopic Scans   A variety of ^{99m}Tc-labeled iminodiacetic acid isotopes that are excreted by the liver and concentrated by the gallbladder have been used to evaluate gallbladder function and pathology. Nonvisualization of the gallbladder is seen with cystic duct obstruction and acute cholecystitis. Visualization of the gallbladder effectively excludes acute cholecystitis. This test can also be used in the jaundiced patient.

Cholangiomanometry   This procedure is used widely in Europe, but rarely in North America. It is an intraoperative technique that determines bile duct pressure and flow of an infused solution into the bile duct.

Choledochoscopy   Both rigid and flexible choledochoscopes can be inserted into the supraduodenal common bile duct to visualize the lumen of the extrahepatic ducts. Stones, tumors, and strictures can be seen. Additionally, choledochoscopy can aid in the extraction of common duct stones at the time of surgery.

TRAUMA

Penetrating and Nonpenetrating Injuries of the Gallbladder

Injuries of the gallbladder occur in 1.9–8.6% of cases of major abdominal trauma. Gunshot and stab wounds are usual causes of penetrating injuries. Much rarer are nonpenetrating injuries occurring after automobile accidents, kicks, blows, and falls. Isolated gallbladder injuries occur much more frequently following penetrating trauma.

Types of injuries include contusion, avulsion, rupture, and traumatic cholecystitis. Contusion presents with vague abdominal symptoms and requires no special treatment unless necrosis and perforation occur. Avulsion usually follows blunt trauma and results in the gallbladder hanging by its neck or cystic duct and artery; volvulus may result. Traumatic cholecystectomy has been reported. Laceration commonly occurs after penetrating injuries. Delayed rupture occurs days to weeks following blunt injury. Traumatic cholecystitis is unusual and is due to bleeding into the gallbladder lumen. Occasionally hemobilia occurs.

Effects of Intraperitoneal Bile   If infected, bile that escapes into the peritoneal cavity causes a fulminant and often fatal peritonitis. If sterile, a much milder chemical peritonitis ensues. Penetrating wounds therefore are potentially more dangerous because of the possibility of secondary infection of the spilled bile. With time, the initially innocuous sterile bile may become encysted or produce ascites. Patients may even develop shock with ongoing chemical peritonitis and third-space fluid losses.

Clinical Manifestations   Diagnosis is usually entertained preoperatively with penetrating injuries in contrast to blunt injuries. Diagnosis following blunt trauma may be delayed up to 36 h, as sterile bile elicits only minimal symptoms. Shock and severe right upper quadrant abdominal pain should make one suspicious of the diagnosis. A fulminant bacterial peritonitis may ensue; or if the leakage is minimal, ascites or an intraperitoneal cyst may develop late. Whereas the finding of bile-stained fluid during diagnostic paracentesis is suggestive, the diagnosis is usually made at celiotomy.

Treatment   Appropriate treatment depends on the severity of the injury and associated injuries. Generally, best to remove the injured gallbladder, as cholecystectomy in an otherwise healthy gallbladder is easy to perform. Cholecystostomy can be used for extensive laceration or traumatic cholecystitis. Simple suture of a laceration may be done.

Injury of the Extrahepatic Bile Ducts

Solitary penetrating wounds to the bile duct are rare; usually there is associated injury to other organs. The clinical manifestations are similar to those of gallbladder injury, and diagnosis is difficult.

Meticulous exploration should be done as well as a Kocher maneuver to exclude perforation of the bile duct behind the duodenum. Treatment depends on the operative findings. Tangential injuries may be treated by primary repair. Partial transection should be treated by primary repair with T-tube drainage of the bile duct. Complete transection of the bile duct may be treated in a similar fashion, although a higher incidence of late stricture formation has been reported with this technique. Therefore, treatment should entail anastomosis of the proximal end of the duct to a Roux en Y limb of jejunum.

Operative Injury of the Bile Duct

Most injuries to the extrahepatic biliary duct system are iatrogenic, occurring during the course of cholecystectomy. Seventy percent are unrecognized at the time of surgery. Various factors have been implicated including cholecystectomy on a contracted gallbladder, intimate association between the ampulla of the gallbladder and the common hepatic duct (as is seen in Mirizzi syndrome), "blind control" of hemorrhage, and excessive tension when ligating the cystic duct. Injuries are also more likely to occur in the setting of an emergency operation such as for acute cholecystitis.

Diagnosis   Injuries are recognized at surgery in only 15%; in the remainder the diagnosis is made postoperatively when either jaundice appears or a biliocutaneous fistula develops. Jaundice usually occurs in 2–3 days but may not appear for several weeks. Ascending cholangitis as well as hepatomegaly may occur. Percutaneous transhepatic cholangiography is the diagnostic test of choice.

Treatment   Preoperative management includes a high-protein, low-fat diet, and fat-soluble vitamins, particularly vitamin K. If present, portal hypertension and bleeding varices preempt repair of the common bile duct.

Operative Approach   If injury is recognized during surgery, immediate reconstruction should be done. End-to-end anastomosis over a T tube may be tried, but late stricture develops in 50%. With complete transection, a mucosa-to-mucosa anastomosis between the proximal bile duct and a Roux en Y limb of jejunum should be done. With late diagnosis, a similar approach should be employed. If not possible, a side-to-side anastomosis between the left hepatic duct and a Roux en Y of jejunum (Hepp-Soupault) is preferable to the Smith transhepatic pull-through technique. The Longmire procedure, with transection of the left lobe of the liver and anastomosis of the jejunum to a dilated intrahepatic duct, has been discouraging.

Operative mortality following stricture repair is 8%. Seventy percent achieve a satisfactory result after one or more operative procedures.

GALLSTONES

Composition   Main elements involved in gallstone formation are cholesterol, bile pigment, and calcium. In Western cultures, most stones are mixed and made up of all three constituents. Pure cholesterol stones are uncommon. Bilirubin pigment stones are also uncommon, and have a smooth glistening green or black surface. Pigmented stones may be "pure," or consist of calcium bilirubinate. "Pure" pigment stones are usually associated with hemolysis, e.g., in sickle cell patients or in patients following cardiac valve replacement.

Formation Gallstones form when solids settle out of solution. Solubility of cholesterol depends on concentrations of conjugated bile salts, phospholipids, and cholesterol in bile. Lecithin is the predominant phospholipid in bile; and in conjunction with bile salts, maintains cholesterol in solution. This relationship can be demonstrated on triangular coordinates by plotting the percentages of cholesterol, lecithin, and bile salts. The limits of micellar liquid in which bile is less saturated with cholesterol is located beneath a small curve on the triangular coordinates. Above this level, solid crystalline cholesterol appears, and gallstones form.

Many factors are implicated in the formation of cholesterol gallstones. These include constitutional elements (an example is the Pima Indians, in whom the incidence of gallstones approaches 70%), bacteria, fungi, reflux of intestinal and pancreatic fluid, hormones, and bile stasis.

Reflux theory is based on presence of pancreatic enzymes such as trypsin and phospholipase A in gallbladders of patients with cholelithiasis. Hormonal influence is implicated on the basis of an associated of gallstones with parity, diabetes, hyperthyroidism, and predominance in females.

Stasis may play a large role in formation of gallstones. Functional disorders or mechanical blockage of the common bile duct may be responsible. Interruption of bile flow into the intestine is associated with interruption in enterohepatic circulation is disturbed, accompanied by a decrease in output of bile salts and phospholipids, reducing solubility of cholesterol.

Dissolution agents such as chenodeoxycholic acid have been investigated as a possible regimen to either prevent stone formation or dissolve stones already formed. This orally administered agent replenishes the bile acid pool and reduces cholesterol synthesis and secretion.

Asymptomatic Gallstones

Rarely reported. Liberal use of ultrasonography and cholecystography has resulted in diagnosis of gallstones in patients without symptoms referable to the biliary tract. In a few series, symptoms developed in 50% and serious complications in 20% of patients. Other studies have shown a much smaller chance of symptoms developing over time. Surgical intervention is *not* indicated in the patient with asymptomatic gallstones.

Cystic Duct Obstruction

Calculi may impact in the cystic duct or neck of the gall-bladder, resulting in a hydrops. The bile is absorbed and gallbladder becomes filled with a mucinous material (white bile). Gallbladder is usually tender and palpable; jaundice may occur if the common duct is encroached upon. Early cholecystectomy is indicated to prevent perforation and complications of biliary tract infections.

Choledocholithiasis

Common duct stones are found in approximately 12% of patients undergoing cholecystectomy. Most originate in the gallbladder and pass into the common duct via the cystic duct. Some form primarily in the bile duct. In patients with parasitic infections such as *Clonorchis sinensis,* and in the Oriental population, stones may form in the hepatic or common duct itself. Both extrahepatic and intrahepatic bile ducts become dilated. Duct walls thicken; and secondary biliary cirrhosis, bile duct proliferation, and fibrosis of the portal tracts occur. Ascending cholangitis and occasionally liver abscesses may also occur, with *E. coli* being the usual offending organism.

Clinical Manifestations   Symptoms are variable. May be asymptomatic for years. Typically, patient has colicky pain in right upper quadrant radiating to right scapula with intermittent jaundice, pale stools, and dark urine. Unlike malignant obstruction, jaundice is usually not intense. In addition, unlike neoplastic obstruction, gallbladder is not distended because of inflammation of its wall (Courvoisier's law).

Elevation in serum bilirubin and alkaline phosphatase occurs. Prothrombin time may be elevated due to poor absorption of the fat-soluble vitamin K.

Charcot's triad of abdominal pain, fever, and jaundice is often seen in ascending cholangitis. The diagnosis can be established with either PTC or ERCP.

Treatment   When surgery is performed on the jaundiced patient, exploration of the common bile duct is usually indicated. Criteria for common duct exploration include: (1) a positive cholangiogram, (2) palpable stones within the common duct, (3) a dilated common bile duct, and (4) significant jaundice or a history of jaundice. Other indications include cholangitis, gallstone pancreatitis, multiple small stones in the gallbladder, and an inflamed gallbladder that is empty of stones. Of course, an intraoperative cholangiogram will dictate the necessity of common duct exploration.

The best time for exploration of the common bile duct is during the initial procedure of cholecystectomy. Acute cholecystitis does not increase the risk. Choledochotomy increases the operative mortality by only 0.2–1.2% in the jaundiced patient. Early operation for gallstone pancreatitis is not associated with a higher morbidity or mortality unless the patient has severe pancreatitis (i.e., three or more of Ranson's criteria).

To avoid a negative duct exploration, intraoperative cholangiography should be performed. Positive findings include an abnormally enlarged duct (greater than 12 mm) or the presence of filling defects such as stones in the common bile duct.

Preoperative antibiotics and vitamin K should be given if indicated. The goal of common duct exploration is the complete removal of stones and sludge from the duct and free passage into the duodenum. Balloon-tipped catheters and special forceps may aid in the extraction of stones.

Intraoperatively, if the stone cannot be extracted, choledochoduodenostomy is indicated if the duct is dilated, or if the stones are felt to represent primary common bile duct stones. Transduodenal sphincteroplasty is indicated when there is no ductal dilatation, when the stone is impacted in the distal duct, or in the face of pancreatitis.

Preoperative endoscopic papillotomy and stone extraction have been employed by some groups with great success. Also indicated in the patient who is medically unfit for surgery.

Retained Common Duct Stones   If stones are noted to be present on the postoperative cholangiogram, many approaches are available. Small stones may be disregarded, as they often pass on their own, and most will remain asymptomatic. Contact dissolution therapy with Capmul 8210, a mono-octanoin, has been used with success.

Another approach employs extraction of the stone or stones through a matured T-tube tract using the Dormia basket under fluoroscopic guidance.

If the T tube has been removed, endoscopic papillotomy and stone extraction may be applied. Operative intervention is indicated if the nonoperative methods fail.

Most intrahepatic stones will pass into the distal ducts, where they are extractable. If not, there have been recent reports of successful disintegration with the biliary lithotripter. If the calculus remains, liver damage may ensue, requiring hepatic resection.

Biliary Enteric Fistula and Gallstone Ileus

Biliary enteric fistulas usually develop between the gallbladder and duodenum. Mechanical obstruction of the intestinal tract occurs rarely. Gallstone ileus (obstruction of the intestinal tract by a gallstone) accounts for only 1–2% of mechanical obstructions.

High predilection for females. Typically occurs in the aged, and associated diseases such as diabetes and cardiovascular disorders are common.

The process usually begins with a gallstone which erodes into an adjacent viscera adherent from previous inflammation or even perforation. The stone may then pass distally and obstruct, usually at the ileocecal valve. Rarely, the stone enters the peritoneal cavity and causes an extrinsic obstruction. The fistulous tract may connect the gallbladder with the duodenum, stomach, jejunum, ileum, or colon.

The cholecystoenteric fistula usually closes. Obstruction occurs with larger stones, and the commonest site is the terminal ileum.

Clinical Manifestations   A past history of cholelithiasis is often present. Sometimes acute cholecystitis immediately precedes the onset of gallstone ileus. Jaundice is uncommon, and the clinical picture is usually dominated by signs and symptoms of small bowel obstruction.

The diagnosis is rarely made preoperatively. Classic radiographic triad of air in the biliary tree, bowel obstruction, and a radiopaque stone lodged in the intestine is seen in only 20% of cases.

Treatment   Biliary enteric fistulas are managed by cholecystectomy and closure of the intestinal opening.

Gallstone ileus is treated with nasogastric decompression and fluid and electrolyte restoration. Operative therapy includes extracting the obstructing stone through a proximal enterotomy, careful search of the remainder of the bowel for other calculi, and cholecystectomy with closure of the fistula if the patient's general condition permits. Interval cholecystectomy and closure of the fistula is indicated if not done at the first operation because of a high recurrence rate, and the association with gallbladder carcinoma.

INFLAMMATORY AND OTHER BENIGN LESIONS

Cholecystitis

Inflammation of the gallbladder, cholecystitis, is associated with calculi in 85–95% of cases. Another cause is stasis with contact between stagnant bile and the gallbladder wall. Bacterial infections have also been implicated, as 60% of patients with cholecystitis have positive bile cultures. *E. coli,* streptococci, *Aerobacter aerogenes, Salmonella,* and clostridia have all been isolated. Pancreatic juice, a known chemical irritant, has also been suggested as a cause of cholecystitis.

ACUTE CHOLECYSTITIS   Most cases are due to stones impacted in Hartmann's pouch obstructing the neck of the gallbladder or cystic duct. The stones cause mucosal ischemia, necrosis, and ulceration with resultant edema and impaired venous return. Perforation may result with pericholecystic abscess formation, fistulization, or free perforation with bile peritonitis.

Acute cholecystitis has been reported in the posttraumatic and postsurgical patient and has also been seen in sepsis, collagen disease, hypertensive vascular disease, and cystic artery thrombosis. Malignancy is rarely a cause.

Clinical Manifestations   Most patients have a history of cholelithiasis or biliary colic. Occurs more commonly in caucasians, with the greatest incidence between the fourth and eighth decades.

Onset of symptoms frequently follows a heavy, fatty, or fried meal. Pain is typically located in the right upper quadrant and midepigastrium with radiation to the scapula or interscapular area. Fever and vomiting may be present. Gallbladder may be palpable, and guarding or rebound may be elicited. Mild icterus, if present, is due to compression of the bile duct by edema or a stone lodged in the ampulla. Choledocholithiasis should be suspected with moderate or marked jaundice.

The differential diagnosis includes peptic ulcer perforation, appendicitis, pancreatitis, hepatitis, myocardial ischemia or infarction, pneumonia, pleurisy, and herpes zoster.

Often a leukocytosis with left shift is present. Flat plate

examination of the abdomen reveals a stone in 20% of cases. Serum bilirubin and amylase should be obtained as well as an electrocardiogram to rule out myocardial disease. Oral cholecystography is not indicated. An ultrasonogram may demonstrate both calculi and gallbladder wall thickening. Radionuclide scanning with DISIDA or PIPIDA is a very effective diagnostic study, although false examinations have been reported.

Treatment There are two major schools of thought concerning treatment and the optimal timing of surgery. Early operation is defined as one performed within 72 h of the onset of symptoms; intermediate operation is one performed between 72 h and cessation of symptoms. Delayed surgery occurs at 6 weeks to 3 months after complete resolution of inflammation.

Advocates of delayed surgery argue the following: (1) Most cases of acute cholecystitis subside on conservative management; (2) early operation may result in the spread of infection; (3) technical errors are more likely to occur in the presence of acute inflammation, and common duct exploration is more difficult; (4) many of these patients have associated medical problems and therefore represent poor surgical risks.

The nonoperative management includes restriction of food and fluids by mouth, nasogastric suction, antibiotics, and analgesics. Demerol is recommended over morphine, since the latter causes more sphincteric spasm. Anticholinergics are used by some.

The advocates of early or intermediate cholecystectomy emphasize that there is a high incidence of exacerbation in those patients who respond initially, as well as a 5% failure rate to respond to medical therapy. The mortality rates are similar to those for the elective procedure. The technical difficulty is not as great as some claim and if performed within the first 72 h, cholecystectomy is very safe.

Early operation is favored in the United States. The mortality rate is comparable between emergency and elective cholecystectomy. Furthermore with early surgery, the period of disability and morbidity is lowered.

Author's Approach Early operation is performed if the patient presents within 3 days of onset of symptoms. If the patient is extremely ill, surgery should be done within 24 h of admission; either cholecystectomy or cholecystostomy under local anesthesia can be done. In the face of severe inflammation, cholecystostomy should be performed. Patients with progressive symptoms under medical management warrant surgery. If the patient presents after 72 h and shows signs of improvement, cholecystectomy is deferred for 6 weeks. If they worsen, there is no hesitation in operating after the "golden" 24-h period.

The indications for common bile duct exploration are the same as in the elective situation. If inflammation compromises a safe exploration and dissection, a cholecystostomy is done and the stones extracted from the gallbladder.

Emphysematous Cholecystitis   This rare form of acute, usually gangrenous cholecystitis, is characterized by the presence of gas in the wall of the gallbladder. It is more common in men and is usually secondary to acute cholecystitis secondarily infected by gas-forming bacilli. Clinically, the presentation is similar to acute cholecystitis. These patients are frequently diabetic. The diagnostic radiographic findings include a gas-filled gallbladder, and gas in the wall of the gallbladder or even outside of the gallbladder. Antibiotics should cover clostridial and coliform organisms. Treatment is cholecystectomy, but if not feasible, cholecystostomy. Perforation occurs frequently, and choledocholithiasis occurs in 9%. Mortality rate is high.

CHRONIC CHOLECYSTITIS   Chronic inflammation of the gallbladder is usually associated with cholelithiasis. Rokitansky-Aschoff sinuses are buried crypts of mucosa dipping into the mucosa. Hydrops of the gallbladder occurs with cystic duct obstruction, and although initially sterile, the bile may become secondarily infected.

Clinical Manifestations   Usually presents with intermittent right upper quadrant and midepigastric abdominal pain radiating to the scapula. Nausea, anorexia, and fatty food intolerance may occur. Pain may occur, with inspiration and tenderness elicited on palpation. The diagnosis can be established by either oral cholecystogram or ultrasound.

Treatment   Cholecystectomy. In the diabetic patient, early cholecystectomy. Seventy-five percent of patients will be completely relieved of their pain, whereas 25% will have residual pain unrelated to the biliary tract.

Postcholecystectomy Syndrome.   Refers to symptoms that develop subsequent to or continue in spite of cholecystectomy. Usually due to hiatal hernia, peptic ulceration, or pancreatitis. Other causes include retained common bile duct stone, residual cystic duct stones, or spasm of the sphincter of Oddi. The etiology is best defined by ERCP.

The cystic duct stump may rarely be the cause of pain, but only if there is a retained stone in its lumen.

ACALCULOUS CHOLECYSTITIS   Frequently complicates burns, sepsis, multiple system organ failure, cardiovascular disease, diabetes, prolonged illness, or a major operation.

The incidence of chronic acalculous cholecystitis is less than 5%. Possible etiologies include kinking, fibrosis, and obstruction of the cystic duct by tumor or anomalous vessels, ischemia and gangrene secondary to vascular thrombosis, spasm or fibrosis of the sphincter of Oddi, diabetes and collagen diseases, and infections.

The treatment is either cholecystectomy or cholecystostomy.

Cholangitis

Usually due to choledocholithiasis, but has been associated with choledochal cysts, carcinoma of the bile duct, and following sphincteroplasty. Multiple liver abscesses may occur as a result of cholangitis. The clinical picture consists of intermittent fever, rigors, upper abdominal pain, jaundice, and pruritus.

Patients should be treated with broad-spectrum intravenous antibiotics directed particularly at *E. coli*. Surgical intervention is indicated when the infection does not respond to antibiotics. If the patient is extremely ill, the common bile duct may initially be decompressed with a T tube, with stone removal occurring at a second operation.

Acute Suppurative Cholangitis   This condition of pus in the biliary tract usually required urgent laparotomy. Currently patients may be managed initially by drainage via ERCP or PTC.

Charcot's triad includes jaundice, chills and fever, and right upper quadrant abdominal pain. Reynolds and Dargan added shock and central nervous system depression to this triad.

The typical clinical picture is that of an elderly patient with fever and jaundice. Hypotension, confusion, and lethargy occur in 20%. Bilirubin, SGOT, and alkaline phosphatase are elevated.

Operative findings include gross distention of the bile duct with frank pus. The obstruction may be due to stones or tumor. Spontaneous bile duct perforation has been reported. Mainstay of treatment is large doses of antibiotics followed by urgent decompression. At laparotomy, T-tube drainage is usually employed; although with ducts greater than 1.5 cm, choledochoduodenostomy has been used by some with good results.

Cholangiohepatitis

Also known as "recurrent pyogenic cholangitis"; seen almost exclusively among the Chinese. In Hong Kong it is the commonest disease of the biliary tract and represents the third most common abdominal emergency.

The etiologic factors include hemolysis associated with malaria, ascariasis, and clonorchiasis-induced stone formation. Spasm of the sphincter of Oddi ensues with bile flow obstruction and resultant cholangiohepatitis.

Pathology The gallbladder wall is thickened, as is the common bile duct. The stones are usually pigmented and may contain an ovum, ascarid, or adult *Clonorchis* worm. The most remarkable finding is that of both dilated and strictured intrahepatic bile ducts. Frank abscess formation may occur.

Clinical Manifestations The diagnosis should be considered when a patient in an endemic area presents with jaundice, pain, and pyrexia. The pain is usually in the right upper quadrant. Reccurrence of symptoms is the rule.

Most patients are toxic at presentation with high fevers. The white blood cell count is often greater than 15,000 and the serum bilirubin is elevated. Routine x-rays may demonstrate air in the biliary tree, representing either infection by a gas-forming organism or a biliary enteric fistula. ERCP, PTC, and intraoperative cholangiograms are diagnostic, revealing intrahepatic stones, strictures, and possibly the parasites themselves.

Treatment Patients should be treated by antibiotics and then surgery.

Cholecystostomy is done for the seriously ill patient showing signs of rupture of the gallbladder. The definitive procedure consists of removal of stones and debris from the bile duct and improving drainage of the duct. This can be accomplished by either choledochoduodenostomy or Roux en Y choledochojejunostomy if the duct is dilated; or transduodenal sphincteroplasty for a nondilated duct. The gallbladder, although not usually involved, is removed. Hepatic abscesses are treated by either drainage or resection.

The prognosis is generally guarded, with recurrence common. In advanced cases, particularly with multiple abscesses, patients eventually die of progressive liver failure or sepsis.

Sclerosing Cholangitis

Involves part or all of the extrahepatic biliary tract. Also called *obliterative cholangitis* and *stenosing cholangitis*.

Associated with ulcerative colitis, Crohn's disease, Riedel struma, retroperitoneal fibrosis, and porphyria cutanea tarda. Most patients in fourth to sixth decades, more common in males.

Cause unknown. Theories postulated include viral infection, autoimmune disorder, and collagen disease.

Pathology Diffuse thickening of the wall of extrahepatic and/or intrahepatic biliary tract, with luminal narrowing. May involve all or only part of the duct system. Gallbladder usually spared. Liver biopsy shows bile stasis, or cirrhosis in long-standing cases. May be confused histologically with cholangiocarcinoma.

Clinical Manifestations Jaundice, right upper quadrant pain, nausea, vomiting, chills and fever. Signs and symptoms of portal hypertension with cirrhosis in long-standing cases. Diagnosis by ERCP. At surgery, severe inflammation in porta hepatis with a cordlike common bile duct.

Treatment Medical therapy first, but both surgery and drug therapy are only palliative.

Asymptomatic patient requires no treatment. Steroids and other immunosuppressive agents have been tried for the symptomatic patient.

If no improvement, or if cholangitis develops, surgery indicated. For a stenotic segment, excision and biopsy indicated with Roux en Y jejunostomy. Stricture of confluence treated by excision and Roux en Y hepaticojejunostomy. For diffuse involvement, T-tube insertion with postoperative steroids and serial cholangiograms to follow progress of disease. For liver failure, cirrhosis, or marked intrahepatic involvement, liver tranplantation is indicated.

Fibrosis or Stenosis of the Sphincter of Oddi

Pathogenesis not known. Factors implicated include longstanding spasm, biliary tract infection, and irritation from stones in common bile duct.

Clinical Manifestations Primarily abdominal pain in right upper quadrant, radiating to shoulder, and intermittent. Many are postcholecystectomy; others are jaundiced.

Treatment Diagnosis often made at surgery when a 3-mm Bâkes dilator is difficult to pass through ampulla of Vater. Surgical therapy involves either transduodenal sphincteroplasty or choledochoduodenostomy. Endoscopic papillotomy may also be very useful.

Pappilitis

Due to acute and subacute inflammatory changes, with stenosis as the final result. Associated with postcholecystectomy syndrome in 30%, common duct dilatation in 50%, biliary disease without stones, obstructive jaundice, and liver damage. Treatment is sphincteroplasty.

TUMORS

Carcinoma of the Gallbladder

Fifth most common GI tract carcinoma. Accounts for 4% of all carcinomas. Eighty percent are female, and many are over age 60.

Pathology Ninety percent of patients with carcinoma of the gallbladder have associated gallstones. Five to ten percent of symptomatic patients over age 65 have carcinoma.

Most are adenocarcinomas, remainder are either squamous or undifferentiated. Metastasize to lymph nodes of common bile duct, pancreas, and duodenum; directly to liver; or to the omentum, duodenum, colon, porta hepatis, and lung.

Clinical Manifestations Signs and symptoms similar to those of cholelithiasis and cholecystitis such as abdominal pain, nausea, vomiting, jaundice, and palpable mass.

Lab data usually noncontributory. In many, carcinoma found incidentally at cholecystectomy.

Treatment Surgery only hope for cure, albeit very small. Long-term survival usually seen only when microscopic disease incidentally discovered on routine cholecystectomy. Some recommend excision of adjacent liver or segment V. Best results seen with cholecystectomy and regional lymphadenectomy, whereby hepatoduodenal ligament is skeletonized from duodenum to porta hepatis. Overall 5-year survival is 2%, for tumor confined to mucosa and submucosa, 64%.

Carcinoma of the Extrahepatic Bile Ducts Exclusive of the Periampullary Region

Occurs more frequently in males and in the sixth and seventh decades. Lesions at the hepatic duct confluence referred to as *Klatskin tumors*.

Pathology Usually a small lesion. One-third occur in

common bile duct, one-fifth at junction of hepatic and cystic ducts, and the rest above this level. Grossly, a firm, circumscribed, grayish tan mass causing a "napkin ring" obstruction. Rarely, polypoid. All are adenocarcinomas. May metastasize to liver, regional lymph nodes, and adjacent structures. Cholelithiasis may be a contributing factor.

Clinical Manifestations Rapid onset of jaundice, preceded by pruritus, weight loss, and abdominal pain. Cholangitis frequent. Liver may be palpable, gallbladder palpable with distal lesions. Serum bilirubin high with fluctuating levels. ERCP may be diagnostic, although transhepatic cholangiography has highest yield.

Treatment Surgery potentially curative. Tumors may be resected or bypassed by anastomosing dilated hepatic duct system to Roux en Y loop of jejunum. Distal third lesions treated by pancreaticoduodenectomy. Middle third tumors treated by resection and reconstruction to a Roux en Y jejunostomy. Upper third lesions treated by resection including hilus and portion of liver if necessary.

Radiation therapy not consistently effective. For unresectable lesions and poor-risk patients, percutaneous transhepatic drainage.

Sclerosing carcinoma arises from major hepatic ducts near hilus and extends into intrahepatic ducts, clinically similar to other carcinomas of the extrahepatic biliary tract. Male/female ratio of 8:1. May progress to hepatic coma, renal failure, or septicemia.

OPERATIONS ON THE BILIARY TRACT

Antibiotic Therapy Patients over age 70 with acute cholecystitis, common bile duct stones, jaundice, or diabetes at increased risk of infection. Antibiotics indicated in this group and also in those undergoing T-tube cholangiogram. *E. coli* and *Klebsiella* most common organisms cultured.

Cholecystostomy Indicated for decompression and drainage of a distended, hydroptic, or empyematous gallbladder in poor-risk patients or those with severe inflammation prohibiting safe dissection.

Technique. Gallbladder decompressed through a pursestring suture in the fundus followed by extraction of calculi and then closure of purse-string around a catheter introduced through a stab wound. If the fundus is necrotic, should excise this part and the remainder of the gallbladder closed around the catheter.

Cholecystectomy Avoid common duct injury and leave a short cystic duct remnant. For the cirrhotic patient, increased bleeding may be anticipated and subtotal cholecystectomy is indicated.

Technique. Incision may be midline, right subcostal (Kocher), or right paramedian. Veil of peritoneum between ampulla and hepatoduodenal ligament incised. Cystic duct isolated and surrounded by a suture, cystic artery isolated and doubly ligated prior to division. Dissection begun from fundus after incising peritoneum close to liver, down to cystic duct pedicle. This duct ligated close to common duct. Drainage not routinely required.

Operations of the Common Bile Duct Include exploration for calculi, repair of injured bile duct, stenosis of the sphincter of Oddi, and bypass procedures for obstructive jaundice.

Initial Exploration for Choledocholithiasis. Indications previously enumerated. Usually done in conjunction with cholecystectomy. After vertical incision is made in common bile duct, calculi are extracted with a combination of stone forceps, scoops, balloon-tipped catheters, and irrigation. Choledochoscopy may be employed if necessary. A #3 Bâkes dilator should easily pass into the duodenum. The choledochotomy is closed over a T tube, which is brought out through a separate stab wound. Completion cholangiogram is obtained to exclude retained stones. After 1 week, a T-tube cholangiogram is obtained; if negative, the tube is removed.

Transduodenal Choledochotomy. Sphincteroplasty. Indicated when a stone is impacted in distal duct, if Bâkes dilator does not pass, or for fibrosis of sphincter of Oddi. Also used for recurrent or multiple stones, especially if common bile duct is not enlarged enough to perform choledochoduodenostomy. Procedure entails division of sphincter of Oddi at "11:00" position to avoid injuring pancreatic duct, removal of stone, and approximating duodenal to common duct mucosa with interrupted absorbable sutures.

Operative Procedures for Recurrent Choledocholithiasis. Choledochoduodenostomy. Indicated for recurrent stones, multiple stones, or following common duct exploration when clearance of duct is not certain. Procedure entails Kocher maneuver (mobilization of duodenum by incising lateral peritoneal reflection) followed by side-to-side anastomosis of common duct to duodenum.

Repair of Injured or Strictured Common Duct. If transection noted at time of cholecystectomy, primary repair with end-to-end anastomosis over a T tube is indicated. If stricture developed following injury to duct, direct repair is still indicated. If stricture is extensive, a decompressive procedure is indicated.

Decompressive Procedures.   Usually obstructed biliary tract is decompressed by anastomosis to a Roux en Y jejunostomy limb. Depending on the level of obstruction, the common bile duct, the hepatic duct, the gallbladder, or the left hepatic duct may be used.

31 PANCREAS

ANATOMY

Lies behind stomach in lesser sac. Composed of head, body, and tail. Uncinate process curls behind head. Superior mesenteric vein and artery lie behind neck of pancreas. Duct of Wirsung is major duct, 3–4 mm diameter, joins common bile duct at papilla of Vater. Minor duct is Santorini; joins main duct in neck, drains via minor papilla into duodenum. 5–10% have Santorini as major drainage of pancreas, with vestigial Wirsung; this is *pancreas divisum*. Arterial supply to head is via anterosuperior and posterosuperior pancreaticoduodenal arcades from gastroduodenal, which anastomose with anteroinferior and posteroinferior pancreaticoduodenal arteries from the superior mesenteric. Splenic, inferior pancreatic arteries supply body. Venous drainage closely parallels arterial supply. In 12% the right hepatic artery arises from SMA and courses behind pancreas and bile duct. Lymphatic drainage is diffuse. Innervation is sympathetic via splanchnic nerves and parasympathetic via celiac branch of posterior (right) vagus.

Anatomic Variants Annular pancreas rare. Duodenum is encircled by head of pancreas. Symptoms are from duodenal obstruction. Cure is duodenojejunostomy. Heterotopic (accessory) pancreas most common in stomach (antrum, greater curvature) or Meckel's.

PHYSIOLOGY

Exocrine Pancreas

FLUID AND ELECTROLYTE SECRETION *Secretin* (and VIP) stimulate bicarb and water secretion from ductal and centroacinar cells. 1500–2500 mL/day, pH 8.0–8.3, isosmotic, clear fluid, 1–3% protein. Vagus, CCK, and gastrin stimulate enzyme secretion that includes amylase, lipase, trypsinogen, chymotrypsinogen, elastase, phospholipase, ribonuclease, deoxyribonuclease, and colipase. Duodenal enterokinase activates zymogens. Islet hormones, pancreatic polypeptide, somatostatin, and glucagon inhibit exocrine secretion (*par-*

acrine effects). Severe malabsorption (especially fats) results from total enzymatic loss or diversion; however, <90% loss can be well tolerated. Gastric hypersecretion also follows loss of pancreatic secretions.

Endocrine Pancreas

Islets of Langerhans are 1.5% weight of pancreas, 75% beta (insulin), 20% alpha (glucagon), and 5% delta cells (somatostatin, gastrin, pancreatic polypeptide). Glucagon causes glycogenolysis, gluconeogenesis. Insulin causes glucose uptake in muscle, fat, and fibroblasts. Brain (neural cells) and erythrocytes metabolize glucose independent of insulin. Insulin inhibits lipolysis and hepatic glucose production and is a major protein anabolic signal. Major stimulus to insulin secretion is hyperglycemia, but fatty and amino acids also play some role.

PANCREATITIS

Acute Pancreatitis

Etiology 40% caused by gallstones. Mechanism unclear. Bile reflux *(common channel theory)* may play a role, but sterile bile in pancreatic duct not under pressure does not cause pancreatitis. Deconjugated bile salts and lysolecithin are toxic to pancreas. Other 40% from alcoholism, probably due to increased pancreatic ductal pressure with hypersecretion and protein precipitation. Dietary-induced hypertriglyceridemia may play a role in alcoholics. *Postoperative pancreatitis,* which may occur after biliary, gastric, or splenic procedures, has high (≈ 50%) mortality. Metabolic factors have been associated, such as hyperparathyroidism, aminoaciduria, hypertriglyceridemia (type IV), and maybe hemochromatosis. Other factors include vascular stasis, drugs and toxins (methyl alcohol, chlorothiazide), and viral illnesses (mumps, coxsackie).

Clinical Manifestations Severe midepigastric pain radiating through to the back, relieved by sitting, accompanied by severe retching. Upper abdominal tenderness and guarding. 90% have fever, leukocytosis, and tachycardia. Ileus is common. Shock from fluid sequestration and myocardial

TABLE 31-1. Signs Used to Classify Severity of Acute Pancreatitis

At admission	
1. Age > 55	4. LDH > 350 I.U./L
1. WBC > 16,000/mm³	5. SGOT > 250 Frankel units %
3. Glucose > 200 mg/dL	
During initial 48 h	
1. Hematocrit fall > 10%	4. Arterial P_{O_2} < 60 mmHg
2. BUN rise > 5% per mg/dL	5. Base deficit > 4 meq/L
3. Ca^{2+} < 8 mg/dL	6. Fluid sequestration > 6 L

depression may be present. Jaundice in 20–30%. Occasionally carpopedal spasm from hypocalcemia.

Laboratory Studies May show hyperamylasemia, which can be very nonspecific. Cholecystitis, cholangitis, perforated peptic ulcer, strangulated small bowel obstruction, salpingitis, renal failure, macroamylasemia, and mumps are among many that may cause elevated amylase. Serum lipase is specific to the pancreas. Urine amylase clearance is not useful. Calcium may fall; values <7.5 indicate a poor prognosis. Radiographs may show a sentinel loop of bowel air. CT scan can be very useful in predicting severity of disease.

Treatment Critical to care are replacement of fluid and electrolyte losses, monitoring vascular volume (Foley, central line), repeated assessment of hematocrit and electrolytes (include calcium), and bowel rest. NG suction is of no proved benefit in uncomplicated pancreatitis without uncontrolled vomiting. Likewise, drugs such as glucagon, Trasylol, and atropine show no benefit. The routine use of antibiotics is not indicated unless abscess or biliary obstruction is suspected. Surgical intervention is of benefit in biliary pancreatitis but of questionable benefit with other causes. Peritoneal lavage does not influence long-term mortality.

Complications, Morbidity, and Mortality Overall mortality can be predicted via Ranson's criteria (see Table 31-1). Across the board, mortality is 10–15%. *Pseudocyst* is most common complication, usually occurs after 2–3 weeks. Abscess is uncommon but has high mortality and demands open drainage, without which mortality is 100%. Most common organisms are coliforms, *S. faecalis,* and clostridia. Biliary obstruction may occur, more often in chronic disease. Hemorrhage may occur from splenic artery or erosion of mesenteric or portal vessels. Likewise, necrosis may lead to biliary or enteric perforation.

Chronic Pancreatitis

Definition vague. Usually changes that result after repeated episodes of acute pancreatitis. Pancreas becomes small, indurated, nodular with acini and islets surrounded by fibrous tissue. There is ductal stricture and dilatation; calcification is common.

Clinical Manifestations Continuous epigastric/back pain, anorexia, weight loss. Vomiting occurs with acute attacks. Steatorrhea, diabetes may be present. Pseudocysts common. *This picture almost never occurs with repeated episodes of biliary pancreatitis,* compared with alcoholism.

Diagnosis Difficult, at best. ERCP, CT scan are useful. Amylase, lipase of little use. Calcification is pathognomonic.

Treatment Recurrent biliary pancreatitis best managed with cholecystectomy and possible bile duct exploration; this is of little use with alcoholics. With chronic alcoholic pancreatitis, chronic pain, and alternating ductal dilatation and strictures (chain of lakes), longitudinal pancreaticojejunostomy (Peustow procedure) is appropriate. With a small duct, 95% pancreatectomy may be of some benefit, but morbidity is high. Abstinence is critical.

TRAUMA

Mechanisms of Injury Penetrating trauma 70–80% of pancreatic injuries. Adjacent organs are also injured in 70–90%. Blunt trauma may contuse or fracture pancreas. Disruption usually at neck, associated injuries less frequent. Consequences of injury usually are result of parenchymal and ductal disruption, leading to fistula, pseudocyst, or abscess.

Clinical Manifestations Blunt injuries may result in delayed presentation. Abdominal findings may be minimal in absence of hemorrhage or other injuries. CT scans may be helpful. Clinical suspicion and mechanism of injury is important. Negative paracentesis does not exclude injury. Hyperamylasemia is very nonspecific in the multiple-trauma patient.

Treatment Careful and total inspection via lesser space exploration and Kocher maneuver is paramount. Hematomas indicate deeper injury. Damaged tissue should be gently debrided. Without ductal injury, or with minor ductal injury, drainage alone usually suffices. Major distal injuries are best treated by resection. Major injury to the head can be treated with debridement and pyloric exclusion. Pancreaticoduodenectomy is rarely indicated, usually for severe proximal blast injuries or major hemorrhage within or behind the head. *Definition of ductal injury is critical.*

Morbidity and Mortality Complications include fistulas, pseudocysts, infection, and delayed hemorrhage. Usually around 30%. More common after blunt injury. Mortality averages 20%.

CYSTS AND PSEUDOCYSTS

True Cysts

Fluid-filled, with epithelial lining. May be congenital, parasitic, retention, or neoplastic. Most are rare. Cystadenoma and cystadenocarcinoma are relatively uncommon.

Pseudocysts

So called because of no epithelial lining. Made of fibrous wall surrounding pancreatic juice. Majority in lesser sac. Etiology is usually ductal disruption from pancreatitis (75%, alcoholism, biliary) or trauma (25%).

Clinical Manifestations Persistent pain, fever, ileus, usually 2–3 weeks after acute pancreatitis or trauma. Pain is usually epigastric or back. May have palpable mass (75%), nausea, vomiting, jaundice. Serum amylase usually remains moderately elevated.

Diagnosis Most readily made with CT scan or ultrasound. ERCP is usually unnecessary.

Morbidity Includes secondary infection, gastric outlet obstruction, erosion into adjacent organs, rupture, or hemorrhage into cyst.

Treatment Enlarging pseudocysts, or those present for >6 weeks should be treated. The cysts should be allowed to mature; usually takes 6 weeks. Most efficacious is internal drainage, usually via cystogastrostomy, but cystojejunostomy, cystoduodenostomy, and distal pancreatectomy are options. External drainage is indicated only for thin, flimsy cysts or true abscesses. Infected mature cysts may be drained internally. Percutaneous, CT-guided drainage is of questionable value at present. Ruptured cysts and pancreatic ascites are treated by internal drainage.

TUMORS

Carcinoma of the Pancreas and Periampullary Carcinoma

Incidence Pancreatic carcinoma most common of periampullary tumors; manifestations similar. Average age is 60, M > F. Etiologies unclear; smoking, coffee links unproved.

Pathology Adenocarcinoma arises from ducts in 90%, acini in 10%. Often major portion of tumor is fibrous stroma with zone of pancreatitis. Most often in head of pancreas, causing biliary obstruction. May invade portal vein, adjacent organs. Lymph nodes positive in 90%, liver metastasis in 80%. Ampullary and duodenal carcinomas may be diagnosed as pancreatic, cause jaundice early, and thus may be small at presentation. Cystadenoma and cystadenocarcinoma are slow growing, have better prognosis, and should be treated aggressively.

Clinical Manifestations Weight loss most common, pain in 80% is dull, aching, midepigastric and back, relieved by sitting hunched over. Cystadenocarcinoma may be asymptomatic. Progressive jaundice in 75% of head carcinoma. Anorexia, fatigue in 50%. Pruritus is common. Exam shows jaundice, palpable liver (50–70%), palpable gallbladder (30%, if nontender and jaundiced, diagnostic for pancreatic cancer, Courvoisier's law.) Diabetes in 10%. With periampullary carcinoma, pain less frequent, often colicky, jaundice intermittent.

Laboratory and Diagnostic Studies Obstructive jaundice, elevated bilirubin, increased alkaline phosphatase, only mild transaminase elevation (contrast hepatitis). 50–60% have radiologic abnormality (antral, duodenal compression, "reverse 3" sign, widened duodenal C loop). CT scan most accurate, especially with needle aspiration cytology. Transhepatic cholangiography better than ERCP with obstructive jaundice. ERCP may be helpful with body/tail neoplasms or duodenal/ampullary lesions. Intraoperative aspiration cytology is useful for difficult cases.

Treatment and Prognosis Rapidly correct nutrition, anemia, volume status, assess renal function. Transhepatic biliary drainage usually unwarranted. Pancreaticoduodenectomy is only hope for cure. Most useful in localized ampullary, duodenal, or distal bile duct carcinoma. May be helpful in small, confined pancreatic head adenocarcinoma. Overall, only 13% of patients with pancreatic carcinoma are potentially curable, with 1-, 2-, 5-year survivals of 54, 29, 8%. Ampullary survival is 2 times that for pancreatic carcinoma. Unresectable patients may benefit from palliative cholecysto- or choledochoduodenostomy and gastrojejunostomy (duodenal obstruction in 20%). Celiac plexus injection may alleviate pain. Rarely, transhepatic drainage may benefit the poor-risk patient. Combined x-ray therapy and 5-FU may be of some value.

Pancreaticoduodenal Resection This includes resection of antrum of stomach with duodenum, distal bile duct, and head of pancreas to neck, just at level of mesenteric vessels. Reconstruction is via choledocho-, pancreatico-, and gastrojejunostomy, with gastric anastomosis below others, to prevent marginal ulceration. Vagotomy is not necessary. Most patients lose weight with some malabsorption postoperatively. Exocrine supplements may be necessary. Total pancreatectomy is of questionable, if any, advantage and has severe morbidity.

Islet Cell Tumors and Hyperinsulinism

Neoplasm of the beta cells is insulinoma. Hyperinsulinemia causes severe hypoglycemia. Leads to convulsions, depression, coma. Glucose promptly reverses symptoms. Whipple's triad: fasting hypoglycemia (< 50 mg/dL), CNS changes brought on by fasting, reversal of changes with glucose; diagnostic for insulinoma. Measurement will show insulin inappropriately high for ambient glycemia. 75% benign adenomas, 13% suspicious for malignancy, 12% overtly malignant. 15% are multiple. Most are 1–3 cm. May be seen in MEA-I syndrome. Preoperative localization is difficult; may be aided by angiography, selective venous sampling, or CT scan. Treatment is surgical except in advanced metastatic disease, where Streptozotocin is helpful (destroys islets). Intraoperative management includes meticulous inspection of entire gland with excision of adenoma. Intraoperative ultrasound can be useful. Resection is performed for malignancy. Distal pancreatectomy may be of benefit when no lesion is located. In children, nesidioblastosis is diffuse islet hyperplasia, usually controlled with ACTH, cortisone, and diet. If necessary, surgical approach is distal subtotal pancreatectomy.

Gastrinoma

Clinical Manifestations Original Zollinger-Ellison triad: fulminant, atypically located peptic ulcers, extreme gastric hypersecretion, non–beta cell pancreatic islet tumor. May start as simple disease and end up with severe complications (perforation, obstruction, hemorrhage, intractability). Unresponsive to standard medical and surgical therapy. May have high-output diarrhea, steatorrhea.

Diagnosis High basal secretory rates BAO/MAO $\geq$ 0.6, hypertrophic gastric folds, hypergastrinemia or paradoxical rise in gastrin after *secretin* infusion, pancreatic mass on CT.

Pathology and Pathophysiology 2-mm to 10-cm non–beta pancreatic islet cell neoplasms. Various reports of malignant potential, although may be $\geq$ 90%. May have lesion in duodenal wall. Lesions are slow growing, metastasize late; death often from ulcer disease. Seen in MEA-I syndrome (Wermer's: pituitary, parathyroid, pancreas).

Treatment Originally treated with total gastrectomy; however, the use of H_2 antagonists with or without parietal cell vagotomy may control patients with unresectable disease. Efforts should be to completely excise lesions in patients without metastatic disease.

Other Islet Cell Tumors

VIPomas may produce diarrhea, "pancreatic cholera," the WDHA syndrome (*w*atery *d*iarrhea, *h*ypokalemia, and gastric *a*nacidity). 40% benign, 40% malignant, 20% islet hyperplasia. Glucagonomas show cutaneous lesions (necrolytic migratory erythema), diabetes, glossitis, anemia, weight loss, depression, and venous thrombosis. Best treated by resection. Somatostatinomas manifest diabetes, diarrhea, steatorrhea, achlorhydria, gallstones, and abdominal pain. Symptoms all attributable to somatostatin excess.

32 SPLEEN

ANATOMY

Arises along the left side of the dorsal mesogastrium. Weight in the average adult is 75–100 g. Located in the left upper quadrant; superior relationship is the left leaf of diaphragm, protected on all sides by the rib cage. Supported by the splenophrenic, splenorenal, splenocolic, and gastrosplenic ligaments. These ligaments are all avascular except the gastrosplenic, which contains the short gastric vessels. Splenic artery arises from the celiac axis; the splenic vein joins the superior mesenteric vein to form the portal vein.

Accessory spleens found in 14–30% of patients, found in decreasing order of frequency in the splenic hilus, gastrosplenic and splenocolic ligaments, gastrocolic ligament, splenorenal ligament, and greater omentum.

Surrounded by a 1–2-mm capsule. Pulp divided into white, red, and marginal zones. Marginal zone surrounds white pulp, and contains end arterial branches of the central arteries. Lymphocytes, macrophages, and red cells found in marginal zone. Red pulp surrounds marginal zone, and consists of cords and sinuses.

Blood traverses the trabecular arteries that enter the white pulp as central arteries. These central arteries either give off vessels at right angles, or cross the white pulp and end in the marginal zone or red pulp, where they collect in splenic sinuses and then into the pulp veins, the trabecular veins, and ultimately the main splenic vein. Splenic cords are located between the sinuses, and red blood cells must deform to pass from sinus to cord. Total splenic blood flow is 300 mL/min.

PHYSIOLOGY AND PATHOPHYSIOLOGY

Spleen forms both red and white blood cells that enter the circulation only between fifth and eighth month of fetal life. Reticuloendothelial tissue removes cellular elements from circulating blood. With splenomegaly, blood elements pool in the spleen.

Abnormal and aged erythrocytes, abnormal granulocytes, normal and abnormal platelets, and cellular debris are cleared from circulation by the spleen.

Pathologic reduction of cellular elements by the spleen may be due to: (1) excessive destruction, (2) splenic production of antibody directed at cellular element, and (3) splenic inhibition of bone marrow. *Hypersplenism* refers to overactivity of splenic function leading to accelerated removal of any or all of the circulating elements.

Howell-Jolly bodies, nuclear remnants of erythrocytes, are removed by the spleen. Postsplenectomy blood smears therefore contain red cells with Howell-Jolly bodies.

Twenty mL aged red cells are removed per day. Hypoxic, acidotic, and glucose-deprived environment promotes further cell injury; compounded by low ATP levels. Red cell surface area is lost with each passage.

Neutrophil is removed from the circulation with half-life of 6 h. Neutropenia occurs in some hypersplenic states because of either accelerated sequestration or enhanced removal of altered granulocytes.

The platelet survives 10 days in circulation. One-third of the total platelet pool is sequestered in the spleen. Postsplenectomy platelet counts may reach as high as 1 million cells/ mm^3. May be transient, but in the extreme situation may result in intravenous thrombosis.

DIAGNOSTIC CONSIDERATIONS

Evaluation of Size   Normally, not a palpable organ except in 2% of adults. With enlargement, may be felt below left costal margin with a notching on its anteromedial surface.

Routine radiographs useful. Splenomegaly suggested by medial or caudal displacement of stomach bubble, and caudal displacement of splenic flexure. CT scan as well as MRI depict abnormalities such as cysts, abscess, and tumor. Radioisotopic scanning with ^{99m}Tc-sulfur colloid also useful.

Evaluation of Function   Hypersplenism manifest by reduction in the number of red cells, neutrophils, or platelets in the peripheral blood smear; marrow production should increase unless there is concomitant marrow disease. The diagnosis of hemolysis, increased red cell turnover, is supported by a reticulocytosis and increase in serum bilirubin.

Spleen's role in hemolytic anemia can be assessed by determining relative uptake of ^{51}Cr-tagged RBCs by the spleen and liver. A 2:1 spleen/liver ratio implicates the spleen, and anticipates beneficial effects of splenectomy. Radioisotope labeling also used to evaluate neutrophil and platelet survival.

RUPTURE OF THE SPLEEN

(See Chap. 6)

HEMATOLOGIC DISORDERS FOR WHICH SPLENECTOMY IS POTENTIALLY THERAPEUTIC

Hemolytic Anemias

Includes disorders in which there is accelerated destruction of mature RBCs. Classified as congential, where there is an intrinsic red cell defect, and acquired. May be demonstrated by measuring disappearance of ^{51}Cr-labeled RBCs.

Hereditary Spherocytosis Autosomal dominant transmission. Erythrocyte membrane defective, with thickened and spherical shape. Increased osmotic fragility; i.e., lysis occurs at a higher than normal concentration of sodium chloride. The abnormal spherocytic red cells are unable to pass through the spleen and are more susceptible to trapping and disintegration with each passage.

Clinical features are anemia, reticulocytosis, jaundice, and splenomegaly. Fatal crises have been reported. Cholelithiasis present in 30–60%. Leg ulcers are uncommon.

Diagnosis by peripheral blood smear; spherocytic cells with a smaller diameter and increased thickness. Increased osmotic fragility is diagnostic, but rarely performed.

Splenectomy is sole therapy; should be delayed until age 4. Intractable leg ulcers mandate early splenectomy. Results are uniformly good. Underlying erythrocyte defect is unchanged, but hemolysis and jaundice resolve, and erythrocyte life span becomes normal. Preoperative ultrasound or oral cholecystogram should be done and if gallstones present, cholecystectomy should be performed concomitant with splenectomy.

Hereditary Elliptocytosis Similar to hereditary spherocytosis. Splenectomy indicated for all symptomatic patients, and cholelithiasis should be treated by cholecystectomy.

Hereditary Hemolytic Anemia with Enzyme Deficiency Includes deficiencies in: (1) anaerobic glycolysis, prototype is pyruvate-kinase deficiency (PK); and (2) hexose monophosphate shunt, prototype is glucose-6-phosphate deficiency (G-6-PD). Spleen enlarged in PK but not in G-6-PD. Most patients have hemoglobins greater than 8 g/dL and do not require therapy. Blood transfusions required for significant anemias. Splenectomy may be beneficial in severe PK, but not in G-6-PD. Postoperative thrombocytosis may occur with hepatic, portal, or caval thrombosis.

Thalassemia   Also known as *Mediterranean anemia*. Autosomal dominant. Defect in hemoglobin synthesis. Heinz bodies present as intracellular precipitates. Classified into alpha, beta, and gamma types, depending on the specific chain involved. Beta thalassemia results in decreased rate of β-chain synthesis and decrease in hemoglobin A (Hb A).

Two degrees of severity: thalassemia major (homozygous) and minor (heterozygous).

Thalassemia major occurs in first year of life with pallor, retarded body growth, and large head. May result in a severe chronic anemia with icterus, splenomegaly, and early death. Most thalassemia minor patients lead normal lives.

Thalassemia major diagnosed by blood smear. Nucleated red cells present. Reticulocyte count elevated. Persistence of Hb F and a decrease in Hb A.

Treatment for symptomatic patients. Transfusions as needed. Splenectomy may reduce transfusion requirements and hemolytic process. Other indications for splenectomy include marked splenomegaly and repeated splenic infarcts.

Sickle Cell Disease   Hereditary hemolytic anemia predominantly in blacks. Hb A is replaced by Hb S, the sickle hemoglobin. Hb F also mildly increased. With reduced oxygen tension, the Hb S molecule crystallizes and the cells elongate and distort. This increases blood viscosity and stasis leading to thrombosis, ischemia, necrosis, and organ fibrosis.

Early in the disease the spleen enlarges, but with repeated infarction, autosplenectomy occurs.

Most patients with the *trait* are asymptomatic. With the *disease,* chronic anemia and jaundice may be interrupted by acute crises related to thrombosis. Symptoms include bone or joint pain, hematuria, priapism, neurologic symptoms, ulcers of the malleolus, abdominal pain, and splenic abscess.

Diagnosis made by blood smear and hemoglobin electrophoresis. Leukocytosis, thrombocytosis, and hyperbilirubinemia may be present.

Treatment is palliative. Sodium cyanate prevents sickling of Hb S. Hydration and exchange transfusions for crises. Splenectomy rarely indicated unless hypersplenism present.

Idiopathic Autoimmune Hemolytic Anemia   Shortened erythrocyte life span secondary to endogenous hemolytic mechanism. Etiology unknown, but presumed autoimmune. Spleen may serve as a source of destructive antibody. "Warm" and "cold" antibodies described; most are hemagglutinins rather than hemolysins. Immunologically altered cells trapped and destroyed by the reticuloendothelial system of the spleen.

More common in women and in those greater than age 50. Mild jaundice present. Splenomegaly in 50% and gallstones present in 25%. Tubular necrosis occurs in severe cases, and the prognosis in this group is grave.

Diagnosis made by demonstrating anemia, reticulocytosis, as well as products of red cell destruction in the urine, blood, and stool; hypercellular bone marrow; and a positive Coomb's test.

Treatment is not necessary for those that run a self-limiting course. Corticosteroids as well as transfusions may be required. With "warm" antibody, splenectomy indicated when steroids are ineffective, required in excess, causing toxic manifestations, or contraindicated. Splenic sequestration as demonstrated by ^{51}Cr-tagged RBCs useful in predicting success following splenectomy. Relapses may occur following splenectomy.

Idiopathic Thrombocytopenic Purpura (ITP)

An acquired disorder whereby platelets destroyed when exposed to IgG antiplatelet factors. The spleen is both the source of antibody and site of sequestration. Features include a bone marrow with normal to increased megakaryocytes and no evidence of systemic disease or drug ingestion known to cause thrombocytopenia.

3:1 F/M ratio. Signs and symptoms include petechiae, bleeding gums, vaginal bleeding, gastrointestinal bleeding, and hematuria. CNS bleeding occurs in 2–4%. Spleen is normal in size.

Laboratory data include platelet count less than 50,000, prolonged bleeding time, and normal clotting time. Bone marrow exam shows normal to increased megakaryocytes in addition to qualitative histologic changes.

Acute ITP resolves in 80% of children less than age 16 without specific therapy. 75–85% of adults with chronic ITP respond permanently to splenectomy without further steroid requirements. Counts should increase to over 100,000 within 7 days.

Treatment begins with 6–8 weeks of steroid therapy. Splenectomy performed if no response; if response, steroids tapered. Splenectomy indicated if thrombocytopenia recurs.

Even if platelet levels approach zero, platelets should not be given until spleen is removed. Accessory spleens may be responsible for recurrence and may be treated effectively by removal.

Thrombotic Thrombocytopenic Purpura (TTP)

TTP is a disease of arterioles and capillaries, but in some patients splenectomy is beneficial. Etiology probably immune; 5% occur during pregnancy. Histologically, widespread occlusion of capillaries and arterioles.

Pentad includes fever, purpura, hemolytic anemia, neurologic manifestations, and renal disease. Lab data include anemia, reticulocytosis, thrombocytopenia, and leukocytosis. Occasionally hyperbilirubinemia, proteinuria, hematuria, or azotemia.

Most cases show a rapid fulminant and fatal course, usually secondary to renal failure or intracranial bleed. Treatment includes heparin, exchange transfusion, plasmapheresis, dextran, antimetabolites, and steroids.

Splenectomy with high-dose steroids have had the best outcome.

Secondary Hypersplenism

Pancytopenia may occur with splenomegaly or splenic congestion. Seen in portal hypertension. However, hypersplenism per se is not an indication for surgery in portal hypertension. If splenectomy should become necessary, it should be combined with splenorenal shunt to decrease the portal pressure.

Myeloid Metaplasia

A panproliferative process with connective tissue proliferation of the bone marrow, liver, spleen, and lymph nodes, as well as simultaneous proliferation of the hemopoietic elements in the liver, spleen, and long bones. Etiology unknown. Splenic enlargement may occur. Portal hypertension may also occur due to either hepatic fibrosis or increased forward flow.

Presenting picture is usually that of anemia and increasing splenomegaly. Symptoms include abdominal pain of splenic infarction, fullness after meals, spontaneous bleeding, secondary infection, bone pain, pruritus, and hyperuricemia. Hepatomegaly is common.

Hallmark is peripheral blood smear. Red cells are fragmented with poikilocytosis, teardrop and elongated forms. White blood cell count usually below 50,000, but may be much higher. Platelet count may be low, normal, or high.

Treatment consists of transfusions, hormones, chemotherapy, and radiotherapy. Busulfan and cyclophosphamide have been used. Although not curative, splenectomy indicated for control of anemia, thrombocytopenia, and symptoms secondary to enlarged spleen. In patients with esophageal varices, splenectomy may require concomitant portal systemic shunt if portal pressures remain high postsplenectomy. Postoperative thrombocytosis and thrombosis of the splenic vein extending into the portal and mesenteric veins occur more commonly in these patients.

Hodgkin's Disease, Lymphomas, and Leukemias

Splenectomy indicated for symptomatic splenomegaly, with anemia and increasing transfusion requirements, or with cytopenia limiting systemic therapy.

Hairy cell leukemia, or reticuloendotheliosis, characterized by malignant cells with filamentous cytoplasmic projections. Splenectomy indicated when neutropenia, thrombocytopenia, and anemia occur. Failures managed with steroids and chemotherapy.

STAGING OF HODGKIN'S DISEASE AND NON-HODGKIN'S LYMPHOMA Diagnosis usually made by biopsy of suspicious lymphadenopathy or splenomegaly. Sternberg-Reed cell is pathognomonic. Four major histologic types: lymphocyte predominant, nodular sclerosis, mixed cellularity, and lymphocyte depletion. Survival related to histology and presence or absence of symptoms. Stage I—limited to one anatomic region; II—two or more regions of disease on the same side of the diaphragm; III—disease on both sides of diaphragm with disease limited to lymph nodes, spleen, and Waldeyer's ring; and IV—involvement of bone marrow, lung, liver, skin, gastrointestinal tract, and any nonnodal tissues.

Reasons for staging laparotomy include: (1) lesion usually starts as single focus and spreads along adjacent lymphatic channels, (2) prognosis related to clinical stage, (3) therapy dependent on stage, and (4) clinical staging by labs and radiographic studies inaccurate.

Staging laparotomy performed in the following fashion: (1) wedge liver biopsy; (2) splenectomy; (3) lymph node sampling from entire periaortic chain, mesentery, and hepatoduodenal ligament; and (4) iliac crest marrow biopsy.

Spleen involvement found in 39%. Following laparotomy, surgical staging upgraded clinical stage in 27–36% and downgraded in 7–15%.

Oophoropexy done in young women to prevent radiation-induced menopause and to permit subsequent pregnancies. Restaging laparotomy done for documentation of residual or recurrent disease.

Indications for staging laparotomy somewhat controversial, but most agree with the following: (1) patients with suspected disease in the upper abdomen provided jaundice is not present, (2) presence of symptoms in clinical stages I and II of nodular sclerosis type, and (3) mixed cellularity or lymphocyte depletion histology.

Regarding non-Hodgkin's lymphoma, routine staging not accepted by many.

Miscellaneous Diseases

Felty's Syndrome Triad of rheumatoid arthritis, splenomegaly, and neutropenia. Mild anemia, thrombocytopenia, and gastric achlorhydria occasionally seen. Corticosteroids and splenectomy used to treat the neutropenia and reduce susceptibility to infection.

Splenectomy indicated for: (1) neutropenic patients with serious or recurrent infections, (2) patients requiring transfusions for anemia, (3) profound thrombocytopenia, and (4) intractable leg ulcers. Course of arthritis usually not altered, while neutrophilic response to infection improved.

Sarcoidosis Disease of young adults with cough, dyspnea, generalized lymphadenopathy, pulmonary and mediastinal involvement, and skin lesions. Splenomegaly in 25%.

No specific treatment. Spontaneous recovery the rule. Splenectomy indicated for splenomegaly with hypersplenism.

Gaucher's Disease Familial disorder, abnormal storage or retention of glycolipid cerebrosides in reticuloendothelial cells. Spleen, liver, and lymph node enlargement occur.

Clinical manifestations include abdominal mass (spleen or liver), yellow-brown pigmentation of head and extremities, bone pain and pathologic fractures, and hypersplenism. Treatment is either splenectomy or partial splenectomy.

Porphyria Erythropoietica Congenital disorder, of erythrocyte pyrrole metabolism. Excessive deposition of porphyrins in the tissues. Splenectomy indicated for splenomegaly and hemolysis.

MISCELLANEOUS LESIONS

Ectopic Spleen Rare condition. Due to lengthening of ligaments and extreme mobility of spleen. Acute torsion may occur requiring surgery.

Splenic Artery Aneurysm Most common visceral artery aneurysm. Incidence is .02–.16%. More frequent in women, atherosclerosis most common predisposing factor. Rupture occurs in less than 10%; 20% occur during pregnancy. Excision with or without splenectomy for enlarging or symptomatic aneurysms, and in women of childbearing age.

Cysts and Tumors Rare. Parasitic cysts usually echinococcal. Nonparasitic are dermoid, epidermoid, epithelial, and pseudocysts (following trauma).

Primary and malignant tumors of the spleen are sarcomatous. Metastases in the absence of widespread disease are extremely rare.

Abscesses Clinical manifestations include fever, chills, splenomegaly, and left upper quadrant tenderness. Diagnosis via CT scan or ultrasound. Splenectomy is treatment of choice. Splenotomy and drainage has been successful in some. Fungal abscesses found in patients on steroids and chemotherapy. Treatment includes antifungal drugs and splenectomy.

SPLENECTOMY

Technique Incision may be either left subcostal or midline. Short gastric vessels are divided. Ligamentous attachments divided to allow mobilization of spleen. Division of splenic artery and vein in hilus, taking care to avoid injury to tail of pancreas. Search for accessory spleens when performing splenectomy for hematologic disease. Drainage of bed not performed routinely unless circumstances dictate.

Postoperative Course and Complications Characteristic blood smear changes include: (1) Howell-Jolly bodies and siderocytes, and (2) leukocytosis and thrombocytosis. Complications include left lower lobe atelectasis, subphrenic hematoma and abscess, pancreatic fistula and pancreatitis, and thrombocytosis.

Overwhelming postsplenectomy infection (OPSI) is a rare occurrence and occurs more frequently following splenectomy for disease than trauma.

Immunologic defects include poor response to immunizations, deficiency in phagocytosis-promoting peptide, decreased serum IgM, and decreased properdin. Most common organisms causing OPSI are diplococcus pneumonia and *H. influenza*.

Pneumococcus vaccine and vaccine against *H. influenza* should be given as prophylaxis; best given 10 days prior to elective splenectomy and preoperatively in anticipation of splenic trauma. Oral penicillin should be given until age 18.

33 PERITONITIS AND INTRAABDOMINAL ABSCESSES

STRUCTURE

The peritoneum is a single layer of mesothelial cells over a fibroelastic base. It is divided into a *visceral* portion, covering the bowel and mesentery; and a *parietal* portion that lines the abdominal wall, in contact with muscular fascia. The *blood* supply comes from underlying structures. *Nerve* supply is more specific. The visceral peritoneum is relatively insensitive, responding only to traction or stretch. The parietal peritoneum has both somatic and visceral components and allows localization of noxious stimuli by leading to guarding and rebound.

FUNCTION

Total surface area is about 2 m, and activity is consistent with that of a biologic membrane. Fluid and small electrolytes can move in both directions, as seen by the efficacy of peritoneal dialysis. Larger molecules are cleared into underlying lymphatics through small stomata. Direct injury leads to rapid regeneration as mesothelial cells migrate into the wound, and free monocytes in the peritoneal fluid stick to the raw surface and differentiate. Adhesions form in response to local hypoxemia or fibrin deposition from infection or foreign material.

PERITONITIS

Inflammation leads to accumulation of fluid as capillaries and membranes become leaky. The general responses to this intravascular fluid loss are outlined in Fig. 33-1. If fluid deficits are not rapidly and aggressively corrected, tissue perfusion is significantly decreased, resulting in cell death and the eventual development of multisystem organ failure. As the body tries to compensate by renal retention of fluid and electrolytes, waste products also accumulate. Tachycar-

GENERAL RESPONSES TO PERITONITIS

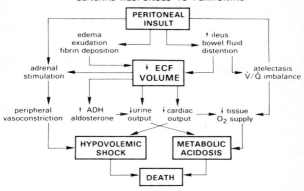

Fig. 33-1 The major general responses to peritonitis are mediated by a decreased extracellular fluid volume that, if not corrected, leads to metabolic acidosis, hypovolemic shock, and death.

dia initially increases cardiac output, but this soon falls off as hypovolemia develops.

The *metabolic* sequelae involve catabolism of muscle to provide amino acid skeletons for energy and acute phase protein synthesis. Hepatic glycogen stores are rapidly depleted early in the course of peritonitis, and a relative insulin resistance develops.

Clinically, the patients appear ill. They are anorectic, sullen, febrile and tend to lie quietly in bed because motion causes pain. Bowel sounds are absent and there is rigidity and tenderness to palpation. *Laboratory studies* are only confirmatory—in fact, *leukocyte count* may be normal or low due to extravascular migration of white blood cells in the peritoneal cavity.

Bacteriology of Suppurative Peritonitis

Four factors determine whether contamination will lead to peritonitis:

1. Virulence of bacteria: In general, single organisms will not cause a fatal peritonitis. The synergism of multiple organisms, however, makes the mixture more harmful. Anaerobic bacteria, especially *Bacteroides* species, are

found in suppurative peritonitis and augment the effects of aerobic bacteria.

2. Extent and duration of contamination: Obviously, the greater the dose of bacteria and the longer untreated leads to more severe peritonitis. Liquids such as found in the ileum and cecum will spread more extensively than solid stool from a perforated sigmoid diverticulum.

3. Influence of adjuncts: Virulence is increased in the presence of foreign bodies, blood, mucus, talc, or barium. These inorganic materials inhibit bacterial clearance by diverting phagocytes to deal with the inert particles rather than organisms. Blood appears to allow elaboration of a leukocyte toxin in the presence of *E. coli*.

4. Inappropriate therapy: Failure to promptly recognize and treat a perforated viscus or the attempt to cure intraabdominal sepsis with antibiotics alone in the face of pus portends a poor outcome.

Therapy There are three key points in preparing the patient:

1. Volume: Vigorous resuscitation with isotonic salt solutions is vital. Restoration of intravascular volume improves tissue perfusion and delivery of oxygen, nutrients, and defense mechanisms. Urinary output and cardiac filling pressures should be monitored.

2. Antibiotics: Broad-spectrum antibiotics are adjunctive to surgical drainage. Adequate levels must be available at the time of surgery, as bacteremia will develop during operation.

3. Oxygen and ventilatory support: Ongoing sepsis leads to hypoxemia due to shunting and chest wall splinting. Adequate oxygen delivery is key.

Other Categories of Peritonitis

ASEPTIC (CHEMICAL) In contrast to polymicrobial peritonitis, the bacterial insult in chemical peritonitis is low. Instead the inflammation is the result of direct irritants such as bile, urine, pancreatic juice, foreign bodies, or barium. The patients will manifest the same third-space losses and peritoneal irritation as in bacterial peritonitis, but may not have fever. Therapy is aimed at stopping ongoing contamination, as in the case of a perforated ulcer, and preventing secondary bacterial infection, as would be seen in a barium-induced colon perforation.

GRANULOMATOUS PERITONITIS   The peritoneum can react to certain insults by granuloma formation, often leading to dense adhesions. In tuberculosis, ascites is often present in the early phase. Although TB peritonitis per se is not fatal, it indicates widespread acid-fast infection and should be treated with triple anti-TB therapy.

Patients may also form granulomas and adhesions in response to talc from surgical gloves. Wiping the gloves prior to incision may ameliorate this problem.

PRIMARY BACTERIAL PERITONITIS   This form is unique because it is monomicrobial in nature, usually from *E. coli* or gram-positive cocci. It occurs in children and cirrhotic patients, and no perforation of a viscus can be identified. Diagnosis is made by peritoneal tap showing only a single organism. Antibiotic therapy is initiated and the patient followed. If there is no improvement, laparotomy is undertaken.

ABSCESS   The body will attempt to wall off infections preventing generalized spread. There are several dependent areas where abscess will form: (1) left and right subphrenic, (2) subhepatic, (3) pelvic, (4) lesser sac, (5) loops of bowel, which can close off infected collections, leading to an "interloop abscess."

Signs and Symptoms   In contrast to generalized peritonitis, patients with an abscess may have vague pain, malaise, and ileus. Leukocytosis and fever are common, and the hyperpyrexia tends to be spiking in nature. Diagnosis involves a high level of suspicion, coupled with confirmation by ultrasound or CT scan. The radioisotope scans may be helpful in situations where CT scan cannot differentiate fluid or phlegmon from frank abscess.

Therapy   "Don't let the sun rise and set on undrained pus." Abscess cavities must be drained. Pelvic collections can be opened per rectum and subphrenic abscesses approached through the bed of the twelfth rib. CT scan–guided percutaneous drainage is achieving comparable success rates, as with open drainage, and may avoid a general anesthetic; however, multiple intraabdominal collections and those that are loculated are best handled by transperitoneal open drainage.

Operative therapy is aimed at drainage of all purulent material, breaking up loculations, and treating the underlying source of contamination. Exudate is debrided cautiously, and large volumes of warm saline are used to lavage the abdomen. There is no clear advantage to topical antibiotic irrigation. Drains should be left in well-walled-off abscess cavities, but it is impossible to drain the abdomen as a whole, per se. The fascia is closed with monofilament, nonabsorbable suture, and the skin left open.

ANTERIOR ABDOMINAL WALL

Rectus Sheath Hematoma

Bleeding into the rectus sheath produces a surgical picture that may simulate the acute surgical abdomen. Bleeding is usually the result of rupture of the epigastric artery or veins and may follow direct trauma or occur spontaneously in patients with debilitating diseases or blood dyscrasia, and in patients on anticoagulation therapy. Bleeding also occurs without obvious trauma or disease following minor straining.

Clinical Manifestations Three times more frequent in women; rare in children; peak age of incidence is fifth decade. The sudden onset of pain is localized to the side of the abdomen where the bleeding occurred. Anorexia, nausea, low-grade fever, and a moderate leukocytosis are frequent. A tender mass may be palpable.

Ultrasonography or CT shows complex lesions within rectus sheath.

Treatment May be managed nonoperatively with bed rest and analgesics. Surgical intervention occasionally is necessary; ideally, the hematoma is evacuated without entering the peritoneal cavity. Bleeding points are then ligated and the wound closed without drainage.

Desmoid Tumor

An aggressive variant within a group of conditions referred to as "fibromatoses." Tumor is of aponeurotic origin and usually is found within or deep to the flat muscles of the anterior abdominal wall. Usually seen in childbearing-age women, often after a recent gestation; may be the result of hemorrhage. Also frequently occurs in patients with familial polyposis coli (Gardner's syndrome) trait. They are locally invasive benign tumors that rarely undergo malignant transformation to a low-grade fibrosarcoma; metastases have not been reported but there is a tendency to recur following local excision. The microscopic appearance varies from an acellular fibroma to that of a cellular, low-grade fibrosarcoma.

Clinical Manifestations Usually a painless, deeply situated mass that is solitary, rarely crosses the midline, and may be fixed.

Treatment Wide surgical excision often necessitates resection of a large portion of the abdominal wall including the skin, muscle, and peritoneum. Recurrences can be treated by reexcision. Tumor is rarely fatal.

DISEASES OF THE OMENTUM

Torsion

A twist on its long axis to an extent causing vacular compromise. Primary omental torsion is relatively rare. Secondary omental torsion associated with adhesions of the free end of the omentum to tumors, foci of intraabdominal inflammation, postsurgical wounds, or internal or external hernias more common.

Clinical Manifestations Pain begins suddenly and is usually localized to the right lower quadrant. Tenderness, rebound tenderness, and voluntary spasm are frequent. The finding of free serosanguineous fluid at the time of celiotomy in the absence of a pathologic condition in the appendix, gallbladder, or pelvic organs should alert the surgeon to the possibility of omental torsion.

Treatment Resection of the involved omentum with correction of any underlying etiologic condition, etc.

Idiopathic Segmental Infarction

An acute vascular disturbance of the omentum not accompanied by omental torsion or an intraabdominal pathologic condition. It is precipitated by thrombosis of omental veins secondary to endothelial injury. The right lower segment of the omentum, which is the most mobile and richest in fat, is the portion usually involved. The involved segment is well demarcated, and serosanguineous fluid in the free peritoneal cavity is a constant finding.

Clinical Manifestations and Treatment Most patients are young or middle-aged adults who present with right-side abdominal pain. There is always tenderness and often rebound tenderness over the region of the infarction. Resection of the infarcted area is indicated to prevent the possible complications of gangrene and adhesions.

Cysts

The cysts have an endothelial lining similar to cystic lymphangiomas. Dermoid cysts are lined with squamous epithelium and may contain hair, teeth, and sebaceous material. Pseudocysts of the omentum probably result from trauma with hematoma formation.

Clinical Manifestations Large cysts present as a palpable abdominal mass or manifestations of torsion, infection, rupture, or intestinal obstruction.

Plain radiographs sometimes show a circumscribed soft tissue haziness. US or CT shows a fluid-filled mass that often contains internal septations. Treatment consists of local excision.

Solid Tumors

The most common solid tumor of the omentum is metastatic carcinoma, which generally involves the omentum by tumor implant. Frequently there is associated ascites. Primary solid tumors of the omentum are rare. Most are tumors of smooth muscle, and about one-third are malignant. Excision is indicated.

MESENTERIC CIRCULATION

ACUTE OCCLUSION OF SUPERIOR MESENTERIC ARTERY This is due more often to an embolus than to thrombosis. Most emboli come from the heart and more often lodge near a major branch where the artery narrows, usually at the egress of the middle colic artery. The initial effect of the embolus on the artery is to cause spasm of its distal branches; secondary thrombosis of the distal artery then occurs. Sudden occlusion of the main stem superior mesenteric artery produces ischemia of the entire small intestine distal to the ligament of Treitz and also ischemia of the proximal half of the colon. Acute thrombosis of the superior mesenteric artery usually occurs in an artery partially occluded by atherosclerosis. The extent of intestinal ischemia or infarction depends on the site of the thrombosis and the status of collateral channels.

Pathology Early the bowel is pale due to intense vasospasm. At this stage, the bowel is hypertonic and contracted. Within 1–2 h the initial vessel spasm subsides and anoxic bowel wall becomes engorged with blood. Thrombosis of the visceral veins follows and the bowel wall becomes inert, boggy, and cyanotic. As the infarction progresses to full-thickness necrosis of the intestine, the bowel wall becomes blood-soaked and cyanotic, and "weeps" serosanguineous fluid into the peritoneal cavity.

Clinical Manifestations The clinical features are usually the same whether occlusion is the result of embolism or thrombosis. Males are affected more often. The peak age of incidence is the fifth and sixth decades. The most striking and constant complaint is sudden extreme abdominal pain initially out of proportion to the physical findings. Muscle spasm may be present, but the rigidity is almost never boardlike. Tenderness and rebound tenderness become severe as intestinal infarction occurs. Bowel sounds are first hyperactive, but within a short time the abdomen becomes silent. As infarction of the intestine progresses, the patient becomes febrile, the pulse rate increases, and the patient becomes hypotensive. Once bowel necrosis and perforation occur, the findings are those of generalized peritonitis and sepsis. The leukocyte count increases to over $20,000/mm^3$ as hemorrhagic infarction occurs. Suspicion of the diagnosis of acute mesenteric ischemia is itself an indication to obtain an immediate mesenteric arteriogram. In addition to demonstrating emboli, thrombosis, and mesenteric vasoconstriction, the arteriogram will define the adequacy of the splanchnic circulation. The angiographic catheter also provides a route for the intraarterial administration of vasodilating agents.

Treatment An occasional patient can be treated successfully by arterial infusion of a vasodilating agent. Early surgical intervention before gangrene and perforation of the intestine has occurred is optimal. The number of patients who present with a situation amenable to arterial reconstruction is small. If the occlusion is limited to a branch of the superior mesenteric artery, or to the superior mesenteric artery distal to the origin of the ileocolic artery, the relatively short segments of affected intestine are best handled by resection with a primary anastomosis. As much as 70% of the small intestine can be removed without creating serious digestive disturbances.

In the situation where the main stem superior mesenteric artery is occluded, the decision to establish arterial flow is based on whether the process in the ischemic intestine is reversible. If the intestines are clearly gangrenous, the only surgical procedure that can be considered is resection. This will usually require removal of the entire small intestine distal to the ligament of Treitz and resection of the right half of the colon. Although this extensive resection is associated with a high operative mortality and late morbidity, it is worth consideration in an otherwise hopeless situation and, with the use of parenteral central hyperalimentation postoperatively, some patients can be salvaged.

If there is any question of the reversibility of ischemia of all or part of the intestine, an attempt at arterial reconstruction is indicated. An embolus can usually be extracted using a Fogarty catheter; a thrombus within a sclerotic vessel will require a thromboendarterectomy. An alternative approach is revascularization with a bypass venous graft between the aorta and the superior mesenteric artery distal to the site of occlusion.

Clinical assessment, such as return of intestinal color and arterial pulsations and the presence of visible peristalsis, is usually reliable in determining that a segment of revascularized intestine will remain viable. Intraoperative use of the Doppler ultrasonic flowmeter to detect pulsatile mural blood flow can give added objective confirmation. Intravenous infusion of a vital dye, usually fluorescein, has also been advocated to define intestinal recovery. If there is any question about the viability of long segments of intestine, leave them and reexamine them at a planned second operation 24–36 h later.

Most patients will have a depleted circulating blood volume resulting from loss of plasma and whole blood into the bowel lumen, bowel wall, and peritoneal cavity. Replacement should be started while readying the patient for the operation. Added intravenous fluids are necessary postoperatively to combat the reactive hyperemia that occurs after revascularization of the intestine. Broad-spectrum antibiotics should be administered in large doses beginning preoperatively and continuing throughout the postoperative period. Anticoagulation, preferably with heparin, has also been recommended for patients who have arterial reconstruction.

The overall mortality following sudden occlusion of the superior mesenteric artery varies between 60–85%. Mortality is higher following acute occlusion by thrombosis than from embolization.

NONOCCLUSIVE MESENTERIC INFARCTION In about 30% of patients with mesenteric infarction, careful examination will reveal no gross arterial or venous occlusion. It has been related to a sustained decrease in cardiac output, such as in prolonged circulatory collapse, and hypoxic states that may accompany septicemia, acute myocardial infarction, and profound hypovolemia. Most patients presenting with non-occlusive mesenteric infarction have received digitalis, an agent that has been shown to induce mesenteric vasoconstriction.

Pathology Outer surface of the bowel is initially mottled, with segmental areas of cyanosis distributed throughout the length of the intestine. Later, gangrenous changes become advanced and lead to perforation.

Clinical Manifestations The clinical picture may be identical to that of patients with acute arterial or venous mesenteric occlusions. There may be prodromal symptoms of malaise and vague abdominal discomfort. Infarction of the intestine is heralded by the sudden onset of severe abdominal pain and vomiting. The patient usually becomes acutely hypotensive with a rapid pulse. Watery diarrhea is frequent and the stools may be grossly bloody. The abdomen becomes diffusely tender and rigid. Bowel sounds are diminished or absent. Fever and leukocytosis are usual, and frequently there is a thrombocytopenia related to intravascular thrombosis. A characteristic early laboratory finding is a markedly elevated hematocrit due to "trapping" of serum in the bowel and seeping into the peritoneal cavity. Selective superior mesenteric arteriograms will demonstrate patent major vessels with multiple segmental areas of narrowing of both small and medium-sized vessels and diminution of absence of mural intestinal circulation.

Treatment The underlying disorder producing the low-flow state should be corrected. An attempt should be made to improve mesenteric artery flow. Direct infusion of a vasodilating drug, such as papaverine hydrochloride, into a catheter positioned in the superior mesenteric artery is used to improve mesenteric arterial flow. Antibiotics should be administered.

If abdominal signs and symptoms persist, operation is mandatory. The process usually involves the entire large and small intestine and may also involve the stomach. For this reason, resection is not usually feasible. With involvement of lesser portions of the intestine, primary resection with anastomosis should be attempted. The reported mortality rates are upward of 80%.

CHRONIC OCCLUSION OF SUPERIOR MESENTERIC ARTERY (INTESTINAL ANGINA)
Intestinal ischemia, "intestinal angina," without infarction is due to collateral blood supply sufficient for life but not for function of the affected bowel. This is analogous to angina pectoris and intermittent claudication.

Etiology Collateral anastomoses among the three main gastrointestinal arteries from the aorta (celiac axis, superior mesenteric, and inferior mesenteric) provide for maintenance of intestinal viability and function when one of these branches is gradually occluded. When one main vessel is occluded and blood flow through one of the remaining patent vessels becomes (or has been) compromised, the now relatively ischemic intestine is unable to respond to the demands of digestion for an increased blood supply.

Chronic occlusion of the major visceral arteries is most often due to atherosclerosis. Less frequently, the stenosis is due to compression of the celiac axis by a celiac ganglion or arcuate ligament of the diaphragm, by involvement of the arteries in an expanding aortic aneurysm, or by an arteritis.

Clinical Manifestations The dominant feature of intestinal angina is generalized cramping abdominal pain that comes on soon after eating. The food–pain relationship soon leads to a reluctance on the part of the patient to eat. Subsequent rapid and severe weight loss characterizes the syndrome. As the intestinal ischemia progresses, a form of malabsorption syndrome contributes to the weight loss. An arteriogram will show stenosis or complete occlusion of one or both the celiac axis and superior mesenteric arteries, usually within 1 cm of their origin.

Treatment Most surgeons prefer improving the circulation with a bypass graft. For a lesion in the celiac artery, a graft is inserted between a major branch of the celiac artery, usually the splenic, and the aorta.

Occasionally, the splenic artery itself may be mobilized and anastomosed to the side of the aorta. Bypassing of a superior mesenteric artery stenosis is best handled by inserting a graft to the side of the artery just beyond the egress of the middle colic artery and to the aorta below the origin of the renal arteries.

MESENTERIC VENOUS OCCLUSION Etiology and Pathology
When visceral venous occlusion produces symptoms, it is almost always due to acute thrombosis. Mesenteric venous thrombosis may be idiopathic or evolve secondarily as a complication of several clinical disorders. Predisposing factors in secondary mesenteric venous thrombosis are (1)

intraabdominal infection; (2) hematologic conditions such as polycythemia vera, the postsplenectomy state, and the hypercoagulability associated with oral contraceptives; (3) accidental or operative trauma to the mesenteric veins. In approximately 25% no associated factor may be implicated.

Depending on the extent and location of the propagating clot, the bowel lesion may be localized or be an extensive infarction.

Clinical Manifestation Frequently, the patient complains of vague abdominal discomfort, anorexia, and change in bowel habits a few days or even weeks prior to the onset of severe symptoms. Early symptoms are followed by sudden severe abdominal pain, vomiting, and circulatory collapse. Bloody diarrhea is more frequent than with arterial occlusion. Rigidity is not present unless gangrene and perforation of the bowel have occurred. A marked leukocytosis and elevated hematocrit are characteristic findings in venous thrombosis. Paracentesis invariably yields serosanguineous fluid.

Treatment Without operation the mortality approaches 100%. Shorter segments of intestine are usually involved than that noted if occlusion is primarily arterial. All devitalized intestine is resected and a primary end-to-end anastomosis is performed. Resection should include adjacent normal bowel and mesentery until all grossly thrombosed veins are encompassed.

Anticoagulation with heparin should be started immediately, and continued for 6–8 weeks. A second-look operation 24–36 h later should be performed because of the frequent recurrence of thrombosis or extension of residual clots. The prognosis is somewhat better than in mesenteric infarction due to arterial occlusion.

ANEURYSMS OF THE SPLANCHNIC ARTERIES Aneurysms of the splanchnic arteries are rare. Arteriosclerosis is the usual etiology in older patients; congenital or acquired defects in the medial wall of the artery are more often incriminated in the young.

Splenic artery aneurysms compromise about 60%. Most occur in women, and in about 40% of patients the aneurysms are multiple. Hepatic artery aneurysms make up 16–20%. Aneurysms of the celiac artery and the superior mesenteric artery and its branches each account for about 3%. Most are due to arteriosclerosis, but a relatively large number of aneurysms of the superior mesenteric artery result from mycotic involvement or necrotizing arteritis.

Most splanchnic artery aneurysms are less than 2 cm in diameter. About 2–10% of splenic artery aneurysms rupture;

the risk of rupture of hepatic, celiac, and superior mesenteric artery aneurysms is high, approximating 50%.

Clinical Manifestations Prior to rupture, most splanchnic artery aneurysms are asymptomatic. When rupture occurs, the major symptoms are related to signs of acute blood loss. A splenic artery aneurysm rarely will rupture into the adjacent stomach or pancreatic duct causing massive gastrointestinal bleeding. Erosion of a hepatic artery aneurysm into the bile duct is an unusual cause of hemobilia with the classic triad of gastrointestinal bleeding, biliary colic, and jaundice.

Treatment A conservative approach is justified for the asymptomatic patient with a small splenic artery aneurysm. There is a hazard of rupture during pregnancy, notably during the third trimester. Operation is indicated for women of childbearing age. The preferred treatment is proximal and distal ligation of the aneurysm with obliteration of all feeding vessels in order to avoid splenectomy. If this is not feasible, resection of the aneurysm and splenectomy will be necessary. Because risk of rupture of other splanchnic artery aneurysms is high, asymptomatic patients should undergo surgical correction as soon as the aneurysm is recognized.

Rupture of a celiac artery aneurysm can be treated by ligation, and although most hepatic artery aneurysms can also be treated safely by ligation, an attempt should be made to reconstruct the hepatic artery with a graft. Rupture of the main superior mesenteric artery aneurysm will require replacement with a graft, preferably of autogenous vein, following excision. Overall mortality following rupture of a splenic artery aneurysm is about 25%, with a 65% maternal and 95% fetal mortality if rupture occurs during pregnancy. The mortality subsequent to rupture of a celiac or superior mesenteric artery aneurysm is between 40–60%, while rupture of a hepatic aneurysm is associated with a 70% mortality rate.

Nonspecific Mesenteric Lymphadenitis

Nonspecific mesenteric lymphadenitis is one of the common causes of acute abdominal pain in young children. The lymph nodes primarily involved are those that drain the ileocecal region.

Clinical Manifestations The disease most commonly occurs in patients under age 18 without sex predilection. The initial pain is usually in the upper abdomen. Eventually the pain localizes to the right side; however, an important point in differentiating the disease from acute appendicitis is that the patient is unable to indicate the exact site of the most intense pain. The usual finding on examination of the abdomen is tenderness in the lower aspect of the right side, which is somewhat higher and more medial and considerably less severe than in acute appendicitis. The clinical similarity to acute appendicitis is marked.

Mesenteric Panniculitis

Mesenteric panniculitis is a process of extensive thickening of the mesentery by a nonspecific inflammatory process. Many consider it a variant of retroperitoneal fibrosis. The cause is unknown. Usually it involves the mesenteric root of the small bowel. Grossly, the normal fat lobulations of the markedly thickened and firm mesentery are lost. Scattered throughout are irregular areas of discoloration that vary from reddish-brown plaques to pale yellow foci resembling fat necrosis.

Clinical Manifestations   Men are affected more often. Rarely described in children. The clinical features are nonspecific; they include recurrent episodes of moderate to severe abdominal pain, nausea, vomiting, and malaise. CT demonstrates mesenteric panniculitis as a localized fat-dense mass containing areas of increased density representing fibrosis.

Treatment   Laparotomy is necessary to establish the diagnosis and to rule out other tumefactions of the abdomen. Widespread involvement of the mesentery precludes more than biopsy. Since neoplasms of the mesenteric lymph nodes may present a similar gross appearance, several biopsies from different sites should be obtained. The inflammatory process is self-limiting and seldom causes any serious complications.

Tumors of the Mesentery

Tumors originating between the leaves of the mesentery are quite rare. In contrast, malignant implants from intraabdominal or pelvic tumors or metastases to mesenteric lymph nodes are relatively common.

Pathology   Primary tumors of the mesentery may be cystic or solid. A classification of these tumors is shown in Table 34-1. The majority of cystic mesenteric tumors are benign. Benign solid tumors of the mesentery are more common than

TABLE 34-1. Classification of Primary Mesenteric Tumors

Origin	Benign	Malignant
Cystic tumors:		
Developmental defects	Chylous cyst	
	Serous cyst	
Lymphatic tissue	Lymphangioma	Lymphangiosarcoma
Trauma	Traumatic cyst	
Embryonic rests	Enteric cyst	
	Dermoid	Malignant teratoma
Solid tumors:		
Adipose tissue	Lipoma	Liposarcoma
Fibrous tissue	Fibroma	Fibrosarcoma
Nerve elements	Neurilemoma	Malignant schwannoma
	Neurofibroma	
Smooth muscle	Leiomyoma	Leiomyosarcoma
	Fibromyoma	Fibromyosarcoma
Vascular tissue	Hemangioma	Hemangiopericytoma

malignant ones. Solid malignant tumors arise near the root of the mesentery; solid benign tumors have a greater tendency to develop peripherally near the intestine.

Clinical Manifestations In most patients, symptoms are few or nonexistent, and the tumor is detected during routine examination. Only rarely will the patient present with symptoms of complete intestinal obstruction or symptoms resulting from complications of the tumor per se such as torsion, hemorrhage, or infarction of the tumor mass. In the absence of intestinal obstruction or these complications, the sole finding will be the presence of a nontender, intraabdominal mass, usually in the lower right part of the abdomen. Mass varies in size from a few inches in diameter to one that may fill the entire abdomen. The extremely large masses are usually cystic, in which case they are tense and fluctuant. Both cystic and solid tumors of the mesentery are laterally mobile; they can be easily moved from side to side but only slightly in an upward and downward direction.

Imaging techniques are the most useful means for diagnosing both cystic and solid mesenteric tumors. On ultrasonography, a mesenteric cyst appears as a well-outlined sonolucent transonic abdominal mass. CT demonstrates a simple mesenteric cyst as a nonenhancing near-water-density mass with a thin wall and a solid tumor as a mass lesion with a soft tissue density.

Treatment Surgical excision is the only treatment for benign and malignant lesions. All mesenteric cysts of a size sufficient to be palpated should be removed if at all possible, since even benign lesions eventually cause pain and compression of neighboring structures. Benign cystic tumors can be removed by enucleation or local excision. Wide excision, together with resection of adjacent intestine, is recommended for benign solid tumors, since these have a tendency toward local recurrence and malignant degeneration. Few patients with malignant primary mesenteric tumors are alive after 5 years.

RETROPERITONEUM

Idiopathic Retroperitoneal Fibrosis

A nonspecific, nonsuppurative inflammation of fibroadipose tissue that produces symptoms by the gradual compression of the tubular structures in the retroperitoneal space. The disease represents one of the manifestations of a widespread entity termed "systemic idiopathic fibrosis." Idiopathic mediastinal fibrosis, Riedel's struma, sclerosing cholangitis, panniculitis, Peyronie disease, and desmoid tumor are other fibromatoses that are considered localized forms of a systemic idiopathic fibrosis.

A plaque of woody, white fibrous tissue that is distributed along the course of the periaortic lymphatics. In about one-third of the cases, it is bilateral. The involved tissue surrounds and constricts but does not invade the regional structures in the retroperitoneum. The pattern varies from a subacute cellular process with polymorphonuclear cells, lymphocytes, fibroblasts, and fat cells to a completely hyalinized, relatively acellular sclerosis.

Clinical Manifestations   Retroperitoneal fibrosis is 2–3 times more common among men, two-thirds of patients are 40–60 years old. The natural history of the disease has been divided into three periods: (1) the period of incidence and development; (2) the period of activity, that is, spread of the cellular and fibrotic process to envelopment of the retroperitoneal structures; and (3) the period of contraction of the fibrotic mass with compression of the involved structures. The disease is apparently self-limiting once the fibrotic stage is reached, a factor of major importance in considering types of therapy. The first complaint is invariably dull, noncolicky pain. It usually originates in the flank or low back and often radiates to the lower abdomen, groin, genitalia, or antero-medial aspect of the thigh. The pain is unilateral at first but may become bilateral later, as the fibrotic process spreads.

Moderate fever and leukocytosis are often present early; the erythrocytic sedimentation rate is elevated. A transabdominal or pelvic mass is palpable in about one-third of the patients.

Symptoms due to compression of the tubular retroperitoneal structures may follow the initial complaints by 1 month to 2 years. The major structures involved are the ureters, aorta, and inferior vena cava. Partial or complete ureteral obstruction occurs in 75–85% of patients. As many as 40% of patients will have oliguria or anuria with laboratory evidence of uremia. Lower extremity edema occasionally occurs. Arterial insufficiency due to fibrous constriction of the aorta or iliac arteries is uncommon.

CT scan shows a homogeneous, soft tissue mass enveloping the ureters, aorta, and inferior vena cava. A triad that is highly suggestive or retroperitoneal fibrosis on the pyelogram is (1) hydroephrosis with a dilated, tortuous upper ureter; (2) medial deviation of the ureter; and (3) extrinsic ureteral compression.

Treatment   Some patients improve with supportive measures. With the onset of urinary infection or depression of renal function, surgical intervention usually becomes necessary. Steroid-induced regression of the inflammatory edema may reestablish urinary patency and thus facilitate elective, rather than emergency, surgery.

Ureterolysis with intraperitoneal transplantation is currently the most effective means of relieving obstruction of the involved ureter. This consists of freeing the ureter from the enveloping mass of fibrous tissue and transferring it into the peritoneal cavity, closing the posterior peritoneum behind it. Aortic or iliac artery obstruction are best treated by arteriolysis or bypass with a synthetic vascular graft.

Symptoms due to venous obstruction are best treated with elevation and elastic support to the lower limbs until a sufficient collateral venous system develops. Release of the obstructed vein from its fibrous encasement may be difficult and hazardous, and bypass procedures for obstruction of the inferior vena cava have been uniformly unsuccessful. Prognosis of the disease is generally good, if appropriate treatment begins before the development of irreversible renal damage.

Retroperitoneal Tumors

The majority occur in the fifth or sixth decades, with a peak incidence at about age 60. Approximately 15% are found in children under age 10. A classification of the benign and malignant tumors according to tissue type is given in Table 34-2.

TABLE 34-2. Classification of Retroperitoneal Tumors

Tissue type	Benign tumors	Malignant tumors
Lymphatic tissue	Lymphangioma	Lymphangiosarcoma
Lymph nodes		Lymphosarcoma
		Hodgkin's disease
		Reticulum cell sarcoma
Adipose tissue	Lipoma	Liposarcoma
Fibrous tissue	Fibroma	Fibrosarcoma
Smooth muscle	Leiomyoma	Leiomyosarcoma
Nerve elements	Neurilemoma	Malignant schwannoma
	Neurofibroma	
	Ganglioneuroma	Sympathicoblastoma
		(neuroblastoma)
		Chordoma
Striated muscle	Rhabdomyoma	Rhabdomyosarcoma
Mucoid tissue	Myxoma	Myxosarcoma
Vascular tissue	Hemangioma	Malignant hemangiopericytoma
Mesothelial tissue		Mesothelioma
Mesenchyme		Mesenchymoma
Extraadrenal chromaffin tissue	Benign pheochromocytoma	Malignant pheochromocytoma
Gland tissue	Adenoma	Carcinoma
Embryonic remnants	Nephrogenic cysts	Urogenital ridge tumor
Cell rests	Dermoid	Teratoma
Miscellaneous	Xanthogranuloma	Synovioma
	Aggressive	Dysgerminoma
	fibromatosis	Undifferentiated malignant tumor

The tumors may be solid, cystic, or a combination of both. Their color varies from white (fibroma), yellow (lipoma), or pinkish to red (sarcoma) depending on the predominant tissue. As a rule, the predominantly cystic tumors are benign; solid tumors are usually malignant.

Clinical Manifestations The tumor may attain large size before producing symptoms. As the tumor grows, it compresses, obstructs, or invades adjacent organs or structures, so that the presenting symptoms are often referable to these organs. The initial manifestations include an enlarging abdomen, backache, a sense of fullness or heaviness, and vague, indefinite pain that later may become more severe and radicular. Pain radiating into one or both thighs is usually late and due to involvement of lumbar and sacral nerve routes; it invariably denotes a malignant tumor. The predominant physical finding is an abdominal mass.

The CT scan can demonstrate the contours of the tumor mass, its size and relationships, as well as its effects on adjacent viscera and other tissues. This information is useful in determining resectability of the tumor and in planning a surgical approach. US differentiates between solid and cystic tumors. Percutaneous needle biopsy directed by CT or US can be used to obtain preoperative histologic diagnosis and for the detection of treatment failures and early recurrences.

Aortography should be an essential part of the workup of patients with a retroperitoneal tumor to define tumor size and can give useful information about the vascular anatomy.

Treatment Some retroperitoneal tumors are benign and can be cured by simple excisions; some are histologically benign but clinically malignant; others grow slowly and tend to recur and invade locally; and still others are rapidly malignant from the start.

Treatment of these growths consists of surgical or irradiation therapy, or a combination of the two. With the exception of treatment for lymphomas, chemotherapy has only limited therapeutic application. Surgical treatment is the most effective and offers the greatest prospect for cure. A cure may be anticipated following complete resection of benign tumor.

As many as one-third of patients with malignant tumors may be inoperable because of distant metastases to liver, lungs, and bone, in order of frequency.

For a malignant tumor, the initial operation offers the best chance of cure. Fewer than 25% of malignant tumors can be completely resected with anticipation of cure.

Malignant retroperitoneal tumors have a high recurrence

rate, 30–50% in most large series. The tumors become more malignant with each recurrence, and reoperation becomes more hazardous. Nevertheless, long-term survival has been reported after multiple resections. 5-year survival free of tumor is less than 10%.

35 ABDOMINAL WALL HERNIAS

DEFINITIONS

1. Hernia: a defect in the muscle-aponeurotic layers of the abdominal wall large enough to permit passage of an intraabdominal structure into hernia sac, a diverticulum of parietal peritoneum
2. Indirect inguinal hernia: protrudes into inguinal canal through the internal inguinal ring inside the cremaster muscle
3. Direct inguinal hernia: protrudes through Hesselbach's triangle between the inferior epigastric artery laterally, the inguinal ligament inferiorly, and the rectus sheath medially
4. Femoral hernia: passes beneath the inguinal ligament medial to the femoral vein to enter the thigh
5. Sliding hernia: intraabdominal organ incorporated in posterior wall of hernia sac
6. Incarcerated hernia: abdominal contents not reducible back into abdomen
7. Strangulated hernia: incarcerated abdominal contents deprived of vascular supply

PREVALENCE

1. Exact figure uncertain, perhaps 5% of adult male population affected
2. Groin hernias more common in males than females
3. Indirect inguinal hernia most common form in both sexes
4. Femoral hernias more frequent in women
5. Direct hernias extremely uncommon in women, children

ANATOMY

1. Indirect inguinal hernia: sac lies within cremaster muscle layers, follows spermatic cord, may enter scrotum
2. Direct inguinal hernia: enters inguinal canal through medial inguinal canal floor, lies behind spermatic cord, rarely passes through external inguinal ring

3. Femoral hernia: passes through inguinal canal floor, leaves groin beneath inguinal ligament medial to femoral vein; opening beneath inguinal ligament small and femoral hernias prone to strangulate
4. Umbilical hernia: occurs as defect in rectus sheath at site where viscera enter extraembryonic coelomic cavity during prenatal period; most umbilcal hernias at this site in newborns close spontaneously but some hernias persist, require closure

ETIOLOGY

1. Generally considered congenital (indirect inguinal hernias and umbilical hernias) or traumatic (direct inguinal hernias); evidence for traumatic origin not conclusive
2. Ventral hernias in postoperative incisions follow wound infections, errors in closure, poor tissue in abdominal wall

SYMPTOMS AND SIGNS

1. Transient local inguinal discomfort may follow acute appearance of groin hernia
2. Large hernia entering scrotum may produce epigastric discomfort from mesenteric stretching
3. Strangulation of abdominal contents within hernia sac accompanied by acute local pain and tenderness
4. Most hernias asymptomatic swellings discovered on physical examination

COMPLICATIONS

Strangulation of abdominal contents within hernia sac, with subsequent tissue gangrene the only common significant complication.

TREATMENT

Expectant management, nonoperative measures, operative repair:

1. Expectant management: allowing hernia to close spontaneously, rational only for infant with umbilical hernia
2. Nonoperative measures: reasonable in elderly debilitated patient with asymptomatic hernia; truss of limited value

with any groin hernia; some large ventral hernias following major postoperative wound infections have minimal residual abdominal wall structures, should be treated by appropriate external support
3. Operative repair indicated for most hernias: at a time of election for hernia with minimal symptoms, several days after reduction for incarcerated hernia, which is readily reduced, immediately for hernia with evidence of strangulation

OPERATIVE REPAIR

1. Many herniorrhaphies now done as ambulatory procedures under local anesthesia
2. Involves two essential steps: management of peritoneal sac and its contents, repair of muscle-aponeurotic abdominal wall defect
3. Concern about peritoneal sac overdone in past; can be treated by simple inversion or excision unless sliding component or strangulated contents must be managed
4. Abdominal wall defect managed by either suture closure or placement of synthetic mesh over weak area
5. With sliding hernia, the sliding component, cecum on right or sigmoid mesocolon on left, should be identified and returned to abdominal cavity without injury
6. With acutely incarcerated hernia, sac must be opened and incarcerated contents examined for viability with resection of gangrenous tissue before reduction

RESULTS

1. With elective herniorrhaphy, morbidity and mortality negligible
2. Wound infection the most frequent complication with groin incision, may lead to recurrence of hernia
3. Possibility of recurrence the major problem with any hernia repair
4. Recurrence rate greater with direct, femoral, or ventral hernia repair than with indirect herniorrhaphy
5. With any herniorrhaphy, injury to bowel or bladder must be avoided to minimize problems
6. With strangulated hernia, significant morbidity and some mortality must be anticipated

SUMMARY

1. Hernia repair not without complications, but elective repair prevents possible bowel obstruction or gangrene
2. Elective hernia repair obviates future problems, should be done in most circumstances unless patient's medical condition contraindicates operation

PITUITARY

Gross Anatomy Nomenclature not well standardized, that of Wislocki recommended. Neurohypophysis composed of infundibulum (median eminence), infundibular stem (pituitary stalk), and infundibular process (posterior lobe, pars nervosa). Adenohypophysis composed of pars distalis (anterior pituitary), pars intermedia, and pars tuberalis.

Human Anatomic Variations In 50% sella turcica is covered by the dura of the diaphragma sella, in 40% the opening in the diaphragma around the stalk is greater than 5mm, in 10% the diaphragma is very thin. Without the barrier, the pituitary tumor may preferentially extend into the suprasellar region; if a barrier is present, a tumor will balloon the sella.

Plain x-rays define only the length of the pituitary. Lateral margins of pituitary may be indented by the carotid arteries.

Vascular Anatomy Neurohypophysis has no blood-brain barrier. Capillaries have fenestrated endothelium and a double basement membrane. No neuronal cell bodies lie within neurohypophysis, only axons projecting from hypothalamus. All elements of neurohypophysis are joined by a common capillary bed; direction of blood flow variable. Adenohypophysis has no arterial supply; all blood reaching it passes first through the capillary bed of neurohypophysis. Neurosecretory material therefore conveyed by portal vessels to adenohypophysis. Distortion of normal vascular relationships by tumor growth important in determining endocrine disturbances that develop with pituitary tumors.

Cellular Physiology

Neurohypophysis Large body neurons project from supraoptic and paraventricular nuclei of hypothalamus into neurohypophysis near capillaries of posterior pituitary. They release the peptides vasopressin (antidiuretic effect), and oxytocin (profound effect on pregnant uterus). Small body neurons project from hypothalamus to median eminence and release TRH, GRH, somatostatin, GnRH, and CRF.

ADENOHYPOPHYSIS   Immunohistochemistry has allowed description of pituitary cells according to their secretory function.

Growth Hormone Cells   Lateral aspect of adenohypophysis. GH effects growth of bone muscle and visceral organs. Resting serum level is 1–5 ng/mL with surges 6–8 times daily. Growth hormone–releasing factor stimulates secretion, somatostatin limits it.

Prolactin Cells   Lateral aspect of adenohypophysis. Promotes lactation. In sleep, basal levels increase 2–3-fold by episodic surges. Hypothalamic control maintained through prolactin-inhibiting factor and prolactin-releasing factor. Pregnancy, lactation, stress, and exercise associated with high levels.

Thyroid-Stimulating Hormone Cells   Central adenohypophysis (basophils). Increases thyroid growth and synthesis of thyroid hormone. Hypothalamic control through thyrotropin-releasing hormone. T3 and T4 inhibit TSH release; cold and stress cause its release.

Adenocorticotropic Hormone Cells   ACTH promotes growth of the adrenal cortex and the synthesis of the adrenal steroid hormones. Biologic half-life 10 min. Circulating levels highest during sleep—circadian rhythm, even in sleep-deprived subjects. Stress, fear, trauma, hemorrhage, and extreme cold cause release, mediated by CRF and vasopressin.

Gonadotrophins   FSH—spermatogenesis and maturation of ovarian follicles and production of ovarian steroids. LH—stimulates testes to produce testosterone and promotes development of corpus luteum. Hypothalamic influence mediated via gonadotropin-releasing hormone.

Pituitary Disorders

TRAUMA   Pituitary stalk traverses the subdural space, may be partially or totally disrupted during deceleration of head trauma. Pituitary necrosis and panhypopituitarism result.

POSTPARTUM PITUITARY ISCHEMIA   In pregnancy pituitary weight increases by 50%. Hemorrhagic shock can cause pituitary necrosis and panhypopituitarism.

CHROMOPHOBE ADENOMAS   Nonsecreting tumors are the most common pituitary tumor. As they enlarge, adjacent secreting cells within sella turcica are compressed and dysfunction results; GH affected first, gonadotrophins next, TSH third, and ACTH last. Visual system may be distorted by larger tumors; the largest impinge on the third ventricle and may cause hydrocephalus and/or hypothalamic dysfunction. Surgical procedures via either transfrontal or transsphenoidal routes are indicated.

ACROMEGALY   Excess growth hormone results in gigantism in children before epiphyses close, and in acromegaly in adults. Enlargement of the heart may result in valvular dysfunction and cardiomyopathy. Hypersecreting tumors may be large (chromophobe) or small. If small, selective transsphenoidal resection is possible; if large, radical hypophysectomy or proton beam ablation is used.

CUSHING'S DISEASE   Although hypersecretion of ACTH by pituitary results in hypersecretion of steroid hormones from adrenal, not all patients with high levels of adrenal steroids have ACTH-producing tumors. Cause can be determined by manipulation of pituitary/adrenal axis with dexamethasone and/or metapyrone. If cause is pituitary tumor, it should be treated directly.

PROLACTIN-SECRETING TUMORS   Forty percent of all pituitary tumors. Excessive prolactin causes amenorrhea and galactorrhea in females and impotence in males. Bromocriptine, an ergot derivative, inhibits prolactin production; may be preferred over operation.

OTHER TUMORS   Hypersecreting tumors of gonadatropic cells or thyrotropic cells are rare but reported. Craniopharyngeoma, a squamous cell tumor arising from remnants of Rathke's pouch, may develop in sella and cause hypofunction, or may develop above diaphragma sella and affect neurohypophysis, and hypothalamus visual and ventricular systems. May be cystic. Treatment: total excision if encapsulated or cyst drainage. Meningiomas or metastases may occur.

Diagnostic Studies

RADIOLOGIC PITUITARY STUDIES   Skull films: lateral views demonstrate sagittal profile of sella; anteroposterior films show floor of sella. CT and MRI most helpful.

FUNCTIONAL PITUITARY STUDIES   Full battery of assays usually essential to understand the functional derangements caused by tumor.

Therapeutic Modalities

TRANSCRANIAL SURGERY   Antibiotics made it possible for surgeons to remove frontal bone and, if needed, open frontal sinus without fear of meningitis.

TRANSSPHENOIDAL APPROACHES   Cosmetically superior, since incision is hidden in gingival mucosa.

STEREOTAXIC TECHNIQUES   Allow accurate administration of ablative isotopes or cryosurgery via transsphenoidal or transethmoidal route.

ADRENAL

Composed of two endocrine tissues merged into a single gland. The cortex synthesizes and secretes the major glucocorticoid cortisol, the primary mineralocorticoid aldosterone, adrenal androgens, and small amounts of estrogen. The medulla synthesizes and secretes catecholamines epinepherine, norepinephrine, and dopamine.

Embryology

The cortex and medulla arise separately. The primitive cortex develops from coelomic mesothelium. The medulla and sympathetic nervous system develop together from primitive neural crest cells. One group migrates along the adrenal vein, invades, and becomes surrounded by cortex. Preganglionic sympathetic fibers synapse directly with these medullary cells. A second group forms the organs of Zuckerkandl lateral to aorta near IMA. They usually atrophy in childhood but are a frequent location of extraadrenal chromaffin tumors.

Anatomy

Bilateral, near upper pole of each kidney, weight 3.5–5 g and bright yellow. Each is supplied by three main arteries, one from the inferior phrenic artery, one from the aorta, and one from the renal artery. The right adrenal vein enters the posterior aspect of vena cava, the left the renal vein.

Adrenal Cortex

PHYSIOLOGY Cortisol *Synthesis, Binding, and Transport.*   Cholesterol is the basic precursor of all adrenal steroids. Circulating cortisol is 90% protein-bound. Free cortisol is the physiologically active form. Cortisol in plasma has a half-life of 70–120 min. Major site of metabolism is liver.

Secretion. ACTH stimulates both synthesis and secretion of cortisol by the adrenal gland. Stimuli that cause release of ACTH include small changes in blood volume without hypotension, tissue damage, hypoxia, deviations in body temperature, and hypoglycemia, pain, and anxiety.

Prolonged administration of cortisol blocks ACTH production and thereby blocks production and secretion of cortisol by adrenal cortex, eventually causing cortical atrophy.

Cortisol secretion follows a diurnal rhythm with peak 4–6 AM and nadir 8–12 PM.

Glucocorticoid Actions. Glucocorticoids tend to cause hyperglycemia, negative nitrogen balance, and lipolysis. Peripheral tissues undergo catabolism, while essential tissues such as the brain and liver are spared.

In supraphysiologic concentrations glucocorticoids inhibit nearly every aspect of the inflammatory reponse.

The effects of glucocorticoids on the cardiovascular system are poorly understood. It is clear that cardiovascular collapse occurs in patients with acute adrenocortical insufficiency. Hypersecretion after injury is essential for cardiovascular stabilization and blood volume restoration.

Aldosterone *Synthesis.* Aldosterone is synthesized from progesterone in the zona glomerulosa.

Protein Binding. 55% of circulating aldosterone is bound to plasma proteins. The unbound portion is physiologically active.

Metabolism. Primarily metabolized in the liver by a series of reduction reactions. Half-life 15 min.

Secretion. Stimulated by two physiologic stimuli: decrease in circulating blood volume leading to salt conservation and restoration of blood volume, or increase in serum potassium concentration. Angiotensin II and ACTH stimulate aldosterone secretion.

Mineralocorticoid Actions. Aldosterone an important regulator of electrolyte and fluid balance. Stimulates renal tubular sodium reabsorption and K^+, H^+, and NH_4^+ secretion by direct action on the tubule. In CHF and cirrhosis, secondary hyperaldosteronism leads to increased salt retention and fluid overload. Spironolactone, a competitive aldosterone antagonist, is helpful.

CUSHING'S SYNDROME   Caused by prolonged exposure to excessive cortisol concentrations. Most common cause is chronic iatrogenic administration. Occurs spontaneously secondary to pathology in hypothalamus, pituitary, or adrenal, or from ectopic ACTH secretion from nonadrenal neoplasm.

Etiology   Cushing's syndrome is caused specifically by a chronic hypersecretion of ACTH (pituitary tumors responsible for 90%). Excessive CRF secretion or vasopressin secretion causes some cases.

Primary adrenal pathology causes 10% of all cases of Cushing's syndrome. Adrenal adenomas and carcinomas secrete independent of ACTH control. Documentation of local tumor invasion or metastatic spread is required to confirm malignancy.

Nonadrenal neoplasms that may secrete ACTH (ectopic ACTH syndrome) constitute 15% of all cases of Cushing's syndrome. These include oat cell carcinoma of lung, tumors of parotid, liver, thymus, islet cells, esophagus, medullary thyroid carcinoma, and pheochromocytoma.

Nodular dysplasia of adrenal is an exceedingly rare cause.

Clinical Manifestations   F/M ratio 4:1, third to fifth decade. Truncal obesity; moon facies; buffalo hump; supraclavicular fat; purple striae on lower abdomen, trunk, and thighs; hypertension; hirsutism; acne; and peripheral edema. Late findings: marked muscle wasting, osteoporosis with pathologic fractures, atherosclerosis and glucose intolerance, emotional lability or psychosis.

Diagnostic Testing   Two phases. Test to confirm diagnosis: plasma cortisol concentration not helpful. 24-h urinary free cortisol excretion of more than 100 μ provides nearly complete distinction between normal and Cushing's syndrome.

Dexamethasone Suppression Test.   Synthetic corticosteroid that blocks ACTH release; 1 mg given orally at 11 PM, plasma cortisol measured at 8 AM—normal suppression to 3.5–10 μg/dL. The two tests are additive in accuracy.

Tests to Determine Primary Pathology   Whether pituitary-dependent, adrenal-dependent, or ectopic ACTH–dependent.

Plasma ACTH Level.   With adrenal pathology, plasma ACTH level usually undetectable. With pituitary or ectopic syndrome, ACTH elevated, ectopic usually highest. (In nodular dysplasia of adrenal, ACTH levels often detectable.)

High-Dose Dexamethasone Suppression Test.   24-h baseline urinary 17-hydroxycorticosteroid excretion measured, then give 2 mg dexamethasone orally every 6 h for 2 days. Supression to 40% base line is positive test, indicates adrenal tumor. (Nodular adrenal dysplasia does not suppress.)

Metapyrone Test.   Metapyrone inhibits cortisol synthesis. Administration to normal individuals and patients with pituitary ACTH hypersecretion causes compensatory increase in plasma ACTH, compared to base line, which does not occur in patients with an adrenal source.

ACTH and CRF Stimulation Tests.   Administration of ACTH to patient with cortical hyperplasia produces a greater rise in plasma cortisol than expected in normals. Adenomas are autonomous and do not respond. Test not always discriminatory. CRF isolated. Response to CRF stimulation may differentiate pituitary from ectopic ACTH production.

Other Tests.   Differentiating pituitary from ectopic source of ACTH may not be easy. With obvious extraadrenal carcinoma, answer is clear. CT scan and sellar radiography may be revealing. Selective venous sampling from inferior petrosal sinus with 2:1 central to peripheral ACTH gradient is diagnostic of pituitary tumor.

Treatment   Termination of cortisol hypersecretion is the goal. Adrenalectomy may be complicated by infection, and lifelong replacement therapy can be complicated. Nelson syndrome: development of large ACTH-secreting pituitary adenoma after bilateral adrenalectomy, the result of continued growth of the underlying microadenoma.

Pituitary Operations.   Most patients with ACTH hypersecretion are best treated by pituitary exploration even if preoperative studies fail to demonstrate adenoma. Microadenectomy is curative in 50–90%. In the absence of adenoma, corticotroph hyperplasia is likely; total hypophysectomy is often curative. Recurrence after microadenectomy is common (13 of 123 patients thought cured).

Pituitary Irradiation.   Has largely been abandoned.

Neuropharmacologic Agents.   Promising, but not yet routine. Primarily indicated in patients unresponsive to pituitary surgery or in Cushing's syndrome proved secondary to CRF hypersecretion. Cyproheptadine blocks release of CRF from hypothalamus. Bromocriptine is a dopamine antagonist that inhibits CRF secretion.

Adrenal Operations.   Surgery should be initial treatment for all patients with Cushing's syndrome secondary to adrenal adenoma or carcinoma. Preoperative radiologic lateralization of the tumor allows resection via a unilateral flank incision.

Adrenalectomy is curative. Postoperative steroid replacement therapy is necessary until the suppressed gland recovers (3–6 months).

Adrenal carcinoma should be approached via a midline incision to allow radical resection, since surgery is only hope for cure.

Mitotane.   Causes selective destruction of normal and neoplastic adrenocortical cells. It is the only chemotherapeutic agent that has proved of some value in the treatment of adrenal carcinoma. Adrenocortical insufficiency is the result of successful mitotane therapy.

Ectopic ACTH Syndrome.   Best treated by complete resection of the primary neoplasm. Bilateral adrenalectomy may be considered when the primary is unresectable and the prognosis is for long-term survival. Chemotherapy with metyrapone or mitotane should be considered.

ADRENOCORTICAL INSUFFICIENCY (ADDISON DISEASE)   Rare in surgical patients, but often lethal. Occurs more commonly in patients on long-term anticoagulation therapy. Signs and symptoms are nonspecific. Adrenal crisis should be considered in any patient who develops sudden or progressive cardiovascular collapse or in any acute illness that does not respond to appropriate therapy. Exact incidence uncertain. Adrenal hemorrhage at autopsy 0.14–1.1%.

Etiology   The most common cause is withdrawal of chronic steroid therapy. Chronic administration of supraphysiologic doses of glucocorticoids suppresses ACTH by feedback. The long-term result is adrenocortical atrophy.

Eighty percent of spontaneous cases are secondary to "Schmidt syndrome," autoimmune destruction of the adrenals. Antibodies to adrenocortical cells occur in high percentage, and histology reveals lymphocytic infiltrate. Autoimmune hypothyroidism is associated in 80%; diabetes, hypoparathyroidism, and ovarian failure also occur. Adrenocortical insufficiency develops gradually in these patients. The adrenal stress response may be impaired during this period. 90% of cortex must be destroyed before basal plasma cortisol levels fall below normal.

Intraadrenal hemorrhage secondary to sepsis, anticoagulant therapy, or coagulopathy can cause acute insufficiency.

Clinical Manifestations   Weakness and fatigue, weight loss and anorexia, a diffuse hyperpigmentation of skin, dehydration. In adrenal crisis, poorly defined upper abdominal or flank pain, fever, nausea, lethargy, disorientation and confusion, hypotension, hypoglycemia, hypokalemia, and prerenal azotemia. These signs with or without cardiovascular collapse in any perioperative or critically ill patient should raise the question of insufficiency.

Diagnostic Testing If clinical condition is rapidly deteriorating, a blood sample for plasma ACTH and cortisol levels should be drawn and 200 mg water-soluble corticosteroid administered with the same needle. Plasma cortisol is often depressed and ACTH is often elevated. Capacity to respond to ACTH stimulation is measured to assess the stress response. Cortisol measured before and at 15, 30, and 60 min after administration of 250 μg ACTH. With confirmed adrenal insufficiency, thyroid function should be tested to screen for Schmidt syndrome.

Treatment After the initial IV bolus, 50–100 mg cortisone acetate should be given IM and steroids are administered in amounts 3–10 times usual endogenous production. Fluid and electrolyte imbalance is corrected with IV fluids, and the underlying cause is sought.

Perioperative Treatment. Patients currently taking steroids or who have taken them within 2 years should be treated perioperatively with hydrocortisone 100 mg IM, on call to OR, 50 mg IM or IV in recovery, and every 6 h for first 24 h, then 25 mg every 6 h for another 24 h, then taper to maintenance over 3–5 days.

Chronic Insufficiency. Chronic treatment must include both glucocorticoid and mineralocorticoid replacement administered 2 times daily in divided doses. Treatment is lifelong, and early medical attention is sought in acute illness, nausea, vomiting, or diarrhea.

PRIMARY HYPERALDOSTERONISM One of the few surgically curable causes of hypertension. Adrenocortical adenoma (80%) or hyperplasia of zona glomerulosa. Adenomas appear sensitive to ACTH, and angiotensin II affects secretion in hyperplasia.

Clinical Manifestations Hypertension with spontaneous hypokalemia. May be asymptomatic or have weakness, fatigue, paresthesias, tetany, or paralysis, particularly with treatment with thiazide diuretics. Polyuria (and polydipsia) may develop secondary to vasopressin resistance from chronic hyperkaluria. More common in women and in third and fourth decades. Hypertension or eclampsia in pregnancy is common. Menorrhagia often leading to hysterectomy is frequent.

Diagnostic Testing Biochemical determinations: Hypokalemia must be corrected with potassium before testing because hypokalemia inhibits aldosterone secretion and may lead to a false-negative workup. Salt loading (9 g NaCl/day for 2 weeks) is used to suppress renin. Hydralazine for severe hypertension. Simultaneous measurement of plasma aldosterone and renin activity. High aldosterone and low renin suggest primary hyperaldosteronism. Fluorohydrocortisone (a potent mineralocorticoid) is given (0.1 mg/day for 3 days) to inhibit the renin system. If aldosterone is still elevated the diagnosis is confirmed.

Only patients with aldosteronoma decrease aldosterone level with change in posture from recumbant to standing.

Localization.   Preoperative radiologic localization of tumor; high-resolution CT scanning (75% accurate). Selective venous sampling for aldosterone indicated when CT scanning fails.

Treatment *Adenoma.*   Unilateral adrenalectomy, posterior approach. Preparation with spironolactone for 6–10 days preoperatively corrects hypokalemia and allows restoration of normal fluid balance. Blood pressure expected to return to normal in 50%; hypokalemia almost always corrected.

Hyperplasia.   Medical management with spironolactone, a competitive antagonist of aldosterone (200–400 mg/day in divided doses). Amiloride, a potassium-sparing diuretic, is useful. Cyproheptadine (blocks CRF release in hypothalamus) and calcium channel blockers may also be useful. If medical management fails, total or subtotal adrenalectomy is indicated, but the response is often poor.

ADRENOGENITAL SYNDROME   Adrenal androgen hypersecretion, pure or mixed (hypersecretion of other cortical hormones). In infants a congenital enzyme deficiency in pathways of cortisol biosynthesis results in decreased cortisol production; causes hypersecretion of ACTH due to loss of feedback inhibition. Secondary adrenocortical hyperplasia develops with overproduction of intermediary compounds including adrenal androgens. 1 in 15,000 live births.

In postnatal children and adults, virilization is almost always caused by tumors of the adrenal. Adrenocortical carcinoma is the most common tumor. Androgen-secreting adenomas are rare.

Clinical Manifestations   Masculinization in females and precocious puberty in young males.

Diagnostic Testing   24-h urine collection for 17-ketosteroids, usually exceeds 30–40 mg. Plasma testosterone increased (due to peripheral conversion of adrenal androgens to testosterone). Dexamethasone suppression distinguishes congenital from adenoma—output of adenoma not suppressed. Suspect carcinoma when 24-h urinary 17-ketosteroid exceeds 100 mg.

Ovarian tumors may secrete testosterone; 24-h urine usually normal and not suppressed by dexamethasone; ovarian tumors may be palpable.

Treatment   Congenital hyperplasia: treated with glucocorticoid to suppress ACTH. Surgical correction of external genital abnormalities required in females.

Tumors.   After localizing studies, transperitoneal adrenalectomy indicated. Resection should include the involved adrenal and, when feasible, local metastatic disease. Recurrence detected by monitoring urinary 17-ketosteroids. Mitotane may be used to treat recurrence.

ADRENAL MASS   Asymptomatic adrenal masses found incidentally on CT scan in up to 0.6%. Patient should be evaluated biochemically for activity of mass (urinary free cortisol and catecholamines and plasma renin, aldosterone, and androgen levels). Small tumor followed by CT scanning. Resection in young and healthy patients.

Adrenal Medulla

PHYSIOLOGY   *Synthesis.*   Adrenal medulla synthesizes and secretes epinephrine, norepinephrine, and small amounts of dopamine. Tyrosine is the precursor of all catecholamines, norepinephrine is the intermediate product, and epinephrine the final.

Inactivation.   Free catecholamines are conjugated before excretion with glucuronide of sulfate.

Secretion.   Catecholamines produced in both sympathetic nerve terminals, and adrenal medullary cells are stored in a highly concentrated form in chromaffin granules. Cell depolarization following stimulation of sympathetic nerves to the adrenal causes exocytosis of the granules. Secretion is analogous to a reflex response.

Response to hemorrhage may be mediated by angiotensin II. Stimuli for secretion of catecholamines: hypoxia, hypoglycemia, changes in temperature, pain, shock, CNS injury, local wound factors, and endotoxin all act via CNS.

Catecholamine Actions.   Major role may be metabolic; synergistic with other metabolically active hormones including cortisol and glucagon. Preparing organism for "flight or fight."

Adrenergic Receptors.   Alpha: activation of alpha receptors in smooth muscle is excitatory, leading to vasoconstriction of most vascular beds, but not coronary or cerebral, and contraction of smooth muscle in other organs. Causes increased systolic, diastolic, and mean arterial pressure.

Beta: inhibition of smooth muscle contraction, leading to vasodilatation and relaxation of other types of smooth muscle and mediates the excitatory effects of catecholamines on the heart (increased rate, output, and oxygen consumption). Beta$_2$ receptors mediate the metabolic actions.

PHEOCHROMOCYTOMA   Derived from chromaffin cells that secrete catecholamines. Secretory crisis in patients with pheochromocytoma may cause sudden death.

Etiology   Most arise in adrenal. 10% bilateral. Extraadrenal pheochromocytoma may be found in any tissue of neuroectodermal origin. Multiple tumors occur in 8–15% of adults and 35–40% of children. 10% are malignant. Malignancy confirmed only by documented metastases to lymph nodes, liver, lungs, or bone or local invasion of surrounding structures.

Morbidity and mortality are secondary to catecholamine hypersecretion. May secrete norepinephrine alone or in combination with epinephrine. Sudden death may occur during stress of pregnancy, surgery, or trauma.

Ten percent are familial, often autosomal dominant, high prevalence of MEN syndromes. Half of these develop bilateral tumors. All family members of patient with pheochromocytoma should be screened to detect asymptomatic tumors.

One to two percent of patients with neurofibromatosis develop pheochromocytoma.

Lindau syndrome: hemangioblastomas of cerebellum, medulla, spinal cord; retinal angiomas; cysts of lung, liver, pancreas, kidney, and epididymis; and hypernephromas.

MEN-IIA, inherited syndrome: pheochromocytoma, medullary thyroid carcinoma, and frequently hyperparathyroidism, autosomal dominant. MEN-IIB: medullary carcinoma of thyroid and pheochromocytoma, with mucosal neuromas and marfanoid body habitus; rarely hyperparathyroidism.

Clinical Manifestations   All age groups. Comprise 0.1–0.2% of patients with sustained diastolic hypertension. Symptoms of catecholamine hypersecretion and complications of hypertension; 50% have paroxysmal hypertensive episodes, headache, generalized diaphoresis, and palpitations. Precipitated by drugs that stimulate secretion, mechanical deformation of tumor, changes in position, invasive tests, anaesthesia, or increases in body cavity pressure. Decreased arterial pressure and tachycardia with postural changes in a hypertensive strongly suggest pheochromocytoma. Mottled cyanosis, mesenteric ischemia, claudication, Raynaud's phenomenon, or livedo reticularis.

Differential Diagnosis. Pheochromocytoma presenting as hypertension during pregnancy may be disastrous. Untreated pheochromocytoma carries a 50% mortality rate for both mother and fetus.

Psychiatric symptoms may range from anxiety to psychosis. Episodes of flushing with hypotension are prominent in carcinoid, urinary hydroxyindoleacetic acid elevated, and injection of small amounts of epinephrine or histamine induce flushing attacks.

Neuroblastoma and ganglioneuroblastoma occur in young patients and are usually asymptomatic.

Diagnostic Testing Test of choice: urinary excretion of free epinephrine, norepinephrine, or metabolites. Plasma concentrations measureable but unreliable because hypersecretion is intermittent.

Provocative tests have no place in initial evaluation of pheochromocytoma, used only with strong suspicion when biochemical tests fail.

CT scanning localizes 90–95% of tumors more than 1 cm in diameter. Nuclear imaging with ^{131}I-metaiodobenzylguanidine (MIBG), available in research facilities, selectively accumulates in chromaffin tissue, very sensitive.

Treatment Surgical resection is the only curative procedure for both benign and malignant pheochromocytoma.

Preoperative stabilization with pharmacologic agents to inhibit synthesis or block alpha and beta receptors usually indicated. Alpha-methyl-1-tyrosine inhibits synthesis, dose starts at 250–500 mg daily and increases until hypertension controlled or daily dose reaches 5 g. Phenoxybenzamine is a noncompetitive alpha blocker. Dose 20–40 mg 2–4 times a day, increasing 20 mg daily until arterial pressure controlled. Time is allowed with liberalized salt intake to restore blood volume. Beta blockers used only for persistent tachycardia (more than 130 beats/min, used only after alpha blockade), begun routinely day before operation, usually propranolol. Steroid prep in case bilateral tumors found. Hydration is most important to maintain blood volume.

Intraoperative Management Monitoring with arterial and central venous catheters, large-bore peripheral lines. Premixed solutions of phentolamine, nitroprusside, levophed, and lidocaine available.

Anterior transabdominal approach required because of the possibility of bilateral and extraadrenal tumors. Changes in arterial pressure and pulse during exploration may help locate tumor foci. Malignant tumors should be aggressively resected.

Operative mortality less than 3%. Continued follow-up important to screen for recurrent disease. Family members require yearly physical examination and screening for elevated catecholamines, calcitonin, and serum calcium.

Neuroblastoma

Incidence Ten new cases per million live births. Third most frequent malignancy in children.

Pathology Highly malignant, derivative of neural crest cells, and found in same locations as pheochromocytoma; 70% intraabdominal and retroperitoneal, 50% intraadrenal. May regress spontaneously or differentiate into a less malignant tumor. Ganglioneuroblastoma is a histologic variant. Ganglioneuromas are benign tumors made up entirely of ganglion cells.

Clinical Manifestations Variable depending on age, site, and size of primary and presence of metastases. Most common is asymptomatic, irregular, firm, intraabdominal mass. May have distention or evidence of bowel or gastric outlet obstruction. Ganglioneuroblastoma may present with a mass in neck, mediastinum, thorax, abdomen, or pelvis. Paraspinal neuroblastomas frequently develop an intraspinal extension with symptoms of cord compression.

Diagnostic Testing Distinguished from pheochromocytoma by clinical presentation, but tissue diagnosis required to distinguish from ganglioneuroblastoma or ganglioneuroma. 98% have elevated catecholamines or their metabolites in urine (VMA and HMA).

Treatment Hydration and nutritional assessment. Emergency operation for bowel obstruction or cord compression. Respiratory compromise from enormous hepatomegaly treated with radiation therapy. Staging is based on size and location of primary and whether primary crosses midline, and on metastases. CT scan superior to other radiologic tests except for detection of bone lesions where bone scan is helpful.

Surgical Therapy. Operation undertaken for complete resection in stages I, II, and III, and to sample lymph nodes, and for life-threatening complications. Also indicated whenever diagnosis or stage in question. Delayed primary resection of stage IV tumor may be possible after radiation or chemotherapy. Anterior transabdominal approach.

Prognosis   Favorable in stages I and II, well-differentiated tumors. Stage IV-S often regresses, even spontaneously. Follow-up every 3 months for 2 years; then annually throughout childhood with measurement of urinary VMA and HMA levels, plasma tumor markers, and bone scan.

Ganglioneuroma

Rare, benign, encapsulated; excised only if symptomatic.

Adrenalectomy

CT scan allows accurate preoperative localization of adrenal tumors in 95%. Posterior approach therefore used more frequently, resulting in fewer complications, for adenomas (and for pheochromocytoma localized to a single adrenal by ^{131}I MIBG scanning). Anterior transabdominal for pheochromocytoma, neuroblastoma, and adrenal carcinoma; preferred in children and in all patients with associated intraabdominal disease that may need correction. Combined thoracoabdominal procedure occasionally indicated for complete resection of large adrenal carcinomas. Bilateral adrenalectomy applicable for bilateral pheochromocytoma and as last resort if pituitary operation, pharmacologic agents, and medical adrenalectomy fail to control hypercortisolism.

37 THYROID AND PARATHYROID

THYROID

Anatomy

Gross Average weight 15–20 g. Consists of lateral lobes that extend along sides of larynx, reaching level of middle of thyroid cartilage and joined by isthmus that crosses the trachea. Pyramidal lobe present in 80%, extends upward from isthmus, and represents remnant of embryonic thyroglossal duct. Arterial supply: superior from external carotid; inferior from thyrocervical trunk.

Microscopic Follicles roughly spherical, average diameter 30 μm store products of cuboidal lining cells. Interfollicular C cells; part of APUD system; secrete calcitonin.

Recurrent Laryngeal Nerves. Injury results in vocal cord paralysis. Located in tracheoesophageal groove 64% right, 77% left. Lateral to trachea 33% right, 22% left. Anterolateral to trachea 3% right, 2% left. Direct (nonrecurrent) $\frac{1}{2}$% right. Anterior to inferior thyroid artery 37% right, 24% left; 50% embedded in ligament of Berry behind upper pole and susceptible to injury from traction on gland.

Superior Laryngeal Nerves. Injury results in paralysis of cricothyroid muscle, which fine-tunes vocal cord. Located adjacent to upper pole vascular pedicle.

ANOMALIES Lingual thyroid, a mass in the region of foramen cecum at base of tongue, may enlarge and cause dysphagia, dysphonia, or dyspnea. Primary treatment should be suppression with thyroid hormone or ablation with radioactive iodine. Surgery indicated for hemorrhage, degeneration, and necrosis, or threatened airway.

Physiology

Principal function to synthesize and secrete thyroid hormone. Calcitonin produced by C cells. No physiologic role. Pharmacologic use in treatment of hypercalcemia and Paget's disease of bone and as tumor marker for medullary carcinoma.

Iodine Metabolism   Exogenous iodine from dietary sources is rapidly absorbed from gut, distributed in extracellular space as iodides, then extracted by thyroid and kidneys; 90% of body iodine stored in thyroid. Partitioning of labeled dose complete within 48 h.

Hormone Synthesis

1. Active transport of iodine from plasma into thyroid cells, gradient 20:1 or more. Influenced by TSH inversely with glandular iodine content.
2. Rapid oxidation of iodides to iodine.
3. Tyrosine radicals iodinated to 3-monoiodotyrosine (MIT) and 3-5-diiodotyrosine (DIT). TSH-sensitive.
4. Coupling to form hormonally active iodothyronines, T4 from two DIT molecules and T3 from one DIT and one MIT.

Storage, Secretion, and Metabolism of Thyroid Hormone   T4 and T3 held in peptide linkage with thyroglobulin, the major component of intrafollicular colloid. Released by hydrolysis (influenced by TSH) bound to plasma proteins. T3 metabolically more active than T4, half-life 3 days.

Thyroid hormone stimulates protein synthesis and affects all aspects of carbohydrate metabolism and some aspects of lipid metabolism.

Regulation of Thyroid Activity   Hypothalamus secretes a thyrotropin-releasing hormone (TRH) that stimulates anterior pituitary cells to secrete TSH, which stimulates all processes leading to synthesis of thyroid hormone. TSH secretion controlled in feedback manner by blood level of thyroid hormone.

Pharmacologic doses of iodide decrease the rate of release of glandular iodine and the formation of active hormone.

Perchlorate and thiocyanate prevent concentration of iodine by thyroid.

Thiourea derivatives propylthiouracil (PTU) and methimazole (Tapazole) block binding of iodine to tyrosine radicals.

Evaluation of Patients with Thyroid Disease

History   Evidence of hyperfunction or insufficiency? Pressure of thyroid on neighboring structures, i.e., dysphagia, dysphonia, dyspnea, or choking sensation? With mass duration, rate of growth and presence of pain? Exposure to low-dose ionizing radiation most important. Ingestion of goitrogenic drugs? Family history?

Examination   Visible mass or enlargement. Deviation of trachea. Palpation from front and back of seated patient for size and consistency and regional lymph nodes. Bruit.

THYROID FUNCTION TESTS

Serum T4	4.9–12.0 µg/dL
Free thyroxine	2.8 ± 0.5 mµg/dL
Serum T3	115–190 mµg/dL
Serum TSH	Varies with lab, 0–6 µU/mL
Serum FTI	Varies with lab, 6.4–10%

Measures of Autoimmunity   Circulating antithyroglobulin and thyroid antimicrosomal antibodies can be measured in serum.

Measures of Thyroid and Pituitary Responsiveness   See Chap. 38 in *Principles of Surgery,* 5th ed, p. 1620.

Thyroid Scanning   Scintillation scanning with ^{123}I or ^{99m}Tc using gamma camera. Nodule may be hotter than remainder of gland, equal to remainder, or hypofunctional or cold.

After total thyroidectomy for papillary or follicular cancer total body scan can detect metastases.

Thyroid Biopsy   Fine needle aspiration is useful in diagnosis of thyroiditis and in separating benign from malignant disease.

Thyrotoxicosis

Etiology and Pathology   Primary excess secretion of active thyroid hormone.

Graves' Disease.   Generally regarded as a systemic autoimmune disease with thyrotoxicosis, exophthalmus, and pretibial myxedema. Thyroid diffusely enlarged, surface smooth, microscopically hyperplastic, with columnar epithelium and minimal colloid.

Toxic Multinodular Goiter.   Usually superimposed on longstanding nontoxic multinodular goiter. The nodules are composed of irregularly large cells and scant colloid. They are autonomous, independent of TSH.

Toxic Adenoma.   Follicular tumor independent of TSH.

Clinical Manifestations   Heat intolerance, increased sweating and consequent thirst, weight loss with increased appetite. Excitable, restless, hyperkinetic and emotionally unstable, insomnia, proximal muscle weakness, tremor of extended and abducted fingers, hyperactive DTRs. Skin warm, moist, flushed, hair fine and falls out, menses scant or absent. Diarrhea. In older patients: tachycardia, frequent atrial fibrillation and poor response to digitalis.

Graves' Disease. Most commonly young, M:F ratio 1:6, gland enlarged, smooth, audible bruit.

Eye signs minimal to severe: (1) spasm of upper lid with retraction and lid lag, (2) external ophthalmoplegia, (3) exophthalmos with proptosis, (4) supraorbital and infraorbital swelling, (5) congestion and edema, a sign of severity.

Toxic Multinodular Goiter. Usually after age 50, several palpable nodules. Exophthalmos rare.

Toxic Adenoma. Age 30–50. History of slowly growing mass; thyrotoxicosis uncommon unless lesion 3 cm in diameter.

Diagnostic Findings T4 and/or T3 levels and free thyroxin index (FTI) all elevated.

Graves' Disease. RAI uptake 45–90%. T3 suppression test applicable; decrease of 50% or less diagnostic.

Toxic Multinodular Goiter and Toxic Adenoma. RAI uptake 40–55%. Scan shows single or multiple hot areas that correspond to palpable nodules.

Treatment *Antithyroid Drugs.* No effect on underlying disease. T4 and/or T3 levels helpful in assessing response to treatment. Treat Graves' disease in hope that natural remission will occur after patient rendered euthyroid. Less than 40% have significant, long-lasting remission. For patients in whom thyrotoxicosis recurs or who are noncompliant, treatment with RAI or surgery is advised.

Radioactive Iodine. Dose of ^{131}I selected to deliver 8500 rad to thyroid; 20% require second dose. Avoids operation with attendant rare complications, and reduces cost. Disadvantages: long time required to control disease, high incidence of permanent myxedema, and development of nodules. Risk of genetic abnormalities following radioiodine treatment is minimal.

Surgery *Preparation.* Antithyroid drugs used initially to control thyrotoxicosis, then iodine added 8–10 drops preoperatively to reduce vascularity. Some prefer 5 to 7 day preparation with propranolol alone.

Results. Mortality less than 0.1%. Subtotal thyroidectomy provides rapid correction in 95%. Recurrent nerve palsy 0–3%, tetany 1–3%, 10–30% hypoparathyroid, 2–12% recurred.

Selection of Therapy. Young, pregnant, or lactating get antithyroid drugs. Failures get thyroidectomy or RAI. Surgery preferred for young with severe disease and large goiters. Older get RAI. Either therapy used in toxic multinodular goiter. Toxic adenoma should be excised.

Hypothyroidism

Failure of the gland to maintain an adequate plasma level of hormone.

Etiology   Ablation by thyroidectomy or RAI therapy for hyperthyroidism accounts for one-fourth of cases. Spontaneous myxedema may result from aplasia or replacement of gland by nonfunctional goiter, adenoma, or thyroiditis.

Clinical Manifestations   Cretinism. Juvenile hypothyroidism. Lymphocytic thyroiditis in adult, 80% female. Course insidiously progressive with tiredness, weight gain, fatigue, and apathy. Skin dry, thickened, puffy; hair dry and brittle, tongue enlarged, voice hoarse. Cardiac output reduced, heart dilated, pulse slow. Constipation, ascites, achlorhydria, pernicious anemia.

Diagnostic Findings   Anemia, bradycardia, flattened T waves. T4, T3, and FTI down; TSH and cholesterol up.

Treatment   Replacement, usually with L-thyroxine. Severe cases sensitive to small doses, so initial doses should be small (50 μg) and increased gradually to avoid myocardial stress.

Thyroiditis

ACUTE SUPPURATIVE THYROIDITIS   Uncommon. Follows acute URI. Signs are those of abscess. Treatment is I & D.

HASHIMOTO'S DISEASE   Most common chronic thyroiditis.

Etiology   Autoimmune: antimicrosomal and antithyroglobulin antibodies measurable. Genetic predisposition?

Pathology   Symmetrically enlarged, pale, and semifirm; may be focal. Lymphoid tissue predominates with disruption of architecture.

Clinical Manifestations   Average age 50. Local swelling, pain, and tenderness. Hypothyroidism may ensue.

Diagnostic Findings Tests biphasic with early signs of hyperfunction, later hypofunction. High titers of thyroid antibodies. Needle biopsy in nodular form if cancer suspected.

Treatment Symmetric and euthyroid—none. Goiter—suppressive doses of hormone. Marked pressure symptoms—subtotal thyroidectomy with clearing of trachea. Nodular—suppression (if cancer ruled out) or thyroidectomy.

Subacute Thyroiditis

Not Hashimoto. Mean age in forties, female predominant. Adherent but not fused. Follicles enlarged, infiltrate mononuclear, lymphocytes and neutrophils with multinucleated giant cells. Onset sudden with swelling and pain, fever, and constitutional symptoms. ESR elevated early. Needle biopsy may be diagnostic. Treatment: steroids.

REIDEL'S STRUMA Rare, chronic inflammatory, involves one or both lobes. Thought a terminal stage of Hashimoto. Follicles small and scant, dense scar tissue permeates. May constrict trachea. Unilateral indistinguishable from cancer. Average age 50. Symptoms from compression of trachea, esophagus, and recurrent nerve. Thyroid function decreased late. Treatment: hormonal replacement. Surgery dangerous because planes fused; may be necessary to relieve compression.

Goiter

Benign enlargement.

Familial Goiter. Inherited enzyme defect, usually autosomal recessive.

Endemic Goiter. Regional environmental; iodine deficiency and ingestion of goitrogens. Prophylactic iodination of table salt.

Sporadic Goiter. Diagnosis of exclusion.

Pathology Diffuse enlargement and smooth, or grossly nodular. Early hyperplasia, reversible. Involution with large, colloid-filled follicles interspersed with normal tissue.

Clinical Manifestations Endemic regions, no sex difference, otherwise F:M ratio 8:1. Most asymptomatic. Dysphagia, or tracheal compression with respiratory distress, particularly with substernal extension. Hemorrhage: sudden pain with rapid expansion. Rarely leads to hypothyroidism, but thyrotoxicosis develops in large percentage with long history.

Diagnostic Findings   Tests of function usually normal. X-ray of chest and neck for trachea and substernal extension.

Treatment   Diffuse goiter: Familial goiter responds to thyroxine. Drug-induced goiter requires the discontinuance of offending drug, if possible; if not, give thyroxine. Surgical indications include respiratory obstruction and cosmesis. Whenever a signficant segment of goiter is removed supplemental hormone therapy is indicated.

Nodules

Four percent of population have palpable thyroid nodules; 40–50 per million develop thyroid cancer; 6 per million die of it.

High-Risk Groups for Cancer   Irradiation to the head and neck: straight-line increase in incidence of both benign and malignant nodules up to dose of 1500 rad, but only after latency of 25 years or more. Was given to enlarged thymus, to tonsils and adenoids, and for acne and hemangiomas. Usually papillary, more often multicentric. Family history of medullary carcinoma: autosomal dominant.

Diagnostic Algorithm   History, physical exam, function tests, radioactive scans (technetium), B-mode ultrasound, needle biopsy.

Benign Tumors

Adenomas are embryonal, fetal, follicular, or microfollicular. Eighty percent of surgical specimens with single nodule prove benign.

Clinical Manifestations   Slowly growing mass. Cold, warm, or hot.

Treatment   When malignancy cannot be ruled out, excisional biopsy is indicated. Postoperative replacement hormone reduces recurrences.

Malignant Tumors

Pathology   Papillary, follicular, medullary, and anaplastic. Lymphoma and metastasis.

PAPILLARY CARCINOMA   Two-thirds of thyroid carcinomas. Peak in third and fourth decades. F:M ratio 3:1.

Pathology   Columnar thyroid epithelium arranged in papillary projections. Psammoma bodies (concentric layered calcium deposits). Some include follicular elements. Slow growing, spread intraglandular (80% multifocal), and to regional nodes.

Clinical Manifestations   Asymptomatic nodule, calcium flecks on x-ray, cold to isotope scan, solid to ultrasound, needle aspiration usually diagnostic.

Treatment   Resection: extent controversial. Lobectomy, frozen section. If benign, stop; if malignant, near total or total thyroidectomy and removal of abnormal lymph nodes performed. Neck dissection only if lateral nodes involved. (Follow-up isotope scans for metastases or RAI treatment. Suppressive doses of hormone for life.)

Prognosis   Excellent. Worse in patients over 50. Overall, 6% die of their disease.

FOLLICULAR CARCINOMA   One-fourth of thyroid malignancies, peak incidence fifth decade, F:M ratio 3:1.

Pathology   Grossly encapsulated. Histologic follicles, but cells may be crowded and look malignant with capsular and vascular invasion. Hematogenous spread to bone, lung, or liver often occurs early.

Clinical Manifestations   Recent change in long-standing goiter. Usually only a solitary nodule. Pain and adherence late. Metastases usually concentrate iodine.

Treatment and Prognosis   Controversy over extent of operation. Some favor removal of lobe and isthmus; others, near total or total thyroidectomy to facilitate later scanning (of body, and treatment with RAI of metastases). More virulent than papillary, 10-year survival 72%.

Other Treatments for Differentiated Cancers   *L-Thyroxine.* Following resection treat with enough L-thyroxine to suppress circulating TSH levels.

Radioiodine Therapy.   Total body scan with RAI, and ablation of residual normal thyroid in neck and to treat any distant metastasis found with ^{131}I. External beam irradiation for invasion of trachea or esophagus.

Chemotherapy.   Adriamycin for widely metastatic lesions that no longer concentrate iodine.

HÜRTHLE CELL TUMORS   Sheets of cells with eosinophilic cytoplasm; some obviously malignant with invasion and nodal spread, others appear benign. Does not concentrate iodine. Total thyroidectomy for obvious carcinomas, for patients with history of radiation, for large lesions, for those with capsular invasion, and when associated with differentiated carcinoma. Lobectomy for small, benign-appearing.

MEDULLARY CARCINOMA   C cells, produce calcitonin, derived from neural crest, APUD. Posterolateral in gland.

Pathology   Microscopic to 10 cm. Bilateral is rule in familial cases. Clusters of cells separated by areas of collagen and amyloid; may be polyhedral and resemble carcinoid or spindle cells. Spreads to regional nodes in neck and superior mediastinum, then distally.

Clinical Features   3.5–11.9% of thyroid malignancies. Familial mean early twenties, autosomal dominant. Single or multiple nodules; 15–20% nodal metastases at diagnosis. Diarrhea common, episodic flushing, 2–4% have Cushing's syndrome from ectopic production of ACTH. Hypercalcemia and pheochromocytomas associated.

Familial Medullary Carcinoma Syndrome.   MEN-IIA: multicentric medullary carcinoma or C cell hyperplasia, pheochromocytomas, or medullary hyperplasia and hyperparathyroidism. MEN-IIB: Medullary carcinoma (particularly virulent), pheochromocytomas and mucosal neuromas of lips, tongue, or conjunctivae; ganglioneuromas of bowel; typical facies, and Marfan-like habitus.

Adrenal medullary hyperplasia or pheochromocytomas are multicentric in 70%. Pheochromocytomas may be malignant, metastases more frequent when primary extraadrenal.

Diagnosis   Elevated serum calcitonin level by radioimmunoassay with thyroid mass diagnostic. Family members should be screened to catch lesions early. CEA also elevated. Return of serum elevations signals recurrence of tumor.

Treatment   Total thyroidectomy because of multicentricity. 50% have positive nodes. Neck dissection if nodes clinically involved. Thallium scanning may locate metastases. Debulking ameliorates APUD effects. Chemotherapy with progressive metastases. Pheochromocytomas should be operated on first; bilateral total adrenalectomy favored because of multicentricity. Parathyroid lesion chief cell hyperplasia.

Prognosis   Survival 80% at 5 years and 57% at 10 years.

ANAPLASTIC CARCINOMA   Ten percent of thyroid malignancies. May arise as transformation of a differentiated tumor. M/F ratio 3:1. 50% in seventh and eighth decades; mean age 66.

Grossly unencapsulated invading adjacent structures. Histology: cell structure variable from spindle to multinucleated giant cells; mitoses numerous.

Present with painful enlargement of thyroid, often fixed; pressure effects common. Metastasizes to lung. Rarely resectable. Diagnose by needle biopsy, then begin ancillary treatment. Seventy-five percent dead in 1 year.

LYMPHOMA AND SARCOMA Rare site for primary lymphoma. Limited procedure for tissue diagnosis indicated, followed by radiation therapy and/or chemotherapy.

METASTATIC CARCINOMA 2–4% of patients dying of malignant disease have metastases in thyroid. Bronchogenic and hypernephroma are most likely sources.

Surgery of the Thyroid

Performed to diagnose a mass within the gland, to remove benign or malignant tumors, as therapy for thyrotoxicosis, and to alleviate pressure symptoms attributable to the thyroid.

Operative Technique Endotracheal anesthesia. Neck extended. Equilateral low collar incision in skin crease. Upper flap raised to upper border of thyroid cartilage, lower flap to manubrial notch. Cervical fascia incised in midline. Sternothyroid and sternohyoid muscles retracted, or if gland large, divided. Lobe rotated medially and middle thyroid veins controlled and divided. Cricothyroid space opened. External branch of superior laryngeal nerve to inferior pharyngeal constrictor and cricothyroid muscles identified and preserved. Upper pole vessels ligated separately and close to lobe and divided. Lobe retracted medially and branches of inferior thyroid artery ligated and divided near capsule to preserve blood supply to parathyroids. Recurrent laryngeal nerve unroofed gently. In operation for Graves' disease 2–4 g of posterior thyroid tissue left and folded against trachea, or lobe may be removed totally. Parathyroids should be identified and preserved with their blood supply. Isthmus separated from anterior trachea leaving no remnant. Wound closed in layers.

Intrathoracic goiter usually represents extension of cervical thyroid tissue into chest and can usually be removed through a cervical incision. Occasionally transsternal resection is necessary.

COMPLICATIONS Thyroid Storm Occurs in patients with preexisting thyrotoxicosis who have not been treated or have been treated incompletely. Manifestations may develop in operating room or in recovery room. Hyperthermia, sweating, tachycardia, nausea, vomiting, and pain. Tremor and restlessness may progress to delirium or coma.

Treat with large doses of sodium or potassium iodide IV, 100 mg cortisol, oxygen and large doses of glucose, balanced fluid and electrolytes, hypothermia blanket, and propranolol or other beta blockers. Mortality approximates 10%.

Wound Hemorrhage Within the first few hours after surgery. Causes respiratory distress, since small amounts of blood in the deep space next to trachea can obstruct airway; 0.3–1% of cases. Treatment: emergency! Open the wound, evacuate the clot, and secure the bleeding vessel.

Recurrent Laryngeal Nerve Injury May be unilateral or bilateral, temporary (3–12 months) or permanent. With abductor laryngeal palsy the vocal cord assumes a medial position. The voice is husky and hoarse. Bilateral vocal cord paralysis can compromise the airway.

Hypoparathyroidism 0.6–2.8%. More common (up to 9%) in procedures for malignant disease. More common in secondary procedures. Devascularized gland may be minced and implanted in pockets in sternomastoid.

Manifest within days of operation. Circumoral numbness, tingling of fingertips, anxiety. Chvostek sign early, followed by Trousseau's sign and carpopedal spasm. May lead to tetany. Serum calcium reduced; phosphorus increased. May be transient (lasting days) or permanent.

Treat with 10 mL 10% calcium gluconate IV slow push, then a drip supplying 2–3 ampules every 8 h. Oral calcium to provide 1.5–2 g calcium ion daily may be started. For permanent hypoparathyroidism, vitamin D will be required.

PARATHYROID

Embryology

The upper parathyroids arise from the fourth branchial pouch along with the thyroid and descending only slightly; they remain close to the upper portion of the thyroid. Their position in adult life remains relatively constant. As adenomas they tend to descend posteriorly along the esophagus, even into the posterior mediastinum. The lower parathyroids arise from the third branchial pouch along with the thymus and descend with the thymus. Because they travel so far in embryologic life, their position in adult life is widely variable (from the hyoid bone to the pericardium). In the mediastinum, they tend to be anterior.

Anatomy

In autopsy series, roughly 80% had four glands, 6% had five, and 13% had three. Seventy-five percent of the upper glands lay on the posterior surface of the upper portion of the thyroid lobe, usually above the inferior thyroid artery. Only 50% of the lower glands lay against or just inferior to the lower pole of the thyroid; 13% were 1 cm below the lower pole in the tongue of thymus that extends into the neck. The average weight of a normal gland is about 35 mg. They may be heavier if they contain much fat. The superior gland is usually supplied by the superior thyroid artery, the lower by the inferior.

Physiology

Calcium   Of the more than 1000 g of calcium in the body, 1 g is in the extracellular fluid, 4 g is exchangeable in bone, and 11 g is in cells. Intake is usually 0.5–1 g. Urinary excretion varies with intake, from 175 mg on a 200-mg restricted diet to 300–400 mg on an unrestricted diet. A small amount is lost in sweat, the remainder is lost in the feces; 600 mg is secreted into the intestines from glands. Most is reabsorbed. Absorption occurs in the duodenum and upper jejunum. Absorption is active and involves vitamin D metabolites.

Normal serum calcium concentration is 8.4–10.2 mg/dL; 47% of serum calcium is ionized. The ionized portion is physiologically active, affecting nerve function and muscle contractility. The kidneys normally resorb 99% of filtered calcium. If the renal threshold for excretion is exceeded, hypercalcemic crisis may ensue.

Phosphorus   The body contains about 500 g phosphate, 0.4 g in extracellular fluid, 425 g in bone, and 75 g in cells. Dietary intake is about 1000 g daily. The serum level changes with diet, age, and hormone secretion. The value ranges 3–4.5 mg/dL in adults and 5–6 mg/dL in children; 70% of dietary phosphate is absorbed, primarily in the midgut. Absorption is increased by PTH, growth hormone, vitamin D, and low calcium intake. Excretion is increased in hyperparathyroidism, decreased in hypoparathyroidism.

Parathyroid Hormone PTH is synthesized within the glands, secreted, then cleaved in the reticuloendothelial cells of the liver into the N-terminal fragment that contains the biologic activity and is metabolized quickly, and the C-terminal fragment that is metabolized slowly and is therefore better measured for determining the serum level of the hormone.

Vitamin D Produced by the irradiation of 7-dihydrocholesterol in the skin, vitamin D is hydroxylated in the liver, then again in the kidney to the metabolically active form, 1,25-dihydroxyvitamin D_3, which mobilizes calcium and phosphorus from bone and enhances their absorption from the intestine. In the presence of PTH, when serum calcium or phosphorus levels are low, synthesis of $1,25\text{-}(OH)_2D_3$ is increased. This mechanism is feedback controlled.

In the treatment of renal osteodystrophy and hypoparathyroidism, microgram quantities of $1,25\text{-}(OH)_2D_3$ are effective.

Calcitonin Calcitonin is a calcium-lowering peptide found in the parafollicular cells of the mammalian thyroid gland (C cells). It lowers calcium by inhibiting bone resorption. Its presence in serum can be measured by radioimmunoassay. Medullary carcinoma of the thyroid is a C cell, calcitonin-producing tumor. Occult medullary carcinoma can be detected by measurement of serum calcitonin levels. Calcitonin is not important in the control of hypercalcemia in human beings.

Serum Calcium Homeostasis Serum calcium concentration is closely regulated, primarily by the parathyroid glands through a negative feedback system. Decreased calcium (or magnesium) stimulates secretion of PTH, which results in a rise in $1,25\text{-}(OH)_2D_3$. These then act peripherally to raise serum calcium to normal. Increased serum calcium level has the opposite effect.

Hyperparathyroidism

Primary hyperparathyroidism may be due to adenoma, which occurs in 70–80% of patients; to hyperplasia, which occurs in familial hyperparathyroidism and MEN syndromes; to carcinoma of the parathyroid glands (fewer than 1% of cases); or to a nonparathyroid tumor that is producing a PTH-like substance.

To judge whether or not a parathyroid gland is normal, size, weight, number of chief cells, and amount of fat contained related to the patient's age must all be evaluated. The major problem for both surgeon and pathologist is to differentiate adenoma (single-gland disease), from chief cell hyperplasia (multigland disease).

Adenomas. Adenomas are diagnosed by recognition of a large, hypercellular gland when the other parathyroid glands are normal. Grossly they are usually reddish brown, though they may be yellowish brown, and they are soft, smooth, and vascular. They may be composed of chief cells, water-clear cells, or oxyphil cells.

Hyperplasia. Almost all cases of hyperplasia are of the chief cell type. (Water-clear cell hyperplasia does occur; the glands are usually very large.) While one expects each of the four glands in hyperplasia to be enlarged, one or more glands may appear relatively normal. The differentiation between hyperplasia and adenoma is important and can be made by inspecting all four parathyroid glands at operation.

Carcinoma. Hypercalcemia and a palpable neck mass should raise the possibility of parathyroid carcinoma. Seventy-five percent of patients have serum calcium levels over 14 mg/dL, 73% have bone disease, 52% a palpable neck mass. Cervical or distant metastases are common, and cervical recurrence is likely. Hypercalcemia may recur months after surgery and can be the first sign of recurrent tumor. The only completely acceptable criteria for malignancy are recurrence of tumor, distant metastases, or invasion of adjacent structures. Morbidity and mortality are due to the complications of persistent and progressive hypercalcemia.

Hypercalcemia with Nonparathyroid Malignancy. The most common cause of hypercalcemia of malignant disease is osseous metastasis. Bone scan is helpful in diagnosing occult metastases. Some malignancies secrete a PTH-like substance that causes hypercalcemia and hypophosphatemia. Serum calcium falls with removal and may rise again with metastases. The most common are squamous and small cell carcinomas of the lung, and hypernephromas. Hyperparathyroidism may coexist. Ectopic hyperparathyroidism is more likely when the serum calcium level exceeds 14 mg/dL, serum alkaline phosphatase is increased, osteitis fibrosa is absent, and significant anemia is present. Primary hyperparathyroidism is more likely with a long history of kidney stones or when osteitis fibrosa is found.

Clinical Manifestations   Hyperparathyroidism most commonly occurs between ages 30 and 70, in women over men 2:1. It is frequently diagnosed in relatively asymptomatic individuals who have elevated calcium levels on routine multiphasic serum chemistry screens. Among patients with renal calcium stones, the incidence is about 5%.

Hypersecretion of PTH results in increased excretion of phosphate and in relative urinary alkalosis, both of which may predispose to calcium precipitation. Calcium excretion is also greatly increased. Calculi, nephrocalcinosis, polyuria, and polydypsia frequently occur.

As a consequence of the increased bone resorption brought about by PTH, the skeleton becomes demineralized and bone cysts, brown tumors, and pathologic fractures may occur. The presence of demonstrable bony change relates to the severity and the duration of the disease. Pseudogout, in which calcium pyrophosphate crystals are present in the joint fluid, may cause joint pain.

If patients with Zollinger-Ellison syndrome (MEN-I) are excluded, it is difficult to demonstrate an increased incidence of peptic ulcer disease in patients with primary hyperparathyroidism. The incidence of pancreatitis associated with hyperparathyroidism has not been definitely established, but one series reported 7%. In carcinoma of the parathyroid and familial hyperparathyroidism, it is somewhat higher.

Hypertension is associated with hyperparathyroidism. The mechanism is uncertain. In almost all instances it may be due to renal damage. Mental changes consisting of depression, fatigue, listlessness, and occasionally confusion are frequent complaints in hyperparathyroid patients, as are muscle weakness, eye changes, and ectopic calcification.

Hypercalcemic crisis is a serious complication. It usually does not occur unless the serum calcium level is above 16 mg/dL. It is much more likely to occur in the presence of severe renal damage. Early symptoms are loss of appetite and weight, nausea and vomiting, constipation, thirst, and polyuria and muscle weakness. These may progress to lethargy, drowsiness, confusion, severe muscle weakness, prostration, and coma. Survival depends on: rapid resuscitation with saline and lasix to rehydrate and lower serum calcium level, correct diagnosis, and early operation with correction of the hyperparathyroid state.

Diagnostic Findings   The diagnosis in most cases rests on biochemical determinations. Most important is elevation of the serum calcium level. The serum level may be close to the normal range or it may fluctuate. Repeated measurements over months or years are often necessary to establish the diagnosis. Serum total protein determination will help in the estimation of the ionized calcium level. Serum phosphate level is low in about 80% of cases. It may rise considerably in patients with significant renal damage. The alkaline phosphatase level is elevated only when there is x-ray evidence of bone disease. It is not specific. Plasma chloride is elevated in patients with primary disease who do not have renal impairment and are not on diuretics. A chloride/phosphate ratio of greater than 33 is virtually diagnostic.

A patient who has hypercalcemia and an elevated serum PTH concentration has hyperparathyroidism—most often due to excessive parathyroid function in the neck but occasionally due to ectopic hyperparathyroidism.

Bone densitometry can detect the demineralization common in hyperparathyroidism. The x-ray appearance of advanced hyperparathyroidism is characteristic. The skull may have a "moth eaten," ground-glass appearance. There may be marked absorption of the distal third of the clavicle. The spine may be markedly decalcified, with wedging of the vertebrae and kyphoscoliosis. There may be osteoclastic tumors of the jaw or metacarpals, metatarsals, and the ends of the long bones. Subperiosteal bone resorption in the middle and distal phalanges is characteristic. Plain films of the kidney may show calculi or nephrocalcinosis.

Ultrasonography has proved useful in locating enlarged parathyroid glands in the neck. Most endocrinologists and surgeons reserve the various localization techniques for patients who have already had a negative neck exploration by a highly competent parathyroid surgeon.

Special Considerations *Familial Hyperparathyroidism.* Mode of inheritance assumed to be autosomal dominant with incomplete penetrance. Usually chief cell hyperplasia. Association with pancreatitis and peptic ulceration. In 11% of patients with primary hyperparathyroidism, other family members have it also.

Familial Hypocalciuric Hypercalcemia (FHH). Hypercalcemia among young family members, without hypercalciuria and which is persistent after standard subtotal parathyroidectomy. Autosomal dominant. Incidence of nephrolithiasis and peptic ulcer not increased. Surgery should be avoided unless symptoms of hypercalcemia are severe.

Pregnancy. The birthweight of infants born to mothers with hyperparathyroidism is low, less than 3000 g in 50%. There is a high frequency of stillbirth, neonatal death, and neonatal tetany. Even borderline high values of serum calcium obtained from the pregnant woman should be followed up with

PTH levels. When the diagnosis is confirmed, parathyroid-ectomy should be performed, preferably in the second trimester so fetal parathyroid development can proceed normally.

Multiple Endocrine Neoplasia (MEN).   In MEN-I, the glands involved are parathyroid, pancreatic islets, and pituitary. With hyperparathyroidism, chief cell hyperplasia is the usual lesion. Recurrence following surgical treatment is frequent. Pancreatic islet cell tumors secrete amines and peptides that can cause a number of clinical syndromes depending on which hormone or combination of hormones are released. While some pituitary tumors in MEN-I syndrome can cause Cushing's syndrome or acromegaly, most are nonfunctioning.

MEN-IIA familial medullary carcinoma of the thyroid is associated with pheochromocytomas or bilateral adrenal medullary hyperplasia and parathyroid gland abnormalities, usually chief cell hyperplasia. MEN-IIB have in addition marfanoid habitus, neuromas of the tongue, or conjunctivae and ganglioneuromas of the plexuses of Meissner and Auerbach. They rarely present with hyperparathyroidism.

Secondary Hyperparathyroidism.   In secondary hypoparathyroidism the increased secretion of PTH is in response to a lowered blood calcium level brought about by renal disease, with impaired production of $1,25-(OH)_2D_3$, or by malabsorption syndromes with impaired intestinal absorption of calcium and vitamin D. There is chief cell hyperplasia of the parathyroids. The skeletal changes are identical to those of primary hyperparathyroidism, except that ectopic calcification in soft tissues is much more common. Severe bone disease is not infrequently seen in patients maintained on chronic hemodialysis. Treatment with the $1,25-(OH)_2D_3$ metabolite is effective in low doses and should be tried before surgery is contemplated. The surgical treatment is subtotal parathyroidectomy or total parathyroidectomy with autotransplantation of parathyroid tissue, usually to the forearm.

Tertiary Hyperparathyroidism.   Tertiary hyperparathyroidism is diagnosed when secondary hyperparathyroidism appears to become autonomous, when elevated serum calcium level develops in the patient with chronic renal failure. True automony rarely occurs. After transplantation hypercalcemia and hypophosphatemia may persist for a long time. If followed carefully over several months, PTH levels and subsequently serum calcium levels in these patients slowly return toward normal if renal function is good. Subtotal parathyroidectomy is seldom necessary.

Differential Diagnosis   If 100 patients with hypercalcemia are evaluated in a hospital setting, the greatest number will be found to have metastatic carcinoma with bone metastases; patients with hyperparathyroidism make up the next group, and thiazide therapy is the third most common cause. Other causes include vitamin A and D poisoning, granulomatous diseases, multiple myeloma, and milk-alkali syndrome.

Treatment Patients with primary hyperparathyroidism should definitely undergo operation if they have either bony or renal manifestations of the disease. Treatment is also indicated if peptic ulcer or pancreatitis is shown to be secondary. Hypertension may or may not be benefited depending on the degree of renal damage. Mild symptoms such as anorexia, arthritis, tiredness, and depression are frequently helped by parathyroidectomy. Depending on the experience of the surgeon, some feel that surgery is correct treatment in most asymptomatic patients with hyperparathyroidism. Hypercalcemic crisis, when due to hyperparathyroidism, is a clear indication for urgent operation when the diagnosis is established and the patient's condition has been stabilized by diuresis with saline and furosemide.

Parathyroid surgery requires an unrushed, meticulous dissection with a bloodless field. Both sides of the neck should be carefully explored in all cases, and the number of glands removed should fit the disease process. Abnormal parathyroid glands are enlarged, more spherical, and often have a darker color ranging from tan to reddish-brown. If a single adenoma is found, it should be removed and one or two normal glands biopsied. If four glands are enlarged, this is hyperplasia. Subtotal parathyroidectomy is necessary. Three glands and part of the fourth are excised, leaving a well-vascularized remnant of 50–80 mg. When two glands are enlarged and the others appear normal, this is probably a variant of hyperplasia and should be so treated.

Management of Persistent or Recurrent Hyperparathyroidism. Hypercalcemia persists after operation when the diagnosis of hyperparathyroidism is incorrect, or when the hyperfunctioning gland or glands have not been adequately removed. This should occur no more than 5% of the time. Recurrent disease means that the calcium returns to normal postoperatively, but that months to years later hyperparathyroidism returns. With recurrence, the disease should be treated as hyperplasia with subtotal resection or removal of all glands with autotransplantation. Recurrence after months should raise the question of carcinoma.

Reoperation. The operation notes and pathology report, or slides, from the first procedure should be reviewed before operation. Localization tests are most applicable to this situation. The recurrent nerve is in greater jeopardy, and the chance of creating permanent hypoparathyroidism is increased. It may be necessary to explore the mediastinum through a sternotomy if careful neck reexploration is unrewarding.

Hypoparathyroidism

Primary idiopathic hypoparathyroidism is extremely rare. The most common cause of hypoparathyroidism is surgical removal, trauma, or devascularization of the parathyroids during parathyroid surgery or, more commonly, during operations on the thyroid. Transient hypoparathyroidism can be noted after removal of adenoma or subtotal resection. The nadir occurs at day 2 or 3. The symptoms of hypoparathyroidism are those of hypocalcemia and have been reviewed above. Alkalosis can produce tetany by lowering the ionized calcium level. Rickets, osteomalacia, and steatorrhea cause a low serum calcium with a normal-to-low phosphate level. Renal failure lowers calcium and raises phosphate and is marked by elevation of the BUN. A low plasma magnesium level can also produce tetany.

Treatment   If postoperative hypocalcemia becomes symptomatic, 1 g calcium gluconate can be given slowly IV and then 1–2 g given by IV drip. If the condition is transient, replacement will be required for only a few days. If it is persistent, oral calcium is given in a dose of 1.5–2 g calcium per day and discharged home when asymptomatic. If the condition is permanent, in addition to the oral calcium therapy, the patient is started on vitamin D.

38 PEDIATRIC SURGERY

GENERAL CONSIDERATIONS

Fluid and Electrolyte Balance Initial intravenous fluids in a newborn should consist of 10% dextrose and water with a volume of 65–100 mL/kg/day. After the first several days of life maintenance fluid is 100 mL/kg/day and the solution should consist of 5% dextrose and $\frac{1}{4}$ normal saline. Daily potassium needs are met by 2 meq/kg potassium chloride. Additional fluid losses are replaced with an equal volume of fluid containing electrolytes equivalent to those lost. Maintenance fluid requirement for children weighing more than 10 kg consists of 50 mL/kg for the next 10 kg and 20 mL/kg thereafter. Hyperosmotic fluids may cause intracranial hemorrhage in the neonate and should be used with extreme caution.

Acid-Base Equilibrium Arterial blood gases permit monitoring of the alveolar ventilation and acid-base equilibrium. A rising P_{CO_2} usually indicates the need for assisted ventilation, and a falling Pa_{O_2} may indicate compromised ventilation-perfusion secondary to parenchymal disease or a right-to-left shunt. In addition, the respiratory or metabolic nature of the imbalance is determined. Correction is made by adjusting ventilation and the possible infusion of sodium bicarbonate.

Blood Volume and Blood Replacement The estimated blood volume of the newborn varies from 85–100 mL/kg/body weight depending on the degree of prematurity. The premature infant has a relatively larger blood volume than does the full-term infant. The transfusion requirement of packed red blood cells is 10 mL/kg. The use of fresh frozen plasma and platelet transfusions should be considered when transfusion exceeds 30 mL/kg.

Hyperalimentation and Nutrition Parenteral hyperalimentation will meet caloric needs for growth and recovery from illness if the alimentary tract cannot. Protein, carbohydrate, and fat, plus minerals and vitamins, may be administered by either a central or a peripheral intravenous route. The latter carries less risk. (The former is used when peripheral access no longer exists.) Prolonged hyperalimentation may lead to intrahepatic cholestasis. Jaundice and cirrhosis may develop, which can be irreversible and lead to the death of the infant.

Thermoregulation   Cold stresses the infant and causes increased glucose and oxygen requirements to meet metabolic needs. The use of overhead radiant warmers regulated by servo-controls and the appropriate wrapping of infants during transport will help protect the infant.

LESIONS OF THE NECK

Cystic Hygroma

Etiology and Pathology   The lesion results from sequestration or obstruction of lymphatic vessels most frequently in the posterior triangle of the neck, axilla, groin, and mediastinum. Adjacent tissues may show lymphatic infiltration and also nests of vascular tissue. Lesions at the thoracic inlet may cause airway obstruction. Sudden enlargement due to infection caused by streptococcus or staphylococcus may also cause airway obstruction.

Treatment   Total excision is the treatment of choice. Radical excision is avoided in this benign lesion. Needle aspiration is worthless because of lack of communication between the cysts.

Thyroglossal Duct Remnants

Pathology and Clinical Manifestations   The thyroglossal duct descends from the foramen cecum in conjunction with the development of the hyoid bone. Remnants from the duct will develop into a cyst, which becomes apparent at about age 2–4. The cyst is located in the midline, over or inferior to the hyoid bone, and moves with swallowing. Occasionally the cyst may become infected, but this usually clears with penicillin therapy. The differential diagnosis includes lymphadenopathy, a dermoid cyst, or, rarely, ectopic thyroid.

Treatment   Infection should be controlled first. Total excision involves removal of the cyst, the central portion of the hyoid bone, and the tract to the foramen cecum.

Branchial Cleft Anomalies

Branchial cleft sinuses and cysts represent remnants from embryologic structures. The most common are from the second branchial cleft. Complete sinuses extend from a fistulous opening in the skin anterior to the sternocleidomastoid muscle and pass superiorly through the bifurcation of the carotid artery, to enter into the pharynx anterior and inferior to the tonsillar fossa. Other remnants may contain cartilage. Sinuses drain a mucoid material and occasionally may become infected. Total excision is necessary to prevent recurrence.

RESPIRATORY SYSTEM

Subglottic Stenosis

This may be congenital or acquired secondarily to prolonged intubation. The former usually resolves with growth of the child. The latter may require laser excision. Severe stenoses may require division of the tracheal rings posteriorly and stenting them with a strip of cartilage.

Subglottic Hemangioma

This lesion can produce inspiratory and expiratory stridor and may lead to airway obstruction. Diagnosis is made by endoscopy, and therapy involves systemic steroids or laser excision. Frequently cutaneous hemangiomata coexist.

Congenital Diaphragmatic Hernia (Bochdalek)

Pathology   The pleuroperitoneal canal in the posterolateral portion of the hemidiaphragm is the last portion to close during embryonic development. The bowel returning from the umbilical cord to the abdominal cavity herniates into the chest when the canal fails to close. This usually involves the left chest. The result is failure of development of the lung on the ipsilateral side by the encroaching intestine and on the contralateral side by the mediastinal shift. The abdomen is scaphoid and the heart tones are shifted away from the side of herniation. A chest x-ray reveals gas-filled loops of bowel in the chest. An antenatal ultrasound will demonstrate the lesion. Symptoms at birth are respiratory distress and cyanosis. The underlying pathophysiology is increased pulmonary vascular resistance and pulmonary artery hypertension, which can lead to a persistent fetal circulation with a right-to-left shunt.

Treatment   Surgical closure via the abdomen is accomplished after the infant is stabilized by endotracheal intubation and ventilation. Sodium bicarbonate may be given intravenously once P_{CO_2} is reduced to further correct a metabolic acidosis. At operation, the posterior rim of the diaphragm must be dissected from overlying peritoneum and a two-layer closure is achieved. A chest tube is placed and put on underwater seal. Suction is avoided to prevent a mediastinal shift with a resultant pneumothorax on the opposite side. Rarely, insufficient diaphragm exists, and a synthetic patch is necessary for closure. The need for a patch or the inability to achieve a Pa_{O_2} greater than 100 torr and a P_{CO_2} less than 40 after correction is a bad prognosis. Pulmonary vasodilators have little therapeutic effect. The use of high-frequency ventilation and extracorporeal membrane oxygenation (ECMO) has resulted in increased survival of these severely compromised infants.

Congenital Lobar Emphysema

The right middle and upper lobes and the left upper lobe are the most frequently involved. Sudden expansion of the involved lobe can lead to respiratory distress and cyanosis because of compression of the remaining lung. Emergent surgical excision of the involved lobe may be needed to relieve the distress. Lobar emphysema developing more slowly may gradually resolve and judicious observation is warranted. Cardiac anomalies may coexist.

Pulmonary Sequestration

This lesion consists of a mass of nonfunctioning lung tissue usually in or adjacent to the left lower lobe. There is no bronchial communication to the respiratory tree and the arterial supply is usually systemic, frequently coming from the aorta below the diaphragm. The condition is revealed as a shadow on chest x-ray. Air may be seen in the intralobar variety if there is communication with adjacent lung alveoli. The latter may present clinically with cough, hemoptysis, and recurrent pulmonary infections.

Bronchiectasis

This is usually associated with an underlying congenital pulmonary anomaly, cystic fibrosis, a foreign body, or immunodeficiency. Symptoms include chronic cough, purulent secretions, recurrent pulmonary infections, and hemoptysis. The diagnosis is made by CT. Treatment is medical, with antibiotic therapy and postural drainage. Lobectomy is rarely indicated.

Foreign Bodies

These are most frequently found in the airways of toddlers. Peanuts or small parts of toys may be aspirated and the child presents with cough and unilateral wheezing. An x-ray of the chest will show atelectasis of the involved lobe and the foreign body if it is radiopaque. Occasionally a clinical diagnosis of asthma will eventually be found to be caused by an unrecognized foreign body in the airway. Bronchoscopy and extraction of the body is the treatment.

ESOPHAGUS

Tracheoesophageal Fistula and Esophageal Atresia

Clinical Manifestations 85–90% of these lesions are made of a blind upper pouch with a tracheal communication to the lower esophagus. An isolated tracheoesophageal fistula occurs in 2–4% of such children. There are frequently associated congenital anomalies that affect the outcome. Imperforate anus and/or congenital cardiac disease occurs in 10–12% of these infants. Excess salivation and attempted feedings result in choking and cyanosis. The diagnosis is made by the inability to pass a stiff catheter into the stomach. Instillation of a minute amount of a contrast material, not injurious to the pulmonary tree, will prove the diagnosis. An x-ray of the infant will reveal air in the intestinal tract if a fistula coexists.

Treatment Sump suction is applied to the upper pouch and broad-spectrum antibiotics are begun. A gastrostomy should be placed immediately to vent the stomach of exhaled air and prevent regurgitation of gastric acid into the tracheobronchial tree. Once the infant has been stabilized, pulmonary infection cleared, and other anomalies assessed, total correction should be performed. Because these infants can be ventilated and provided intravenous nutrition delayed repair is rarely indicated. A thoracotomy on the side opposite the aortic arch will expose the anomaly. The fistula is severed and the tracheal defect closed. The upper pouch is dissected and the distal tip excised. A primary anastomosis is performed. A chest tube is placed adjacent to the anastomosis to afford egress of any leakage and drainage of air and serum. If the gap is too great to anastomose the two ends, additional length in the upper pouch may be achieved by a circular myotomy. A colon interposition can bridge a gap too long to permit a primary anastomosis. This is performed as a delayed procedure when the child is larger and has greater reserve.

ISOLATED ESOPHAGEAL ATRESIA This is diagnosed by a film demonstrating a nasogastric tube coiled in the blind upper pouch and no air in the intestinal tract. A cervical esophagostomy is performed and a feeding gastrostomy will permit feeding the infant. When the child is approximately 1 year old, the defect is bridged by a colon interposition or a reversed gastric tube.

ISOLATED (H-TYPE) TRACHEOESOPHAGEAL FISTULA The symptoms may be delayed and confusing. There is usually choking on feeding, especially with liquids. Gaseous abdominal distention develops, and frequently there is a history of repeated aspiration pneumonia. The diagnosis is made by a careful contrast study via the esophagus, or, more safely, by fiber-optic tracheoscopy. Surgical division of the fistula, usually through the neck, is curative.

Corrosive Injury of the Esophagus

These are caused by the ingestion of strong alkaline or acid substances. All children suspected of swallowing a corrosive agent should have esophagoscopy within 24 h of the injury. The scope is passed only to the first evidence of injury; further insertion may lead to perforation of the injured esophagus. If the injury is circumferential, a string is passed for future guidance during dilatations, and a gastrostomy is performed. Steroids are generally begun to modify stricture and they are continued for 3 weeks. Antibiotics are administered for 3 weeks. Dilatation is started after 3 weeks and continued as needed until any stricture has resolved.

Esophageal Substitution

There are two indications for this procedure: unrelenting stricture of the esophagus or a large defect in esophageal atresia. The connection is achieved with either colon based on the middle colic vessels or a reversed gastric tube fashioned from the greater curvature of the stomach or a jejunal graft. The conduits are usually placed in the anterior mediastinum but can be brought up behind the lung root in the left chest.

Gastroesophageal Reflux (GER)

This has been termed *chalasia*. Failure to thrive is the usual presentation in children over 1 year old, and esophagitis and stricture may develop in the adolescent or mentally retarded.

Clinical Manifestations These children usually have a history of repeated vomiting. There may be symptoms of asthma. Esophagitis can lead to chronic blood loss and anemia. A barium swallow will reveal the anatomy of the esophagus, but may not reveal reflux. A pH probe placed in the distal esophagus should reveal the reflux. Esophagoscopy and biopsy may reveal esophagitis.

Treatment Most children respond to medical therapy: propping, and thickened feedings. Drugs such as metaclopromide or bethanacol may relieve the reflux. If medical therapy fails and the reflux is life-threatening or causing esophagitis and stricture, surgical correction is indicated. The most frequently used procedure is the transabdominal Nissen fundoplication.

GASTROINTESTINAL TRACT

Pyloric Stenosis

Clinical Manifestations Vomiting, progressing to explosive (projectile), begins after the first 2–3 weeks of life. The vomitus is nonbilious. Most infants are males and the disease is hereditary but penetrance is low. A metabolic alkalosis develops with a depressed serum chloride and potassium and elevated sodium bicarbonate. Most tumors are palpable, and can be demonstrated by ultrasonography or contrast study.

Treatment Metabolic alkalosis is corrected by intravenous 5% dextrose and $\frac{1}{2}$ normal saline with 30 meq/L of potassium chloride at 2 times maintenance until the urine specific gravity is less than 1.010, the chloride is greater than 95%, and the bicarbonate is less than 30 meq/L. A Fredet-Ramstedt pyloromyotomy is then performed. Before operation a nasogastric tube is passed to empty the stomach and prevent vomiting during induction of anesthesia. 4 h after operation, small, frequent feedings of an electrolyte solution are begun; the volume is gradually increased to maintenance and then formula is given. Discharge is usually 24–36 h postoperation.

Pneumoperitoneum

This is usually a surgical emergency. The radiographic finding is seen in the setting of sudden increase in abdominal girth, often with respiratory distress due to elevation of the diaphragm. It is usually caused by a perforated hollow viscus in necrotizing enterocolitis, idiopathic gastric perforation, or perforation of the colon due to distal obstruction as in Hirschsprung disease. Occasionally, respiratory high ventilatory pressures will lead to pneumomediastinum and retroperitoneal air dissection and pneumoperitoneum. Aspiration of the abdominal cavity and microscopic examination of the fluid will help to reveal the cause of the free air. Abdominal distention can be relieved temporarily by aspiration. Rapid exploration following adequate resuscitation is necessary when there is perforation of a hollow viscus.

Gastrostomy

This provides a means for feeding when the oral route is not appropriate, and for gastric drainage when prolonged drainage is necessary and a nasogastric tube cannot be passed. A Stamm gastrostomy consists of the placement of a mushroom catheter through a gastrotomy bounded by two concentric purse-string sutures. The stomach is sutured to the anterior abdominal wall to prevent leakage. The use of a gastrostomy for feeding brain-damaged children is often met with vomiting from gastroesophageal reflux. These children should be evaluated for that condition prior to gastrostomy. An antireflux procedure (Nissen fundoplication) should be performed if reflux is present. (A healing gastrostomy wound requires periodic cauterization with silver nitrate to destroy excess granulation tissues that cause purulent drainage and leakage of gastric contents. Cultures, antibiotic treatment, and the insertion of larger gastrostomy tubes do not correct this condition and are inappropriate.)

Intestinal Obstruction in the Newborn

Bilious vomiting in the newborn means intestinal obstruction until another cause is proved. An abdominal x-ray will help determine the level of obstruction. A barium enema is useful to look for malrotation, a microcolon signifying ileal obstruction, colonic atresia, Hirschsprung's disease, meconium plug, or small left colon syndrome.

DUODENAL MALFORMATIONS Obstruction may be complete, as in atresia; or partial as in annular pancreas, stenosis, or bands associated with malrotation. The abdominal x-ray classically shows the "double bubble" of air in a distended stomach and duodenum. Intrinsic obstructions are managed by a duodenoduodenotomy. If obstruction is secondary to volvulus from a malrotation, timely surgery is needed to prevent infarction of the midgut secondary to occlusion of the superior mesenteric vessels. Duodenal webs usually contain the common bile duct and must be approached with extreme caution. One-third of all such infants have Down's syndrome.

JEJUNOILEAL ATRESIA This condition is believed to be due to an antenatal vascular accident or volvulus. There may be simple atresias or loss of considerable amounts of intestine with a deep cleft in the mesentery and resulting short-gut syndrome. Multiple atresias exist in about 10% of such patients. An x-ray will usually determine the level of atresia, and a barium enema will detail the rotation of the colon and its caliber. The disparity in caliber of the two atretic ends can be managed by an end-to-oblique anastomosis using a single layer of nonabsorbable sutures. A complementary gastrostomy aids greatly in the management of these children, who may have a prolonged period before enteric function is restored. About 10% will have cystic fibrosis. All should have sweat test at about 6 months of age. The "apple peal" or "Christmas tree" deformity is a type of jejunal atresia resulting from occlusion of the superior mesenteric artery distal to the middle colic artery. The small bowel distal to the occlusion is short and spirals about a longitudinal vessel supplied by the middle colic and marginal vasculature of the colon.

MALROTATION AND MIDGUT VOLVULUS This condition arises during the tenth through twelfth week of embryonic development. In a complete malrotation, the duodenum and ascending colon are attached to each other by bands of peritoneal tissue (Ladd's bands). These bands may pass over the duodenum to the right upper posterior peritoneum, causing extrinsic compression. In addition, the mesentery is stalk-like containing the superior mesenteric vessels.

If the viability of the gut is compromised by a midgut volvulus, the infant shows evidence of third-space fluid loss and the abdomen becomes tender. Stools may become bloody. Urgent celiotomy is required to relieve the volvulus (counterclockwise untwisting), divide the peritoneal bands, and place the duodenum in the right gutter and the ascending colon in the left gutter. This prevents a recurrence of the volvulus. An incidental appendectomy removes the dislocated appendix.

MECONIUM ILEUS Infants born with this condition almost always have cystic fibrosis. Inspissated meconium caused by a lack of pancreatic enzymes and viscid mucus obstructs the distal ileum. The infant presents with late bilious vomiting, palpable loops of bowel with maleable meconium, a low small bowel obstruction on x-ray, and a microcolon on contrast enema. Antenatal perforation of the intestine will be revealed by calcific densities noted on abdominal x-ray. Uncomplicated obstruction can be relieved by the detergent in Gastrografin given as an enema with fluoroscopic control. The hyperosmolality of the solution must be diluted to prevent diarrhea and dehydration. Complicated conditions are managed surgically by the creation of temporary ileostomies and irrigation of the obstructed bowel with N-acetyl cysteine.

NECROTIZING ENTEROCOLITIS (NEC) This condition almost exclusively affects the stressed premature infant. There is a breakdown of the mucosal barrier, and endogenous bacteria invade the bowel wall. This causes poor feeding, vomiting, abdominal distention, and bloody stools. Sepsis, metabolic acidosis, and third spacing soon follow. There is a left shift in the white blood cell count and the platelet count falls. The diagnosis is made by the palpation of tender loops of bowel on abdominal examination and the demonstration of pneumatosis intestinalis on an abdominal x-ray. Gas may also be noted in the hepatic portal veins.

The disease may be corrected in most infants by medical therapy: decompression of the intestinal tract by a nasogastric tube, giving adequate amounts of intravenous fluids (both electrolyte and colloid) to restore circulating volume, and the administration of broad-spectrum antibiotics to treat the sepsis. Frequent observation and abdominal x-ray examination is needed to document improvement or progression of the disease, which then requires surgical management. Free air on abdominal x-ray is a specific indication for surgery. Necrotic bowel is excised and enterostomies fashioned. The latter are closed after the child recovers. Thought may be given for primary anastomosis of the small bowel to prevent the large caustic fluid losses that occur with small bowel fistulae. Postoperative parenteral hyperalimentation is needed to provide adequate calories for healing and continued growth of the infant. Occasionally, intestinal stenosis may develop with signs of obstruction in infants recovering on medical management. This condition requires surgical correction.

INTUSSUSCEPTION This is a common cause of intestinal obstruction in the infant. The usual age range is 3 months to 3 years. The lead point is a hypertrophied Peyer's patch in the terminal ileum, which then intussuscepts into the cecum and ascending colon. If intussusception occurs in the child over age 5, a different cause must be suspected that may include malignant disease. Such lead points include polyps, Meckel's diverticulum, Henoch-Schönlein purpura, and non-Hodgkin's lymphoma.

Clinical Manifestations The onset is sudden and consists of severe, crampy abdominal pain lasting a minute. There is usually marked pallor suggesting shock. A period of ease follows, only to have the brief episode of pain recur. Vomiting usually follows, and during a period of relaxation, a soft elongated mass can be felt in the right upper quadrant. The absence of bowel in the right lower quadrant (Dance's sign) may be noted. A bloody mucoid stool may be passed (currant jelly stool), and a guaiac test of the smear from a rectal glove is usually positive. A barium enema will reveal the "coiled-spring" appearance of the intussuscepted bowel.

Treatment The barium enema will reduce the intussusception by hydrostatic pressure 60–70% of the time. The cannister should be no higher than 3 ft, and no manipulation of the abdomen should be performed. Reduction is watched until barium fills the distal 2–3 ft of terminal ileum. The child is hydrated with intravenous fluids and observed for 4–6 h. If all symptoms are relieved, oral fluids are begun and the child is discharged. If reduction is not achieved, it must be accomplished by celiotomy. The intussusceptum is gently milked out of the intussuscipiens by distal pressure until reduction is complete. An incidental appendectomy is usually performed. If the serosa of the intussuscipiens begins to split during reduction, resection of the intussuscepted bowel is carried out with primary anastomosis. The recurrence rate is about 3% for both hydrostatic and operative reduction.

DUPLICATIONS, MECKEL'S DIVERTICULUM, AND MESENTERIC CYSTS

Duplication

These may occur anywhere in the intestinal tract but are usually in the ileum. They are usually cystic masses, but also may be long tubular structures. They lie in the leaves of the mesentery and share a common wall with the adjacent bowel. They usually present as a palpable movable mass or as an acute abdomen if torsion and infarction occur. If the duplication communicates with the intestinal tract and contains gastric mucosa, gastrointestinal bleeding may be the presenting sign. Diagnosis is made by sonography or a technetium pertechnetate scan. The lesion should be excised with the adjacent bowel if it is short. Longer lesions may be treated with multiple enterotomies in the duplication with mucosal stripping or the creation of a distal connecting anastomosis if no ectopic gastric mucosa exists.

Meckel's Diverticulum

This is a persistent portion of the omphalomesenteric duct and occurs in about 3% of the population 2–3 ft from the ileocecal valve. It is usually asymptomatic, but may present as appendicitis, intestinal obstruction, or, most commonly, as intestinal hemorrhage. The latter occurs if there is aberrant gastric mucosa within the diverticulum. The stools are maroon, and the hematocrit drops appreciably. Diagnosis may be made by technetium scan. The treatment is surgical excision.

Mesenteric Cysts

These also lie in the leaves of the mesentery, but, unlike duplication cysts, contain no mucosa or muscular wall. They are believed to result from obstructed lymphatic channels. They present as a palpable movable mass and may cause intestinal obstruction. The diagnosis is suspected by sonography. Excision is the treatment, and adjacent bowel may need to be resected. If the lesion is large, marsupialization to the peritoneal cavity is indicated.

HIRSCHSPRUNG'S DISEASE

This usually is a disease of male infants and consists of the absence of ganglion cells with hypertrophied nerve fibers in the sigmoid colon and rectum including the internal sphincter. Longer segments may be involved and in the long segment disease the sex incidence is equal. There is an increased incidence in children with Down's syndrome. The aganglionic segment is spastic and causes obstruction. This presents as constipation in the newborn with abdominal distention and vomiting. Occasionally, it may present with diarrhea and toxicity from an enterocolitis that carries a serious mortality rate when fully developed.

Diagnosis A barium enema usually shows a megacolon in the innervated bowel, and the distal aganglionic colon has a normal caliber. This may not be apparent during the first 2–3 weeks of life. Definitive diagnosis is made by a biopsy of the distal rectum to search for the presence or absence of ganglion cells. This can be a suction biopsy of the mucosa and submucosa or a full-thickness biopsy of the rectal wall as a surgical procedure.

Treatment Initially a sigmoid colostomy is performed through ganglionated bowel. A pull-through procedure is accomplished when the child is 9–12 months old. If the child is older and has a megacolon, pull-through is delayed until the bowel has returned to normal caliber. The colostomy may be closed at the time of the pull-through or as a third stage depending upon the surgeon's judgment. The various procedures used are a Swenson, Duhamel, or Soave endo-rectal pull-through.

IMPERFORATE ANUS

This congenital anomaly occurs equally in both sexes. It results from the failure of normal development of the urorectal septum, which divides the cloaca and separates the urinary from the hind-gut systems. The lesion is considered "high" when the rectal pouch ends above the levator ani muscles, and "low" when it ends below. High lesions usually have fistulas to the vagina in the femal and to the prostatic urethra in the male. Low lesions usually have fistulas to the perineum. There are frequently associated anomalies involving other systems.

Diagnosis The diagnosis is determined by physical examination. The level is determined either by a fistulogram or by a perineal injection of contrast material into the blind pouch under fluoroscopic control. A cystourethrogram should be performed to look for an associated fistula or ureteral reflux.

Treatment Initially, a sigmoid colostomy is performed if the lesion is high. If the lesion is low, a perineal proctoplasty can be done in the newborn. High lesions are best managed by a posterior sagittal anoproctoplasty using a muscle stimulator to identify the anal sphincters, vertical fibers, and the levator ani muscles. The rectum is detached from the fistula without sacrificing any of its distal length and placed precisely through the above muscle complex. The colostomy is closed several months later following complete healing of the pull-through. The caliber of the cutaneous anastomosis is maintained during the healing phase with the daily insertion of Hegar dilators.

BILIARY ATRESIA

Neonatal jaundice is usually physiologic. It becomes abnormal if it persists beyond 2 weeks, especially if the direct fraction of bilirubin is elevated. Biliary atresia affects both the extrahepatic biliary tree and the liver.

Etiology and Pathology The cause is unknown but an infectious etiology is suspected. Atresia or hypoplasia may involve all or part of the extrahepatic biliary ducts and also the intrahepatic ducts.

Clinical Manifestations Jaundice is present from birth, but may not be marked until after the first several weeks. The urine becomes dark and stools acholic. The abdomen may gradually become distended by the enlarging liver or ascites. Eventually, the spleen enlarges also.

Diagnosis The serum bilirubin gradually elevates and the direct fraction is at least half of the total. After a month of observation, a nuclear scan using technetium 99m IDA (DISIDA) is performed after pretreatment with phenobarbital. If there is no excretion of the radionuclide into the intestinal tract, atresia is virtually assured. A sample of duodenal contents may be assayed for the presence of bile. An ultrasound may reveal a choledochal duct cyst. The intrahepatic ducts are never dilated in biliary atresia. Screening tests for infectious and metabolic causes should be negative.

Differential Diagnosis These include physiologic jaundice, hemolytic disease, sepsis, neonatal hepatitis (a probable variant of biliary atresia), α-trypsin deficiency, the inspissated bile syndrome, infection with different viruses, or metabolic defects.

Treatment Surgical exploration should be performed. A cholecystogram is obtained. If no ductal system is seen, a dissection of the portahepatis is carried out to see if any proximal duct is present. If there is none, the portahepatis is excised between the right and left hepatic arteries and a portoenterostomy, Roux en Y, is performed. If a duct is present, it is anastomosed to a Roux en Y loop of jejunum. If the operation is performed prior to the third month of life and the diameter of the bile ducts in the resected portahepatis greater than 100 μm in diameter, there is an excellent chance for prolonged bile excretion into the intestinal tract. Inflammation of the liver may continue with the development of fibrosis and portal hypertension. If portoenterostomy fails, liver transplantation becomes the treatment of choice.

Choledochal Duct Cyst

There are a variety of such cysts. The most common type is the fusiform dilatation of the common bile duct with the cystic duct opening into it. The F:M ratio is 4:1. The symptoms may include pain, a palpable mass, and jaundice.

Diagnosis This is accomplished by ultrasound or CT. Occasionally endoscopic retrograde cholangiopancreatography (ERCP) will be required.

Treatment Surgical excision and anastomosis of the proximal duct to a defunctionalized loop of jejunum is preferable to drainage of the cyst into a loop of bowel. The latter will lead to stasis, recurring symptoms of jaundice and cholangitis, and possibly malignant degeneration of the cyst.

DEFORMITIES OF THE ABDOMINAL WALL

Embryology

Four separate embryologic folds contribute to the formation of the abdominal wall: cephalic, caudal, and the right and left lateral folds. These coalesce at the umbilical ring. The developing gut herniates into the umbilical cord during the fourth through the eighth week of gestation and returns to the enlarging abdominal cavity from the ninth to the tenth week. Failure of the cephalic fold to close results in sternal defects and the pentalogy of Cantrell. Caudal fold abnormalities include extrophy of the bladder or the cloaca. Lateral fold defects result in omphalocele. Gastroschisis results from an antenatal rupture of the umbilical cord while the gut is extruded into the cord.

Umbilical Hernia

These hernias result from failure of closure of the umbilical ring. They frequently are small, less than 1 cm, and will close spontaneously. Larger ones may not close and sometimes are so disfiguring that early closure is justified. Supraumbilical hernias produce a protrusion of the umbilical skin, but the defect is adjacent and superior to the umbilicus. The pigmented portion of the skin points inferiorly. These defects do not close spontaneously, and early repair is justified. Repair of an umbilical hernia is done through a skinfold incision within the navel; the navel is not excised. Incarceration is extremely rare.

Patent Urachus

During development of the abdominal cavity, the bladder communicates to the umbilical cord through the urachus. If this tract persists, urine will be observed emanating from the navel. Incomplete closure may result in a urachal cyst, demonstrated by sonography. These are rare abnormalities and are treated by surgical excision.

Patent Omphalomesenteric Duct

During fetal life, this duct connects the ileum to the yolk sac via the umbilical cord. Normally the duct involutes, but a portion may persist as a Meckel's diverticulum seen in about 5% of the population. If the entire duct persists, ileal contents will spill from the umbilicus. The diagnosis is made by intubation of the duct and instillation of contrast material. An x-ray will reveal the material flowing into the terminal ileum. Complete excision is the definitive treatment.

Omphalocele

These present at birth as herniation of abdominal contents into the umbilical cord. They may be small and contain only a small amount of intestine, or large and contain liver in addition to intestine. There may be rupture of the cord and herniation of the contents into the amniotic cavity. Associated anomalies are noted in about two-thirds of these children. Primary closure of the abdominal wall is the surgical goal. If the mass of the contents is small, closure is easy. In large omphaloceles, the intestine and liver have lost the "right of domain," and primary closure is frequently not possible. If other life-threatening severe anomalies are present, escharification of the cord may be accomplished using povidone. This will allow epithelialization over the defect. If the child's condition will permit closure, this can be accomplished as a staged repair. A pouch of silastic mesh is sutured to the medial borders of the recti and covers the herniated viscera. The size of the pouch is decreased by taking multiple tucks every 2–3 days. This returns the contents to the enlarging abdominal cavity. Once reduction is complete, the pouch is removed and a primary repair accomplished. Severe associated anomalies account for the 20–30% mortality in this malformation.

Gastroschisis

This condition was once thought to represent a ruptured omphalocele, but now is believed to represent rupture of the umbilical cord at the site of the resorbed right umbilical vein. The intestine herniates through a small defect to the right of the umbilical cord. Fallopian tube may also herniate. Intestinal atresia is the only associated abnormality and occurs infrequently. The intestine may appear normal but more frequently is covered by a thickened peel. Often primary closure is possible by manually stretching the abdominal wall. This will require intubation and mechanical ventilation for several days following surgery to allow the abdominal cavity to stretch and relieve the subdiaphragmatic pressure. If pressures are too great, staged closure with a silastic pouch is accomplished as in giant omphalocele. There may be considerable delay in return of intestinal function, and central venous hyperalimentation should be initiated early.

Exstrophy of the Cloaca (Vesicointestinal Fissure)

This is a severe congenital malformation involving the inferior abdominal wall. Included are omphalocele, exstrophy of the bladder separation of the symphysis publis, foreshortened colon, imperforate anus, prolapse of the distal ileum through the bifid bladder, and epispadias in the male. Many of these children do not survive. The operation involves a distal ileostomy, closure of the omphalocele, and closure of the bladder or creation of an ileal loop with transplanted ureters.

Congenital Deficiency of the Abdominal Musculature (Eagle-Barrett Syndrome; Prune-Belly Syndrome)

This is a rare syndrome affecting males. There is usually minimal muscular development in the abdominal wall. In addition, there are undescended testes and hydroureters and a megacysticus. Treatment involves antibiotics to prevent or treat urinary tract infections. An operation involves reduction cystoplasties and excision of the inferior portion of the abdominal wall. Mesh may be incorporated in the repair, or an external shield may be constructed to protect the weakened abdominal wall. Orchidopexy is performed at 2–3 years of age.

Inguinal Hernia

Indirect inguinal hernias result from failure of closure of the processus vaginalis, which usually occurs by 2–3 months of age. Incarceration is particularly likely in young infants, and surgical correction is recommended early after diagnosis. Gentle maneuver reduction by taxis usually is successful. If this maneuver is unsuccessful, immediate surgery is necessary to prevent necrosis of the involved loop of intestine. A hydrocele of the cord may mimic an incarcerated hernia, but there is no pain and no vomiting, as intestinal obstruction does not exist. Hydroceles of the tunica vaginalis may herald an associated hernia and, in children over the age of 2, usually does. In infant females, an ovary may incarcerate in the hernia sac. These usually are associated with sliding hernias, and, at surgery, the sac must be opened in all such cases to prevent ligating the fallopian tube.

Treatment involves a high ligation of the sac. No repair of the floor of the inguinal canal is indicated unless the internal ring is so stretched that the transversalis fascia is incompetent. If the hernia is a slider, the sac is ligated distal to the sliding component. A purse-string suture is placed at the base of the sac, and following excision of the sac, the stump is inverted and the purse-string tied.

There is controversy over repairing the opposite asymptomatic side. Many advocate repair if the child is under 1 year of age or if the presenting hernia is on the left side.

GENITALIA

Cryptorchidism

The testes develop from the urogenital ridge and by the seventh month of gestation, lie in the pelvis. They then begin their descent along with the developing processus vaginalis into the scrotum. The undescended testis may lie in the abdominal cavity or the inguinal canal. An ectopic testis that has passed through the external ring may lie in the subcutaneous tissue of the abdominal wall, the thigh, or the perineum. There is increased risk of malignancy in the gonads of the patient with an undescended testis, probably due to the character of the testes themselves rather than to their position. Histology of the undescended testis reveals decreasing spermatogonia after 2 years of age. Therefore, orchidopexy is recommended prior to that age. The rationale for orchidopexy is to protect spermatogenesis, place the testis in a less vulnerable position, make early detection of malignancy possible, and most important, make the child feel the equal of his peers.

Ambiguous Genitalia (Intersex Syndromes)

Normal sexual differentiation of the gonad occurs in the sixth fetal week and is dependent upon a gene located on the Y chromosome. Wolffian (male) and müllerian (female) ducts exist in the embryo until sexual differentation. The fetal testis secretes testosterone and müllerian-inhibiting substance. Testosterone stimulates maturation of wolffian duct structures into epididymis, vas deferens, and seminal vesicles. Müllerian-inhibiting substance produces regression of the female structures. In the absence of the fetal testis, the müllerian system proceeds to full maturation. Any disruption of the orderly steps of sex differentiation may present as an intersex problem. These may be classified as a true hermaphrodite, a male pseudohermaphrodite, a female pseudohermaphrodite, or mixed gonadal dysgenesis. Most of these present with ambiguous external genitalia.

The true hermaphrodite is the rarest and usually has an XX karyotype. They usually have an ovary and a testis or an ovotestis. The male pseudohermaphrodite has bilateral testes, but there is a persistence of müllerian duct structures due to a defect in androsynthesis or müllerian-inhibiting substance. Female pseudohermaphrodites usually have a defect in adrenal cortisol synthesis, resulting in adrenal hyperplasia and increased ACTH production. The latter stimulates the production of adrenal androgens and masculinization of the developing female infant. Mixed gonadal dysgenesis may result in malignant degeneration of the gonad. Determination of the sex of rearing must be made early. This involves studies of urinary and serum biochemical factors, physical and radiologic examination, chromosomal studies, and occasionally celiotomy and study of the gonads with biopsy.

The appearance of the external genital abnormalities may be surgically modified by reducing and recessing an enlarged clitoris, repairing and elongating the hypospadius penis, vaginoplasty, or insertion of testicular prostheses.

NEOPLASTIC DISEASE

Cancer is the second leading cause of death after trauma in children 1–14 years of age. Improved survival over the past two decades is due to several factors: better diagnostic imaging; new chemotherapeutic drugs; collaboration between surgeons, chemotherapists, and radiation therapists; and multi-institutional studies that evaluate new treatments and protocols.

Wilms' Tumor

Wilms' tumor is an embryonal neoplasm of the kidney and usually presents as an asymptomatic mass in the flank and upper abdomen. The peak age of incidence is 1–3 years. Associated conditions include familial aniridia, Beckwith-Widemann syndrome, urinary tract defects, hemihypertrophy, and chromosomal deletion, suggestion genetic influences. Bilateral involvement occurs in 5–10% of series.

Evaluation consists of CT scans to study the tumor-containing kidney, the status of the contralateral kidney, and the rest of the abdominal viscera. CT scan of the chest will reveal any pulmonary metastases, the most likely site of the metastic disease. Ultrasound examination of the abdomen will reveal any tumor extension into the renal vein or vena cava.

Treatment Surgical excision is performed through a wide transabdominal incision. The entire kidney and tumor is removed along with the attached ureter. Invasion of the tumor into adjacent viscera is treated by excision of the involved tissue in continuity with the tumor. Paraaortic nodes are sampled for staging, biopsy of any suspicious areas is taken, and the opposite kidney is evaluated for tumor. Chemotherapy is given to all children; the mainstays are actinomycin-D and vincristine. Adriamycin is added to children with more advanced disease, as is radiation therapy.

If the tumor is of "favorable" histology and all the tumor is removed at surgery, cure rate approaches 95%. A small percentage of tumors are of "unfavorable" histology and their cure rates are diminished.

Neuroblastoma

Following central nervous system tumors and lymphomas, neuroblastoma is the next most common solid neoplasm in children. Therapy has not been nearly so successful as in Wilms'. Neuroblastomas arise from neural crest cells and are seen most frequently in the adrenal medulla. Less frequently noted sites include the posterior mediastinum, neck, or pelvis. Ninety percent of children present before age 9, and 40% are younger than 4. Two-thirds will present as asymptomatic abdominal masses and the majority will have metastases at diagnosis. Most frequently noted site of metastases is bone. Prognosis is age-related. About 85% of children under 1 year will be cured even with metastatic disease to skin, liver, or bone marrow. Only 15% of children over age 2 are cured.

Evaluation consists of CT scans of the involved body cavity plus bone marrow examination and bone scans. Catecholamines and their metabolites will be elevated in serum and urine.

Treatment   Total surgical excision in children over 1 year of age is the only hope of cure. This may include laminectomy, especially in posterior mediastinal tumors where extension may occur through the vertebral foramina. The tumor is radiosensitive and responsive to chemotherapy, but these adjunctive treatments have not altered the dismal prognosis associated with metastatic disease in patients over age 2.

Rhabdomyosarcoma

This is an embryonic tumor arising from a variety of mesenchymal tissues. Common sites of origin are the head and neck, extremities, and the genitourinary tract. Diagnosis is made by incisional or excisional biopsy. Extent of disease is determined by radionuclide scans, CT scans, and bone marrow biopsy.

Wide local excision, sparing mutilating surgery, is accompanied with radiation therapy and chemotherapy. Commonly used drugs include actinomycin-D, vincristine, and cyclophosphamide.

Prognosis is affected by site of origin and the pathologic type. Embryonal pathology is more favorable than alveolar histology.

Teratoma

These tumors are composed of all three embryonic germ layers. They are usually benign, but can harbor malignant elements. Sites are varied, with the most frequently noted site being the sacrococcygeal area (40%). Other sites include the anterior mediastinum, ovary, retroperitoneum, testis, and neck. Therapy involves total surgical excision. Newer chemotherapeutic agents including *cis*-platinum have improved the outlook in higher staged malignant disease. Radiation is used without proven effect on survival.

Liver Tumors

More than two-thirds of all liver tumors in children are malignant. Hepatoblastoma is the most common malignant tumor of the liver; 65% of these are diagnosed before age 2. Hepatocellular carcinoma is the next most common lesion, with a peak incidence between ages 10 and 15. Most present with an upper abdominal mass. There may be weight loss, fever, and anorexia. Alpha-fetoprotein levels are elevated in 90% of children with hepatoblastoma and serve as a good marker for follow-up evaluation. Double contrast CT scan of the abdomen and chest, and celiac axis angiography are required for adequate evaluation of the tumor.

Preoperative chemotherapy to debulk massive tumors along with complete surgical extirpation results in cure of the majority of hepatoblastomas. Half of these tumors are completely resectable, and 80% are curable with adjunct chemotherapy. Children with hepatocellular carcinoma have a more dismal prognosis because fewer are completely resectable. Their survival is only 15%.

TRAUMA

Accidents account for 46% of all pediatric deaths, more than cancer, congenital anomalies, pneumonia, heart disease, homicide, and meningitis combined. Motor vehicle accidents account for 20%, drowning 8%, burns 5%, and firearms 1% of all trauma deaths. The establishment of major trauma centers skilled in the management of child trauma has improved survival statistics. Most fatal cases have associated head trauma, and the management of those injuries affects survival rates. By virtue of their soft, pliable skeletons, growing bodies, and immature emotional development, children constitute a special trauma patient where injuries and the management differ markedly from those in the adult.

Battered Child Syndrome   Injuries that are bizarre or histories that are inconsistent should raise the suspicion of this type of trauma. It is imperative for the examining physician to recognize this form of trauma because it is repetitive and frequently ends in death secondary to head injury.

39 UROLOGY

ANATOMY

Kidney The kidneys are paired organs that lie in the retroperitoneum enveloped in Gerota's fascia and variable amounts of fat. Dorsally, lower ribs, quadratus lumborum, and the psoas muscle are in close proximity. Ventral relationships of the right kidney include adrenal, liver, colon, and ileum; the left kidney include, adrenal, stomach, spleen, pancreas, colon, and ileum.

The renal arteries arise from the aorta and approximately two-thirds of kidneys will have single renal artery. The main renal artery divides into five major branches, which represent an end artery supplying a renal segment. Thus occlusion of the renal artery branches will cause infarction of the renal segment. The renal veins empty into the inferior vena cava. The renal lymphatics empty into the hilar trunks, and the capsular lymphatics empty into infradiaphragmatic periaortic nodes. The renal nerves contain vasomotor and pain fibers and receive their contributions from T_4–T_{12} segments. The renal pelvis lies dorsal to the renal vessels and has transitional epithelium.

Ureter The ureters are muscular tubes that travel through the retroperitoneum and connect the renal pelvis to the bladder. The normal adult ureter is 28–30 cm long and about 5 mm in diameter. The ureter transmits urine from the renal pelvis to the bladder by active peristalsis. The blood supply of the ureters originates from the renal, aortic, iliac, mesenteric, gonadal, vasal, and vesical arteries. Pain fibers transmit stimuli to the T_{12}–L_2 segments. The ureter can be deviated medially in retroperitoneal fibrosis and laterally by retroperitoneal tumor or aortic aneurysm.

Bladder The urinary bladder is a muscular organ located in the bony pelvis. The blood supply originates from the superior, middle, and inferior branches of the hypogastric arteries. The lymphatics drain into the perivesical, hypogastric, and periaortic nodes. Autonomic nervous system enters via the sacral cord and the presacral and epigastric plexus.

Prostate and Seminal Vesicles The prostate encases the proximal urethra and is attached to the bladder neck and the symphysis pubis. Distally, the prostate sits on the pelvic diaphragm, which contains the voluntary urinary sphincter. The blood supply is derived from inferior vesical, middle hemorrhoidal, and internal pudendal arteries. The prostate receives secretory and motor (parasympathetic) innervation from S_3 and S_4 and vasomotor (sympathetic) fibers from the hypogastric plexus. The lymphatics drain into the obturator nodes and the external, internal, and common iliac nodes. The seminal vesicles are situated behind the bladder, lateral to the ampullae of the vasa deferentia.

Penis and the Urethra The penis is composed of two erectile bodies called *corpora cavernosa* and a single body, which the urethra travels through, called *corpus spongiosum*. The latter terminates with glans penis, which is also erectile. Urethra in the male is divided into pendulous, bulbous, membranous, and prostatic segments. Female urethra corresponds to the prostatic and membranous urethra in males.

Testis and Epididymis The testes are ovoid firm organs that reside in the scrotum. They are covered by tunica albuginea. The epididymis and the vascular pedicle lie posteriorly. The epididymis is a crescent-like structure located around the dorsal portion of the testis. The vas deferens is a tubular structure that originates from the inferior portion of the epididymis. The arterial blood supply of the testis originates from the aorta. The venous drainage of the left testis is into the left renal vein; the right testis is into the inferior vena cava.

DIAGNOSIS

Gross Hematuria Any amount of gross blood in the urine warrants further evaluation. The common causes are inflammation, tumors, calculi, and trauma. In young patients gross hematuria is more likely to be the result of infection; while in older patients it is more likely to be the result of tumor or prostate disease. It is also important to determine if the hematuria is initial, terminal, or total. This may help to localize the exact site of the pathology.

Acute Postrenal Retention of Urine This term reflects inability to empty the bladder. A variety of afflictions can cause this condition.

Benign prostatic hypertrophy is the most common cause of acute retention in men. There is usually a long-standing history of difficulty in voiding. In carcinoma of the prostate, the symptoms are more acute. Carcinoma of the prostate usually coexists with benign prostatic hypertrophy. In young males, prostatic inflammation may lead to acute urinary retention. This is usually due to urethritis and/or prostatitis. Acute urinary retention may also be due to a urethral stricture that can be due to urethritis or trauma.

Neurogenic bladder dysfunction may lead to increase in residual urine and finally to complete urinary retention. This may be the first indication of spinal cord disease. Other causes of neurogenic retention include trauma, pelvic surgery, general anesthesia, drugs that influence the innervation of the bladder and the sphincter mechanism. Acute urinary retention in females is usually due to neurogenic and psychogenic factors, or urethral obstruction.

Incontinence   True incontinence is the situation in which a patient is not aware of the loss of urine. Enuresis is nocturnal bed wetting, usually affecting children. Urgency occurs when the sensation of urination cannot be controlled before reaching a bathroom. Certain urinary cutaneous or urinary genital fistulas can lead to incontinence. Stress incontinence is due to ineffective sphincter muscle tone. Overflow incontinence represents small amount of urine leakage from a bladder carrying large amount of residual urine.

Ureteral Colic   This is related to a sudden increase in the hydrostatic pressure of the upper urinary tract. Typically, there is a sudden, increasing pain at the costovertebral angle. This may be associated with nausea or vomiting.

Frequency   This refers to voiding an excessive number of times, whereas *polyuria* refers to excessive amount of voiding. Frequency may be related to reduction in bladder capacity or to reduction in the effective bladder capacity that is seen with high residual urine. Frequency may also be a symptom of psychologic stress.

Nocturia   This may be caused by excessive fluid intake, generalized restlessness, cardiac decompensation, diuretic intake, and prostatic hypertrophy.

Urgency   This symptom is due to bladder or bladder outlet inflammation.

Dysuria   This is difficult or painful urination. It is usually described as a burning sensation. Severe pain at the termination of urination is called *strangury*. *Hesitancy* indicates delay in voiding following mental command. *Intermittency* is involuntary stopping or starting of the stream.

Urinary Stream   Lack of force of the urinary stream may reflect obstructive uropathy.

Erectile and Ejaculatory Dysfunction   The etiology may be endocrinologic, vasculogenic, or neurogenic. Certain drugs can lead to erectile and ejaculatory disturbances. In some instances the problem may be situational psychogenic. When anatomic abnormalities are found, they can be corrected. When directly injected into the corpora cavernosa, certain pharmacologic agents such as papaverine can result in adequate erections. In selected cases, insertion of penile prosthesis may be indicated.

Physical Examination

Renal Areas   The renal areas are first examined with the patient in the upright position. Attention should be made to bulging or asymmetry of the costovertebral region. Gentle palpation of the costovertebral region is followed by sharp percussion. Palpation is performed by bimanual examination of the area below the rib cage.

Ureters   Due to their location in the retroperitoneum the ureters cannot be palpated.

Bladder   The bladder is examined with the patient in the supine position and when empty cannot be palpated. With high residual urine the bladder can present as a lower abdominal mass.

Penis   Penis can be examined with the patient in the upright position or the supine position. If the patient is not circumcised, the foreskin should be retracted. The urethral meatus, foreskin, and the glans should be examined.

Scrotum   Examination of the scrotum is carried out in conjunction with examination of the penis. The use of flashlight to transilluminate lesions may help in diagnosis.

Scrotal Masses.

1. *Epididymitis.*   Acute epididymitis is a result of retrograde infection from the prostate, urethra, or the bladder. Scrotum is very tender; overlying skin is red and erythematous. There may be a mass in the scrotum. Nonspecific chronic epididymitis represents an incompletely resolved acute epididymitis. There may be an indurated scrotal mass that can be tender. Tuberculous epididymitis is nontender, stony hard, and associated with indurated vas deferens. A sterile or chemical epididymitis can occur with retrograde extravasation of urine into the epididymis secondary to abdominal strain.

2. *Varicocele.* This is more common on the left side, because the left spermatic vein drains into the left renal vein, which is usually higher. Characteristically there is a "bag of worms" appearance in the scrotum. The acute onset of a varicocele after the age of 40 may be due to an invasive kidney tumor. If the patient is being evaluated for infertility, the finding of a varicocele may be significant. These patients may have low sperm count with reduced motility and change in the sperm morphology.

3. *Hydrocele.* Primary hydrocele may be unilateral or bilateral, which represents fluid between the tunica vaginalis. It presents as a nontender, fluid-filled scrotal mass. Secondary hydrocele is the consequence of serous effusions in the vicinity of disease process. Acute hydrocele may be due to testicular tumor. A communicating hydrocele is present in a patient with a patent processus vaginalis.

4. *Spermatocele.* This is a cyst of an efferent ductule of the rete testis. It is located at the head of the epididymis as a cystic mass.

5. *Testis tumor.* A nodule within the testis is a malignant tumor unless proved otherwise. These are usually firm and nontender. Ultrasonic examination can help define the lesion. Prompt surgical approach is indicated.

6. *Mumps orchitis.* This lesion occurs following acute parotitis. Marked testicular swelling without scrotal edema is noted.

7. *Torsion of the testis and appendages.* "Torsion of the testis" refers to torsion of the spermatic cord. The patient presents with sudden onset of pain associated with scrotal swelling and edema. The testis is elevated in the scrotum and is very tender to palpation. Cremasteric reflex is usually absent. This may be confused with acute epididymitis; isotopic testicular scanning may aid diagnosis. Detorsion and bilateral orchidopexy should be performed as soon as possible. Appendix testis, which is an embryologic remnant above the testis, can undergo torsion. It can be detected as a black dot on transillumination.

Prostate Prostate is examined transrectally by digital palpation. This could be done with patient in a lateral recumbent or standing flexed position. The normal prostate is two finger breadths wide with a sulcus in between two lobes. The consistency of normal prostate and benign hypertrophy is similar to the thenar eminence. In contrast, carcinoma of the prostate feels stony hard. Crepitations are due to prostatic calculi. Acute inflammation of the prostate is accompanied by tenderness or fluctuations that require gentle examination.

Female Urethra   Pelvic examination of the female is necessary to evaluate the lower urinary tract. Presence of urethral lesions, cystocele, or urethrocele can be determined. A urethral diverticulum can be detected by expressing purulent material by pressure.

Urinalysis

Optimal urine collection from males is fresh two-glass specimen and in females a catheterized collection. However, carefully obtained midstream urine in both sexes is usually satisfactory. The specimen should be examined while fresh.

Cloudy urine is not normal. This may be due to phosphaturia, which will clear with acetic acid. Certain foods and drugs can alter the color of urine. The degree and the origin of bleeding can be determined by gross inspection of urine. Screening examination includes test for the presence of blood, albumin, sugar, acetone, and pH. With microscopic examination of the centrifuged urinary sediment one can detect casts, crystals, epithelial cells, white blood cells, red blood cells, and bacteria. Cytologic examination of the exfoliated cells may help in detecting malignancy in the urinary tract. Flow cystometry may give additional information about malignancy.

Genital Secretions

Urethral Discharge   The discharge is collected on a glass slide before the patient urinates. Gonococcal urethritis is diagnosed by the presence of gram-negative intracellular diplococci. Wet specimen is adequate for the diagnosis of *Trichomonas* infections. Noninfected secretions are usually whitish and opalescent; infected secretions are purulent.

Prostatic Secretions   The specimen is obtained by gentle massage. Normal prostatic fluid contains 3–5 white blood cells per high-power field. In the presence of infection secretions become granular and contain large amounts of white blood cells.

Semen Analysis   The semen specimen should be obtained by masturbation. After 1 h the semen will liquefy and should contain more than 20 million spermatozoa per milliliter, with 80% motility and 60% normal morphology.

Instrumentation

Insertion of any instrument into the urethra carries a risk of trauma, introduction of infection, sepsis, stricture formation, and the exacerbation of the preexisting condition.

Cystourethroscopy   This can be performed in the office with local anesthetics with either flexible or rigid instruments. Not only can very small lesions be detected but also small calculi, ureteral orifices, prostate size, urethral strictures or valves, and other lesions.

Ureteropyeloscopy   The entire upper urinary tract can be visualized with flexible or rigid ureteroscopes. Certain procedures can be performed with these instruments.

Therapeutic Instrumentation   An indwelling catheter affords temporary relief of obstruction. If the catheter is left in for over 3 days there is associated infection. Bladder drainage can also be obtained with suprapubic tap and insertion of a polyethylene tube. Drainage of an obstructed upper urinary tract can be accomplished by percutaneous nephrostomy tube or a retrograde ureteral catheter placement.

Therapeutic instrumentation may be applied in the endoscopic removal of calculi or foreign bodies, biopsy or excision of tumors, drainage of prostatic abscesses, dilatation or incision of urethral strictures or valves, and transurethral removal of prostatic obstruction.

Special Diagnostic Studies

Excretory Urography   Certain intravenously administered organic molecules are excreted and concentrated by the kidneys. When they are rendered opaque by iodinization, renal parenchyma and the collecting system can be visualized by x-ray. Since these agents are hyperosmotic they can lead to diuresis and dehydration. These agents can also cause severe allergic reactions.

Renal Size, Location, and Axis.   The adult male kidney is about 13 by 6.2 cm on pyelography. Female kidney is approximately 5 mm smaller. The right kidney is about a half vertebral body lower than the left. The longitudinal axis of the kidneys follows the lateral margin of the psoas muscle, and any deviation may indicate a pathologic condition. The calyces and the infundibulae should be delicate. The pelvis and the ureter should be smooth without redundancy.

Nephrotomography A more detailed visualization of the kidney is obtained by taking slices posteriorly and advancing anteriorly.

Retrograde Pyelourethrography This is indicated to further evaluate the pyelocalyceal system. This study requires cystoscopy, insertion of ureteral catheters, and injection of contrast material.

Antegrade Pyelography Percutaneous insertion of a small catheter into the pelvocalyceal system may be both therapeutic and diagnostic. An infected and obstructed kidney can be drained while injection of contrast material allows the collecting system to be visualized. Following percutaneous access to the kidney, stones can be fragmented (nephrolithotripsy), strictures dilated or incised, and lesions biopsied using nephroscopes.

Renal Arteriography Transfemoral renal arteriography is useful in the evaluation of renal vascular hypertension and therapeutic dilatation of narrow arteries (angioplasty). This is also useful in evaluating renal masses and renal vascular anatomy.

Digital Subtraction Angiography Following intravenous or intraarterial injection of contrast material, a computerized subtraction system provides clear visualization of the renal vasculature.

Vena Cavography Inferior vena cava can be visualized by injection of contrast through a catheter placed from the femoral vein. This is especially helpful in evaluating renal or testicular neoplasms.

Lymphangiography Pedal lymphangiography may provide information regarding lymph node involvement in certain genitourinary cancers.

Renography and Renal Perfusion Scan The ^{131}I hippurate renogram provides information regarding function and drainage of the kidneys. The use of different isotopes may provide further information about renal perfusion, drainage, morphology, and differential renal function.

Ultrasonography Using this noninvasive test, cystic renal lesions can be differentiated from solid lesions. Hydronephrosis can also be determined with this technique. Transrectal ultrasound can also aide in the detection of prostate cancer. Using ultrasound as a guide, biopsies and cyst aspirations can be performed.

Computed Tomography   This is one of the most useful and accurate means of evaluating intraabdominal pathology, and in some instances it has replaced other tests. It can be performed with and without contrast. Along with detailed anatomy, the extent and the size of the tumors can be detected.

Cystometrics, Urethral Pressure Profiles, and Sphincter Electromyography   These studies are useful in evaluating micturition dysfunction due to a variety of clinical problems.

Percutaneous Renal Cyst Puncture   Aspiration of fluid from a renal mass may aid in differentiation of cysts from tumor.

Biochemical and Radioimmunoassay (RIA)   Evaluation of renal function, hypertension, electrolyte disturbances, calculus disease, impotence, and genitourinary neoplasms requires the use of biochemistry and radioimmunoassay.

BLADDER FUNCTION

Physiology of Micturition   Gradual bladder filling under normal circumstances is accompanied by a voiding reflex at certain volume. This can be inhibited by cortical centers. If the conditions are socially acceptable, voiding results by contraction of the detrusor and relaxation of the sphincter. In patients with bladder outlet obstruction, the pressure required to empty the bladder exceeds normal, and detrusor hypertrophy ensues. In long-standing obstruction muscle fibers may decompensate and result in atonia, which can be accompanied with high residual urine.

Bladder Innervation   Sensations are mediated by sensory fibers accompanying the sympathetic and parasympathetic nerves. They arise from T_9–L_2 segments of the spinal cord. Motor pathways originate in the S_2–S_4 segments and reach the bladder via the pelvic nerves. Parasympathetics are responsible for reflex contractions of the detrusor. The external sphincter is innervated with motor nerves from the S_2–S_4 segments via the pudendal nerve. Sympathetic nerves play an important role in detrusor function and outlet resistance.

Motor pathways can be evaluated by bulbocavernosus reflex. Cystometry is the best method for evaluating motor function. This is performed by installation of either gas or water at a certain rate into the bladder and recording pressure changes. Intravesicle pressure rarely exceeds 20 cmH$_2$O.

Neurogenic Bladder Dysfunction

Uninhibited Neurogenic Bladder   This condition presents as urgent voiding that is without voluntary control. Cerebral vascular accidents and multiple sclerosis are classic examples. Treatment is with parasympatholytic drugs.

Reflex (Automatic) Neurogenic Bladder   A well-functioning reflex bladder results if the spinal cord is transected. The lesion must be between T_7 and C_7. With rehabilitation the bladder can provide adequate emptying.

Centrally Denervated Neurogenic Bladder   This dysfunction is the result of the lesions involving the sacral segments of the cauda equina. Meningomyelocele or occult spina bifida are the most frequent lesions. The symptoms are overflow incontinence with high residual urine and infections. Surgical therapy is directed toward facilitating bladder emptying. When bladder rehabilitation is unsuccessful, clean intermittent catheterization may be employed. Cholinergic drugs may enhance detrusor tone, whereas sympatholytic agents can decrease urethral resistance.

Sensory Paralytic Bladder   This results from sensory loss of bladder innervation such as tabes dorsalis or cord degeneration. The patient is unable to sense bladder filling that results in overflow incontinence. Treatment is similar to condition described above.

Motor Paralytic Bladder   Dysfunction may be seen with poliomyelitis or infectious polyneuritis. Loss of motor activity results in large capacity bladder. This may be reversible depending on the disease process.

Bladder drainage is required in the immediate posttrauma stage. This can be done with either indwelling catheters or intermittent catheterization. Chronic indwelling bladder catheterization is almost always accompanied by bacterial colonization. The specific complications of catheter drainage include acute cystitis and pyelonephritis, acute epididymitis, urethral abscess and fistula formation, and bladder or kidney stones. A regimen of intermittent catheterization should be used as soon as possible in these patients.

Rehabilitation of Bladder   During the first months following trauma attention is directed to prevention of infection. Following stabilization of the spine the patient can resume the upright position and begin rehabilitation. Patient's bladder function is assessed with a thorough urodynamic evaluation, and every attempt is made to remove any indwelling catheters. Cholinergic agents can be tried at this time. Clean self-intermittent catheterization may also be instituted. It may be necessary to reinsert an indwelling catheter and to reevaluate at a later date. Certain patients may require antibacterial suppressive therapy.

ACUTE INFECTIONS

Pathogenesis The most common entry site for urinary tract infections is the urethra. When there is obstruction, inflammation, or ulceration in the urinary tract, the defense mechanism is inadequate. Most urinary tract infections occur in the female because of the short urethra. In older age groups incidence of urinary tract infections increases in the male. Recurrent urinary tract infections in children are most likely associated with congenital malformations of the urinary tract. Urinary tract infections can also result from hematogenous spread.

Bacteriology The most common urinary pathogen is *E. coli*. Other common pathogens include *Proteus, Klebsiella,* the enterococci, and *Pseudomonas*.

Treatment The kidneys enhance the efficacy of certain antibacterial agents by increasing their concentration in the urine. Drug selection is facilitated by culture and sensitivities. Drugs that are rapidly excreted by the kidneys are preferred in the treatment of uncomplicated lower urinary tract infections. Patients with acute pyelonephritis or urinary sepsis are treated with drugs that yield high blood and tissue concentration. These patients usually require parenteral combination therapy for an extended period of time.

Urinary tract infection is sometimes a result of anatomic abnormality. Upper tract infections may need further evaluation after the treatment of the infection. These patients are also at risk for recurrence, and close follow-up is mandatory. Occasionally long-term, low-dose suppressive therapy is required.

Gram-Negative Bacteremia This syndrome is considered a urologic disease because the source is usually from the urinary tract. Bacteremia can result from instrumentation. The patients show signs of sepsis with hemodynamic alterations. Bacteria can be resistant to common antibiotics.

Acute Staphylococcal Infections of the Kidney

Staphylococcal pyelonephritis or abscess is of hematogenous origin and usually results from metastatic infection. The patients are usually very ill with fever, flank pain, frequency, and dysuria. Complications include renal carbuncle or perinephric abscess. Treatment consists of parenteral antibiotic therapy.

Perinephric Abscess This usually follows perforation of renal infection or abscess into the perinephric space. The patient presents with high fever and rigid abdomen. Radiographs reveal absent psoas shadow and concavity of the spine to the site of the lesion. Treatment requires drainage and long-term antibiotics.

Acute Papillary Necrosis

Necrosis of renal papillae occurs in patients with diabetes, sickle cell disease, tuberculosis, and excessive ingestion of phenacetin. Along with symptoms of infection, renal colic may be seen. Diagnosis is made on intravenous pyelogram by demonstrating sloughed renal papillae. Treatment is conservative unless there is obstruction.

Acute Urethritis

Acute urethritis is usually venereal in origin. Most common organisms include gonorrhea, *Ureaplasm urealyticum, Chlamydia,* and *Trichomonas vaginalis.* Diagnosis is established by Gram's stain of the discharge and appropriate cultures. Gonorrhea is a common venereal disease that presents with symptoms of acute urethritis. Diagnosis can be made with identification of intracellular gram-negative diplococci. Unless resistant, they are best treated with penicillin-type drugs. Nonspecific urethritis (NSU) is the more common venereal disease in the male. *Chlamydia trachomatis* and *U. urealyticum* are the usual organisms. These can be treated with tetracyclines, while *Trichomonas* infections are treated with metronidazol (Flagyl).

Acute Bacterial Prostatitis

This is usually caused by the same organism that produces urinary tract infections. Infection is usually ascending from the urethra and the prostatic ducts. Symptoms consist of perineal pain, dysuria, frequency attended by fever, chills, and malaise. Liquefaction necrosis may lead to abscess formation. Parenteral antibiotics should be instituted pending appropriate cultures. Rectal examination should be performed gently and reveals warm, tender prostate. Persistence of the symptoms suggests an abscess that requires drainage.

Acute Epididymitis

This is characterized by rapid swelling of the epididymis and the testis along with pain. Urinary tract infection is usually present with associated symptoms. It may be difficult to identify the pathogen if urinary tract infection is not present. Differential diagnosis includes acute torsion of the spermatic cord. Radioisotope and scrotal ultrasound may aid in diagnosis. Treatment consists of symptomatic measures such as scrotal elevation, and broad-spectrum antibiotics. Abscess formation may occur and may require surgical drainage. Traumatic epididymitis can be seen following strain in lifting or scrotal trauma. Antibiotics are usually administered because infection cannot be ruled out.

CHRONIC INFECTIONS

Chronic Bacterial Prostatitis

Chronic bacterial prostatitis is characterized by recurrent urinary tract infections, low back and perineal discomfort, urinary frequency, and dysuria. The duration of the symptoms can be variable; recurrence is common. Expressed prostatic secretions reveal many white blood cells although prostate is usually nontender. Majority of the drugs that are effective in urinary tract infection are unable to penetrate the prostate. Trimethoprim, tetracyclines, carbenicillin, and quinolones seem to be effective. In nonbacterial prostatitis, although symptoms and findings are the same, cultures are usually sterile. Therapy in these cases is usually empirical and often unsuccessful.

Chronic Cystitis

Chronic cystitis can be the end result of recurrent bacterial cystitis. Infiltration of the bladder with the inflammatory process can impair detrusor function. There are often predisposing factors such as tumors, stones, or indwelling catheters. Irritating voiding symptoms are usually present. Diagnostic workup is directed toward identifying the predisposing factors. Chronic antibacterial therapy is often required.

Interstitial cystitis is a form of abacterial cystitis usually seen in females in their later years. Etiology is unknown, and the symptoms are that of cystitis. This must be differentiated from tuberculous cystitis and carcinoma in situ of the bladder. Treatment is very difficult. Periodic instillations of dimethyl sulfoxide (DMSO) may relieve symptoms.

Chronic Epididymitis

This is characterized by persistent induration of the epididymis. Epididymis is minimally tender and there usually is a history of acute epididymitis. Ultrasound examination may aid in differential diagnosis. Treatment consists of empirical antibacterial therapy.

Chronic Pyelonephritis

Histologically this represents a nonspecific inflammation with fibrosis and scarring. Radiologic findings include loss of parenchyma, calyceal blunting, and cortical scars. Treatment is usually directed at correcting the predisposing factors and antibacterial therapy.

Urinary Tuberculosis

Renal tuberculosis is the result of hematogenous spread from other lesions. This infection is usually cortical and bilateral and becomes symptomatic when it ulcerates into the collecting system. Symptoms are similar to cystitis. There is abacterial pyuria on Gram's stain. Special cultures reveal *Mycobacterium tuberculosis*. Radiographic findings include calcification of caseous abscess, ulceration, and stenosis of the collecting system. Therapy is usually medical with combination of isoniazid (INH), ethambutol, rifampin, and pyridoxine.

Genital tuberculosis may accompany renal tuberculosis or may exist alone as a result of hematogenous spread. Epididymis is the most frequent site of infection.

URINARY CALCULI

The consequences of urinary calculi are responsible for many hospital admissions. Primary metabolic stones result from excessive excretion of insoluble substances like uric acid or cystine. In hyperparathyroidism, increased calcium and phosphorus excretion may result in stone formation. Idiopathic hypercalciuria may be the result of increased intestinal absorption, or a renal tubular defect that can lead to stone formation. Excessive absorption of oxalate can produce hyperoxaluria and result in urinary calculi. Secondary stones arise as a result of foreign bodies, obstruction, reflux, or prolonged recumbency. Infections with urea-splitting organisms result in ammonium-magnesium phosphate calculi.

Composition   The calcium oxalate stones make up approximately 75% of calculi. Ammonium-magnesium phosphate is found with infected urine and accounts for approximately 15% of calculi. Uric acid stones constitute approximately 8% of all calculi. Cystine stones represent only 1% of stones.

Diagnosis   Calculi within the ureter usually present with typical colic. Some stones can be asymptomatic, however, and urinalysis may be negative. Approximately 90% of the urinary calculi are radiopaque. Intravenous pyelogram generally will diagnose the stone and reveal additional information about obstruction. Retrograde pyelogram, ultrasonography, and CT may aid in the differential diagnosis.

Management   Analgesics are usually necessary to relieve severe renal colic. Radiologic evaluation will assist in selecting treatment. Ninety-three percent of all ureteral calculi less than 4 mm in diameter will pass spontaneously. Those patients who are treated expectantly should have serial renal function evaluations.

Indications and Methods for Removal.   The mere presence of a stone within the urinary tract does not warrant intervention. Recent technologic developments significantly changed the indications. The technique with which stones can be pulverized by directing shock waves was developed in Germany. Extracorporeal shock-wave lithotripsy (ESWL) is currently the treatment of choice for most urinary stones. This procedure is noninvasive and morbidity is significantly less. A major disadvantage is the fate of the fragments following treatment. These may cause ureteral obstruction and colic. Stones within the urinary tract can also be approached by endoscopic techniques. A variety of energy sources can be applied directly to the stones for their removal; with the combination of ureteroendoscopy, percutaneous nephrolithotripsy, and ESWL the need for open surgical procedures is significantly decreased.

Open Surgery. The techniques described above should be the initial approach to most urinary calculi. Surgical removal of staghorn calculi still represents a clinical challenge. Open surgical approach is still recommended by some authors. Occasionally large bladder stones have to be removed by cystolithotomy. Certain urinary calculi can be dissolved by direct irrigation. Uric acid stones dissolve with alkalinization. Infection stones can be dissolved with Renacidin.

Radiologic Procedures. By placing percutaneous nephrostomy tubes obstruction can be relieved and an emergency situation may become more elective.

Prevention of Recurrence. Stones usually recur, and most patients have a previous history of stones. Hydration is the single most important factor in preventing stone formation. Since some stones rapidly form at certain pH levels, this could be easily adjusted. Urinary tract infections should be treated. Regulation of diet is particularly important in some situations. A low-protein diet is useful in lowering uric acid levels excreted in the urine. Low-oxalate diet may be effective in preventing calcium oxalate stones. Furthermore, low-calcium diet may be beneficial in eliminating calcium-containing stones. Urinary calcium can be decreased by hydrochlorthiazides or cellulose phosphate binders. Allopurinol may reduce the uric acid stone formation.

Hyperparathyroidism Majority of patients with hyperparathyroidism present with urinary calculi. Patients with recurrent urinary calculi should be investigated for increased serum calcium and alkaline phosphatase and decreased phosphorus. Serum parathormone level should be assayed. Treatment consists of surgical removal of parathyroid adenoma.

PEDIATRIC UROLOGY

The genitourinary system should be evaluated in all instances of "failure to thrive" syndrome, undiagnosed febrile illnesses, externally apparent congenital anomalies, and abdominal masses. Wilms' tumor of the kidney and neuroblastoma of the adrenal gland are the most common solid tumors in children.

Congenital Anomalies

Phimosis (Redundant Prepuce) Due to poor hygiene this condition predisposes to infection and carcinoma of the glans penis. Circumcision is generally recommended.

Urethral Meatal Stenosis   This condition can be congenital or acquired in the male. It is easily detected by inspection, and treatment consists of meatotomy.

Urethral Valves   These are usually seen in boys and produce variable changes due to obstruction. Diagnosis is established by voiding cystourethrography and endoscopy. Along with dilatation of the posterior urethra, hydroureteronephrosis is common. Endoscopic incision or fulguration of the valves is usually done early. However, in some cases, excessive dilatation may require a supravesical diversion such as a cutaneous vesicostomy.

Neurogenic Bladder   This is usually due to autonomic dysfunction accompanying meningomyelocele. The patient presents with overflow incontinence, infection, and impaired voiding. Diagnosis is established by cystourethrogram and cystometry. Mild cases can be treated by bladder rehabilitation and preventing infections. Severe cases are treated for reducing residual urine with either surgery or intermittent catheterization.

Ureterocele   This is cystic dilatation of the intravesicle portion of the ureter. The ureteral orifice may or may not be stenotic. This may become large enough to obstruct the urethra. Diagnosis can be made with the cystogram phase of the intravenous pyelogram. The contrast-filled intravesicle mass is referred to as "cobra head deformity." Treatment is usually surgical.

Hydronephrosis   This is often a result of a congenital obstruction at the ureteropelvic junction. This can result in significant dilatation and atrophy of the renal parenchyma. Children commonly present with a palpable abdominal mass. Intravenous pyelogram and ultrasound will establish the diagnosis. Pyeloplasty is the treatment of choice; however, nephrectomy may be required for poorly functioning kidneys.

Congenital Nonobstructive Renal Disease   Congenital or neonatal glomerular disease is usually fatal. There are many forms of cystic disease of the kidney. In medullary cystic disease collecting ducts are ectatic, whereas in polycystic disease there is a failure of communication between tubules and glomeruli. Nonfunctioning multicystic disease may be the failure of the development of the metanephric blastema. Detailed renal function studies and close follow-up are required.

Hypospadias   This is a fusion defect of the urethra. The anomaly consists of a dorsal hood (absent ventral foreskin), chordee (ventral curvature of the penis), and proximal location of the urethral opening. Hypospadias can be associated with abnormal urinary stream, and infertility. Hypospadias with urethral opening in the scrotum can be accompanied with bilateral undescended testicles; this must be differentiated from adrenogenital syndrome or pseudohermaphroditism. Treatment consists of surgical correction.

Epispadias   This is associated with a dorsally cleft urethra, which is very rare.

Exstrophy of the Bladder   In this anomaly the bladder that is open is the part of the abdominal wall. Several procedures are usually required for total reconstruction.

Ectopic Ureteral Orifice   This is usually associated with duplex ureters, and the ectopic orifice drains the upper collecting system. The condition is more common in females. When the opening is in the vagina, incontinence is the rule. Treatment is surgical.

NEOPLASMS

Renal Tumors

Incidence and Etiology   Renal tumors account for 2% of all cancer deaths. Tumor probably arises from tubular cells. Etiology is unclear.

Pathology   There are three major types of malignant tumors of the renal parenchyma. Granular cell carcinoma and tubular adenocarcinoma account for 60%. Wilms' tumor (adenomyosarcoma), which is commonly seen in children, accounts for 14%. These are followed by sarcomas and tumors of the collecting system.

Clinical Manifestations   The classic triad of pain, mass, and hematuria is seen in fewer than half the patients. Hematuria is a late manifestation. Passage of blood clots can mimic renal stone colic. Mass can be palpated if the lesion is in the lower pole. Fever may be seen, which can be due to necrosis. Hypertension may be the result of compromised renal perfusion from the tumor compression. Renal tumors can secrete excessive erythropoietin, which will result in erythrocytemia. Metastases involve the lung, bone, lymph nodes, liver, and skin.

Diagnosis   Excretory urography is frequently diagnostic. Nephrotomography is helpful in differentiating cysts from tumors. Calcified cysts are more suggestive of tumor. Ultrasound is also very helpful in differentiating cyst from tumor. Renal arteriography is occasionally needed, and inferior vena cavography may be necessary to rule out tumor extension into the venous system. CT not only is diagnostic but also gives valuable information regarding the extent of the tumor. MRI can also be diagnostic and may be more sensitive for showing venous extension.

Treatment   Removal of the kidney with perinephric fat and lymph nodes offers the best chance of cure. Radiation therapy or chemotherapy is generally not effective. Recently there have been some promising results with adaptive immuno-therapy.

Prognosis   This depends on grade and the extension of the tumor. Overall survival rate for renal tumors is about 50% for 5 years.

CARCINOMA OF THE RENAL PELVIS   Tumors of the pelvo-calyceal system are usually transitional cell types. Squamous cell carcinoma is rare and generally associated with chronic infection or calculous disease. Gross hematuria and colic is a common mode of presentation. Intravenous pyelogram is diagnostic, showing the filling defect in the pelvis or the ureter. Cytology is also helpful in establishing diagnosis. Treatment is by removing the kidney and the ureter.

Tumors of the Urinary Bladder

Incidence and Etiology   This tumor is more commonly seen after the fifth decade of life. The usual lesion is transitional cell carcinoma and it is more common in males. Papillary bladder tumors have been linked to certain chemicals, ciga-rette smoking, schistosomiasis, and bladder calculi.

Clinical Manifestations   Gross or microhematuria is the initial sign present in almost all cases. When the tumor is confined to the bladder, physical findings are minimal. The tumor can be visualized on excretory urography; however, cystoscopy and biopsy are confirmatory. Local extension and metastasis can occur. Bimanual examination may reveal fixed bladder in the pelvis. Urine cytology and flow cysto-metry are also helpful in diagnosis.

Treatment and Prognosis   Endoscopic resection is suitable for superficial lesions. Most tumors recur with superficial lesions; very few patients will eventually have invasive lesions. For locally invasive tumors, the best treatment is total cystectomy with urinary diversion. Definitive radiation therapy and combination chemotherapy may provide satisfactory results. Intravesicle administration of certain chemotherapeutic agents or BCG may reduce the recurrence rate of superficial lesions.

Prostatic Tumors

BENIGN PROSTATIC HYPERTROPHY   Incidence and Etiology
Benign prostatic hypertrophy (BPH) is a benign tumor that originates from the periurethral prostatic tissue. It is more commonly seen after the fifth decade of life.

Clinical Manifestations   The symptoms are related to mechanical obstruction. The onset is usually insidious, and nocturia is the most common symptom. Hematuria can be seen, in which case other pathology must be ruled out. Acute urinary retention is the result of detrusor decompensation. On examination most patients present with a smooth, enlarged prostate. However, a normal-size gland does not rule out obstruction. Occasionally the bladder can be palpated, indicating urinary retention. Radiographically there may be thickening of the bladder wall, increased postvoid residual urine, and ureteral dilatation.

Residual Urine   The amount of residual urine can be determined by catheterization after voiding. Normally postvoid residual urine is a few cubic centimeters. Residual urine is the result of stretching of the detrusor; as a result urine retention increases with time. Functionally reduced bladder capacity is manifest by multiple voiding. Anesthesia, anticholinergics, and sympathomimetics will increase the likelihood of acute urinary retention. The presence of residual urine also predisposes to bladder stone formation and infection.

Treatment   The obstructed or symptomatic patient is best treated by prostatectomy. However, some patients without urinary tract infection and compromised renal function can be followed conservatively. Patients with deteriorating renal function are initially treated with an indwelling urethral or a suprapubic catheter, followed by prostatectomy. Poor surgical risk patients may be treated with chronic indwelling catheters. As the adenoma grows in BPH it compresses the true prostate, and during operation the true prostate is usually left behind.

Transurethral Prostatectomy.   This is performed by electroresection of the prostate through the urethra. Multiple pieces of the obstructing tissue are removed under direct vision.

This procedure can be combined with endoscopic lithotripsy (crushing and removal of a bladder calculus). This technique is also applicable in carcinoma of the prostate which is not amenable to curative or palliative measures. Because of the excellent results obtained with transurethral resection of the prostate, open prostatectomy is rarely performed. The indications for open prostatectomy include large adenoma, and associated bladder stone or tumor.

Prognosis   Over 90% of the patients have complete relief or improvement of their symptoms. Approximately 10–20% of the patients will have recurrent obstruction in 5 years.

CARCINOMA OF THE PROSTATE   Incidence and Etiology   The etiology of prostate cancer is not known; it is rare before age 50 and not seen in eunuchs. It is the second most common cancer in males in the United States.

Early Carcinoma   This is the stage in which the carcinoma is localized to the gland. More than 50% of the nodules palpated on rectal examination are positive for cancer on biopsy. Patients with localized cancer are best treated with prostatoseminalvesiculectomy. Careful dissection will preserve continence and sexual function. Ultrasound guided transrectal biopsy is the most accurate diagnostic technique. On rectal examination carcinoma usually feels rock hard; however, this could be seen in prostatitis, BPH, calculus, and bladder or rectal cancer extension. Bony metastasis can be evaluated with bone scan. Serum acid phosphatase may be elevated in metastatic cancer.

Histologically, prostatic malignant tumors are adenocarcinomas. Prognosis depends on the degree of differentiation and the stage of the disease.

Alternative treatment of early carcinoma is radiation therapy. Some centers report similar survival rates with surgery and radiation therapy. Cure can be achieved only by total removal of the lesion. Patients who are not candidates for radiation therapy or surgery can be treated with antiandrogen therapy.

Advanced Carcinoma   Patients can present with bladder outlet symptoms. Weight loss, extremity pain, gross hematuria, and lower extremity lymph edema can be seen. Rectal examination reveals fixed, stony hard prostate. Acid and alkaline phosphatase and prostatic-specific antigen is elevated. Prostatic-specific antigen can also be elevated in localized carcinoma. Treatment of symptomatic advanced carcinoma is with anti-androgen therapy. This could be done with bilateral orchiectomy, administration of estrogens, ketoconazole, flutamide, cyproterone acetate, amino glutethimide, and luteinizing hormone-releasing hormone (LHRH). Palliation is obtained in approximately 90% of the patients. Local radiation therapy for painful bone metastasis is also effective.

Testicular Tumors

Incidence and Etiology Testicular tumors account for 1% of cancers in the male. The average age at diagnosis is 30. They occur more frequently in undescended testis. Testicular cancer is infrequently seen in the black race.

Clinical Manifestations These patients usually present with a lump in their testis. The examination usually finds a firm, nontender, solid mass. These must be differentiated from hydroceles and epididymitis. Late symptoms of metastasis include weight loss, fatigue, lymph node enlargement, and ureteral obstruction.

Diagnosis and Treatment When a testicular tumor is suspected, an inguinal exploration is required. The testis, along with the spermatic chord, is usually removed and a radical orchiectomy is performed. Prior to orchiectomy, a beta HCG and AFB tumor marker should be obtained. Seminomas represent approximately 40% of malignant testis tumors, embryonal cell carcinomas and teratocarcinomas about 25% each, and teratomas 8%; choriocarcinoma is limited to approximately 1–2%. Benign tumors of the testis are very rare. Because seminomas are usually very radiosensitive, further operation is usually not indicated. However, nonseminoma testicular tumors will require bilateral retroperitoneal lymph node resection for accurate staging of the disease. The use of combination chemotherapy has markedly increased the survival of these patients with advanced metastatic tumors. Survival depends on the cell type and the stage of the disease at the time of diagnosis.

Carcinoma of the Penis

Carcinoma of the penis develops in the squamous epithelium of the glans and foreskin and is almost eliminated by circumcision at infancy. This lesion is uncommon in the United States, and the average age of onset is over 60. Patients usually present with an ulcerated lesion on the penis, and the diagnosis is obtained by biopsy. Local excision and x-ray therapy is associated with a 90% 5-year cure rate when there is no distant metastasis. When there is lymph node involvement, the 5-year survival is reduced to 30%.

GENITOURINARY TRACT INJURIES

Renal Injury

Blunt renal trauma is more common than penetrating kidney trauma. Rapid deceleration such as impact following falls may result in renal vessel injury. Patients who suffer renal injury will usually have gross hematuria or microhematuria. Diagnosis of renal injury is confirmed by excretory urography or CT scan. Abdominal CT may be the single most important diagnostic test. It will give not only adequate visualization of the renal structures, but also an idea about other intra-abdominal organs. Patients with renal contusions and lacerations without extravasation of urine may be treated conservatively. When there is failure to visualize a kidney on a CT scan and arteriography or when there is significant extravasation, surgical treatment is considered. Every effort should be made to preserve renal parenchyma. In massive trauma to the kidney, nephrectomy may be a life-saving procedure. Most cases of renal trauma can be treated conservatively.

Bladder and Urethral Injury

The full bladder is more vulnerable to trauma. Direct blows and penetrating injury by spicules of bone, stab wounds, and gunshot wounds may all result in rupture of the bladder. Direct blows usually cause intraperitoneal rupture; the penetrating injuries are usually extraperitoneal. Urine can be grossly bloody and the patient may not be able to void. When there is suspicion of bladder trauma, a retrograde urethrogram and cystography should be performed. Blood at the meatus suggests urethral injury; a retrograde urethrogram should be done prior to any instrumentation of the urethra. Treatment of severe bladder trauma usually consists of surgical repair and cystostomy drainage. In most cases of bladder injury, conservative management without an operation may be satisfactory. This is especially true in extraperitoneal rupture of the bladder, in which catheter drainage may result in adequate healing. If the urethra is avulsed, this may be repaired at the time of repairing the bladder rupture. However, if the trauma is extensive and the patient's condition is poor, cystostomy under local anesthesia may be the procedure of choice and this would allow second-stage repair.

Ureteral Trauma

Ureteral injuries occur mainly as a result of surgery. If the injury is recognized, direct repair over an indwelling stent can be performed. If it is not recognized, the patient may present with anuria, urinary fistula, or urinoma. Ureter also can be injured by penetrating objects such as bullets and knives. In this case, exploratory laparotomy and surgical repair usually are indicated.

OPERATIONS ON GENITOURINARY ORGANS

Nephrectomy

Nephrectomy can be performed either by retroperitoneal flank approach or by transabdominal anterior approach. Flank approach is usually preferred in the treatment of inflammatory disease, calculi, perinephric abscess, hydronephrosis, and renal cystic disease. Nephrectomy for renal carcinoma is carried out through the transperitoneal approach where the vascular ligation is carried on early.

Cutaneous Ureteroileostomy (Ileal Conduit)

This is the most popular method of supravesicle urinary diversion. The major indication for this procedure is urinary diversion following removal of the bladder. The patient has an ileal conduit that is continuously draining urine to the skin and requires carrying drainage bags. Recently there have been modifications of the conduit in which the stoma has been made into a continent-drainage system. In these select cases the patients have to catheterize their conduits. There is also research developing continent neobladders using small or large bowel segments. Ileal loop is usually performed through a midline abdominal incision. The stoma is created before the creation of the conduit on the appropraite area of the abdomen. Following this, a segment of ileum is mobilized and the bowel is reanastomosed end to end. After that, the ureters are anastomosed to the conduit in one end and the conduit in the other end is brought out through the skin as a stoma.

Cystostomy, Cystolithotomy

The bladder is usually approached with a lower abdominal incision and the detrusor muscle can be incised longitudinally. If stones are present, these are removed. Drainage can be provided by a large catheter. In the urinary tract it is important to use absorbable sutures such as chromic catgut. Any foreign bodies such as silk sutures will result in formation of stones.

Prostatectomy

Transurethral Prostatectomy This is the most common operation to remove prostatic obstruction. This is done endoscopically using a resectoscope. Using electric current and a cutting loop, prostatic tissue is resected and hemostasis is secured with electrocoagulation. Catheter is inserted for several days for hemostasis and this is removed and patient's voiding is observed.

Suprapubic Prostatectomy This operation is performed through a cystostomy approach as previously described. The adenoma is mobilized and enucleated using finger dissection. The surgical capsule of the prostate is left behind. Hemostasis is obtained and a suprapubic tube as well as a urethral Foley catheter is left indwelling. The urethral catheter is removed in 5–7 days and the patient is observed voiding.

This is also accomplished through an incision intraabdominally. However, the bladder is not entered during this operation. An incision is made on the bladder neck and the capsule of the prostate is incised. Following this, the adenoma is exposed and dissected through the capsule of the prostate and removed. Hemostasis is established and again the capsule is closed with absorbable sutures. Adequate drainage of the urinary tract is established by a Foley catheter and a suprapubic tube.

Hydrocelectomy

A vertical scrotal incision is used; the hydrocele sac is approached and dissected. Then the sac is entered and fluid evacuated. The excess tunica is excised, and hemostasis is established. The layers are then reapproximated with absorbable sutures. Hydrocelectomy in children is carried out through an inguinal incision. At this time, hernia repair usually is undertaken.

Inguinal Orchiectomy

This is performed when a testicular tumor is suspected. It provides access to the spermatic vessels before manipulation of the testis. The spermatic cord is identified and ligated. The spermatic cord and the testis are then removed and sent to pathology.

Orchiopexy

This is performed through an inguinal incision and permits mobilization of the spermatic cord and correction of the indirect hernia. The testis is then brought to the scrotum and placed in a dartos pouch and fixed. No tension is placed on the spermatic cord.

Bilateral Vasectomy

This is a male sterilization procedure generally carried out under local anesthesia in an outpatient setting. The vas deferens on each side of the scrotum is identified and these are dissected, tied, and coagulated. A small portion of the vas is then sent to pathology for identification.

Vasovasostomy

This procedure is carried out on an in-hospital basis and can be done under local or general anesthesia. The incision is made in the scrotum on both sides of the vas. The granulomatous areas of the vas are excised until the sperm is noted from the testicular portion of the vas. Following this, using magnification with either surgical loops or a microscope, the anastomosis is performed in an end-to-end fashion.

FEMALE REPRODUCTIVE TRACT

Embryology

An embryo cannot be distinguished as male or female until the eighth week of development. An ovary or estrogen is not essential for development of a female phenotype, as müllerian structures develop in agonadal individuals. Androgens are required to promote wolffian duct (male) development and the testis produces müllerian inhibiting factor (MIF) to suppress development of müllerian structures.

Anatomy

The cardinal (Mackenrodt's), round, and uterosacral ligaments form the supporting ligamentous attachments to the uterus. The ovarian arteries originate from the aorta below the celiac plexus and reach the ovaries through the infundibulopelvic ligament, which forms a portion of the broad ligament. The uterine arteries originate from the internal iliac arteries and reach the uterus through the cardinal ligaments, after passing over the ureter. The autonomic nerve supply to the pelvis is twofold: the sympathetic pathway originates from L_1–L_4 and is distributed to the pelvis via the presacral plexus, the parasympathetic supply is from spinal cord level S_2–S_4 and reaches the pelvis via the nervi erigentes.

ENDOCRINOLOGY

The hypothalamic pituitary axis modulates ovarian steroid production through the production of GnRH, FSH, and LH. Estradiol is the principal estrogen secreted by the ovary. Progesterone, which is thermogenic and transforms endometrium from proliferative to secretory, is produced only after ovulation by the corpus luteum.

The prepubertal female has low levels of FSH and LH, and ovarian estrogen production is low. At puberty increased FSH/LH levels occur with increased estradiol production, and ultimately initiation of the ovulatory cycle occurs. At menopause increased levels of FSH and LH occur in association with cessation of ovulation and declining estrogen production by the ovary.

GYNECOLOGIC EXAMINATION

In addition to a complete history relevant information specific to a gynecologic history includes information about presenting symptoms, menarche, past obstetric history, contraception, and menstrual history.

Physical Examination

A thorough gynecologic examination, in addition to a thorough history and physical examination, includes a Pap smear of the cervix; inspection of the vulva, vagina, and cervix; and bimanual examination of the uterus and adnexae with rectovaginal examination to detect cul-de-sac abnormalities or disease of the rectum.

Radiologic Investigation

Ultrasound is useful in determining the nature of a pelvic mass and is used routinely in the evaluation of patients with suspected ectopic pregnancy. Transvaginal ultrasound is particularly well suited to the evaluation of pelvic abnormalities.

A CT scan may also be useful in the evaluation of an undiagnosed pelvic mass, especially if contrast is used so that information regarding the GU and GI tract is also obtained.

SYMPTOMS Pain Cyclic pain occurring with menses is termed *dysmenorrhea,* and when no other cause is found is designated *primary* dysmenorrhea, which has been attributed to abnormal prostaglandin levels in the uterus. *Secondary* dysmenorrhea may be due to endometriosis, adenomyosis, cervical stenosis, an IUD, or malformations of the uterus or vagina.

The differential diagnosis of acute pelvic pain includes both surgical and medically managed conditions. *Mittelschmerz* is the occurrence of midcycle pain related to ovulation. Pelvic inflammatory disease is usually associated with diffuse pelvic pain and an exquisitely tender cervix. An ectopic pregnancy, ruptured or twisted ovarian cyst, appendicitis,

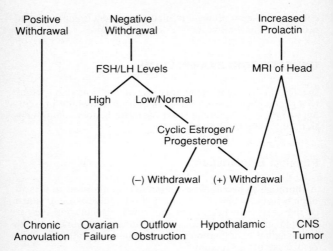

Fig. 40-1 Evaluation of amenorrhea. HX and PE, B-HCG, Prolactin, if β-HCG negative progestin test (progesterone in oil 100 mg im).

or leaking tuboovarian abscess may all cause acute lower abdominal pain.

Chronic pelvic pain may occur with endometriosis, pelvic inflammatory disease, or a variety of benign and neoplastic growths of the ovary, tube, or uterus.

When a definitive diagnosis is not established by clinical evaluation, laparoscopy is necessary to determine the cause of pelvic pain.

Amenorrhea Amenorrhea is primary when initiation of menses has not occurred by age 16. *Secondary* amenorrhea refers to the absence of menses for 6 months in a patient who previously had regular cycles. *Primary* amenorrhea is most frequently related to inherited abnormalities in sexual development. Causes of secondary amenorrhea include hypothalamic-pituitary disorders, gonadal failure, and outflow tract obstruction. Pregnancy must always be excluded. Amenorrhea may be evaluated according to the schema outlined in Fig. 40-1.

Bleeding Vaginal bleeding in the prepubertal female is always abnormal and may be due to a foreign body, a hormone-producing ovarian tumor, or a malignancy of the genital tract.

Abnormal vaginal bleeding in reproductive-age women has

a variety of forms and a multiplicity of causes. *Oligomenorrhea* refers to infrequent menstruation and occurs with irregular ovulation due to polycystic ovarian syndrome or oligoovulation around puberty or the menopause. *Metrorrhagia* is the occurrence of bleeding at times other than during menses. *Menorrhagia* refers to abnormally heavy menses. *Menometrorrhagia* may be due to abnormalities of pregnancy such as spontaneous, incomplete, or threatened abortion, ectopic pregnancy, or a molar gestation. Other causes include leiomyomata, neoplasms, infection, trauma, blood dyscrasias and coagulopathies, and dysfunctional uterine bleeding.

Postmenopausal bleeding is always abnormal and requires biopsy of the endometrium. Causes include neoplasms, endometrial or cervical polyps, endometritis or cervicitis, other infections, atrophic vaginitis, and trauma.

Mass The presence of an adnexal or pelvic mass in the prepubertal female is always abnormal and requires radiologic and frequently surgical investigation. The most frequent ovarian neoplasms in adolescents are germ cell tumors of the ovary such as dysgerminoma and endodermal sinus tumor.

In reproductive-age women functional ovarian cysts occur frequently, so that evaluation of an asymptomatic mobile adnexal mass depends on the clinical characteristics (see Fig. 40-2). Pregnancy, intrauterine or ectopic, should always be considered. Routine tests with a symptomatic cyst include a CBC, ESR, β-HCG, and pelvic ultrasound.

A pelvic mass in a postmenopausal female is always abnormal and may be due to neoplasms of the uterus, ovary, or other pelvic structures (see Table 40-1).

CONTRACEPTION

The most frequently used contraceptive method currently is male or female sterilization. Vasectomy is accomplished easily under local anesthesia, and laparoscopic tubal ligation, the most frequently employed method of surgical sterilization in the female, is usually performed under general anesthesia and has a failure rate of approximately 1:1000.

Reversible contraceptive methods include oral contraceptives, the IUD, and barrier methods such as the condom or diaphragm. Oral contraceptives afford the greatest protection, with an intrauterine device next in efficacy followed by barrier methods.

A wide variety of oral contraceptives are available, but

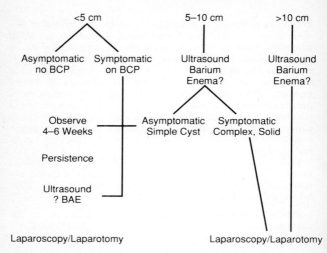

Fig. 40-2   Evaluation of adnexal mass Premenopausal patient.

most use a combination of an estrogen, either ethinyl estradiol or mestranol, and one of several different progestins. Oral contraceptives probably should not be used in women over age 40. Absolute contraindications include a history of estrogen-dependent neoplasia, thromboembolic disorders, cerebrovascular disease, undiagnosed uterine bleeding, and pregnancy.

SPECIFIC GYNECOLOGIC DISORDERS

See Chap. 41 in *Principles of Surgery,* 5th ed.

OUTFLOW TRACT OBSTRUCTION

Imperforate hymen and congenital absence of the vagina (Kuster-Rokitansky-Hauser syndrome) are the most commonly encountered problems, both causing primary amenorrhea. Imperforate hymen is treated by incision, and an absent vagina is treated by vaginal reconstruction. Other causes of outflow tract obstruction that may cause secondary amenorrhea are Asherman syndrome (intrauterine synechiae) and cervical stenosis, which both may occur following infection or surgical injury.

TABLE 40-1.   Differential Diagnosis of Adnexal Mass (Nonovarian Causes)

Nonneoplastic
  Pregnancy
  Tuboovarian abscess
  Diverticular or appendiceal abscess
  Hydrosalpinx
  Stool in colon
  Full bladder
  Pelvic kidney
Neoplastic
  Leiomyomata
  Carcinoma of tube, colon, or appendix
  Retroperitoneal tumor
  Lymphoma
  Krukenberg tumor

PREGNANCY DISORDERS

Spontaneous Abortion

Refers to the natural termination of pregnancy before the fetus is capable of extrauterine life and occurs in about 40% of all pregnancies, although about one half are not clinically significant. The majority of first-trimester abortions have detectable chromosomal aberrations, the most frequent being autosomal trisomy. Subgroups of clinical importance are threatened, inevitable, incomplete, complete, missed, septic, and habitual spontaneous abortion. In Rh⁻ patients management includes administration of RhoGAM.

Threatened abortion is diagnosed with any uterine bleeding in the first half of pregnancy when the conceptus is still viable, and occurs in about 20% of pregnancies. Bleeding is usually scanty and without cramps, and the cervical os is closed. About one half of those with threatened abortion will go on to miscarry. The differential diagnosis includes inevitable or incomplete abortion, ectopic pregnancy, a molar gestation, and cervical or vaginal neoplasia. Useful diagnostic tests include a quantitative HCG and pelvic ultrasound. When fetal viability is demonstrated ultrasonically there is only a 10% risk of subsequent abortion. Management of threatened abortion is expectant.

Inevitable abortion is diagnosed when progressive cervical dilatation occurs with pain and bleeding. An ultrasound should be obtained to exclude a twin pregnancy with abortion of a single conceptus. As there is no fetal survival in first-trimester inevitable abortion, management is by suction curettage of the uterus.

Incomplete abortion is diagnosed when the products of conception have been partially expelled from the uterus. A pelvic ultrasound is sometimes diagnostic, and management is by suction evacuation of the uterus.

Complete spontaneous abortion refers to those cases in which all the products of conception have been spontaneously expelled from the uterus. When the diagnosis is certain, further therapy is unnecessary. Otherwise, suction evacuation of the uterus should be performed. Rh⁻ patients should receive mini-RhoGAM (50 µg).

Missed abortion refers to those cases in which the conceptus dies but the products of conception are not expelled. Diagnosis is usually by ultrasound. Although most will eventually spontaneously abort, the recommended management is suction evacuation of the uterus.

Septic abortion refers to any subtype of spontaneous or induced abortion complicated by infection. Abdominal and uterine pain usually occur in association with fever and leucocytosis. Initial management includes the administration of parenteral broad-spectrum antibiotics followed by careful evacuation of the uterus. Complications that can lead to death include septic shock and ARDS. If septic shock does not respond to conservative measures, hysterectomy may be necessary and lifesaving.

Habitual abortion is the occurrence of three or more consecutive first-trimester abortions. Evaluation includes hysteroscopy to exclude uterine defects and chromosomal evaluation of the conceptus, when possible, and of the parents. In addition, cervical culture for *Ureaplasma urealyticum* and *Mycoplasma* is commonly performed, although an etiologic relationship remains unproven.

Ectopic Pregnancy

The fallopian tube is the most common site of an ectopic pregnancy, and ectopic pregnancy still accounts for 10% of maternal deaths.

The etiology is multifactorial, with the common denominator a delay in ovum transport. Pelvic inflammatory disease is most commonly implicated. When a pregnancy occurs with an IUD in place, 6% are ectopic. Also, progestin-only (minipill) contraceptives are associated with a *fivefold increase* in risk of ectopic pregnancy.

Symptoms include pain in virtually all cases, with a history of irregular bleeding and amenorrhea less frequent. Syncopal symptoms occur in those cases presenting with hemorrhagic shock.

Signs include adnexal tenderness in nearly all cases. An adnexal mass occurs in 50%, and the uterus is normal in size in most cases. Temp $> 37°$ is infrequent.

Laboratory tests useful diagnostically and for management include determination of β-HCG, CBC, culdocentesis, and transvaginal ultrasound. A serum HCG > 6500 with an empty uterus by ultrasound is presumptive evidence of an ectopic pregnancy, although this constellation of findings may occur following a spontaneous abortion. In some instances pathologic findings from D&C may be helpful in diagnosis.

The differential diagnosis includes corpus luteum cyst, pelvic inflammatory disease, threatened or incomplete abortion, appendicitis, and degenerating uterine fibroids.

Laparoscopy may be necessary to make a definitive diagnosis, and in unruptured ectopic pregnancy linear salpingotomy, with removal of the ectopic pregnancy via the laparoscope, is the preferred treatment. When necessary, salpingectomy may be performed either laparoscopically or by laparotomy.

DISORDERS OF PELVIC SUPPORT

Pelvic support is weakened through childbirth, trauma, and the aging process. Disorders of pelvic support include cystocele, rectocele, enterocele, uterine prolapse, procidentia, and urinary stress incontinence.

Symptoms due to pelvic relaxation relate to the organs affected. A cystocele causes a sense of vaginal fullness, and when severe, the bladder may protrude from the vagina. Without an accompanying urethrocele, the patient is usually continent. A rectocele may cause difficulty with defecation, sometimes requiring insertion of a finger in the vagina to effect complete evacuation. Severe uterine prolapse or procidentia is accompanied by eversion of the bladder and rectum and is noted by the patient as a mass protruding from the vagina.

Disorders of pelvic relaxation are easily diagnosed by physical assessment. Distinguishing between a rectocele and enterocele may be difficult prior to operation. When urinary incontinence is part of the symptomatology, a cystometrogram should be included in the diagnostic evaluation in order to exclude other causes of urinary incontinence.

Treatment of cystocele, rectocele, and uterine prolapse is usually by vaginal hysterectomy with anterior/posterior colporrhaphy. Sometimes the vaginal vault must be suspended by sacrospinous ligament fixation. When surgery is not desirable mild cases may be managed by insertion of a pessary. Urinary stress incontinence requires suspension of the vesical neck, which can be accomplished by an abdominal procedure (Marshall-Marchetti), or vaginally by anterior colporrhaphy or percutaneous needle (Stamey, Peyrera) urethropexy.

GYNECOLOGIC INFECTIONS

VAGINITIS   Vaginal discharge is the most frequent symptom associated with vaginitis, although postmenopausal patients may complain of vaginal bleeding. The etiology of vaginitis includes infection with *Trichomonas, Monilia,* and *Gardnerella vaginalis.* Other conditions associated with vaginal discharge are foreign bodies, cervicitis, and atrophic vaginitis.

Specific diagnosis requires cervical culture with wet and KOH prep of the discharge. A patient with chronic monilial vaginitis should be screened for diabetes.

Treatment of trichomonal and *G. vaginitis* is with metronidazole 1 g every 12 h for 2–4 doses. Monilial vaginitis is treated with topical miconazole or clotrimazole 100 mg pv twice daily pv for 3 days. Treatment of atrophic vaginitis is with estrogen replacement therapy.

BARTHOLIN'S ABSCESS AND CYST   Bartholin's glands are usually nonpalpable and located at the vaginal orifice at 5 and 7 o'clock. Obstruction of the glandular duct leads to cystic dilatation and cyst or abscess formation. Bartholinitis is usually polymicrobial, and is not often due to gonorrhea as was previously thought.

Most Bartholin's cysts are asymptomatic. Abscess formation leads to vulvar pain, dyspareunia, and sometimes difficulty walking.

Treatment of Bartholin's cysts is by marsupialization. Simple incision and drainage of an abscess is frequently inadequate, so that placement of a Word catheter or marsupialization is necessary in order to ensure adequate drainage of the abscess. Antibiotics are unnecessary unless there is an associated cellulitis. Necrotizing fasciitis has been described in diabetic patients stemming from bartholinitis. A women over 40 with a Bartholin's cyst should undergo excision of the cyst or biopsy of Bartholin's gland to exclude an underlying carcinoma.

PELVIC INFLAMMATORY DISEASE (PID)   *PID* refers to inflammation of the upper genital tract (salpingitis, oophoritis, etc.) resulting from ascending infection from the vaginal and cervical microbial flora. Usually a polymicrobial infection.

Frequent isolates include *N. gonorrhea, Chlamydia trachomitis,* and endogenous aerobic and anaerobic organisms. Spontaneous cases occur in 85%, with the remainder occurring following endometrial biopsy, D&C, hysteroscopy or a hysterosalpingogram, or an IUD insertion.

A wide spectrum of symptoms occur, ranging from lower abdominal pain with fever and a vaginal discharge to diffuse peritonitis and septic shock. Physical findings include fever (38°C) and cervical and adnexal tenderness. An adnexal mass, when present, frequently is due to a tuboovarian complex or abscess. Although bilateral adnexal tenderness is characteristic, unilateral pain and abscess may occur when an IUD is in place.

Routine tests include Gram's stain and culture (Thayer-Martin) of the cervix, an erythrocyte sedimentation rate, CBC, and β-HCG. A pelvic ultrasound is useful in cases where adequate examination is not possible.

The differential diagnosis includes appendicitis, endometriosis, corpus luteum bleeding, ectopic pregnancy, rupture or torsion of ovarian cysts, and neoplasia of the genital tract.

The diagnosis of PID is frequently clinical, but laparoscopy may be necessary to make a definitive diagnosis. All atypical cases should undergo diagnostic laparoscopy, as the clinical diagnosis is incorrect in about 25%.

Indications for in-hospital treatment include nulliparity, abscess formation, pregnancy, uncertain diagnosis, peritonitis, an IUD in place, gastrointestinal symptoms, and an inadequate response to outpatient therapy.

Treatment *Outpatient.* Cefoxitin 2 g IM, or amoxicillin 3 g orally, procaine penicillin 4.8 million units IM, or Ceftriaxone 250 mg IM, followed by doxycycline 100 mg orally twice daily for 2 weeks or tetracycline 500 mg orally four times daily for 2 weeks.

Inpatient. Regimen A: doxycycline 100 mg IV twice daily plus cefoxitin 2 g IV six times daily. Regimen B (preferred for abscess, IUD-related): clindamycin 900 mg IV eight times daily, gentamicin 2 mg/kg IV load then 1.5 mg/kg eight times daily.

Operative. Required for abscess rupture or drainage, persistent mass, or failure to respond within 72 h to parenteral antibiotics. Procedures necessary range from simple incision and drainage of a loculated abscess laparoscopically or through the cul-de-sac to total abdominal hysterectomy and bilateral salpingo-oophorectomy in those cases not responsive to more conservative measures.

Sequelae of PID include an increased risk of ectopic

pregnancy, infertility, and chronic pelvic pain. Recurrent acute PID occurs in 25%.

OTHER INFECTIONS

Herpes Vulvitis

Usually herpes simplex type II. Presents with painful vesicles that ulcerate; may become secondarily infected. Diagnosis by culture, Tzanck prep, or clinically. Treatment for primary infection is acyclovir 200 mg orally five times daily for 10 days. Treatment of recurrences is symptomatic, nonsteroidal. Anti-inflammatory agents are helpful.

Syphilis

Due to *T. pallidum*. Symptoms of primary infection relate to chancre (usually painless); secondary infection has nonpruritic macular rash and condylomata lata. Diagnosis by darkfield examination, VDRL. Treatment is benzathine penicillin 1.2 million units times 2 or tetracycline 2 g orally four times daily for 2 weeks.

ENDOMETRIOSIS

Endometriosis is defined as heterotopic endometrial glands and stroma and is found in about 10% of reproductive-age women undergoing laparotomy. Although the typical patient is in her midthirties, nulliparous, and has symptoms of secondary dysmenorrhea, 5% of cases are diagnosed in postmenopausal women.

Etiology   Uncertain; theories include retrograde menstruation, metaplasia of the peritoneum, and vascular dissemination.

Symptoms   Cyclic pelvic pain (secondary dysmenorrhea) and infertility. About one-third of patients are asymptomatic, with diagnosis made incidentally at laparoscopy/laparotomy for an unrelated problem. Catamenial hemothorax is a rare manifestation.

Physical Findings   Include a fixed retroverted uterus with nodularity of the uterosacral ligaments and cul-de-sac. Adnexal enlargement secondary to endometrioma may occur.

Laboratory Tests None are specific for endometriosis. CA 125 levels may be elevated with endometriosis as well as other benign and malignant disorders of the female genital tract.

Diagnosis Requires diagnostic laparoscopy or laparotomy. An intravenous pyelogram, CT scan of the abdomen and pelvis, or barium enema may be appropriate based on the patient's symptoms and physical findings. The ovaries are most frequently involved (usually bilateral). Other frequent sites are the pelvic peritoneum, uterosacral ligaments and, rarely, the cervix and vagina. The rectosigmoid is involved in 15% of cases. Appearance of "powder burns," "chocolate cysts," and "raspberry spots" are characteristic, but biopsy is required for definitive diagnosis.

Treatment *Medical.* Danazol 400–800 mg/day orally for 6–9 months: Superior to treatment with oral contraceptives. Side effects are acne, edema, flushing, GI disturbance, and hirsutism. Oral contraceptives: Treat continuously. Side effects are alleviated in two-thirds. Side effects are weight gain, breast tenderness, nausea, and chloasma. Other hormones for treatment include medroxyprogesterone (Depo-Provera) and LH-RH agonists.

Surgical. Mandatory for diagnosis, ruptured endometrioma, ureteral obstruction, bowel obstruction, and with endometrioma >1 cm. Conservative surgery in childbearing-age patients performed by either laparoscopy or laparotomy includes excision of endometriomas, fulguration by laser or cautery of endometrial implants, and uterine suspension with or without presacral neurectomy. Definitive surgical treatment is total abdominal hysterectomy and bilateral salpingo-oophorectomy and appendectomy. Indications include advanced disease, failed medical therapy, failed conservative surgery, or completion of childbearing. GI involvement: Majority of cases involve rectosigmoid and are not of clinical significance. No specific radiologic appearance on BaE. Advanced cases causing obstructive symptoms require intestinal resection. Urinary tract involvement: ureteral obstruction occurs in 1%. Ureterolysis or ureteroneocystotomy may be required.

BENIGN DISORDERS OF THE CERVIX AND UTERUS

Cervix

MUCOPURULENT CERVICITIS Causes yellow vaginal discharge and is diagnosed by >10 PMNs/HPF on Gram's stain of cervix. Cervical culture should be performed, and shows *Chlamydia* in up to two-thirds. Treatment is guided by culture, but doxycycline 100 mg orally twice daily for 1 week is recommended.

CERVICAL POLYPS   Most common benign growths of the cervix. Smooth, soft, friable protrusion from the cervix that may cause intermenstrual bleeding. Usually easily removed by grasping with forcep and twisting off. Pathologic evaluation mandatory to exclude a malignancy.

NABOTHIAN CYSTS   Retention cysts of the endocervical glands. Size varies but most are less than 3 cm in size. Asymptomatic and so common they are considered normal variant. No treatment necessary.

Uterus

Leiomyomata (fibroids), the most frequent pelvic tumor, are composed of whorls of benign smooth muscle. Symptoms vary according to location (submucosal, intramural, pedunculated), but most common are pelvic pain and pressure, dysmenorrhea, and abnormal bleeding. Physical findings such as an enlarged, firm, and irregular uterus may be characteristic, but often pelvic ultrasound or laparoscopy may be necessary to confirm the diagnosis. Neoplasms of the uterus, ovary, or other pelvic structures must be excluded. Small asymptomatic fibroids are managed expectantly. Hysterectomy or myomectomy for those desiring to bear children are indicated for enlarging fibroids, persistent symptoms, or complications such as torsion, degeneration, or habitual abortion.

MALIGNANCY OF THE CERVIX AND UTERUS

Cervical Carcinoma

Etiology/Epidemiology   Formerly the most common tumor of the female genital tract, currently comprises 40% of female genital malignancies. Risk factors include early age at initiation of sexual intercourse and multiple sexual partners. Squamous cancers occur in 85%; the remainder are adenocarcinomas. HPV types 16 and 18 are frequently associated with squamous cancers, but an etiologic relationship has not been established.

TABLE 40-2. Staging of Cervical Carcinoma (FIGO)

Stage I	The carcinoma is confined to the cervix
Stage IA	Preclinical carcinoma, diagnosed only by microscopy
IA1	Minimal microscopically evident stromal invasion
IA2	Lesions detected microscopically that can be measured. The depth of invasion measured from the basement membrane, either surface or glandular, is less than 5 mm. A second dimension, the horizontal spread, must not exceed 7 mm. Larger lesions should be classified as stage IB
IB	Lesions of greater dimensions than stage IA2, whether seen clinically or not
Stage II	Extension beyond cervix but not to the pelvic wall and not the lower one-third of the vagina.
Stage IIA	No obvious parametrial involvement
IIB	Obvious parametrial involvement
Stage III	Extension to the pelvic wall. On rectal examination, there is no cancer-free space between the tumor and the pelvic wall. The tumor involves the lower one-third of the vagina. All cases with hydronephrosis or a nonfunctioning kidney (unless due to other causes)
Stage IIIA	No extension to pelvic wall
IIIB	Extension to pelvic wall
	Hydronephrosis or nonfunctioning kidney
Stage IV	Extension beyond true pelvis or mucosal involvement of the bladder or rectum
Stage IVA	Spread to adjacent organs
IVB	Spread to distant organs

Symptoms Classical symptoms are intermenstrual bleeding, postcoital bleeding, and abnormal vaginal discharge. May be discovered on routine examination. Late symptoms include pain, weight loss, sciatica.

Physical Findings Exophytic, endophytic, and ulcerative lesions on the cervix require biopsy, as a normal Pap smear does not exclude malignancy. Endophytic tumors may cause an expanded, "barrel-shaped" cervix that is firm but has no visible tumor.

Diagnosis Preclinical cases detected by cytology require colposcopic evaluation of the cervix with biopsy of suspicious areas. Conization of the cervix is required for unsatisfactory colposcopic examination. Cervical biopsy is all that is required for diagnosis in clinically apparent cases. Occasionally with an adenocarcinoma D&C may be helpful in distinguishing between cervical and endometrial adenocarcinoma.

Staging Based on clinical and radiologic evaluation (Table 40-2). Cystoscopy, proctoscopy, IVP, and CXR are useful in staging. A CT scan is frequently performed to detect nodal

TABLE 40-3.   Cervical Carcinoma, 5-Year Survival

Stage	Survival, %
IA1	100
IA2	95
IB	78
II	57
III	31
IV	8

enlargement, but surgical staging (paraaortic and pelvic node biopsy) is most accurate for assessing nodal spread in advanced cases.

Treatment   Cervical intraepithelial neoplasia I–III: Local ablative measures such as cryocautery, laser ablation, and conization of the cervix are highly effective.

Microinvasive carcinoma (Stages IA1 and IA2).   Stage IA1/ IA2: Further childbearing desired: Cases with <3 mm invasion may in selected instances be managed by conization of the cervix. Further childbearing not desired: Cases with <3 mm invasion are usually managed by hysterectomy. *Stage IA2 (3–5 mm invasion):* Treated by modified radical hysterectomy and pelvic/paraaortic node dissection. When surgery is undesirable, pelvic radiotherapy with external beam followed by an intracavitary implant is appropriate.

Stage IB/IIA.   Radical hysterectomy with pelvic and paraaortic lymphadenectomy or external pelvic radiotherapy (4500–5500 cGy) is followed by intracavitary radiotherapy.

Stages IIB–IVA.   Advanced cervical cancers are usually managed by radiotherapy with external beam and an intracavitary implant with 6000–8000 cGy to point A and 5000 cGy to point B. Extended field (paraaortic) radiotherapy is used for cases with documented paraaortic nodal spread. New treatment approaches utilizing neoadjuvant chemotherapy are being investigated.

Stage IVB.   Metastatic cervical carcinoma is treated palliatively. Chemotherapy or local radiotherapy may be helpful to control symptoms.

Treatment results   See Table 40-3.

Complications of Disease and Treatment   Radiation proctitis, cystitis, GI, and GU fistula.

TABLE 40-4.   Staging of Endometrial Carcinoma (FIGO)

Stage IA G1-3	Tumor limited to endometrium
IB G1-3	Invasion < ½ of myometrium
IC G1-3	Invasion > ½ of myometrium
IIA G1-3	Endocervical glandular involvement
IIB G1-3	Cervical stromal invasion
IIIA G1-3	Tumor invades serosa/adnexae/or positive peritoneal cytology
IIIB G1-3	Vaginal metastasis
IIIC G1-3	Pelvic or paraaortic lymph node metastases
IVA G1-3	Tumor invasion of bladder or bowel mucosa
IVB	Distant metastases including intraabdominal and/or inguinal lymph nodes

ENDOMETRIUM

Adenocarcinoma

Etiology/Epidemiology Most common malignancy of the female genital tract, affects 1 in 100 women. Age 50–65 most common, but 5% of cases occur in women <40. Risk factors include unopposed estrogen stimulation from exogenous (hormone replacement) or endogenous [polycystic ovaries (PCO), obesity, feminizing ovarian tumors] sources. Most are adenocarcinomas, although squamous elements (adeno-acanthoma, adenosquamous carcinoma) may be present.

Symptoms Postmenopausal bleeding is the hallmark symptom and occurs early in most cases. In younger patients menorrhagia or metrorrhagia may occur. Rarely a Pap smear showing atypical endometrial cells leads to the diagnosis in an asymptomatic patient.

Physical Findings Usually there are no abnormal findings. Uterine enlargement may occur but is nonspecific. In advanced cases the cervix, vagina, adnexa, or GI or GU tract may be involved by tumor.

Diagnosis Endometrial biopsy, D&C, or hysteroscopy are required to establish the diagnosis in most cases.

Staging See Table 40-4.

Treatment The mainstay of therapy is total abdominal hysterectomy with bilateral salpingo-oophorectomy with pelvic/paraaortic node sampling in all suitable patients. Occasional severe coexistent medical problems preclude surgery, in which case radiotherapy may be curative.

Treatment *Stage I/II.*   TAH and BSO with pelvic/paraaor-

TABLE 40-5.   Endometrial Carcinoma, 5-Year Survival*

Stage	Survival, %
I	75
II	58
III	30
IV	11

* FIGO staging prior to 1988 revision.

tic node sampling; adjuvant pelvic radiotherapy recommended when myometrial invasion $>\frac{1}{3}$ or with grade 3 tumor. Pelvic radiotherapy alone in cases unfit for surgery.

Stage III.   TAH and BSO with pelvic/paraaortic node sampling with adjuvant pelvic radiotherapy for adnexal or pelvic node or vaginal involvement. Extended field radiotherapy with paraaortic nodal spread. Therapy of positive peritoneal cytology is controversial; some advocate instillation into the abdomen of P32.

Stage IV.   TAH and BSO with pelvic/paraaortic node sampling and removal of intraabdominal tumor if resectable. Pelvic radiotherapy when disease confined to the pelvis. Whole abdominal radiotherapy may be useful for intraabdominal spread if no gross residual exists following surgery. For patients with distant metastases palliative treatment with progestational agents or chemotherapy with adriamycin is useful.

Treatment Results   See Table 40-5.

Complications of Disease and Treatment.   As obesity, old age, diabetes, and associated medical problems are commonplace, the most frequent complications include wound infection, postoperative MI, and pulmonary emboli. Antiembolic prophylaxis with pneumatic compression boots or heparin is used routinely.

BENIGN AND MALIGNANT DISORDERS OF THE VULVA

Benign

LICHEN SCLEROSIS   A form of vulvar dystrophy usually associated with chronic vulvar pruritus. The vulvar skin appears atrophic and whitish, and is frequently excoriated from itching. Biopsy by Keyes punch is required for diagnosis. Treatment with topical testosterone is effective.

SQUAMOUS CELL HYPERPLASIA (FORMERLY HYPERPLASTIC DYSTROPHY) Itching is the most prominent symptom. White hypertrophic areas are noted on the vulvar skin. Biopsy required for diagnosis and shows hyperkeratosis and acanthosis with atypia. Treatment with topical steroids (triamcinolone 0.1%) is effective.

Premalignant Disorders

VULVAR INTRAEPITHELIAL NEOPLASIA (VIN) Vulvar pruritus is the most common symptom. Lesions may be multifocal and appear as white, red, or pigmented areas on the vulva. Biopsy is required for diagnosis. Unifocal lesions may be treated by wide local excision. Large or multifocal VIN may be treated by skinning vulvectomy with skin graft or partial vulvectomy by laser ablation. Although the propensity for invasive cancer is low compared to cervical CIS, careful follow-up is mandatory.

PAGET DISEASE OF THE VULVA An uncommon cause of vulvar pruritus. Lesions appear as erythematous, eczematoid areas with scales and crusts. Biopsy is mandatory for diagnosis and shows an intraepithelial adenocarcinoma with characteristic Paget's cells. An underlying invasive adenocarcinoma must be excluded. Treatment consists of wide local excision, but recurrences are common, as the skin is frequently involved well beyond the area clinically apparent.

Vulvar Malignancy

Etiology/Epidemiology An infrequent malignancy, accounting for 5% of female genital malignancies; the majority are squamous. Affects predominantly postmenopausal women, with median age of 63. An association with condylomata acuminata (HPV infection), lymphogranuloma venereum, and prior vulvar dystrophy has been noted.

Symptoms Majority seek medical attention because of pruritus or the discovery of a mass. Other less frequent symptoms include bleeding, dysuria, and discharge.

Physical Findings Most carcinomas are located on the labia majora, less frequently the labia minora or clitoris. Exophytic, ulcerative, or infiltrating lesions may be noted. Spread to the inguinal/femoral lymph nodes may cause a firm mass in the inguinal region that may become fixed or ulcerated with extensive involvement.

TABLE 40-6.   Staging of Vulvar Cancer (FIGO)

Stage I	Tumor confined to vulva or perineum, less than 2 cm, no nodal metastasis
II	Tumor confined to vulva or perineum, more than 2 cm, no nodal metastasis
III	Tumor of any size with (1) Adjacent spread to lower urethra and/or vagina, or anus, or (2) Unilateral regional lymph node metastasis
IVA	Tumor invades any of the following: Upper urethra, bladder or rectal mucosa, pelvic bone, and/or bilateral regional lymph node metastasis
IVB	Any distant metastasis including pelvic lymph nodes

Diagnosis   The cornerstone of early diagnosis is vulvar biopsy for any abnormality noted on the vulva. Performed easily using a Keyes dermatologic punch or by excisional biopsy under local anesthesia. In early cases inspection of the vulva with a magnifying glass or colposcope following application of 3% acetic acid may be helpful. In most cases inspection of the vulva is all that is necessary for diagnosis.

Staging   The staging of vulvar carcinoma is shown in Table 40-6. Although the International Federation of Obstetricians and Gynecologists (FIGO) has not defined "microinvasive" carcinoma of the vulva, patients with tumors less than 1 mm thick have <1% chance of having lymph node metastases.

Treatment   Varies from wide local excision for very superficial cancers to radical vulvectomy and groin dissection with total pelvic exenteration for advanced cases. The treatment according to stage is shown below.

Stage I.   Tumor < 1 mm thick: wide local excision. tumor > 1 mm thick: modified radical vulvectomy with groin dissection (ipsilateral or bilateral if midline lesion or ipsilateral nodes have metastases).

Stage II.   Radical vulvectomy with groin dissection through separate incisions.

Stage III.   Radical vulvectomy with groin dissection.

Stage IV.   Preoperative radiation therapy followed by radical vulvectomy, or if necessary radical vulvectomy and pelvic exenteration.

Treatment Results   Patients with lymph node metastases have a poorer prognosis (50% 5-year survival) vs. those without lymph node metastases (85% 5-year survival). See Table 40-7.

TABLE 40-7. Vulvar Carcinoma, 5-Year Survival*

Stage	Survival, %
I	91
II	80
III	48
IV	15

* Prior to FIGO 1989 revision of staging system.

Complications of Disease and Treatment Complications include wound breakdown, groin lymphocyst, lymphedema, stress urinary incontinence, introital stenosis, dyspareunia, and anorgasmia. Operative mortality is about 2%.

BENIGN AND MALIGNANT DISORDERS OF THE OVARY

Benign

FUNCTIONAL CYSTS Include follicular and corpus luteum cysts. Women in the reproductive age range develop follicular cysts and a corpus luteum as part of the normal ovulatory cycle. If ovulation does not occur, a follicular cyst may persist, enlarge (usually less than 8 cm), and cause pain. Similar symptoms along with irregular bleeding may be caused by persistence of a corpus luteal cyst. Asymptomatic cysts that are less than 8 cm in diameter and that are unilocular on ultrasound may be observed. Persistence or acute symptoms require ovarian cystectomy by laparoscopy or laparotomy.

ENDOMETRIOMAS So-called chocolate cysts of the ovary are formed with extensive involvement of the ovary by endometriosis. Although some patients are asymptomatic, many have secondary dysmenorrhea, and a leaking endometrioma may cause peritoneal signs consistent with an acute abdomen. Although small (<1 cm), cyst may resolve with danazol treatment; larger endometriomas require excision.

CYSTIC TERATOMAS (DERMOID) Composed of tissue from all three germ layers, the ectoderm and skin structures frequently predominate, giving rise to the classic features of sebaceous material with hair. One of the most frequent neoplasms of the ovary, accounting for 33% of benign tumors of the ovary. Bilateral ovarian involvement occurs in 15%. Although frequently asymptomatic, torsion may cause an acute abdomen, and rupture or leakage has been associated with granulomatous peritonitis, which can be mistaken for carcinomatosis. Abdominal x-ray may show teeth or calcification, and ultrasound appearance may be characteristic. Treatment consists of ovarian cystectomy or oophorectomy. Malignant degeneration of a dermoid cyst occurs in 1% and is more common in postmenopausal patients.

FIBROMAS Notable due to association with Meig's syndrome, consisting of a pelvic mass, ascites, and hydrothorax, which resolves with excision of the fibroma but can be confused with an ovarian malignancy.

CYSTADENOMAS Serous tumors occur more frequently and are bilateral more often than mucinous tumors. Mucinous cystadenomas may be associated with a mucocele of the appendix and the syndrome of *Pseudomyxoma peritoneii*. Psammoma bodies (calcific concretions) may be seen in serous tumors and may be visible radiologically. Treatment consists of ovarian cystectomy or oophorectomy.

Malignant

EPITHELIAL CARCINOMA (SEROUS, MUCINOUS, ENDOMETRIOID, CLEAR CELL) Etiology/Epidemiology The fifth leading cause of death from cancer in women, ovarian malignancies have the highest mortality of gynecologic cancers, with only 35% of patients with this diagnosis surviving 5 years. Affects predominantly peri- and postmenopausal women, with higher risk in nulliparas. Oral contraceptives reduce the risk of developing ovarian carcinoma. Familial aggregation in some families suggest that heredity may play an etiologic role, as women with two or more first-degree relatives with ovarian cancer have a 50% risk of developing an ovarian malignancy.

Symptoms Abdominal pain and swelling are the most frequent. Pelvic discomfort and irregular vaginal bleeding may also occur. Vague GI complaints, bloating, heartburn, and anorexia frequently lead to evaluation of the GI tract. Unfortunately, symptoms usually become manifest only with an advanced stage of disease.

Physical Findings A pelvic mass is the most frequent finding, and irregularity and firmness suggest malignancy, as does nodularity in the cul-de-sac. Abdominal swelling and a fluid wave are noted when ascites is present. A pleural effusion is associated with dullness and decreased breath sounds at the lung bases.

Diagnosis Ultimately the diagnosis of ovarian carcinoma

TABLE 40-8. Staging of Ovarian Cancer (FIGO)

Stage I	Growth limited to ovaries
IA	Growth limited to one ovary; no tumor on surface, capsule intact, no ascites
IB	Growth limited to both ovaries: no tumor on surface, capsule intact, no ascites
IC	Tumor on surface of ovary, capsule ruptured, malignant ascites, or peritoneal washings
II	Growth involving one or both ovaries with pelvic extension
IIA	Involvement of uterus or tubes
IIB	Involvement of other pelvic structures
IIC	Tumor on surface of ovary, capsule ruptured, malignant ascites, or peritoneal washings
III	Peritoneal implants outside the pelvis and/or positive retroperitoneal or inguinal nodes. Superficial liver metastasis equals stage III, as does histologically proven involvement of small bowel or omentum
IIIA	Tumor grossly limited to true pelvis with negative nodes but microscopic seeding of upper abdomen
IIIB	Negative nodes but implants in upper abdomen < 2 cm in diameter
IIIC	Positive nodes or implants > 2 cm in upper abdomen
IV	Distant metastases, parenchymal liver involvement, malignant pleural effusion

requires exploratory laparotomy and biopsy. The workup of a patient suspected of having an ovarian malignancy usually includes BaE, CT scan of the abdomen and pelvis, chest x-ray, and, if symptoms warrant, a UGI with small bowel follow-through.

Staging Based on surgical findings. The current FIGO staging system is shown in Table 40-8.

Treatment Surgical extirpation of all visible tumor is the foundation of treatment for all ovarian malignancies. In advanced cases adjunctive chemotherapy with a regimen containing *cis*-platinum is standard. In young patients conservation of fertility is possible with early stage tumors. The surgical treatment of ovarian cancer according to stage is shown below.

Stage IA, IB, Grade 1 or 2. Removal of the tumor by unilateral or bilateral oophorectomy with or without hysterectomy, according to the patient's desires regarding future fertility. Biopsy of the opposite ovary should be performed in those cases in which fertility is being preserved. If fertility is not an issue, TAH and BSO with omental and nodal biopsies is standard treatment.

TABLE 40-9. Ovarian Carcinoma, 5-Year Survival

Stage	Survival, %
I	73
II	46
III	17
IIIA	31
IIIB	32
IIIC	14
IV	5

Stage IC. TAH and BSO with omental biopsy and nodal sampling is followed by adjunctive chemotherapy.

Stages II–IV. TAH and BSO, omentectomy, nodal sampling, and removal of all gross tumor (cytoreductive surgery) followed by adjunctive chemotherapy.

Treatment Results Survival correlates with stage, grade of tumor, and residual tumor following surgery. Survival figures are shown in Table 40-9.

Complications of Disease and Treatment Cachexia, GU and GI obstruction, respiratory compromise, hypercalcemia, and paraneoplastic syndromes. Chemotherapeutic agent side effects include the following: *cis*-platinum: renal compromise, peripheral neuropathy, ototoxicity, hypomagnesemia, myelosuppression, nausea, and vomiting. Cytoxan: myelosuppression, hemorrhagic cystitis, alopecia. Adriamycin: cardiotoxicity (dose-related), alopecia, myelosuppression, extravasational injury.

41 NEUROLOGIC SURGERY

GENERAL CONSIDERATIONS

Loss of consciousness as a presenting symptom requires not only consideration of central nervous system (CNS) pathology but also evaluations of cardiac output, vascular competence, metabolic or toxic aberrations, alterations in body temperature, and the myriad causes of each. Small lesions in the reticular core, or the *reticular activating system,* can also cause loss of consciousness, and sudden isolation of the spinal cord from descending influences of the reticular core by cervical-medullary transection produces a reflexic paralysis or *spinal shock* followed by mass withdrawal reflexes when spinal shock ceases. Isolation of the reticular core from descending hemispheric influences by midbrain section produces a facilitation of antigravity musculature known as *decerebrate posturing.* Lesions above the midbrain produce *decorticate posturing,* with flexion of upper extremities and extension of lower extremities.

Surgical diseases of the CNS are frequently manifestations of *space-occupying lesions* (i.e., tumor, hemorrhage, abscess, edema, spinal fluid, or foreign body), and the fact that the intracranial space and spinal canal are confined spaces determines a set of mechanical conditions through which mass lesions affect nervous system functions. CNS tissue is deformable but not compressible, and rapid deformation by masses causes (1) flow toward sites of decompression including the falx (*subfalcine herniation*), the incisura of the tentorium (*transtentorial* or *uncal herniation*) and the foramen magnum (*tonsillar herniation*) and (2) compression, obstruction, and rupture of small blood vessels causing tissue ischemia and infarction, which produces further mass by edema. The *incisural syndrome* of altered consciousness followed by oculomotor (III) nerve paralysis, decerebrate rigidity, and death reflects the cycle in supratentorial mass lesions. With *tonsillar herniation,* altered consciousness followed by depression of respiration and reflexes, cessation of respiration, and death represent progression of the cycle. The early recognition of these patterns and the initiation of appropriate treatment is a sine qua non of neurologic surgery.

Diagnostic Studies Advances in neuroimaging, including computed tomography (CT), magnetic resonance imaging (MRI), digital angiography, and ultrasound have revolutionized our diagnostic abilities and preoperative preparation. Other new modalities, including single photon emission tomography (SPECT) and positron emission tomography (PET), are yielding benefits of diagnostic and therapeutic relevance. With these advances, myelography and electro-encephalography (EEG) subserve diminished functions.

Computed Tomography (CT). Widely employed in the workup of intracranial mass lesions, hydrocephalus, acute traumatic injuries, and acute hemorrhage, and in situations where the requirement for accurate bone detail cannot be compromised. ''Infusion CT'' in which intravenous contrast is infused during the scan, is occasionally employed in the acute preoperative setting of a ruptured vascular malforma-tion or aneurysm. CT with and without the subarachnoid infusion of contrast has proved valuable in the evaluation of nerve root or cord compression in spine or intervertebral disc disease; as a tool to localize posttraumatic CSF fistulae; and as a means of evaluation of intracranial CSF cisterns.

Magnetic Resonance Imaging (MRI). Combines startling anatomic precision with resolution equivalent to CT, and with the exception of acute trauma in which bone imaging is important, and hemorrhage in which acute blood must be accurately visualized, MRI is the diagnostic procedure of choice for the majority of intracranial processes. With the addition of gadolinium DTPA as an intravenous contrast agent, all intracranial tumors are well visualized. MRI is also invaluable in the evaluation of diseases of the spinal region including Chiari malformations, spinal cord tumors, syrin-gomyelia, and intervertebral disc abnormalities.

Myelography. Involves the introduction of contrast into the spinal subarachnoid space and outlines radiographically the spinal cord, nerve roots, and soft tissue of the spinal canal. This study is helpful especially in conjunction with CT in the evaluation of ruptured intervertebral discs in the cervical and lumbar regions.

Cerebral Angiography. The principal method of demon-strating vascular lesions such as arteriovenous malformations (AVMs), aneurysms, and vascular occlusive (i.e., carotid) disease, as well as normal and abnormal vessels associated with brain tumors. Angiography is performed by a transfem-oral artery puncture; with fluoroscopic positioning of a catheter into the carotid, vertebral, and intracranial arteries; and by serial x-rays of the injection of contrast material. *Digital enhanced angiography* uses computer techniques to decrease the amount of contrast material required. Thera-peutic angiographic techniques include microballoon dilatation of vasospastic intracranial arteries, occlusion of carotid-cavernous fistulae, and small-particle embolization of AVMs and vascular brain tumors either as definitive treatment or as a preamble to surgical resection.

Ultrasonography. In infants with an open fontanel or patients with a skull defect, ultrasonography can yield information regarding ventricular size and position, and the presence of hemorrhage, tumor, or foreign bodies. Ultrasound is also used intraoperatively to localize masses for biopsy or excision, to identify the lateral ventricles for catheter placement, to outline a syringomyelia cavity, or to check for retained disc fragments during discectomy.

HEAD INJURY

In the immediate care of patients with head injury, primary consideration must be given to respiratory exchange, control of hemorrhage, and maintenance of peripheral vascular circulation. During the initial period of treatment, as vital functions are stabilized, a preliminary evaluation of nervous system is essential, followed by careful repetitive neurologic examinations to detect improvement or deterioration in function. Management decisions are then made based upon the information obtained from these examinations and other diagnostic studies.

Scalp Lacerations. These are treated by the attainment of hemostasis, and by transforming a contaminated open wound into a closed clean wound. Hemostasis is obtained by compression of the scalp against the intact skull, or when the skull is not intact, by traction on the galea with a clamp that grasps the galea and pulls it back over the dermis. Care of a scalp wound includes shaving hair in the immediate vicinity, debriding devitalized tissue, and removal of foreign bodies. Closure of the galea is essential, either as a separate layer or as a layer included with the dermis. If a major portion of the galea is separated from the subgaleal tissue, a compression dressing will reduce the likelihood of formation of a subgaleal hematoma or infection.

Subgaleal Hematomas. These can attain considerable size, and may constitute a significant percentage of the circulating blood volume in infants. Early treatment involves pressure and a firm dressing. If the overlying skin is intact, natural absorption is permitted to occur, but if the circulation of the scalp appears compromised, or if there is a question of infection, total evacuation of the hematoma with obliteration of dead space via a compression dressing is indicated.

Scalp Infections. These may spread into the epidural or subdural space through emissary veins causing epidural and subdural abscess, cerebral thrombophlebitis, cerebritis, or brain abscess, requiring treatment with antibiotics and/or surgical evacuation.

Skull Fractures. These are described on the basis of pattern (*linear, stellate, comminuted*), inward displacement (*depressed*), as *basilar* when fractures traverse the skull base, and as *compound* when associated with a break in the scalp or mucous membrane. Many simple fractures may be handled conservatively, with observation. Compound fractures should be cleansed and debrided, and the wound closed. Replacement of large skull fragments depends upon the degree of contamination, intactness of the dura, and the area of the skull involved. Depressed fractures are elevated if they are depressed more than 1 cm, are located over the motor strip, or if they appear sharp on x-ray, since they may tear the dura and damage the brain. Compound depressed fractures require elevation to be certain that neither the subarachnoid space nor the brain have been contaminated. Fractures that traverse paranasal sinuses, mastoid air cells, or the middle ear are often heralded by the presence of CSF drainage from the nose or ear. Patients with posttraumatic CSF fistulae should be closely observed for signs of intracranial infection, with head elevation until drainage ceases; and if otorrhea or rhinorrhea continues for more than 10–14 days, surgical repair of the offending dural tear is indicated.

Mechanisms of Brain Injury. These involve direct disruption by a penetrating object, focal tissue injury from rapid deceleration or rotation of the brain vis à vis the rigid skull, or "diffuse axonal injury" caused by rotational/shear stresses. The brain responds to traumatic injury by alterations in fluid content, dysautoregulation of blood flow, hemorrhage, and massive swelling. Diffuse elevation of intracranial pressure (ICP) and alterations in vasomotor tone may further compromise the brain's blood supply.

HISTORY Taking into account the setting of head injury, history must include detailed information about the mechanism of injury. Information concerning the level of neurologic and autonomic function and vital signs at the scene of the accident and during transport may suggest additional complicating factors of hypoxia or ischemia.

TABLE 41-1.   Levels of Consciousness

Responds to spoken word, is alert, cooperative, and oriented

Responds to spoken word, is confused, and obeys simple commands

Responds to spoken word only after receiving painful stimuli of supraorbital pressure; obeys commands only while receiving painful stimuli

Does not respond to auditory stimuli before or while receiving painful stimuli but has purposeful, effective motor response to painful supraorbital and sternal pressure

Responds to painful supraorbital and sternal pressure with purposeful but noneffective motor movements

Responds to painful supraorbital and sternal pressure with nonpurposeful movement

Responds to painful stimuli only with alteration in pulse and respiratory rate or with decerebrate posturing

No response to painful stimuli, but cough and gag reflexes are present

No response to stimuli

Lowest level is unconsciousness; the only step below this is death

Care of the Head-Injured Patient

Resuscitation.   This involves immediate attention to adequate respiratory exchange, control of hemorrhage, and cardiovascular stabilization, and the neurologic status may improve remarkably when hypoxia and ischemia are reversed. Endotracheal intubation may be indicated, even in the adequately exchanging patient, to prevent delayed airway compromise and to facilitate transportation to another facility. Attention must also be directed toward the possibility of spinal injury or occult bleeding in the chest or abdomen, which if unrecognized in an unresponsive patient can result in drastic consequences.

Evaluation   Evaluation of neurologic function following initial resuscitation must include serial assessments of the level of consciousness, via a description of the patient's responses to various stimuli (Table 41-1) or more quantitatively using the Glasgow coma scale (Table 41-2). In the unconscious patient the examiner must rely upon serial evaluations of brainstem reflexes to determine what level of the brain is compromised (Table 41-3). These serial evaluations can alert the surgeon to subtle changes in status that may be the early signs of impending problems warranting further investigation.

Diagnostic Studies   These may not be required in stable, conscious patients without severe head trauma who may be observed for 6 h with serial neurologic examinations. Any patient, however, who has had a significant alteration in the level of consciousness following head trauma should receive

TABLE 41-2.   Glasgow Coma Scale

Best motor response	Obeys	M6
	Localizes	5
	Withdraws	4
	Abnormal flexion	3
	Extensor response	2
	Nil	1
Verbal response	Oriented	V5
	Confused conversation	4
	Inappropriate words	3
	Incomprehensible sounds	2
	Nil	1
Eye opening	Spontaneous	E4
	To speech	3
	To pain	2
	Nil	1

NOTE: The coma scale score is the sum of the sectional scores. See *Principles of Surgery*, 5th ed., for details.

a CT scan of the brain, for the detection of parenchymal injury, hemorrhage, or skull fracture.

Treatment   This should include adequate oxygenation and brain circulation, removal of mass effect, control of ICP, prevention of infection, and rehabilitation. Frequent monitoring of vital signs, arterial blood gases, and fluid intake and output is a routine necessity. As a rule, any focal mass from hemorrhage, devitalized brain, or swelling that alters the patient's level of consciousness should be removed. ICP can be monitored using an intraventricular catheter, through which spinal fluid may be removed when ICP is elevated; or with subdural monitors and tissue pressure devices. These monitors alert the surgeon to changes in ICP and lead to expeditious medical or surgical interventions. Nonsurgical methods of lowering ICP include hyperventilation (P_{CO_2} 25–30 torr), osmotic diuresis to reduce cerebral edema, judicious fluid restriction, and avoidance of hyponatremia. If these methods prove inadequate, *barbiturate coma* and *neuromuscular blockade*, which obviate the neurologic exam, may be employed as a last resort. Attention must also be paid to pulmonary hygiene, venous stasis, and skin care, in an effort to prevent pneumonia, pulmonary embolism, and skin breakdown.

Traumatic Intracranial Hemorrhage

Subarachnoid hemorrhage following head injury has little acute significance but may contribute to the development of communicating hydrocephalus weeks or months after injury.

TABLE 41-3. Brainstem Reflexes

Pupil reaction to light	Midbrain
Decorticate posture	Midbrain
Corneal reflex	Pons
Oculocephalic reflex	Pons
Decerebrate posture	Pons
Caloric stimulation	Pons
Spontaneous respiration	Medulla
Cardiovascular function	Medulla

SUBDURAL HEMATOMA (SDH) In the setting of head trauma, SDH usually is caused by rupture of veins traversing the subdural space from the brain to the dural sinuses. *Acute SDH* causes significant, rapidly progressive neurologic deficits, since it may have both arterial and venous bleeding. It is often accompanied by significant primary brain injuries, which are compounded by the mass effect represented by the enlarging hematoma and swelling of the injured brain, threatening brainstem compression and death within hours. CT is diagnostic and defines contiguous intracerebral hematomas, facilitating surgical removal via a large craniotomy. Without prompt surgical care, mortality approaches 100%, and even with the best care it remains quite high. *Subacute SDH* causes significant neurologic deficits more than 48 h but less than 2 weeks following injury, usually as the result of venous bleeding into the subdural space. CT or MRI is diagnostic, and treatment usually involves surgical removal via craniotomy, craniectomy, or burr holes. *Chronic SDH* occurs most frequently in the infant and the elderly, and is often unaccompanied by any history of trauma. Typically, a progressive alteration in mentation and level of consciousness occurs over 4–6 weeks, out of proportion to the focal neurologic deficit, which may or may not be present. CT or MRI is diagnostic. These thin, liquefied hematomas may be drained at the bedside or in the operating room through simple twist drill or perforator openings followed by closed-system drainage, with rapid recovery of neurologic function; and removal of accompanying membranes is unnecessary.

Subdural Hygroma This is caused by a tear in the piarachnoid with leakage of CSF into the subdural space. These can rapidly increase in size, mimicking an acute or subacute SDH. Following a diagnostic CT scan, treatment involves burr holes with external drainage or artificial subarachnoid/subdural fistula formation.

EPIDURAL HEMATOMA (EDH) EDH from arterial bleeding most commonly occurs following rupture of the middle meningeal artery, caused by a fracture of the temporal squama overlying the artery or at the foramen spinosum, where the artery enters the skull. The typical history is that of a young adult who receives a minor blow to the head causing a momentary alteration in consciousness, followed by a lucid interval extending from a few minutes to a few hours, terminated by a rapidly progressive loss of consciousness, with dilatation of the ipsilateral pupil, evidence of upper midbrain compression (hemiparesis or decerebrate posturing), and ultimately global brainstem compromise and death. Treatment is lifesaving, and consists of early recognition, emergent temporal craniectomy, evacuation of the hemorrhage, and control of the bleeding artery.

INTRACEREBRAL HEMATOMA   This occurs at points of brain/skull impact, especially in the anterior temporal lobe and less frequently in the tips of the frontal or occipital lobes. Some patients are relatively asymptomatic and the hematomas may resolve spontaneously. Surgically significant hematomas present with a progressive decrease in consciousness and/or focal neurological deficit (hemiparesis, III nerve palsy) secondary to increasing mass effect, which may develop within a few hours or days following the injury. Following CT localization, treatment involves craniotomy, cortical incision, and evacuation of clot and devitalized brain.

Posttraumatic Epilepsy   This develops in 30–45% of patients with cortical lacerations, in 5% with simple closed-head injury, and only rarely following less than 4 h of altered consciousness or focal neurologic deficit. EEG may be diagnostic, but occasionally trials of anticonvulsants are required to rule out seizures.

SPINAL CORD INJURIES

Mechanism of Injury   This usually involves cord compression, commonly following fracture/dislocation in the cervical region (50–60%) or thoracolumbar junction (20–30%). Cord injuries are caused by motor vehicle accidents, diving into shallow water, and accidental falls, with a M:F ratio of 3:1 and a mean age between 15 and 30. Fifty percent experience immediate and total loss of function below the level of the injury at initial exam, with the remainder demonstrating some sensory/motor preservation. Penetrating injuries include gunshot wounds, stabbings, and foreign bodies from explosions. The concussive energy delivered by a bullet usually abrogates significant functional recovery, and patient management is directed toward surgical debridement of the spinal cord, closure of CSF leaks, and stabilization of an unstable spine.

Spinal Cord Injury Syndromes. These include *transverse injury,* which, if complete, is followed by a loss of reflex activity, autonomic function, and motor/sensory activity (spinal shock), with a return of deep tendon reflexes and some autonomic tone within days to weeks. *Central cord syndrome,* following contusion and compression of the cord, begins as a central gray matter hemorrhage that spreads centrifugally with preservation of peripheral white matter. Sacral fibers of the lateral corticospinal and spinothalamic tracts are less affected, resulting in "sacral sparing," with retained motor power and pain and temperature sensation in the legs and sacral area with plegia and anesthesia in the arms and thorax. *Brown-Séquard syndrome* is observed following compressive or penetrating injury to the lateral half of the spinal cord, producing ipsilateral plegia and loss of vibration and position sense with contralateral loss of pain and temperature sensation. *Anterior spinal artery syndrome* affects the anterior two-thirds of the spinal cord including all the gray matter except for the dorsal horns, and most of the lateral and anterior funiculi. Symptoms include motor plegia and loss of pain and temperature sensation, with preservation of vibration and position sensation subserved by the dorsal columns.

Patient Management This always involves immobilization on a firm surface with neck stabilization in a cervical collar and/or sand bags, and attention to respiratory and autonomic function, which may be compromised. A detailed initial neurologic examination will localize the area of injury, following which the appropriate radiographic studies of the spine may be obtained.

Radiologic Examination. This consists of initial AP and lateral views of the area of injury, supplemented with additional plain films (obliques, flexion/extension, etc.), and CT with or without intrathecal contrast to assess instability, fracture and dislocation, cord compression, and the presence of extradural masses. MRI provides parenchymal and soft tissue detail in cord injury, and sagittal images of extradural soft tissue masses (i.e., disc, hematoma) impinging upon the cord.

Treatment In the acute phase, treatment includes stabilization of unstable bony injuries and decompression of the cord. Reduction of cervical dislocations involves progressive axial traction using a halo or skull tongs, under x-ray control to a maximum of 50 pounds, followed by surgical realignment if this is unsuccessful. Thoracic or lumbar injuries cannot be reduced with skull traction and are treated by immobilization on a firm surface. While early surgical decompression of the cord is generally advocated, emergent decompression does not appear to improve neurologic recovery in patients with complete transverse deficits; even in patients with residual function, it may not improve recovery. Emergent decompression is usually indicated in patients with progression of deficits. When appropriate, stabilization via external bracing or casting or internal (surgical) fixation or fusion will facilitate patient care. Loss of bowel and bladder control, skin ulceration, thrombophlebitis, peptic ulceration, and respiratory and cardiovascular instability also require constant attention.

Prognosis   For neurologic recovery, prognosis is poor in patients with complete deficits and improves when residual sensory/motor function is detected at the time of the initial exam. In these patients progressive deterioration noted on serial neurologic examinations mandates careful reevaluation and expeditious intervention to prevent loss of retained function.

PERIPHERAL NERVE INJURIES

Acute peripheral nerve injuries from penetrating wounds or from compressive, stretch, electrical, or chemical insults encompass three pathophysiologic processes: (1) *neuronopraxis* following compression injury, in which axons cannot reestablish membrane potentials, characterized by an incomplete sensory/motor deficit and spontaneous recovery in days to weeks; (2) *axonotmesis,* in which axonal loss occurs with preservation of myelin sheaths, a complete sensory/motor deficit, and a proximal to distal recovery (1–2 mm/day) concomitant with axonal regrowth; (3) *neurotmesis* following the partial or complete severing of a nerve requiring surgical repair in which nerve regeneration occurs at a rate of 1 inch per month.

Treatment   This includes (1) careful serial exams, and monitoring of return of sensory/motor function, (2) suture repair of the nerve, or (3) resection and reconstruction of damaged segments with or without interposition grafts. Little is lost by a delay of 3–6 weeks if a nerve is thought to be in continuity following injury.

Focal Laceration.   This requires immediate repair except when: (1) the nerve is contused for more than a few millimeters on either side of the injury; (2) blood loss from arterial injury jeopardizes the life of the patient; and (3) the wound is older than 5–6 h, and dissection might spread bacterial contamination. Significant motor return cannot be expected in any muscle more than 15 inches from a nerve suture.

Focal Contusion.   Following gunshot wounds, focal contusion is often extensive and mitigates against immediate repair. These wounds are initially treated to prevent infection with exploration 4–5 weeks later, if no function has returned, and resection and resuturing undertaken as indicated.

Stretch.   These injuries are common in the brachial plexus following a shoulder injury, and are usually treated conservatively by careful recording of motor/sensory loss in serial exams, with radiographic evaluation if the pattern of loss suggests a radicular avulsion. Since root avulsions are not surgically reparable, no immediate exploration is indicated. Ultimately orthopaedic reconstruction and rehabilitation may be appropriate.

BRAIN TUMORS

Classification   This is done on the basis of cells of origin; includes *glial* (astrocytoma, oligodendroglioma, ependymoma, microglioma, and choroid plexus papilloma), *neuronal* (ganglioglioma), *leptomeningeal* (meningioma), *vascular* (hemangioblastoma, AVM), or *metastatic* (lung, breast, renal, melanoma). Histologic characteristics predict patient survival; therefore glial tumors are classified from grade I to grade IV, with grade IV the most malignant; or alternatively in three categories, (1) low-grade (astrocytoma), (2) intermediate-grade (anaplastic astrocytoma), and (3) high-grade (glioblastoma). Seventy percent of adult brain tumors are supratentorial, and 75% of childhood tumors occur in the posterior fossa. The most common adult primary tumor is malignant astrocytoma, followed by meningioma, pituitary tumor, and neurilemmoma. In childhood the most common primary tumor is the astrocystoma of the posterior fossa, followed by medulloblastoma, ependymoma, and craniopharyngioma.

Clinical Manifestations   These range from progressive focal deficits to a more generalized neurologic dysfunction secondary to elevated ICP, by one or more of the following mechanisms:

1. Compression of neural tissue
2. Infiltration/invasion/destruction of neural tissue

3. Alteration in blood supply to neurons
4. Alteration in neuronal excitability (seizures)
5. Increased intracranial mass (tumor, edema, cyst, blood)
6. Alteration in CSF circulation (hydrocephalus)

Compression, invasion, and altered blood supply compromise cerebral cortical functions causing both focal deficits and seizures, which are presenting signs of brain tumor. Elevated ICP from increased mass or hydrocephalus may engender cloudy mentation and consciousness, headache, papilledema, vomiting, bradycardia, and systolic hypertension. A patient's family may notice altered personality, behavior, or recent memory, or inattention to details. As intracranial compensatory mechanisms are exhausted by the expansion of the mass, these patients may experience a precipitous clinical demise at the time of presentation.

Evaluation   Evaluation of these patients requires the recognition of a history of progressive and often subtle neurologic deficits or behavioral/cognitive symptoms. A thorough examination followed by CT or MRI with and without intravenous contrast usually provides diagnostic information, with arteriography as an aid in making surgical decisions.

Treatment   This does not always involve surgical removal, since resulting neurologic deficits may leave a patient seriously impaired. Histologically benign tumors (i.e., meningiomas or schwannomas) are curable if totally removed; however, proximity to vital brain structures may preclude total removal. Solitary metastases are removed if located in an accessible area of the brain and if the patient's systemic cancer is under control or treatable. Primary malignant brain tumors are not usually curable, but significant palliation may be obtained with a combination of surgery, irradiation, and chemotherapy. The spread of malignant cells in the CSF (meningeal carcinomatosis) commonly occurs in aggressive cancers and may cause hydrocephalus, cranial nerve palsies, and elevated ICP, and is treated with intrathecal chemotherapy.

Pituitary Tumors

The pituitary gland within the sella turcica is surrounded by structures that may be compressed by enlarging tumors, including the optic chiasm and cavernous sinuses, which contain the carotid arteries, and the III, IV, V_1, and VI cranial nerves. Pituitary tumors are generally benign adenomas of anterior lobe origin, and cause symptoms by hormone overproduction, mass effect, or compromised anterior pituitary functions. Tumors less than 1 cm are referred to as *microadenomas*, while those greater than 1 cm are *macroadenomas*, and may exhibit suprasellar or parasellar extension.

Diagnosis Involves identification of neurologic deficits from compression of contiguous structures, which include bitemporal hemianopsia (optic nerve), extraocular motor loss (cavernous sinus), hypothalamic dysfunction (suprasellar extension), or frontal or medial temporal lobe signs (parasellar extension). Endocrine symptoms resulting from pituitary tumors, in order of frequency include: (1) *hyperprolactinemia*, causing amenorrhea and galactorrhea in females; (2) *hypopituitarism*, caused by endocrine-inactive tumors, which present with infertility or impotence, fatigue, temperature intolerance, diminished hair growth, pallor, and headache; (3) *acromegaly/gigantism*, with enlargement of distal parts and altered glucose and fat metabolism in adults, excessive body growth in children, and elevations of serum growth hormone and somatomedin C; (4) *Cushing disease*, caused by hypersecretion of ACTH, hypercortisolism with myriad clinical manifestations, and diagnosed with low-dose/high-dose dexamethasone suppression tests, MRI, and occasionally surgical exploration.

Treatment Treatment of prolactin-secreting tumors with bromocryptine effectively reduces tumor volume and serum prolactin; transnasal transsphenoidal microsurgical excision may also normalize serum prolactin in many patients. Medical therapy for non-prolactin-secreting tumors is less effective, and transsphenoidal excision and adjunctive radiation therapy remain the standard of care. Emergent surgical intervention is often required following hemorrhagic infarction of the pituitary, or *pituitary apoplexy*, especially in large adenomas, which may present with subarachnoid hemorrhage, acute headache, oculomotor paresis, visual loss, and decreased consciousness that can lead to death.

SPINAL CORD TUMORS

Classification This is done according to the compartment in which they appear: (1) *intramedullary* (ependymoma, astrocytoma, hemangioblastoma, epidermoid/dermoid); (2) *intradural, extramedullary* (neurofibroma, schwanomma, meningioma, metastasis of brain tumor, ependymoma, lipoma); and (3) *extradural* (metastasis, myeloma, lymphoma, cordoma, sarcoma, neuroblastoma). Ninety percent of extradural tumors are malignant, while 60% of intradural tumors are benign. Seventy five percent of extradural tumors are metastatic (lung, breast, lymphoid, prostatic, kidney, thyroid), while 98% of intradural tumors are primary tumors. Metastatic and primary spinal tumors occur with equivalent frequency.

Clinical Manifestations Manifestations of extradural tumors reflect rapid compression of the cord either by tumor or by collapsed vertebrae, with progressive paraparesis and sensory loss, while intradural tumors present with slowly evolving spastic paraparesis and partial sensory loss. The clinician should always consider this diagnosis when any bilateral progressive neurologic loss occurs below any transverse level of the body. The neurologic exam reveals local *motor signs* (weakness, hyporeflexia) and *sensory signs* (local or radicular pain, spinal tenderness, dermatomal sensory loss) that localize the lesion along the rostral = caudal axis, as well as *tract signs* (loss of pain and temperature, loss of position and vibratory sensation, paraparesis, hyperreflexia, Babinski sign).

Diagnostic Studies Include MRI as well as postcontrast CT. Since extradural metastatic tumors frequently involve the adjacent vertebrae, close attention should be paid to the integrity of the vertebral bodies and pedicles, and the potential for instability of involved spinal segments.

Therapy For malignant extradural tumors that usually compress the anterior or lateral aspects of the cord, treatment involves removal via an anterior or posterolateral approach followed by radiotherapy. Occasionally vertebrectomy and insertion of strut grafts of autogenous bone or acrylic may be required. Intradural-extramedullary tumors (neurofibroma, meningiomas) are approached posteriorly with total excision when possible, occasionally followed by radiation therapy. Intramedullary tumors, (ependymomas, astrocytomas) present in the central region of the spinal cord, and posterior microsurgical approaches in conjunction with radiotherapy have increased the frequency with which these tumors can be completely removed and prolonged palliation or cure provided.

VASCULAR DISEASE

A cerebral blood flow (CBF) of 55 mL/100 g min is required to maintain CNS metabolism (20% of the body's oxygen supply), and when CBF falls below 20 mL/100 g per min, cerebral ischemia and neurologic dysfunction occur. Adequate CBF (750 mL/min) is normally provided by the paired internal carotid (80%) and vertebral (20%) arteries, which supply "anterior" and "posterior" cerebral circulations, respectively, by anastomoses within the circle of Willis, and by intrinsic cerebral autoregulatory mechanisms.

Cerebral Ischemia and Infarction

This may result from (1) cardiac disorders, (2) atherosclerotic stenosis of major vessels, (3) thromboembolic events, or (4) thrombosis of large or small vessels. Thromboembolic events of vascular or cardiac origin are manifest by abrupt ischemia and alterations in neurologic function, including (1) *transient ischemic attack (TIA),* with recovery in 24 h; (2) *reversible ischemic neurologic deficit (RIND),* with recovery in 1–7 days; and (3) *infarction,* with a fixed neurologic deficit. TIAs are characterized by symptoms typical of carotid (monocular blindness, hemiparesis, dysphasia, hemisensory loss) or vertebrobasilar (homonymous field defect, diplopia, dysarthria, quadraparesis, drop attacks) circulations, and portend infarction within 5 years in 33% of affected patients. Workup includes history, neurologic and cardiac evaluation, auscultation for bruits, carotid Doppler studies, oculoplethysmography, and angiography. High-grade stenoses and ulcerated plaques in symptomatic patients receive endarterectomy, while other patients are managed medically with aspirin or anticoagulants. Superficial temporal to middle cerebral artery bypass and emergency revascularation procedures have more limited applications.

Hypertensive Hemorrhage

This is most common in the basal ganglia, pons and cerebellar hemispheres, with initial symptoms of headache, dizziness, paresthesia, or mild speech disturbance followed by a rapidly progressive neurologic demise and death as the hematoma enlarges. Surgical removal is reserved for patients with (1) larger, accessible supratentorial lesions and retained neurologic function; (2) progression of deficits; and (3) cerebellar hemorrhage or infarction with mass effect, where surgery can be lifesaving. Small lesions in asymptomatic patients, inaccessible hematomas and large hematomas in patients without retained neurologic function are managed medically.

Aneurysmal Hemorrhage

Aneurysmal hemorrhage presents with the explosive onset of severe headache and may progress rapidly to neurologic compromise, with death occurring in 30% of patients prior to receiving medical attention. Morbidity and mortality are associated with (1) the severity of initial hemorrhage; (2) rehemorrhage within hours or days; and (3) vasospasm of intracranial vessels with neurologic decline, ischemia, or infarction 5–20 days posthemorrhage. Outcome of medical and surgical therapy is directly related to neurologic status at presentation (grades I–V), with higher-grade patients (I–III) experiencing the best outcome. Diagnostic workup involves history, neurologic exam, lumbar puncture to detect subarachnoid hemorrhage, CT, and four-vessel angiography for precise localization of the offending aneurysm. Therapy is directed at early surgical repair in higher-grade patients, which eliminates rebleeding, and postoperative volume expansion therapy, and calcium channel blockage (nimodipine) to minimize vasospasm, ischemia, and infarction.

Arteriovenous Malformations (AVMs)

AVMs involve congenital abnormal arterio-capillary-venous anastomoses which tend to enlarge with time and present with minor focal deficits, seizures or hemorrhage. The morbidity of individual lesions corresponds to the size and location of the lesion and the associated hemorrhage. While life-threatening hemorrhage demands surgical intervention for clot evacuation and AVM obliteration, careful consideration must be given to the natural history of individual asymptomatic lesions along with the risks of surgical therapy. Complete surgical removal remains the cornerstone of therapy, with adjunctive preoperative intraluminal embolization to reduce flow. Small, surgically inaccessible AVMs may be successfully obliterated with high-energy irradiation.

EPILEPSY

Epilepsy affects over 1% of the population, and surgical treatment is increasingly considered for those who are inadequately controlled by medical therapy. The objective of surgical therapy is to identify with scalp or intracranial electrodes the irritable tissue or "focus," to ascertain with functional brain mapping techniques that this tissue lies within "dispensable" (resectable) brain, and to subsequently resect this electrographically abnormal tissue. MRI is used to identify mass lesions (15%) and structural abnormalities, and memory and language functions are assessed preoperatively during the amytal or Wada test. With this approach, significant or total relief of seizures is attained in over 80% of patients.

INTRACRANIAL INFECTIONS

These infections occur following (1) infections of contiguous structures (middle ear, sinuses, scalp), (2) hematogenous spread (cardiac), and (3) contamination via penetrating trauma, and are considered for surgical therapy when localized infections are refractory to antibiotics, or present as mass lesions or hydrocephalus. *Osteomyelitis* of the skull and *epidural abscess* are treated by removal of affected bone and drainage; *subdural empyema* represents a surgical emergency, since rapid speed of infection and neurologic demise may occur, and requires immediate evacuation of pus through a craniotomy or craniectomy; *brain abscess* is usually refractory to antibiotic therapy and requires surgical evacuation following radiographic localization. Broad-spectrum antibiotic therapy is always initiated pending culture results, and in the acute stage of encephalitis and brain swelling, steroids, judicious fluid restriction, and even hyperventilation may be required to control ICP.

PAIN

Chronic pain may arise from nociceptive stimuli attendant to malignancy, or from injury to peripheral nerves or CNS structures; or it may be symptomatic of an underlying psychiatric disorder. Although narcotics provide relief when life expectancy is less than 2 months, other patients with chronic pain are best treated with a variety of surgical therapies including (1) section of peripheral and CNS pathways subserving pain neurotransmission, (2) CNS lesions to alter the affective response to pain, (3) section of the efferent limb of the vasomotor reflex arc, (4) electrical stimulation in brain or spinal cord to suppress pain, and (5) intrathecal narcotic infusion pumps.

STRUCTURAL ABNORMALITIES OF THE AXIAL SKELETON

Craniovertebral Border Abnormalities

These abnormalities are often congenital and asymptomatic until adult life when minor trauma causes neurologic symptoms of cervicomedullary compression including cranial nerve dysfunction and long tract signs. In *platybasia* and *basilar impression* the volume of the posterior fossa may be reduced, with distortion and compression of the hindbrain and cervicomedullary junction and hydrocephalus; and in *atlantoaxial dislocation,* cervicomedullary compression may induce a severe, progressive deficit. In patients with progressive or significant symptoms, following diagnostic CT or MRI, decompression and occasionally fusion may be required.

Intervertebral Disc Disease

This disease involves the degeneration and herniation of intervertebral discs with compression of nerve roots or spinal cord; greatest frequency is in the lower cervical and lumbar areas. Signs and symptoms of "radiculopathy" or nerve root compression include segmental sensory (pain, paresthesias) or motor (hyporeflexia, atrophy, weakness) deficits. *Lumbar herniation* occurs predominantly at the L4 and L5 interspaces, generally with compression of the nerve root of the level below, i.e., L4 disc herniation associated with L5 radiculopathy (weak foot dorsiflexion and dorsal foot hypesthesia), and L5 disc herniation with S1 radiculopathy (calf weakness and lateral foot hypesthesia). Radiculopathy is manifest by intermittent pain in the back and in the distribution of the sciatic nerve (sciatica), which is exacerbated by coughing or sneezing, prolonged sitting, or physical activity. On exam, radiculopathy is accompanied by axial muscle spasm and reproduction of the typical pain when tension is placed on the affected nerve root (i.e., straight-leg-raising or femoral stretch test). Treatment is initially conservative and involves 1–2 weeks of bed rest, local heat, and analgesics, followed by a graded program of exercises designed to strengthen abdominal and back muscles. Diagnosis is made with CT and MRI or myelography, and early surgery is considered when major deficits (foot drop or incontinence) are observed. Back pain alone is not an indication for surgery.

CERVICAL DISC HERNIATION This occurs predominantly between C5 and C6 (C6 radiculopathy) and C6 and C7 (C7 radiculopathy), with diminished biceps reflex and strength and C6 hypesthesia and pain and diminished triceps reflex and strength and C7 hypesthesia and pain, respectively. Central herniation is rare, causing cervical cord compression and quadraparesis. Cervical myelography, CT, and MRI assist in diagnosis, and lateral herniations are usually treated conservatively, with posterolateral or anterior surgical approaches to disc removal, if conservative therapy is ineffective. Emergent removal of central herniation with quadraparesis requires an anterior approach.

SPONDYLOSIS Characterized by extensive bony proliferation and canal narrowing, spondylosis often coexists with disc herniation, and may occur both in the cervical and lumbar spine, causing compression of the spinal cord, cauda equina, or nerve roots. Diagnosis involves history, neurologic examination, and radiographic procedures (myelography, CT, or MRI). Cervical spondylosis or stenosis may present with radicular symptoms and/or signs of spinal cord compression (myelopathy) and is treated surgically using posterior or anterior decompressive techniques. Lumbar stenosis presents with back pain and "neurogenic claudication" in which leg pain and paresthesias are exacerbated by standing or walking, and gratifying results are obtained following posterior surgical decompression.

PEDIATRIC NEUROSURGERY

Intraventricular Hemorrhage Occurs in 40–50% of preterm infants (less than 1500 g) and may lead to hydrocephalus and compromised neurodevelopmental outcome. Diagnosis is made with ultrasound, and treatment involves serial lumbar punctures and placement of a ventriculoperitoneal shunt if this is ineffective.

Myelomeningocele Expressed as a failure of closure of the neural tube in the lumbar or thoracolumbar region and is associated with Arnold-Chiari II malformation in 100%, and hydrocephalus in 80–90% of patients. Therapy involves closure of the dural and cutaneous defect within 24–48 h of birth and VP shunt insertion when appropriate.

Craniosynostosis Identified clinically by the abnormal morphology of the cranium, which occurs due to premature fusion of various sutures (metopic, coronal, sagittal, lambdoid). Surgery must be undertaken early in life, and involves craniectomy of prematurely fused sutures, and repositioning of cranial structures to allow a normal subsequent pattern of cranial growth.

Hydrocephalus   With ventricular dilatation, hydrocephalus may reflect a disorder of absorption of CSF by arachnoid granulations (*communicating hydrocephalus*) or of movement of CSF through the ventricular system (*obstructive* or *noncommunicating hydrocephalus*). Following diagnosis with ultrasound or CT, a pressure-regulated shunt system consisting of a ventricular catheter, valve, and distal peritoneal catheter is inserted. While these systems often fail, and have inherent disadvantages, the natural history of hydrocephalus is so devastating that this operation represents a true benefit for these patients, in 60% of whom normal IQs are preserved.

42 ORTHOPAEDICS

MANIFESTATIONS OF MUSCULOSKELETAL DISORDERS

Pain

Pain is the most common symptom of musculoskeletal disorders. Stimulation of peripheral receptors by noxious agents produces a spatiotemporal pattern of nervous impulses that is interpreted as pain within the higher cerebral centers. Neural pain activity is modulated by analgesics, as well as by neurohormones called *endorphins,* which function as endogenous pain-inhibiting substances.

Pain may be described as localized, diffuse, radicular, or referred. Local pain occurs at the site of the pathologic process, while diffuse pain appears to be more characteristic of deep tissues. Radicular pain involves the anatomic distribution of a peripheral nerve and is generally due to pathology involving the nerve or nerve root, as in sciatica. Pain is referred when manifested at a location remote from the site of pathology. Examples of referred pain include knee pain as a manifestation of hip joint pathology, or pain in the flank or gluteal area secondary to a spinal problem. Muscle pain may result from direct injury or from muscle spasm, a sustained reflexive contraction of muscle. Peripheral nerve pain can be caused from external pressure (neuralgia) or internal compression of a nerve between anatomic structures (compression neuropathies), ischemia, infection (e.g., herpes zoster), metabolic disturbances, or toxins such as lead or arsenic.

Bone lesions in the vertebrae such as metastatic carcinoma, multiple myeloma, infections, or osteoporotic compression fractures can also cause persistent local and occasionally radicular pain.

Cervical Disc Disease Cervical disc herniation can cause neck or radicular pain, neurologic symptoms, and compression of either the spinal cord or nerve roots. Thus, motor weakness or sensory abnormalities can occur either in a nerve root distribution or diffusely below the level of the lesion. Myelography or MRI can demonstrate the lesion. The C4–C6 levels are most commonly involved, and patients usually present with relatively acute pain, with neurologic

TABLE 42-1. Causes of Low Back Pain

---

1. Structural (anomalous or transitional vertebrae, spina bifida, spondylolysis, spondylolisthesis, facet anomalies)
2. Functional (scoliosis, leg-length discrepancy, work or postural attitudes, pregnancy, hip or knee flexion contractures)
3. Infections (pyogenic osteomyelitis, tuberculosis, etc.)
4. Inflammatory (arthritis, ankylosing spondylitis, myositis, fibrositis, etc.)
5. Degenerative (osteoarthritis, osteoporosis, degenerative disc)
6. Neoplastic (multiple myeloma, giant cell tumor, eosinophilic granuloma, or metastases such as breast, prostate, lung, kidney, thyroid)
7. Traumatic (compression fracture, transverse process or posterior element fracture, ligament sprain or muscle strain, disc herniation)

---

findings depending on the level and extent of the herniation. Cord compression will cause motor weakness and hyperreflexia in the lower extremities, and occasionally incontinence. Treatment consists of cervical traction, followed by anti-inflammatory medication and a cervical collar. If neurologic deficit does not respond promptly to traction, surgical discectomy and fusion of the involved level may be necessary.

LOW BACK PAIN "Low back syndrome" refers to a disease or injury of the lumbosacral spine which may be acute or chronic in nature. Table 42-1 lists causes of low back pain. Clinically low back pain may be activity-related, aggravated by sneezing or coughing, or associated with muscle spasm. Referred pain may occur in the buttocks or leg, and nerve root compression can cause radicular pain and/or sensory and motor symptoms in a given nerve root distribution.

Examination of the patient should include assessment of spinal range of motion, straight-leg-raising test (for sciatic irritability; produces radicular pain if positive), and a complete neurologic examination. Most often low back syndrome is due to traumatic or mechanical causes, and will usually respond to conservative treatment of bed rest, anti-inflammatories, local heat, and occasionally antispasmodics for muscle spasm. With subsequent mobilization, isometric back and abdominal exercises are helpful, and occasionally a corset or back brace.

Spondylolisthesis Spondylolisthesis is a forward subluxation of one vertebral body on another, and can be caused by (1) spondylolysis (a defect in the pars interarticularis), (2) fracture of posterior elements, (3) facet deficiency (congenital), (4) facet deficiency due to degenerative disc disease, or (5) isthmic (elongation of the pars). Clinically, spondylolisthesis may be asymptomatic, although back pain may be present along with variable degrees of hamstring tightness, sciatica, and rarely, neurologic symptoms. Lateral radiographs will best demonstrate the displacement, and oblique views will show any defect in the pars (spondylolysis). Treatment is conservative, with rest and abdominal exercises, unless progression of the subluxation or of symptoms occur, in which case a posterolateral fusion usually is done.

Sciatica Sciatica is a symptom and not a disease, and is used to describe radicular type of pain. Sciatica can be caused by nerve root compression by a herniated disc, tumor, abscess, or foraminal narrowing due to degenerative arthritis with facet hypertrophy. Occasionally an intrapelvic or gluteal tumor or abscess can cause sciatica, as can inflammatory or toxic processes. Disc herniations or degenerative arthritis are by far the most common causes. Disc herniations occur most commonly at the L5/S1 and L4/L5 levels, when a tear in the annulus fibrosus allows herniation of the soft, gelatinous, interior nucleus pulposus posteriorly into the spinal canal. The herniated disc then impinges on nerve roots, causing back and radicular pain (sciatica), and sometimes neurologic symptoms. Disc herniations are uncommon in children or older adults, and occur most often in middle-aged individuals. Pain is usually aggravated by sitting, coughing, and sneezing, and forward flexion. Symptoms will also be elicited by straight-leg raising, particularly with additional dorsiflexion of the foot (Lasegue's sign). The lesion can be demonstrated by CT scan, although generally visualization is better with myelography or MRI. Treatment is generally conservative initially, with 80–90% of patients improving spontaneously and not requiring surgery. Surgical excision of the extruded portion of the disc or digestion by percutaneous injection of chymopapain or collagenase into the disc can be effective invasive treatments.

Spinal Stenosis Spinal stenosis is a narrowing of the spinal canal or neuroforamina, and can be either acquired, as with degenerative disc disease, or congenital, as in achondroplasia. Currently the disorder is most readily diagnosed with MRI or CT scans. Patients present with back or leg pain, generally exacerbated by standing and walking and relieved by sitting, in contradistinction to discogenic back pain. Neurologic signs and symptoms may be present, including hyporeflexia. Treatment is conservative, with flexion exercises and bracing, anti-inflammatories, or epidural steroids. Refractory cases are treated by wide posterior surgical decompression, with or without fusion.

TABLE 42-2.   Clinical Grading of Muscle Strength

Grade	Muscle Power
0	Paralysis—no muscle contraction
1	Flicker of contracton without joint excursion
2	Some joint motion, but not against gravity
3	Full joint motion against gravity with no resistance
4	Less than normal strength, but full motion against resistance
5	Normal muscle strength

Pyogenic Osteomyelitis of the Spine   The most common organism responsible for this condition is *Staphylococcus aureus*, which spreads hematogenously from other sites of infection. Patients have back pain, radiographic destruction of the disc space, and sometimes neurologic deficit. They may or may not have fever or other systemic symptoms of infection. Usually leukocytosis and elevated sedimentation rate are present. Treatment usually involves intravenous antibiotics, immobilization, and frequently surgical debridement often with anterior bone grafting.

Chest Wall Pain

Causes of chest wall pain include infections (e.g., herpes zoster), spinal cord tumors, vertebral disease (infection, nerve root impingement), referred pain from visceral disease, or inflammation of the costochondral junctions (costochondritis, or Tietze's syndrome).

Disorders of Muscle

MUSCLE PARALYSIS AND SPASTICITY   *Motor paralysis* is loss of voluntary control of muscular contraction. Normally muscle has some resting tone, which is absent with lower motor neuron lesions, causing flaccid paralysis. Tendon reflexes are also abolished with interruption of the lower motor neuron pathway. *Spasticity* refers to abnormal increases in muscle tone with passive stretch, and is seen with upper motor neuron lesions. Loss of inhibitory control of tendon reflexes with upper motor neuron lesions also causes hyperreflexia. Electrical diagnosis of disorders of nerve and muscle is assisted by electromyography (fine needles inserted into muscles record intrinsic electrical activity of the muscles), and by nerve conduction velocity studies (electrical stimulation of a peripheral nerve with recording of the distally induced muscle action potentials). The clinical grading of muscle strength is shown in Table 42-2.

INTRINSIC DISEASES OF MUSCLE Muscular Dystrophies Hereditary disorders of muscle with progressive degeneration. Types: Duchenne (fatal), fascioscapulohumeral(benign), and limb girdle.

Myotonias Hereditary progressive disorders, including myotonic dystrophy and myotonia congenita (Thomsen disease).

Myositis An inflammation of muscles, and may be caused by a virus, parasite, or spirochete, as well as occurring in association with the various collagen vascular diseases such as dermatomyositis, systemic lupus erythematosus, scleroderma, and rheumatoid arthritis.

Poliomyelitis An acute viral disease that invades the central nervous system, causing destruction of the anterior horn cells in the spinal cord, which results in flaccid paralysis. In the acute phase, patients have a febrile illness with malaise and headache, and may recover or go on to a paralytic phase within a few days. The convalescent phase follows, and some motor improvement may occur for up to 2 years. Treatment is with physical therapy to maintain joint range of motion and prevent contractures. In the final residual stage, surgeries may be needed to stabilize flaccid joints by arthrodesis, correct leg-length inequalities, and transfer tendons to restore lost functions. In tendon transfers a loss of one grade of muscle strength will occur, so only muscles of grade 4 or 5 are suitable. Foot deformities are common, and can be corrected by bracing initially, and by combinations of tendon transfers and, near skeletal maturity, arthrodesis. With quadriceps paralysis, patients may be able to stabilize the knee adequately for walking if the gluteus maximus and gastrocnemius are functional; occasionally anterior transfer of the hamstrings is needed. Muscle transfers about the hip are generally not as successful, and occasionally arthrodesis may be needed. Paralysis of the deltoid and rotator cuff can be benefited by arthrodesis of the shoulder, and paralysis of the hand is treated by various tendon transfers, depending on the particular muscles involved.

Cerebral Palsy Cerebral palsy occurs in about 3 births per 100,000. It can be caused by head injury or birth trauma, anoxia, or viral diseases (such as measles or cytomegalovirus). Fifty percent of patients are spastic, 25% are athetoid, 5% ataxic, 5% rigid, and 15% have a mixed clinical picture. Sixty percent of spastic patients have hemiplegia (ipsilateral upper and lower extremity involvement). The next most common form is diplegia (lower extremities), and finally quadriplegia (all extremities involved). Treatment is directed toward prevention of contractures, gait training, and surgical correction of deformities that develop from muscle imbalance. Bracing may help prevent equinus deformities of the ankle, adduction and flexion contractures of the hip, and flexion contractures of the knees. Adductor spasticity of the hip can cause painful hip subluxation or dislocation, and may require treatment with adductor tenotomies, obturator neurectomies, or varus/de-rotation osteotomies of the proximal femur. Hamstring releases and tendo achilles lengthening may be necessary to correct contractures; occasionally, spinal fusion is needed to control progressive neuromuscular scoliosis.

Myelodysplasia (Spinal Dysraphism) *Myelodysplasia* describes a developmental defect in the vertebral column associated with a neurologic lesion. Failure of midline fusion of vertebral elements may occur without cord involvement (spina bifida occulta), or with a myelomeningocele, a neural tube defect at the level of the lesion. Antenatal screening for the alpha-fetoprotein can aid in diagnosis. Eighty percent of patients have associated hydrocephalus. Patients with myelomeningocele generally have paralysis below the level of the defect, and are treated shortly after birth by surgical closure of the cystic defect and shunting for hydrocephalus. Functional prognosis varies with the level; with lesions below the L4 level, patients will usually be ambulatory, although lower extremity deformities such as talipes equinovarus and hip subluxation may occur, requiring surgical correction. Additionally, lack of sensory function makes pressure sores a common recurring problem.

Degenerative Diseases of the Nervous System with Skeletal Deformity *Peroneal muscle atrophy* (Charcot-Marie-Tooth) is an inherited progressive process usually beginning in the first or second decade and involving initially the peroneal nerve, with foot drop, cavo-varus foot deformities, claw toes, and later intrinsic atrophy in the hands. Treatment involves surgical correction of deformities. *Friedreich's cerebellar ataxia* is a familial disease that begins in childhood; it involves the spinocerebellar tracts, corticospinal tracts, and posterior columns. Patients have progressive gait disturbance, speech disturbance, and also scoliosis and foot deformities, with a steady downhill course. Finally, *syringomyelia* is a degenerative condition of the spinal cord with neuronal destruction centrally resulting in a cavity or syrinx, usually in the cervical area. Onset is usually in the second or third decade, and involves intrinsic muscles of the hand initially, followed by progressive loss of both motor and sensory function in the upper and lower extremities. Orthopaedic treatment is directed at bracing for prevention of contractures and deformities, or arthrodesis of neuropathic joints.

Requirements for Efficient Locomotion

1. Stability of joints, normal bone length, normal skeletal relationships
2. Normal joint range of movement and normal muscle power
3. Cortical control of voluntary muscle action
4. Normal muscle tone, including coordination as well as postural tone
5. Normal sensory modalities
6. Cerebellar control of muscle action, and intact ocular and auditory balance mechanism

Gait disturbances can result from neurologic disorders such as ataxia (from cerebellar lesion, posterior column lesion, Guillain-Barré, or Friedreich's ataxia), or from spastic paraplegia (upper motor neuron lesion, stroke, or cerebral palsy). Mechanical causes include limb-length discrepancy, hip joint pathology (congenital dysplasia or dislocation, slipped femoral capital epiphysis, Legg-Calvé-Perthes disease, arthritis), or knee joint problems (arthritis, osteochondritis dissecans, genu valgum or varus, etc.).

SPINAL DEFORMITIES "Kyphosis" refers to an increase in the normal posterior convexity of the thoracic spine involving a number of vertebral bodies. A gibbus deformity is an acute kyphotic angular deformity, and can be congenital, traumatic, or due to infection such as tuberculosis. In adolescence, kyphosis can be the muscular or postural type (benign, and treated with exercise) or discogenic (Scheuermann's disease). Scheuermann's disease tends to be progressive, and is associated with abnormalities of the vertebral end plates with disc herniations into the vertebrae (Schmorl's nodes). It is treated with exercises, and occasionally with bracing or spinal fusion in refractory cases with severe deformities. Senile kyphosis occurs most commonly with osteoporosis, where multiple compression fractures cause wedging of the vertebrae.

Scoliosis "Scoliosis" refers to any lateral deviation of the spine from its usually straight form. Congenital scoliosis is associated with vertebral anomalies such as hemivertebrae or complete or partial fusions of vertebral bodies. Progression

of these types of scoliosis is treated by early limited fusion.
Paralytic or neuromuscular scoliosis usually is associated
with a long C-shaped thoracolumbar curve and often requires
instrumentation and fusion if bracing does not prevent progression. Idiopathic scoliosis progresses during adolescence,
and important factors are the age of onset and site of the
curve. Thoracic curves starting before age 10 have a poorer
prognosis. After skeletal maturity progression is minimal.
The most common curve is the right thoracic curve, usually
seen in girls. Generally rotation of the vertebral bodies occurs
in addition to lateral curvature. The rotational component is
accentuated with forward flexion causing an obvious asymmetry or prominence of the ribs or transverse processes on
the convex side of the curve. Lateral bending radiographs
help to determine the flexibility of the curve. Treatment
consists of regular follow-up to determine progression radiographically, and postural exercises. With progression, bracing
is used such as a Milwaukee brace or plastic thoracolumbar
sacral orthosis (TLSO). Alternatively, electrical muscle stim-
ulators on the convex side of the curve have been also used.
For progressing curves greater than 40°, surgical correction
with Harrington rods or Luque instrumentation (sublaminar
wiring) and posterior fusion is generally indicated. For rigid
thoracolumbar curves or adult degenerative scoliosis, anterior fusion with Zielke instrumentation may be used.

FOOT AND ANKLE DEFORMITIES Pes planus (flatfoot) can
be flexible or rigid. Congenital flexible flatfoot is the most
common type and is usually painless and benign. Rigid
flatfoot (peroneal spastic flatfoot) is usually due to a tarsal
coalition or congenital fusion between the calcaneus and the
navicular, talus, or cuboid, and is frequently painful and
treated by insoles or often resection of the coalition bar.
Acquired flatfoot may result from trauma with rupture of
midfoot ligaments, posterior tibialis tendon rupture, or muscle
imbalance from a neurologic disorder such as poliomyelitis.

Contracture

"Contracture" refers to a permanent shortening and rigidity
of muscles, joints, and fascial structures, and may be congenital or acquired. Congenital examples include clubfoot,
and arthrogryposis multiplex congenita. Acquired contractures of joints can result from periarticular trauma, muscle
imbalance (as previously discussed with cerebral palsy),
burns, or idiopathic conditions such as Dupuytren's contracture of the palmar fascia. Volkmann's ischemic contracture

results from a compartment syndrome of the forearm muscles following trauma. Swelling within muscle compartments bounded by fascia leads to ischemia with permanent muscle necrosis and later fibrosis. A similar problem can occur in the lower extremities. Clinical signs include diminished perfusion or pulses, pain with passive stretch of involved muscles, paresthesias, and motor weakness. Diagnosis is made by measurements of muscle compartment pressures using a special catheter and monitor, and treatment consists of prompt surgical decompression of involved compartments.

EPIPHYSEAL DISORDERS (OSTEOCHONDRITIS OR OSTEOCHONDROSIS)

The term "osteochondritis" refers to an abnormality of the secondary ossification centers of the long bones. Generally the pathologic changes are most consistent with avascular necrosis of the epiphysis. The most common locations of osteochondritis are the lunate (Kienböck), scaphoid (Preoser), tarsal navicular (Köhler), vertebral epiphyses (Scheuermann), capitellum (Panner), femoral head (Legg-Calvé-Perthes), patella (Sinding-Larsen), tibial tubercle (Osgood-Schlatter), calcaneus (Sever), and metatarsal heads (Freiberg). Patients usually present with pain and radiographic abnormalities in the associated epiphysis.

Legg-Calvé-Perthes of the hip usually occurs in males between 5 and 9 years of age, and is bilateral in 10% of cases. Patients present with hip or knee pain and limping in the initial or prodromal stage. This becomes associated with loss of motion in the hip and flattening of the femoral head (coxa plana). Later, with revascularization of the epiphysis, symptoms and signs diminish, although limitation of motion and deformity of the femoral head may be permanent. The key to treatment is containment of the femoral head within the acetabulum, usually with ambulatory abduction bracing, until the restoration or revascularization stage is completed (about 1–2 years). In some cases with severe involvement, varus osteotomy for containment is necessary.

Osgood-Schlatter disease of the tibial tubercle presents in patients in the 13–15 age range, sometimes with history of an antecedent injury. Pain, tenderness, and enlargement of the tibial tubercle occur, with a fragmented appearance radiographically. Treatment is symptomatic, with restriction of activities, and for more severe cases a plaster cylinder cast or knee immobilizer for 6 weeks. The disease is self-limited, although prominence of the tibial tubercle is permanent.

Köhler's disease involves the tarsal navicular in young children between the ages of 3 and 6. Symptoms consist of pain and swelling, and diagnosis is made by radiographs demonstrating sclerosis of the navicular. Treatment consists of a plaster cast for a few weeks, and a molded arch support subsequently.

CONGENITAL ORTHOPAEDIC DEFORMITIES

Deformities Present at Birth

Metatarsus adductus, valgus hindfoot, unilateral externally rotated leg, internal tibial torsion, or an adducted thigh with external rotation of the leg are thought to result from in utero position, and this may also be a contributing factor to talipes equinovarus (clubfoot) deformity. These conditions generally respond to passive stretching exercises, with corrective casts occasionally being used in refractory cases.

Congenital dislocation of the hip consists of partial or complete displacement of the femoral head from the acetabulum, with an incidence of 0.67 per 1000 births. Treatment is most successful if undertaken early, and all babies must be examined carefully for CDH. On exam, a hip click (Ortolani's sign) can be elicited, as the hip reduces in abduction and flexion. Also, limitation of abduction to 75° or less, apparent shortening of one thigh (Galeazzi's sign), and asymmetric gluteal creases may be present. If undetected in infancy, the child will have a noticeable limp or waddle when beginning to walk. Radiographically, delay in ossification of the epiphysis will occur, and the acetabular index (angle of the acetabulum from horizontal) will be greater than normal (22°). An arthrogram of the hip or MRI scan will also demonstrate the dislocation. Treatment of subluxation in the neonate can usually be accomplished with a Pavlik harness for 3–6 months. If the hip does not reduce in abduction or in older infants, a period of skin traction followed by closed reduction in an abduction spica cast may be needed. Open reduction is generally unnecessary in children under 1 year of age, but may be needed in cases of late diagnosis. In the older child, femoral shortening and innominate osteotomies may be necessary to ensure a stable concentric reduction with containment of the femoral head by the acetabulum.

Congenital talipes equinovarus (clubfoot) is a deformity involving flexion of the ankle, inversion of the foot, adduction of the forefoot, and medial rotation of the tibia. Incidence is about 4 per 1000 births. Without treatment the deformity is permanent and ambulation difficult. Treatment begins immediately after birth with passive stretching exercises followed by application of serial corrective plaster casts. The forefoot adduction is corrected first, then the hindfoot varus, and only then the equinus. If the deformity recurs or correction is incomplete, surgical release of the hindfoot must be done with open reduction of the deformity and subsequent casting. In the older child, mild degrees of recurrence can be treated by lateral transfer of the tibialis anterior and/or tendo achilles lengthening.

Congenital convex pes valgus (vertical talus) involves a dislocation of the talonavicular joint, with the talus in a vertical position, and the navicular articulating with the dorsum of the talus. The sole of the foot has a rocker-bottom flatfoot deformity, and is rigid. Early manipulation with plaster casting may be successful, but most cases will require operative reduction and pinning with tendo achilles lengthening. Triple arthrodesis may be indicated in the older child.

Arthrogryposis multiplex congenita is associated with fibrous tissue replacement of muscles at birth causing loss of joint mobility, and associated deformities such as CDH, clubfoot, knee dislocation, which are treated as previously described.

Sprengel's deformity (congenital high scapula) is caused by embryonic failure of the scapula to migrate to its normal position. Occasionally the scapula is attached to the vertebral column by an abnormal band of fibrous tissue or cartilage called the *omovertebral mass*. Mild cases need no treatment, but in more severe cases surgical correction may be undertaken, although it is generally delayed until age 3–6 years.

Klippel-Feil syndrome, or congenital short neck, is caused by multiple fusions of cervical vertebrae, and is generally not treatable. Congenital wryneck (torticollis) is caused by unilateral contracture of the sternocleidomastoid causing a lateral inclination of the head, and is thought to be posttraumatic, with a tender swelling in the muscle preceding the deformity. Treatment consists of stretching exercises, and in refractory or late-diagnosed cases, by surgical release of the muscle.

Other congenital deformities include: radioulnar synostosis (fusion of the proximal radius and ulna), Madelung's deformity (bowing of the distal radius with subluxation of the radioulnar joint), and congenital aplasia or dysplasia of long bones (most commonly, absence of the radius with radial "clubhand," fibula, or proximal femoral focal deficiency).

GENERALIZED BONE DISORDERS

Bone Composition

Organic components: 90% type I collagen; the remaining constituents include phosphoproteins, bone-specific proteoglycan, sialoprotein, osteonectin, osteocalcin, and growth factors such as transforming growth factor-beta, fibroblast growth factor, and bone morphogenetic proteins.

Inorganic components: calcium phosphate in the crystalline form of hydroxyapatite, and 8–9% water.

Bone cell enzymes: Osteoclasts contain acid hydrolases, collagenase, and acid phosphatase, while osteoblasts contain alkaline phosphatase and collagenase activity.

There are two primary forms of ossification, or mineral deposition within skeletal tissues. The long bones form developmentally by mineralization of cartilage initially, with subsequent conversion of this mineralized tissue to bone. This process is called *endochondral ossification,* and in addition to embryonic bone formation, gives rise to the growth plates of long bones, secondary ossification centers of the epiphyses, and callus formation in fracture healing. The other form of ossification is called *intramembranous ossification,* and involves mineralization of osteoid by osteoblasts directly without a cartilage phase. Bone remodeling occurs when osteoclasts resorb bone, which is followed by a tightly coupled formation of bone by osteoblasts, and occurs constantly throughout the skeleton.

Developmental Disorders of Bone

1. Achondroplasia: The most common form of dwarfism, is associated with relatively normal trunk height but shortened extremities, and is autosomal dominant in inheritance.
2. Ollier's disease (also called *dyschondroplasia*): Multiple abnormal rests of cartilage in the metaphyses lead to deformities of the long bones.
3. Multiple exostoses: This autosomal dominant hereditary disorder is characterized by numerous cartilaginous outgrowths from the metaphyses of the pelvis and long bones. These require surgical excision only when symptomatic or occasionally when malignant degeneration into a chondrosarcoma occurs.
4. Polyostotic fibrous dysplasia: This disease usually appears in childhood, and results in dysplastic bone formation by

fibroblastic-like cells in the metaphyses and diaphyses of long bones. Pathologic fractures or bowing of the bones can occur and may require surgical treatment.

5. Osteogenesis imperfecta: A familial disorder of the type I collagen gene with several subtypes. Patients may have blue sclera and deafness, and all have fragile bones which fracture easily. The fetal form is severe and lethal. The infantile form is less severe, and the adolescent form, called *osteogenesis imperfecta tarda,* is the least severe. In children, intramedullary rodding and osteotomies are often used to prevent long bone fractures.

6. Osteopetrosis (Albers-Schönberg, marble bones, congenital osteosclerosis): A rare hereditary disease with defective osteoclasts incapable of bone remodeling, characterized by dense bones radiographically, anemia, and frequent fractures and infections.

7. Melorheostosis: This disease involves regional asymmetric osteosclerosis of cortical bone with the radiographic appearance of candle drippings, local pain, and adjacent joint fibrosis.

Metabolic Diseases

1. Scurvy: Vitamin C deficiency results in defective cross-linking of collagen, and therefore weakness of vascular endothelium. Subperiosteal hemorrhages occur, and increased density of the calcification zone of the growth plate due to defective remodeling and bone formation. Treatment with vitamin C is rapidly curative.

2. Rickets: Vitamin D deficiency can be caused by a number of diseases, and results in inadequate absorption of calcium in the intestine. Nutritional deficiency and intestinal malabsorption syndromes cause inadequate vitamin D absorption, while renal or hepatic diseases result in inadequate hydroxylation of vitamin D to the active form. In children, the long bones are soft and bowed, with widening of the growth plate and enlarged and tender epiphyses. Treatment is with vitamin D repletion. Vitamin D–resistant rickets is a hereditary disease that requires massive doses of vitamin D plus phosphate to treat the bone disease.

3. Hypophosphatasia: This rare hereditary disorder is characterized by low levels of alkaline phosphatase and urinary excretion of phosphoethanolamine.

4. Osteomalacia: This disease is the adult equivalent of rickets, and is caused by any derangement of vitamin D

metabolism as noted above. Pathologic fractures can occur, and treatment is with vitamin D.

5. Osteitis fibrosa (parathyroid osteodystrophy): Multiple bony lesions and areas of bone resorption are caused by excessive secretion of parathyroid hormone. Hypercalcemia may be present in the case of primary hyperparathyroidism, and pathologic fractures or bowing of long bones can occur. Parathyroidectomy is generally the treatment of choice.

6. Osteoporosis: This condition results from an inadequate amount of bone that is otherwise biochemically normal. It is seen in association with Cushing's syndrome, thyrotoxicosis, chronic steroid therapy, and most commonly in postmenopausal women as a consequence of estrogen loss. Treatment is with calcium and physiologic doses of vitamin D (to offset any component of superimposed osteomalacia), exercise, estrogen supplementation when appropriate, and occasionally calcitonin or fluoride.

7. Pituitary disturbances: Hypopituitarism in childhood can cause dwarfism, while hyperpituitarism in childhood leads to gigantism. In adulthood, onset of hyperpituitarism (usually due to a pituitary adenoma) causes acromegaly, with enlargement of the skull, thorax, and digits.

8. Hypothyroidism (cretinism): Delayed ossification results in short stature, and the bones are short with a thick cortex. Epiphyseal ossification is delayed and irregular, resembling osteochondroses such as Legg-Perthes disease. Thyroid replacement is curative if begun in infancy.

9. Mucopolysaccharidoses: A series of 12 hereditary disorders of mucopolysaccharide (glycosaminoglycan) metabolism have been identified, including Hurler, Hunter, Scheie, Sanfilippo, and Morquio syndromes. These vary in severity and are variably associated with spinal deformities, mental retardation, osseous abnormalities, corneal opacities, and joint stiffness.

10. Paget's disease (osteitis deformans): This disorder of bone turnover is thought to be caused by a slow virus infection of osteoclasts. Early in the disease there is excessive osteoclastic resorption and vascularity, followed by abnormal bone formation and sclerosis, with trabecular and cortical thickening. In the late phase, dense sclerotic woven bone and inactive fibrous marrow replacement predominate. The disease begins between ages 35 and 50 and is painful in about 30% of patients. Pathologic fractures occur, and bowing of long bones also occurs. Serum alkaline phosphatase and urinary hydroxyproline levels are elevated and correlate with activity of the disease. Diphosphonates or calcitonin are

useful in controlling the disease by inhibiting bone resorption.

Reticuloendothelial Disorders

1. Lipoid granulomatosis: Results from any disturbance of lipid metabolism. In Gaucher's disease, a cerebroside lipoprotein accumulates; in Niemann-Pick disease, a phosphatide lipoid; in Hand-Schüller-Christian disease, cholesterol; in Tay-Sachs, a cerebroside protein. Radiographs show lytic skeletal lesions.
2. Eosinophilic granulomatosis: May present as a solitary skeletal lesion in childhood, or multiple lesions that are then referred to as Hand-Schüller-Christian disease. HSC disease is also associated with hepatosplenomegaly, exophthalmos, and diabetes insipidus. Solitary EG may cause vertebrae plana or pathologic fracture in long bones, and generally responds to conservative treatment, being a self-limited disorder. The most severe form of disease is Letterer-Siwe, which presents in infancy and is generally fatal. The systemic forms of eosinophilic granulomatosis respond to treatment with vinblastine and prednisone.
3. Hodgkin's disease: A form of malignant lymphoma that may present with lytic lesions in bone secondary to bone marrow involvement. Symptomatic lesions respond to radiation therapy, and the systemic disease is responsive to chemotherapy.
4. Leukemia: May produce bone lesions, most commonly in lymphoblastic leukemia, which can demonstrate lucencies adjacent to the growth plate in the metaphyses.
5. Multiple myeloma: A proliferation of malignant plasma cells, and produces sharply demarcated, "punched-out" lesions in bone. The skull, ribs, and long bones are all affected, and diagnosis can be made on bone marrow biopsy or by demonstration of an abnormal monoclonal immunoglobulin on serum immunoelectrophoresis.
6. Hemolytic anemia: Can cause bone marrow changes in the vertebrae and skull, with a "hair on end" or "sun ray" appearance, particularly in the skull.

FRACTURES   (See Tables 42-3, 42-4, and 42-5)

A fracture is by definition a deformation or discontinuity of bone produced by forces exceeding the strength of the bone. Fractures are classified according to pattern (transverse, spiral, oblique, segmental, comminuted), location (diaphy-

TABLE 42-3. Fractures and Joint Injuries in the Upper Extremity

Injury	Type	Diagnostic aids	Treatment	Complications
Sternoclavicular dislocation	1. Anterior 2. Posterior	P. exam; AP x-ray	Closed reduction; figure-of-8 strap	Airway or neurovasc. compromise (posterior only)
Clavicle fracture	Usually middle ⅓	AP x-ray	Figure-of-8 strap	Nonunion rare
Acromioclavicular dislocation	1. Grade I or II sprain 2. Grade III (tear of conoid/trapezoid lig.)	AP x-ray ± weights	Sling Sling or ORIF*	AC arthritis or prominence of distal clavicle with sling Rx
Scapula fracture		Routine x-rays	Sling/swathe	
Shoulder dislocation	1. Anterior 2. Posterior	AP and axillary or transcapular x-rays	1. CR*, sling/swathe 2. Or abduction pillow (posterior)	Neurologic injury, esp. axillary nerve; recurrent dislocation
Proximal humerus	1. Surgical neck 2. Comminuted	Routine x-rays	Sling Surgical repair	Shoulder stiffness, esp. in elderly
Humeral shaft		Routine x-rays	CR with cast or splint	Radial neurapraxia
Supracondylar	Children	Comparison views of normal elbow	CR; percutaneous pinning	Neurovasc. injury; compartment synd.
Radial head/neck	1. Minimally displaced 2. Comminuted	Routine x-rays; fat pad sign on lateral	1. Sling/splint 2. Excision of r. head	1. Elbow stiffness; 2. Late instability

618

Lateral condyle	Children	Comparison views	ORIF usually needed	Growth disturbance
Olecranon fracture		Routine x-rays	ORIF usually needed	Elbow stiffness
Elbow dislocation	Usually posterior	P. exam; x-rays	CR; splint/sling	Elbow stiffness
Montegia fracture	Ulna fracture with radial head dislocation	Routine x-rays	ORIF or ulna often necessary	
Radius/ulna fractures	1. Incomplete (child) 2. Adult	Routine x-rays	1. Complete fracture; CR/cast 2. ORIF	Loss of pronation and supination if not anatomic
Distal radius (Colles)	1. Extraarticular 2. Intraarticular	AP, lateral and oblique views	1. CR; cast or splint 2. CR; pins or ext. fix.	Residual deformity common
Scaphoid		AP, lat., navicular view	CR; cast	Nonunion common
Metacarpal		Routine x-rays	CR; cast—occ. pinning	
Bennett's fracture (CMC joint thumb)	Usually intraarticular and unstable		CR; percutaneous pinning	
Phalanges	Intraarticular or extraarticular		Splinting with IPs in extension, MPs in flexion	IP or MP joint stiffness
Mallet finger	Avulsion fracture of extensor		Splint DIP in hyperextension	

* ORIF = open reduction and internal fixation; CR = closed reduction.

TABLE 42-4. Fractures and Joint Injuries in the Lower Extremity

Injury	Type	Diagnostic aids	Treatment	Complications
Femoral neck fracture	1. Minimally displaced 2. Displaced	AP and tube; lateral x-rays needed	1. Pinning 2. Pinning; prosthesis in older patients	Nonunion and avascular necrosis; esp. in displaced
Intertrochanteric fracture	May be comminuted	"	ORIF, screw & plate	Loss of fixation
Subtrochanteric fracture	"	"	ORIF	Nonunion common
Femoral shaft	"	"	Skeletal traction or IM rodding	Malunion, limb-length discrepancy
Knee injuries	ACL tear MCL tear LCL tear PCL tear	+ Lachman; drawer + Valgus stress test + Varus stress test + Posterior drawer	Isolated tears may be treated by brace or cast; ACL & multiple may require repair	Symptomatic instability, stiffness
Meniscal tears	Medial or lateral; can be peripheral or in body of meniscus	MRI; arthrogram; diagnostic arthroscopy	Peripheral tears repaired; otherwise fragment removed arthroscopically	Recurrent tears; late degenerative arthritis
Patella fracture	Transverse or comminuted	Routine x-rays	ORIF; or excision of smaller fragments	Knee stiffness; patellofemoral DJD

Tibial plateau fracture	1. Min. depressed 2. Displaced and/or comminuted	Varus/valgus stress views; tomograms	1. Cast, crutches 2. ORIF, occ. bone grafting	Late DJD; knee stiffness
Tibial shaft fractures	1. Closed 2. Open and/or comminuted	Routine x-rays	1. CR; long leg cast 2. Debridement, external fixator	Delayed or nonunion common; infection in open fractures
Ankle sprain	Inversion most common	Stress mortise views may be helpful	Ace wrap, splint, or cast, depending on severity	Recurrent instability
Ankle fracture	Medial, lateral, and/or posterior malleoli ± Subtalar dislocation	AP, lat., and mortise views needed	CR, cast; if not anatomic, ORIF	DJD if nonanatomic result
Talus fracture	± Subtalar dislocation	Routine x-rays	CR if nondisplaced; ORIF if displaced	Avascular necrosis of talus
Calcaneus fracture	± Subtalar joint involv.	"	CR, cast; occ. ORIF	Poor prognosis if subtalar joint involved
Metatarsal fractures		AP, lat., oblique views	usually short leg cast	Nonunion in Jones type (5th MT shaft)
Phalangeal fractures			Buddy taping	

TABLE 42-5. Fractures and Joint Injuries of the Pelvis and Spine

Injury	Type	Diagnostic aids	Treatment	Complications
Hip dislocation	1. Anterior (rare) 2. Posterior	1. Leg abducted 2. Leg adducted	CR: light traction	Sciatic nerve injury; avascular necrosis
Acetabular fracture	Displaced or nondisplaced	45° obliques; CT scan	Displaced—ORIF; non-displ., traction	DJD common
Pubic ramus fracture	Isolated		Bed rest, crutches	
Pelvic ring disruption		CT scan; pelvic inlet and outlet views	Bed rest, ext. fixator, or ORIF, depending on severity	SI joint disruption may lead to DJD
Cervical spine	Facet dislocation; compression fracture	Important to see all 7 vertebrae on x-ray; CT scan helpful	CR: halo traction and/or fusion if unstable	Neurologic deficits, including quadriplegia
Thoracolumbar spine	1. Compression 2. Burst fractures 3. Fracture/dislocation	AP and lat x-rays; CT scan	1. Brace 2. Cast or ORIF 3. ORIF/fusion	Neurologic deficits

seal, metaphyseal, epiphyseal), and integrity of the surrounding skin and soft tissue (open or compound vs. closed). A pathologic fracture is one through bone that is abnormally weakened by a pathologic process such as metabolic bone disease or a tumor. Clinical manifestations include pain, swelling, deformity, ecchymosis, instability, and crepitus. Diagnosis requires two orthogonal radiographs as a minimum, including views of the joint above and below the fracture site. Evaluation should include assessment for other injuries, as well as assessment of the neurologic and vascular function in the injured extremity. Open fractures represent orthopaedic emergencies, requiring immediate debridement in the operating room setting to prevent occurrence of osteomyelitis. Debridement should be carried out within 6–8 h, and wounds are generally not closed primarily. Any devitalized tissue is removed, and the fracture is stabilized in either an external fixator or a plaster cast.

Associated vascular injuries require early recognition and treatment, as irreversible muscle ischemia will occur within 6–8 h. Also in the presence of ischemia, prophylactic fascial compartment releases are necessary to prevent compartment syndrome on reperfusion of the limb. Fat embolism syndrome, a form of adult respiratory distress syndrome (ARDS), occurs in some patients, particularly with multiple long bone fractures. This syndrome occurs 2–3 days postinjury, and is attended by hypoxemia, confusion, fever, and transient petechiae. Treatment is with respiratory support and corticosteroids.

Nerve injuries may be associated with fractures, and range from neurapraxia (a transient, reversible impairment of nerve function), to axonotmesis (axons transected but nerve sheath intact; can regenerate), to the most severe irreversible form of neurotmesis in which the entire nerve is transected. Transected nerves should be repaired primarily when possible at the time of fracture fixation or debridement.

DELAYED UNION AND NONUNION   ''Delayed union'' refers to a fracture that takes longer than average to heal, and is somewhat poorly defined. ''Nonunion'' refers to a fracture that fails to progress toward healing. Causes of nonunion include excessive motion at a fracture site, excessive distraction, infection, and severe soft tissue disruption.

STRESS FRACTURES   Stress or fatigue fractures are a result of repeated stress to a bone that would not be injured by isolated forces of the same magnitude. They can occur on long marches, after jogging, or other activities. X-ray findings may be subtle, but eventually show periosteal reaction. Treatment is with immobilization.

EPIPHYSEAL PLATE INJURIES   Longitudinal growth occurs from the growth plate adjacent to the epiphyses of the long bones. The zone of provisional calcification of the plate is a mechanically weaker area of the bone, and it is through this zone that fractures about the epiphysis usually occur. The Salter-Harris classification of growth plate injuries is in wide use:

Type I: Transverse fracture through metaphyseal side of growth plate; excellent prognosis after closed reduction.

Type II: Fracture through growth plate partially, exiting through the metaphyseal bone; also excellent prognosis with closed reduction.

Type III: Fracture longitudinally through the articular surface and epiphysis, and then transversely through the metaphyseal side of the growth plate; prognosis good with anatomic reduction only.

Type IV: Longitudinal fracture through epiphysis, growth plate, and exiting through metaphyseal bone; open reduction generally necessary, and has higher risk of late growth disturbance.

Type V: Crush injury to the growth plate; high incidence of late growth disturbance.

Fractures in children generally heal more rapidly than in adults, with nonunions being extremely rare. Greater capacity for remodeling also allows acceptance of greater angular deformities. However, limb-length discrepancies can occur with growth after fractures, as can progressive angular deformities, unlike the adult.

Closed treatment of fractures generally involves application of plaster casts. Complications of cast treatment include swelling, which can impair circulation and cause ischemic limb damage; pressure sores; and neurapraxias. Casts should include the joint proximal and distal to the fractured bone. Body casts can be used for spinal fractures.

External fixation is used in open fractures associated with soft tissue injury or loss. Pins inserted into the bone above and below the fracture are connected to an outrigger and stabilize the fracture, while allowing access to wounds. Another method of stabilizing a fracture is with traction. In children, skin traction with adhesive tapes can be used, although with older children and adults skeletal traction through a transverse percutaneous pin is necessary.

Electrical stimulation can be used through either percutaneous pins or externally applied coils to stimulate a high percentage of nonunions or delayed unions to heal without surgery.

DISEASES OF JOINTS

Joints consist of hyaline articular cartilage bounded by a fibrous capsule that has a lining of synovial cells, which secrete the synovial fluid that provides nourishment and lubrication of the articular surface. Articular cartilage matrix is composed of 40% type II collagen, 40% proteoglycan, and 20% glycoproteins as the organic components. Normal synovial fluid contains hyaluronate and up to 200 nucleated cells, as well as glucose and electrolytes.

Clinical examination of a joint includes measurement of range of motion, presence of effusion, synovial thickening, warmth, erythema, and tenderness. Radiographic examination includes standard biplanar x-rays, and occasionally, arthrography if meniscal or capsular pathology is suspected. Synovial fluid analysis is helpful. Normal synovial fluid is clear and straw-colored. When the cell count is increased or crystals present, turbidity results. Viscosity is decreased due to breakdown of hyaluronate when inflammation is present. A poor mucin clot is another indication of inflammation. Normal synovial fluid contains about 10mg/dL less glucose than serum, and this gradient is increased in the presence of large numbers of inflammatory cells.

"Pyogenic arthritis" refers to a bacterial infection, or septic arthritis, and can result in rapid and irreversible destruction of the articular cartilage. *Staphylococcus aureus* and hemolytic streptococci are the most common organisms, but many organisms are possible agents. Patients may have fever, effusion, pain with motion of the joint, and an elevated white blood cell count and sedimentation rate. The white blood cell count in the synovial fluid is generally greater than 50,000, with 90% PMNs. Organisms may be identified by Gram's stain or culture of the fluid aspirated. Treatment is generally by surgical drainage of the joint in conjunction with appropriate intravenous antibiotics. Some infections may be treated with daily aspirations rather than surgery. Infections of the hip joint must all be treated by prompt surgical drainage to prevent avascular necrosis. The knee joint frequently can be drained arthroscopically. Early motion after subsidence of the acute infection is important to prevent joint stiffness, and antibiotics are usually continued 3–6 weeks.

Tuberculosis is now an uncommon infection in this country, but can cause severe destruction of bone and joints. Most commonly the spine is involved, with destruction of adjacent

TABLE 42-6.   Criteria for Diagnosis of Rheumatoid Arthritis

1. Morning stiffness present for longer than 15 minutes
2. Pain with motion or direct tenderness in at least one joint
3. Swelling unrelated to bony overgrowth of at least one joint for at least 6 weeks
4. Swelling observed in a second joint within a 3-month interval
5. Symmetric joint swelling excluding DIP joints
6. Presence of subcutaneous nodules over bony prominences
7. X-ray changes consistent with rheumatoid arthritis
8. Positive sheep cell agglutination or latex fixation test
9. Poor mucin clot on synovial fluid analysis
10. Characteristic histopathologic changes in the synovial membrane on biopsy
11. Characteristic histopathologic changes in nodules
12. Elevated sedimentation rate
13. Iritis

vertebrae, kyphosis, and abscess formation. In peripheral joints, the subchondral bone is eroded and destroyed early, while the articular cartilage is relatively well preserved until late in the course. The end result is fibrous ankylosis of the joint. The clinical course may be insidious, and diagnosis depends on recovery of organisms from the bone or joint by biopsy or aspiration. Synovial fluid usually contains less than 20,000dL leukocytes. Patients are treated by surgical debridement of involved joints, supportive therapy, and triple-drug therapy (isoniazid, ethambutol, rifampin) for 6 months to 1 year. Surgical arthrodesis of destroyed joints may be necessary. Tuberculous spondylitis (Pott's disease) is treated by anterior debridement, decompression, and fusion with rib grafts, in conjunction with triple-drug therapy.

Gonococcal arthritis is more common in females. Symptoms start with migratory polyarthralgia, followed by localization in one or two joints. The knee, elbow, and wrist are the most common sites of involvement. Infection may be clinically subacute or chronic, and treatment is with aspiration and penicillin.

Lyme arthritis is a tick-borne illness caused by a spirochete *Borrelia burgdorferi.* A skin eruption may herald the onset of a rheumatic syndrome resembling rheumatoid arthritis with oligoarticular presentation. Cardiac and neurologic symptoms can also occur. Penicillin or tetracycline therapy will eliminate the infection.

Rheumatoid arthritis is a systemic disease affecting many organs of the body, characterized especially by proliferative synovial destruction of multiple joints. The proliferative synovium that destroys the articular cartilage is called *pannus,* and radiographically periarticular osteopenia and concentric joint space narrowing occur. Table 42-6 lists the criteria for diagnosis of rheumatoid arthritis.

Classic RA would have 7 of the listed criteria with continuous joint swelling for 6 weeks. Diagnosis requires at least 5 criteria with 6 weeks of continuous swelling; 90% of rheumatoid patients have the anti-γ-globulin factor, called *rheumatoid factor,* measured by latex fixation test. X-rays show soft tissue swelling, osteoporosis, and periarticular erosions, followed by complete joint destruction.

Medical management includes anti-inflammatory drugs (both steroidal and nonsteroidal), gold salts, methotrexate, and antimalarials. Surgical treatments include synovectomies of involved joints and tenosynovectomies to prevent tendon ruptures; joint replacements for end-stage disease (hip, knee, shoulder, elbow, wrist, MCP and PIP joints); metatarsal head resections (Hoffman procedure) for forefoot deformity; and various procedures on the hand for correction of deformity.

Osteoarthritis, or degenerative arthritis is a noninflammatory form of progressive joint destruction. Cartilage wear is manifested by loss of proteoglycans, which then causes fibrillation of the articular surface. Marginal osteophytes form as part of the injury and repair process, and the cartilage surface eventually becomes denuded to subchondral bone. Radiographs demonstrate asymmetric joint space narrowing, subchondral sclerosis, subchondral cysts, and osteophytes. Joints deranged by any process such as trauma, Legg-Perthes disease, septic arthritis, gout, or hemophilia can undergo changes of osteoarthritis. Effusion tends to be minimal, and the arthritis is only slowly progressive. Treatment involves limitation of activities, anti-inflammatory medications, walking aids, osteotomy to correct deformity or realign joints, and, as a last resort, joint arthrodesis or total joint replacement.

Gout is a metabolic disease in which crystals of sodium urate are deposited in and around joints, with severe episodic arthritis, classically involving the MTP joint of the great toe in males over age 30. Diagnosis can be confirmed by aspiration of the joint with demonstration of urate crystals by polarized light microscopy. Treatment is with colchicine or indomethacin acutely, and chronically with allopurinol to decrease serum urate levels.

Pyrophosphate arthritis (pseudogout or chondrocalcinosis) is an episodic arthritis resembling gout, and most commonly affects the knee or wrist. The diagnosis rests on finding pyrophosphate crystals in the synovial fluid; radiographs may also demonstrate calcification of menisci. Treatment is with anti-inflammatory medication.

Hemophilic arthritis results from acute recurrent bleeding

into synovial joints, usually after minor injury. The knee, elbow, shoulder, and ankle may be involved. Contractures develop, with synovial thickening and hemosiderin deposition, and progressive destruction of the articular cartilage. Minimization of hemorrhages is the key to preventive treatment, along with dynamic splinting for contractures. In end-stage disease, total joint reconstruction or arthrodesis may be necessary under protection of large infusions of factor VIII.

Synovial Lesions

Pigmented villonodular synovitis is a proliferative inflammatory process of synovium of unknown etiology. Patients have a thickened, brownish proliferation of synovium that causes progressive joint destruction. Effusions aspirated from the affected joint will be brown in color due to the hemosiderin content. Treatment consists of early synovectomy, by either arthrotomy or arthroscopy.

Synovial chondromatosis is a condition of cartilaginous metaplasia of synovium that may become detached and form loose bodies within the joint. This condition, like PVNS, is monarticular and slowly progressive, and is best treated by synovectomy.

Toxic or transient acute synovitis of the hip occurs in childhood, and mimics septic arthritis or Legg-Perthes disease. It frequently follows a viral illness, and usually presents with a limp or refusal of the child to walk. One must exclude septic arthritis, and hip aspiration is generally necessary to accomplish this. Treatment is symptomatic with bed rest, skin traction, and protected weight-bearing until the condition resolves.

Slipped Capital Femoral Epiphysis

This condition affects adolescents ages 10–15 and is more common in males. It presents with hip pain and a limp, and involves slippage of the epiphysis medially and posteriorly on the femoral neck. Patients have a loss of internal rotation of the hip and an antalgic gait. The condition is bilateral in 25% of cases. Diagnosis is by orthogonal radiographs of the hip. The condition is treated by pinning in situ (subacute or chronic slips) or by closed reduction and pinning (acute slips). Chondrolysis is a complication of this disease, more common in blacks and females. Patients can develop secondary degenerative changes later in life.

Hypertrophic Pulmonary Osteoarthropathy

This syndrome affects bones and joints of the extremities, with new periosteal bone formation, and clubbing of the digits. It is associated with pulmonary pathology, but the mechanism is not known.

Neuropathic (Charcot) Joints

A Charcot joint results from any denervating process affecting the extremities. Tabes dorsalis, syringomyelia, leprosy, diabetes, or spinal cord injury may lead to neuropathic joints. It is generally thought that joint destruction results from repeated trauma to joints with impaired sensation. The joint may undergo very rapid and severe destruction, with gross instability and swelling, but minimal inflammation. Arthrodesis is difficult to achieve, so usually conservative methods such as bracing are employed.

Painful Shoulder

The rotator cuff consists of the common tendinous insertions of the supraspinatus, infraspinatus, teres minor, and subscapularis. Tendinitis or bursitis is common, and usually results from an impingement of the rotator cuff on the coracoacromial ligament (impingement syndrome). Acute episodes may be relieved by injection of the subacromial bursa with corticosteroid. Chronic cases are treated with anti-inflammatories, rest, ultrasound or heat, and exercises, and refractory cases occasionally are treated by resection of the coracoacromial ligament with anterior acromioplasty. Rotator cuff tears present with acute pain and difficulty with active shoulder abduction. Diagnosis can be made with arthrography, MRI, or ultrasound, and treatment is usually conservative with rest and exercises. Large tears with persistent symptoms, particularly in younger patients, may require surgical repair.

TUMORS OF THE MUSCULOSKELETAL SYSTEM

Primary bone tumors are relatively rare, but a variety of both benign and malignant types occur. *Primary bone-forming tumors* are listed below:

1. Osteoma: This is a small, benign, sessile lesion of dense

bone usually occurring in the skull bones and generally asymptomatic. No treatment is necessary.

2. Osteoid osteoma: A benign, sclerotic bone-forming tumor of children and young adults that is usually painful and less than 1 cm in diameter. Aspirin often relieves the pain, and adjacent bone may show sclerotic thickening. Excision must include the radiolucent central nidus of the lesion to prevent recurrence.

3. Osteoblastoma: A benign, bone-forming tumor of children and young adults, common in the spine, which is histologically identical to osteoid osteoma but larger in size. Curettage and bone grafting is the treatment.

4. Osteosarcoma: This is the most common aggressive malignant bone tumor, generally involving the metaphyses of long bones about the knee, and predominantly found in adolescents. Pulmonary metastases are frequent, and treatment consists of amputation or radical resection with limb reconstruction, in conjunction with systemic chemotherapy. Occasionally seen in older patients as a secondary malignancy arising in Paget's disease or following radiation treatment. Parosteal osteosarcoma is a less aggressive variant arising extraosseously adjacent to the periosteum, usually near the knee in young adults.

Cartilaginous tumors include the following:

1. Osteochondroma (exostosis): A benign exophytic growth from the metaphyses of long bones with a cartilage cap. Multiple form is hereditary. Secondary malignant change can occur in older adults (chondrosarcoma). Simple excision when indicated is curative.

2. Enchondroma: A benign, sometimes expansile cartilaginous tumor of the metaphyses of long bones or the tubular bones of the hands that exhibits calcification radiographically. Pathologic fractures can occur, as can late secondary malignant change. Treatment when necessary consists of curettage and bone grafting.

3. Chondroblastoma: A benign tumor of the epiphyses of children, which may cause joint pain or effusion, and is treated by curettage and bone grafting.

4. Chondrosarcoma: A malignant tumor of cartilage, most commonly seen in the metaphyses of long bones and in the pelvis of adults age 30–60. Wide resection or amputation is needed, and chemotherapy or radiation is of little benefit. Secondary tumors can arise in older individuals from an enchondroma or osteochondroma.

Fibrous tumors of bone include:

1. Nonossifying fibroma (metaphyseal fibrous cortical defect): A benign fibrous lesion of childhood that is usually an incidental x-ray finding. Large lesions may cause pathologic fractures. Lesions spontaneously regress at skeletal maturity.
2. Fibrosarsoma: An aggressive malignancy, rare as a primary tumor in bone. Radical surgical removal or amputation with radiation usually needed for treatment.

Other musculoskeletal tumors include:

1. Giant cell tumor (osteoclastoma): An aggressive, destructive, benign epiphyseal tumor of young adults, with high recurrence rate with local treatment. A small percentage are frankly malignant and can metastasize to the lungs. Treatment is with resection and limb reconstruction or thorough curettage and cementation with methylmethacrylate bone cement, which seems to reduce local recurrence incidence.
2. Unicameral bone cyst: This is a metaphyseal, expansile benign lesion of childhood, most commonly seen in the upper humerus or femur, and consisting of a fluid-filled cavity in the bone. Pathologic fractures are common, and the lesion spontaneously resolves after skeletal maturity is reached. Steroid injections into the lesion may effect healing, and occasionally curettage and bone grafting is necessary, but recurrence rate is 50%.
3. Ewing's sarcoma: An aggressive malignancy of childhood affecting the diaphyses of long bones, with permeative bone destruction and periosteal reaction, which must be differentiated from solitary eosinophilic granuloma and osteomyelitis. Treatment is with systemic chemotherapy and radiation, with 50–70% 5-year survival.
4. Reticulum cell sarcoma (primary histiocytic lymphoma of bone): A malignant tumor of bone occurring in the diaphyses of long bones in patients age 20–40. Treated by radiation unless metastases present in which case chemotherapy is used.
5. Aneurysmal bone cyst: An aggressive, benign, expansile lesion of the metaphyses in children or young adults. Lesion is vascular, with blood-filled cystic spaces, and is treated by curettage or resection, except for inaccessible lesions in the spine or pelvis, which may respond to intermediate-dose radiation.
6. Hemangioma: A benign vascular tumor of bone that is usually asymptomatic and most commonly diagnosed as an incidental finding on spine films; generally no treatment needed.

7. Adamantinoma: A low-grade malignancy resembling an epithelial tumor; arises in the diaphyses or metaphyses of long bones (usually the tibia) in young adults. Wide resection or amputation is the usual treatment.
8. Chordoma: A slow-growing malignancy derived from notochordal remnants, usually occurring in the sphen-ooccipital or sacrococcygeal areas of middle aged adults. Recurrence incidence is high after surgical resection.
9. Soft tissue sarcomas: Include fibrosarcoma, malignant fibrous histiocytoma, rhabdomyosarcoma, liposarcoma, neurofibrosarcoma, synovial sarcoma, and epithelioid sarcoma. All are treated by aggressive surgery or amputation, often in conjunction with radiation and chemotherapy.
10. Metastatic tumors of bone: A number of cancers which do not arise primarily in bone have a propensity to metastasize to bone, including breast, prostate, lung, kidney, and thyroid carcinoma, and neuroblastoma. Patients may present with pain or pathologic fractures. The lesions generally are controlled by radiation treatment, and fractures are stabilized surgically with rods or plating and bone cement, followed by radiation treatment for the lesion.

43 AMPUTATION

INDICATIONS

1. Nonreconstructible peripheral vascular disease with intolerable ischemic pain or infection
2. Intolerable pain or infection in a nonambulatory patient with peripheral vascular disease
3. Extensive spreading infection not responsive to conservative measures
4. Tumors poorly responsive to nonoperative measures
5. Trauma sufficiently extensive to preclude repair

Patients with severe medical problems and a severely ischemic limb have frequently been offered amputation rather than revascularization. There is little data to substantiate this position, and poor medical condition should no longer be considered a contraindication to revascularization.

PROCEDURES

1. Toe amputation: A transphalangeal level may be used if necrosis is distal to the proximal interphalangeal joint.
2. Transmetatarsal amputation: This procedure is used when necrosis extends proximal to the proximal interphalangeal joint, but distal to the metatarsal head on the plantar surface. A long plantar flap is frequently used, cutting the metatarsal bones at their midportion.
3. Syme amputation: This procedure is usually performed when the foot has been destroyed by trauma. This amputation preserves the limb length, removing the foot between the talus and calcaneus.
4. Below-knee (BK) amputation: This procedure is generally performed in end-stage peripheral vascular disease. It provides excellent rehabilitation because it preserves the knee joint. Contracture of the knee or hip represents a contraindication to this procedure. A long posterior flap technique is generally used, and immediate prosthesis is sometimes used postoperatively.
5. Above-knee (AK) amputation: This amputation holds the highest healing rate in patients with peripheral vascular disease. An AK amputation that does not heal is an ominous situation with extremely high mortality. Anterior

and posterior skin flaps are generally fashioned of equal length, using a fishmouth incision.

6. Hip disarticulation and hemipelvectomy: These procedures are usually performed for malignant tumors of the leg. They may be performed occasionally in peripheral vascular disease, but usually with poor results.

7. Amputations of the upper extremity: Most amputations of this nature are performed in trauma cases. Malignant diseases represent the next most common indication. It is rare for arterial occlusive disease to necessitate a major upper extremity amputation; however, digital amputations are frequent in patients with collagen vascular diseases and Buerger's disease.

PRINCIPLES

1. Transmetatarsal amputations are usually unsuccessful in the absence of a palpable foot pulse.

2. BK amputations are best performed at the junction of the upper and mid-third of the calf. Patients with BK amputations are more easily fitted with a prosthesis and ambulate better than patients with more distal leg amputations.

3. Nonambulatory patients are better managed with an AK rather than a BK amputation.

4. Nonhealing of AK amputations is an ominous, usually premorbid condition.

5. Extremities involved with extensive infection are best managed with early open guillotine amputation followed by closure at a later date after the infection has been cleared.

6. If the great toe must be sacrificed proximal to the metatarsal head, the patient is most quickly rehabilitated if a standard five-digit transmetatarsal amputation is accomplished.

44 HAND

BASIC PRINCIPLES

CLINICAL ASSESSMENT *History* The patient's age, hand dominance, occupation, mechanism of injury, and previous hand injury or impairment should be obtained.

Physical exam *Circulation.* Ulnar, radial pulse, and capillary refill

Sensibility. Essential to assess before local anesthesia. Light touch and two-point descrimination are better than pinprick. Autonomous zones for testing: median nerve—flexor surface over the distal phalanx of the index finger; ulnar nerve—flexor surface over the distal phalanx of the little finger; radial nerve—dorsal web space of the thumb.

Coverage. Notation of any loss of soft tissue.

Bones. Radiologic examination including AP, lateral and oblique views.

Joints and ligaments. Notation of stability and instability.

Flexor tendons. Flexor digitorum profundus and flexor pollicis longus flex the distal segments and are tested by holding the proximal and middle segments in extension and attempting to flex the distal segment. Flexor digitorum superficialis flexes the proximal interphalangeal joints and are tested by holding the other fingers in extension and attempting to flex the entire finger.

Extensor tendons. Extensor digitorum communis to each of the four fingers, extensor digiti minimi to the little finger, and extensor inducis proprius to the index fingers are the main extensors.

Intrinsic musculotendinous function. The entire muscle-tendon complex is within the hand. The median nerve innervates the intrinsics of the thenar eminence on the radial side of the flexor pollicis longus and the first two lumbricals. The ulnar nerve innervates the hypothenar muscles, the interossei muscles, the ulnar two lumbricals, the ulnar head of the flexor pollicis brevis, and the adductor pollicis. The median nerve is tested by palmar abduction of the thumb and opposition. The ulnar nerve is tested by finger abduction and adduction.

DISTAL BLOCK ANESTHESIA Median nerve The needle is placed at the palmaris longus tendon at the wrist flexion crease.

Ulnar nerve The needle is placed to the dorsal aspect of the flexor carpi ulnaris, 1 cm deep and perpendicular to the forearm.

Radial sensory nerve The needle is placed three finger breadths proximal to the radial styloid.

Digital The needle is placed a few millimeters into the web space on both sides of the digit. Examination of sensory function must be done before any block, and epinephrine should never be combined with the anesthetic agent.

TREATMENT OF THE ACUTELY INJURED HAND Acute wounds should not be probed for diagnostic purposes in the emergency room. More can be acertained by covering the wound and performing an organized systematic exam.

Hemorrhage is controlled with gentle local pressure and elevation. Attempts to "clamp a bleeder" may damage tendons and nerves.

RECONSTRUCTIVE HAND SURGERY The goal is function, not cosmesis. Reconstruction is usually staged and the tissues involved usually treated in the following sequence: (a) coverage, (b) stability of skeletal framework, (c) joint reconstruction for mobility with stability, (d) reconstruction of musculotendinous units, and (e) repair of innervation.

TOURNIQUET USE Tourniquets ensure a near bloodless field, which facilitates repair. The limb should have the blood present reduced by compression applied in a distal-to-proximal direction first. The tourniquet should be placed as proximal as possible. Axillary blocks allow $1\frac{1}{2}$ h of tourniquet time. Distal blocks allow 20 min of tourniquet time. Penrose drains are used for digital tourniquets, never rubber bands.

INCISIONS *Palm.* Parallel to the skin creases.

Digits. (a) Side—midaxial (area of skin change from volar to dorsal skin); (b) flexor—avoid flexor crease, incisions should angle from segments to lateral edge of flexor crease; (c) dorsal—should cross skin creases transversely or obliquely.

DRESSINGS AND SPLINTS The hand should be immobilized in a "safe position"; wrist in 20–30° of extension, metacarpophalangeal joints in 60–90° of flexion, interphalangeal joints extended and the thumb projecting from the hand.

Dressings should be moist, smooth gauze or a single layer

of Xeroform. Additional layers should be soft, absorptive gauze.

HAND THERAPY Exercises should be gentle and active or active with assist, never passive. Whirlpool and heat are rarely indicated and tend to produce increased edema.

TRAUMA

COMMON FRACTURES AND JOINT INJURIES Colles' fracture Fracture of the distal radius with dorsal angulation. Commonly seen in older women after a fall on an outstretched hand. Evaluation needs to rule out median nerve injury. Treatment is usually with closed reduction.

Smith's fracture Also known as a "reverse Colles'," with volar angulation of the radius fracture. Usually occurs secondary to a fall on the dorsum of the wrist. Usual treatment is closed reduction.

Ligamentous injuries of the wrist Most commonly injured are the ligaments between the radius, scaphoid, and lunate. Most common radiologic findings are an increased gap between the scaphoid and lunate and a decreased scaphoid height on AP view. Satisfactory results usually require acute surgical repair.

Scaphoid fracture Usually seen in young adults from a fall on an outstretched hand. Physical exam reveals pain in the anatomic snuff box. X-rays may not show the fracture and therefore if a fracture is suspected, the patient is immobilized in a plaster cast for 3 weeks, at which time repeat x-rays will usually show the fracture if present. If the fracture is still not visible, the patient is left in the plaster cast and the films are repeated again in another 3 weeks. Fractures are treated with casting for 4 months from thumb tip to and including the elbow.

Lunate and perilunate dislocations Occur with wrist hyperextension. X-rays show disruption of the axial alignment of the radius, lunate, and capitate. Treatment is closed reduction and plaster immobilization.

Metacarpal fractures The digit is immobilized with MCP flexed 60–70° and IP fully extended. An adjacent digit should be included in the immobilization. Unstable fractures are managed with internal support (Kirschner wires, screws, or plates) and plaster immobilization.

Carpometacarpal dislocations Diagnosis is with lateral x-ray and usual treatment is with internal fixation.

Bennett's fracture Fracture of the base of the proximal phalanx of the thumb into the joint space. May be managed with closed reduction but often requires open reduction and internal fixation with a Kirschner pin.

Thumb metacarpophalangeal joint Disruption of the ulnar collateral ligament from forced abduction of the thumb. "gamekeeper's thumb" results is valgus instability. Open repair is indicated.

Proximal phalanx fracture Stable fractures are managed with immobilization in "safe position." Unstable fractures require internal fixation and plaster immobilization.

Proximal interphalangeal joint Incomplete ligament tears and dorsal dislocations are treated with reduction and dorsal splint for 2–3 weeks followed by "buddy taping." Dislocations with small fracture avulsion fractures can be treated in the same fashion. Fractures involving more than 20% of the articular surface require open treatment.

Middle phalanx Managed with closed reduction and external immobilization.

Distal phalanx Crush injuries are common. Associated nail matrix injuries must be repaired. Subungual hematomas with intact matrix and nail plate should be drained through the nail. Fracture fragments need not be removed.

TENDON INJURIES Flexor tendons Repairs are not attempted in the emergency room. The wounds are irrigated, the ends of cut tendon are tagged with suture if visible, and the skin is closed. Antibiotics are given and the hand is elevated. The tendons are then repaired in the operating room within 7 days. If wound contamination or delayed treatment prevents primary repair, free tendon transfer can be performed. With tendon lacerations in the center of the palm, both superficial and profundus tendons are repaired. With tendon injuries in the wrist or in the midline of the proximal palm, the profundus tendons are repaired. The area of the distal palm and proximal phalanx are considered "no-man's land," and treatment is controversial except in children in whom profundus tendons are always repaired.

Extensor tendons Primary repair usually can be performed in the emergency room with simple or mattress sutures.

Boutonniere deformity Disruption of the central extensor tendon just proximal to its insertion at the base of the middle phalanx. The intact lateral bands result in flexion at the proximal interphalangeal joint and extension at the distal interphalangeal joint. Management involves immobilization of the PIP joint in a dorsal splint with 0 degrees of extension for 6–8 weeks. Surgical repair does not shorten the healing time.

Mallet finger Disruption of the insertion of the extensor tendon into the base of the distal phalanx with or without fracture of the distal phalanx. These injuries usually result from blunt trauma to the tip of the finger. Treatment involving no fracture or a small fracture is dorsal splinting of the PIP joint in 0° of extension for 8 weeks. If the fracture is greater than 30% of the articular surface, open reduction and internal fixation are required.

NERVE INJURIES Injuries may be secondary to stretching, compression, or nerve transection. Stretching and compression injuries have a better prognosis. Operative repair is required for nerve transection. Nerve repair can be done at the time of injury or may be delayed, but for no more than 6 months. Epineural repair is accomplished under magnification without tension. Regeneration proceeds at 1 mm/day and is faster in children.

FINGERTIP INJURIES Tuft fractures rarely need internal fixation. Soft tissue loss can be covered with split-thickness skin graft if the pulp is intact or full-thickness skin graft if the pulp is absent. Severely crushed or mangled tips are often best managed with shortening or amputation of the terminal phalanx.

INFECTIONS *S. aureus* accounts for 80% of hand infections with *E. coli,* β-hemolytic streptococci, *Proteus,* and *Pseudomonas* accounting for the rest.

Cellulitis Treated with antibiotics and elevation. This may be done on an outpatient basis for mild cases but may require IV antibiotics and hospitalization for more severe infections.

Subcutaneous abscess Incision and drainage along with antibiotics and elevation should proceed without delay, as spread to vital structures of the hand can occur quickly.

Paronychia Infection around the nail margin. Antibiotics and soaks may arrest mild infections, but removal of a portion of the nail is often required for more severe infections.

Felon Infection of the distal pulp. If untreated, this can cause distal necrosis and osteomyelitis. Incision and drainage is performed via an incision over the midline of the pulp or at the lateral edge of the nail.

Tenosynovitis The index, long, and ring fingers have individual flexor tendon sheaths. The flexor tendon sheaths of the little finger and the thumb communicate via the ulnar and radial bursas in the palm. Patients present with pain, which is increased with either active or passive motion of the involved digit. Treatment is prompt surgical drainage and IV antibiotics.

BURNS   Full-thickness burns rarely occur on the palm but do occur over the digital tips and dorsal aspects. Early treatment includes splinting of the hands in a "safe position." If the extensor tendons are destroyed, joints need to be fixed to prevent flexor contraction.

CRUSH INJURIES   Nerve involvement is common, arterial pulses are often intact, and fasciotomies are often necessary. Myoglobinemia and myoglobinuria should be ruled out.

COMPARTMENT SYSDROMES   Volkmann's contracture results from ischemia of the deep flexor compartment of the forearm and may occur despite bounding radial pulses. Tenderness over the muscle and pain with passive extension of the fingers are the most reliable signs. Early treatment is fasciotomy from the elbow to the wrist and epimyosotomy of the involved muscle bellies.

REPLANTATION   Guillotine amputations are more easily replanted than avulsion injuries. Crush injuries are often not suitable for replantation. Parts should be placed in a sterile dressing and placed in a plastic bag, which is then placed in ice water at 4°C. The part is never placed directly in the ice. Proximal parts with smooth muscle must be replanted within 4 h. Distal parts with little or no smooth muscle can tolerate ischemia for 24 h.

AMPUTATIONS   Once replantation has been ruled out as a possibility or the attempts to replant have failed, completion amputation is often needed. The thumb is the most important digit for hand function, and all possible length should be perserved. Amputations at the midportion of the four fingers can be shortened for coverage. Amputations through the proximal phalanx should have all possible length saved to preserve hand grasp.

NONTRAUMATIC CONDITIONS AND RECONSTRUCTION

CARPAL TUNNEL SYNDROME   Neurapraxia of the median nerve from compression within the canal. Patients present with pain and numbness in the distribution of the median nerve, often referred to the neck and shoulder; positive Tinel's sign over the median nerve in the wrist; and increased symptoms with forced wrist flexion. Treatment involves splinting, nonsteroidal anti-inflammatory agents, and possibly a single injection of cortisone into the canal. Failure of conservative treatment necessitates operative intervention; release of the median nerve from the flexor retinaculum at the wrist.

DEQUERVAIN'S DISORDER Idiopathic tenosynovitis with entrapment of the abductor pollicis longus and extensor pollicis brevis tendons within the first extensor compartment of the wrist resulting in pain over the radial styloid. Management is with nonsteroidal anti-inflammatory agents and splinting combined with a change in the pattern of hand use. Failure of conservative treatment is the indication for surgical decompression, with care to avoid the sensory branch of the radial nerve.

TRIGGER FINGER Swelling or tenosynovitis of the flexor tendon within the fibroosseous tunnel results in a "snapping" or "locking" of the involved finger as it moves within the pulley system. Treatment involves nonsteroidal anti-inflammatory drugs and steroid injections or surgical intervention with partial release of the proximal portion of the involved pulley.

DUPUYTREN'S CONTRACTURE Contracture of the palmar aponeurosis. Patients have dimpling of the skin in line with the tendon, and flexion contracture most commonly involving the ring and little fingers. Conservative management is with nonsteroidal anti-inflammatory agents. Surgical treatment consists of open fasciotomy and/or radical excision of the involved palmar fascia with or without skin grafting.

TENDON GRAFT Tendons may be harvested from the palmaris longus, plantaris, or other sites. Proximal repair is in the forearm or the palm, and the distal repair is at the insertion onto the volar aspect of the distal phalanx. If the bed as well as the tendon requires reconstruction, a two-stage procedure is performed, reconstructing the bed first using a silastic rod.

NERVE GRAFT Nerve gaps Nerve injuries with a gap of nerve substance may be closed by mobilization of the ends and anastomosis without tension. If primary repair is under tension, it is best to perform an autograft using a portion of the sural nerve.

Neuroma Occurs secondary to unrepaired peripheral nerve. Patients usually experience electric shock–like sensations with palpation or percussion over the neuroma. Treatment is by nerve repair or bearing the nerve end deep in soft tissue or into bone.

MUSCULOTENDINOUS TRANSFERS When there is irreversible paralysis of muscles not suitable for nerve grafts, muscle still innervated may be transferred to replace lost function (e.g., flexor superficialis tendon of the ring finger to insert into the abductor pollicis longus).

CONGENITAL ANOMALIES Syndactyly Webbing of the fingers. Repair is performed at 1 year of age if digits of different growth rates are involved, to prevent retardation of the longer digit's development. If there is no difference in the growth rates, repair is delayed until the second or third year. If more than one side of a digit is involved, only one side is repaired at a time to decrease the risk of compromise of the blood supply.

Polydactyly Extra digits may be supernumary phalanx or duplication of the entire digit. X-rays are mandatory before surgical repair. Care must be taken to preserve sensory nerves and tendons to the digits left in situ.

THUMB RECONSTRUCTION Congenital absence of the thumb can be managed by rotation of the index finger into the thumb position. Traumatic amputation can be reconstructed by pollicarization of the index finger or free toe transfer.

TUMORS Ganglion Occurs in four locations: dorsal side of the wrist extending into the joint, flexor aspect of the wrist extending into the joint, at the base of the digit arising from the flexor sheath, and from the distal interphalangeal joint called a *mucous cyst*. Excision needs to include the entire extent of the cyst, including its origin.

Giant cell tumor Originates from the flexor tendon at the interphalangeal joints. Treatment is surgical.

Inclusion cyst Implantation of epithelium with or without a foreign body. The cyst is lined with a squamous epithelium and contains a creamy white substance.

ARTHTITIS Rheumatoid arthritis Initial treatment is nonoperative and includes nonsteroidal anti-inflammatory agents, splinting, and exercise programs. With loss of function despite maximum conservative therapy, surgery is often needed. Surgical procedures include: wrist—procedures on extensor tendons, flexor tendons, and the joint itself; thumb—procedures are a combination of joint fusion, joint arthroplasties, and tendon transfers; MCP—implant arthroplasties are often needed. All operations are combined with postoperative exercise and splinting.

Osteoarthritis Commonly affects multiple joints in the hand, most often the interphalangeal joints of the fingers and thumb and the base of the thumb. Initial management is conservative, nonsteroidal anti-inflammatory drugs. With failure of conservative therapy, surgical management is often indicated. For distal interphalangeal joint involvement arthrodesis is usually performed. With involvement of the proximal interphalangeal joints, implant arthroplasty is often needed. Involvement of the base of the thumb is extremely disabling. The usual treatment is arthroplasty, though arthrodesis may be used in the younger patient.

45 PLASTIC AND RECONSTRUCTIVE SURGERY

BASIC PRINCIPLES

SKIN INCISIONS Incisions should be planned parallel to the skin lines. Elliptical incisions have a long axis 4 times the length of the short axis to prevent dog ears.

WOUND CLOSURE Wound preparation includes debridement of the skin edges and the use of noncrushing instruments. Excess tension produces a wide scar. Undermining and subcutaneous absorbable sutures reduce wound tension. Early suture removal reduces scarring. Facial sutures should be removed at 3–5 days, others at 7 days.

SKIN GRAFTING Split-thickness skin grafts include epidermis and a portion of the dermis. Full-thickness skin grafts include the epidermis and the entire dermis. "Take" of a skin graft requires an adequately vascularized recipient bed. Skin grafts will "take" on paratenon and periosteum but not bare tendon or bone.

Skin grafts may be stored for up to 21 days soaked in sterile saline at 4°C. Meshing of a skin graft allows an increased area to be covered, irregular contours to be covered more easily, and escape of fluid that would normally accumulate under the graft and could compromise graft survival. Grafts to the face and hands should not be meshed. Not meshing a graft will require fluid to be removed by syringe and needle as it accumulates under the graft.

Grafted areas must be kept immobilized, as motion may disrupt the graft. Grafts to the extremities should not be allowed to hang dependent.

Antibiotics need be given no longer than 24 h after grafting. Grafted skin is more fragile than normal tissue and will darken with sun exposure.

Composite grafts contain several tissue layers such as ear skin and cartilage grafted to the nose. Take is usually accomplished if no portion of the graft is more then 1 cm from the vascular bed.

FLAPS *Random flaps.* Z-plasty, advancement, rotation, transposition, and interpolation flaps are based on a skin pedicle and used for altering scars or covering defects.

Axial flaps. Forehead flaps, deltopectoral flaps, and omental flaps are all examples of axial flaps. They are based on specific vessels, and are better vascularized and more reliable than random flaps.

Fasciocutaneous flaps. These include the underlying fascia as well as the subcutaneous tissues. A good vascular supply allows greater length to the flap.

Free tissue transfer. Many myocutaneous and some fasciocutaneous flaps have a consistent vascular pedicle, which may be divided and reanastomosed in a distant site.

TISSUE EXPANSION The tissue expanders are placed under the skin and subcutaneous tissue. After 3 weeks the tissue expander is filled with sterile saline over a number of weeks. Once enough tissue is expanded, the tissue expander is removed and the defect is closed with transposition of the expanded skin.

TISSUE TRANSPLANTATION Autogenous tissue—rib, iliac crest, dermis, fat, cartilage, tendon, and fascia have all been used for successful reconstruction.

SYNTHETIC MATERIALS Various plastics and metals may be used when acceptable autogenous tissues are not available.

LIPOSUCTION Through one or more small incisions a metal cannulae is inserted into the area of fat deposition. The cannulae cuts the fat, which is then aspirated via a vacuum device attached to the cannulae.

RECONSTRUCTIVE SURGERY

BREAST *Macromastia.* An abnormal enlargement of the breast. Reduction is achieved with resection of the redundant breast tissue and nipple preservation by pedicle or full-thickness nipple areolar graft. Risks include nipple necrosis, decreased sensation at the nipple, and an inability to lactate or breast feed.

Ptosis. Occurs when the nipple has descended below the inframammary crease. Repair involves nipple repositioning with either reduction or placement of implants depending on the cause of the ptosis.

Hypomastia. Insufficient volume in one or both breasts. Augmentation is performed with a prosthesis placed in either the submuscular or subcutaneous position.

Reconstruction with mastectomy. Can be accomplished with either tissue expanders and subsequent prosthesis or myocutaneous flap (e.g., latissimus dorsi or rectus abdominis). Repair is delayed until after any radiation therapy or chemotherapy. There is no known increased risk in recurrence or failure to identify recurrence after reconstruction. Reconstruction is often needed on the nonmastectomy breast to obtain symmetry.

Gynecomastia.   An enlargement of the male breast secondary to increased ductal tissue. The most common form is idiopathic and occurs in adolescence. Treatment in adolescence is expectant, as the process usually resolves spontaneously within 2 years. For excessive enlargement or enlargement of greater than 2 years' duration excision through a circumareolar incision is the treatment of choice.

CHEST AND ABDOMINAL WALL   Defects may be secondary to trauma, tumor resection, radiation necrosis, infection, or congenital abnormalities. Repair is usually accomplished with one of several myocutaneous flaps (e.g., latissimus dorsi or deltopectoral). Pressure sores often appear small externally and are usually located over a bony prominence. Their presence may indicate a more extensive involvement of underlying subcutaneous tissue, fascia, and muscle.

LYMPHEDEMA   May be secondary to regional lymph node dissection or congenital malformation. Nonoperative treatment consists of elevation and compression. Surgical management (reserved for those failing medical therapy) includes excision of involved tissue either under skin flaps or with split-thickness or full-thickness skin grafts. Microvascular lymphaticovenous anastamosis has inconsistent results.

LOWER EXTREMITY DEFECTS   Small tissue defects, those less than 1 cm, can be expected to heal on their own. Venous stasis ulcers need treatment of venous disease prior to reepithelialization or STSG. Large defects such as compound tibial fractures with soft tissue injury are best managed with fasciocutaneous, muscle, or musculocutaneous flaps. Local muscle transposition is usually the preferred treatment except for wounds in the distal third of the tibia, where free muscle transfer is most often used.

GENITOURINARY SYSTEM   *Hypospadias.*   Occurs when the urethral meatus opens on the ventral surface of the penis, on the scrotum, or in the peritoneum. These patients should not be circumcised, as the foreskin is used in the repair.

Epispadias.   Occurs when the urethral meatus opens on the dorsum of the penis. This is often associated with extrophy of the bladder. Primary treatment is the establishment of unobstructed renal function.

Vaginal agenesis.   May be idiopathic or secondary to testicular feminization syndrome, adrenogenital syndrome, or gonadal dysgenesis. Management consists of dissection of a perineal pocket and STSG to create a vagina.

Vaginal and vulvar resections.   Resections for carcinoma result in large defects often closed with skin flaps and gracilis myocutaneous flaps.

AESTHETIC SURGERY

FACIAL AGING *Rhytidectomy (facelift).*   Involves an incision in the hairline at the lateral aspect of the forehead, continues in front of the ear, inferior and then posterior to the lobe. The skin is undermined from the frontalis muscle to the platysma in order to free it from the underlying structures. The skin is then advanced toward the ear and secured to the fascia anterior to the ear. The redundant tissue is excised. Rhytidectomies may be performed more than once.

Dermabrasion.   Improves fine wrinkling.

Chemical face peel.   Tightens skin and flattens fine wrinkles.

EYELID   Bagging of the eyelids or ptosis can be corrected by blepharoplasty (excision of redundant lid skin and fat) or brow lift, respectively.

NOSE   Rhinoplasty, performed under local or general anesthesia, can be done with incisions hidden inside the nose to minimize visible scarring.

ABDOMEN, THIGHS, BUTTOCKS, AND UPPER ARM   Redundant skin secondary to aging or significant weight loss may be surgically excised; however, resulting scars are often fairly prominent.

HEAD AND NECK SURGERY

CONGENITAL DEFORMITIES Cleft lip   These deformities may be unilateral or bilateral and incomplete (skin bridge connecting the cleft and noncleft sides) or complete (no skin bridge). Repair is usually timed according to the "rule of tens"; at least 10 weeks of age, 10 lb, and a hemoglobin of 10%. Unilateral repairs are often done in one stage, while bilateral clefts may be done in two stages. Associated nasal deformities may be repaired at the same time or at a later date.

Cleft palate   Occurs from a malformation of the primary plate (anteriorly) or the secondary plate (posteriorly) or a combination of both. Repair is usually performed by the age of 12–14 months before speech patterns, often hypernasal if the cleft is not repaired, develop.

Craniofacial anomalies   Craniosynostosis—Apert syndrome and Crouzon syndrome involve premature closure of one or more cranial sutures. Repair involves separation and repositioning of the involved bone and the use of bone grafts and interosseous wiring for support.

Maxillomandibular disproportion   Abnormal size, shape, and position of the mandible or maxilla can result in malocclusion. Less severe disproportioning can be corrected with orthodontia. More severe disproportioning: micrognathia, retrognathia, and prognathia require surgical correction by splitting, advancing, or resecting a portion of the mandible depending on the specific deformity. Small chins not associated with any malpositioning can be treated with silicone prosthesis to improve projection. Repair of severe maxillary deformities, hypoplasia or hyperplasia, involves surgical fracturing of the maxilla with repositioning.

Ear deformities   *Microtia.*   Congenitally small, malformed ears; repaired in stages beginning at the age of 5 or 6 years. Uses rib cartilage for the structural framework.

Prominant ears.   Corrected by elevating and excising a portion of the skin from the posterior aspect of the ear and scoring the underlying cartilage. Closure results in a more normal contour.

Hemangioma and lymphangioma   *Strawberry hemangiomas.*   Abnormal collections of small vessels. These become prominent at 1–3 weeks of age, often increase in size over the first 6 months, and usually disappear spontaneously over the next several years. Surgical excision may be performed for compromised vision or respiration or for failure to resolve spontaneously.

Port wine stains.   Uniformly darker and do not resolve spontaneously. Treatment of choice is laser coagulation.

Cystic hygroma.   Most often involves the head and neck. Swelling often accompanies upper respiratory infections and may compromise the airway. Should surgical excision be required, partial excision may be all that is possible in order to preserve local vital structures.

Thyroglossal duct and brachial cleft anomalies   *Thyroglossal duct cysts.*   Present as a midline mass. If infected, incision and drainage is performed. Resection, which should include the entire tract and the midportion of the hyoid bone, requires preoperative thyroid scan or palpation of normally located thyroid tissue, as the cyst may represent the patient's only functioning thyroid tissue.

Brachial cleft cysts and sinuses. Remnants of the first or second brachial pouches. Infected cysts require incision and drainage. Excision of the fistula requires removal of the entire tract.

ACQUIRED DEFORMITIES Skull and scalp deformities *Avulsions of the scalp.* May be closed by microvascular replantation, STSG, or multiple scalp flaps transposed into the defect.

Loss of scalp and calvarium. Requires early coverage to decrease the risk of infection. Transposition flaps can cover small defects. Free tissue transfer or STSG to the dura may be necessary to cover larger areas of loss.

Eyelid and eyebrow reconstruction The upper eyelid is more important than the lower for protection of the cornea. Loss of one-fourth or less of either lid can be closed directly. Larger defects in the upper lid are closed with composite tissue from the lower lid. Local flaps from a portion of the upper lid or the cheek can be used to recreate the lower lid.

Loss of the hair-bearing eyebrow can be replaced using hair-bearing tissue from the scalp.

Eyelid ptosis. Moderate ptosis is managed by resection of a portion of the levator aponeurosis. Severe forms are treated by suspension of the eyelid by a portion of the frontalis muscle.

Nasal reconstruction Following loss of part or all of the nose, support framework is supplied by bone graft and skin coverage by nasolabial, forehead, or scalp flaps.

Lip reconstruction Full-thickness lip defects are usually reconstructed with various local lip flaps.

Facial palsy Lacerated or resected facial nerves should be repaired or grafted promptly. Long-standing palsy traditionally was treated with static suspension of the cheek and/ or eyelid. Newer techniques include muscle transfers and nerve grafts.

Parotid duct laceration May be repaired over a stent or can be tied off proximally.

Facial fractures *Examination.* Proceeds from upper to lower face and includes an ophthalmologic exam, intraoral as well as extraoral examination of the mandible and maxilla, evaluation of dental occlusion, and assessment of midface stability by grasping the upper incisors and gently attempting to displace the structures anteriorly and posteriorly.

Radiographic Studies. Fractures are diagnosed by visible fractures, blood in the sinuses, or subcutaneous air.

Mandibular fractures. Mandible is often fractured in more than one place, and displacement is common secondary to the pull of the muscles of mastication. Treatment is early reduction and restoration of normal dental occlusion and firm immobilization. These may be managed by intermaxillary fixation (IMF) or open reduction and internal fixation (ORIF) using plates and screws. Antibiotics should be given to control infection.

Zygomatic fractures. Often displaced. Significant deformities require manditory ORIF.

Orbital fractures. ''Blowout'' fractures may trap the inferior rectus muscle and are often associated with double vision. Surgical repair involves returning of the herniated tissue to the orbit and reinforcing the orbital floor with a silastin sheet if the bony fragments are unstable after anatomic reduction.

Nasal fractures. Obvious deformities are corrected immediately. With nasal edema, reduction of the nasal fracture is delayed several days until the swelling subsides. Septal hematomas should be drained and the nose packed.

Maxillary fractures. Classified as *LeFort I* (transverse)—separation of the lower maxilla, hard palate, and pterygoid processes from the rest of the maxilla; *LeFort II* (pyramidal)—separation along the nasofrontal suture, floor of the orbit, zygomaticomaxillary sutures, and the pterygoid processes; *LeFort III* (craniofacial disjunction)—separation of the midface from the rest of the cranium by fracture through the zygomaticofrontal sutures, nasofrontal sutures, and the floor of the orbit. Treatment for LeFort fractures is ORIF and IMF.

Reconstruction after tumor excision *Intraoral defects.* Many can be managed with STSG. Larger defects can be closed with forehead, deltopectoral, platysma, sternocleidomastoid, and pectoral flaps or free tissue transfers.

Bony deficits. May be managed with bone grafts or composite bone and soft tissue grafts (e.g., pectoralis major with attached rib).

Reconstruction of the cervical esophagus. Can be achieved by numerous musculocutaneous flaps, gastric transposition, or intestinal interposition with microvascular anastomosis.

INDEX

Note: Figures are referenced in italic numbers and tables with a lowercase t after the number.

NOTES

NOTES

NOTES

NOTES

NOTES

FREQUENTLY USED PHONE NUMBERS

Name   **Number**

FREQUENTLY USED PHONE NUMBERS

Name   **Number**

_____

_____

_____

_____

_____

_____

_____

_____

_____

_____

_____

_____

FREQUENTLY USED PHONE NUMBERS

Name   **Number**

_____

_____

_____

_____

_____

_____

_____

_____

_____

_____

_____

FREQUENTLY USED PHONE NUMBERS

Name   **Number**

FREQUENTLY USED PHONE NUMBERS

Name   **Number**

FREQUENTLY USED PHONE NUMBERS

Name   **Number**